Controversies in Cardiology

John A. Ambrose • Alfredo E. Rodríguez

Editors

Controversies in Cardiology

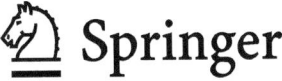 Springer

Editors
John A. Ambrose
UCSF Fresno
Fresno, CA
USA

Alfredo E. Rodríguez
Department of Interventional Cardiology
Otamendi Hospital
Buenos Aires
Argentina

ISBN 978-3-319-20414-7   ISBN 978-3-319-20415-4   (eBook)
DOI 10.1007/978-3-319-20415-4

Library of Congress Control Number: 2015949472

Springer Cham Heidelberg New York Dordrecht London

Printed on acid-free paper

Springer International Publishing AG Switzerland is part of Springer Science+Business Media (www.springer.com)

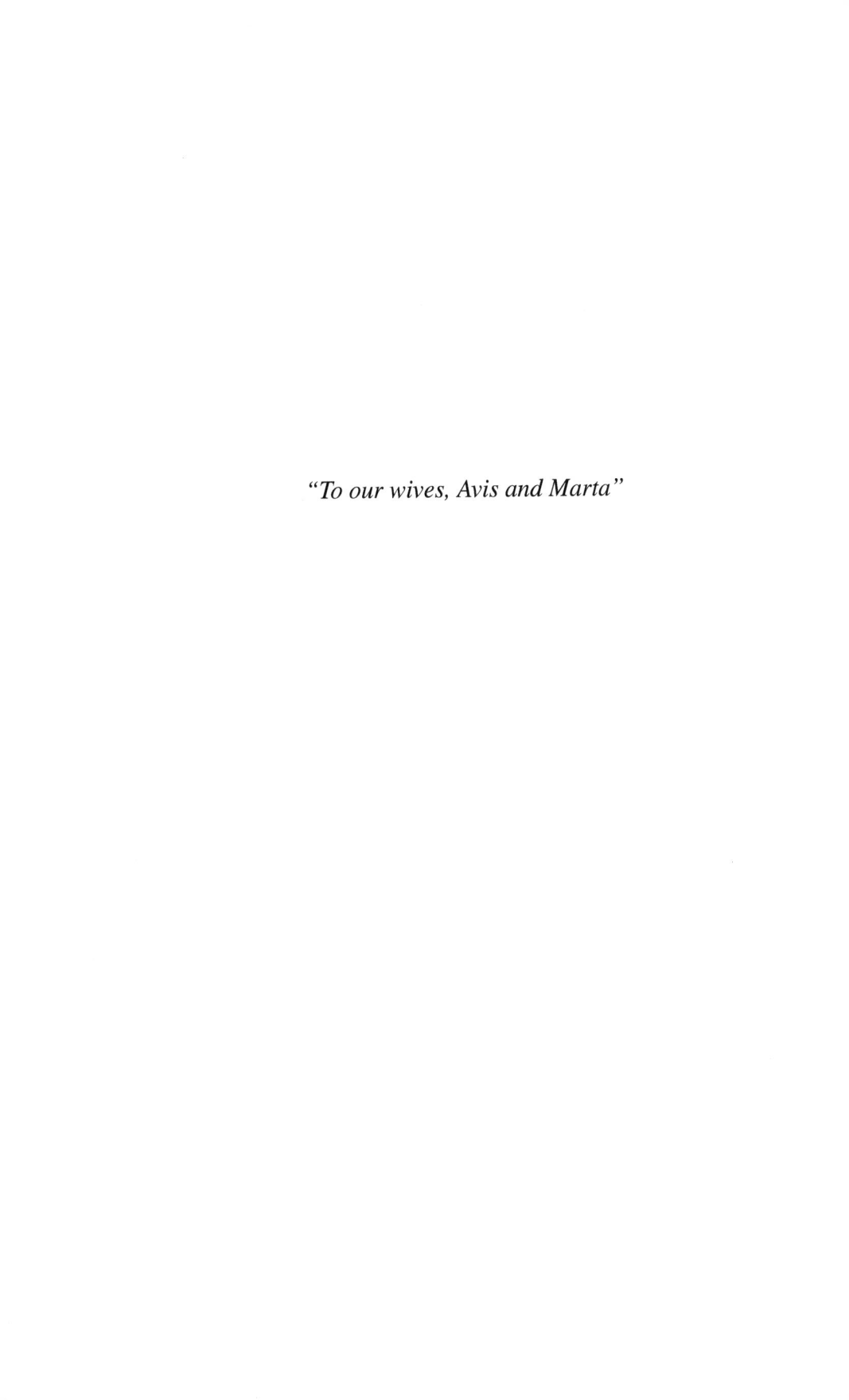

"To our wives, Avis and Marta"

Foreword

As a clinician, I have always been attracted to the problem-oriented method not only for patient care but also for education. My mentor at Emory, Dr. J. Willis Hurst, was a great advocate of the problem-oriented approach to patient care, and 30 or more years ago my university, Mercer University, established a medical school with the problem-oriented method of education as a centerpiece. The idea of identifying problems and then addressing all aspects of those problems in order to answer specific questions is attractive to many clinicians. In medical education, this approach certainly keeps the attention of the student better than the traditional digesting of all the basic sciences and ultimately applying them to clinical problems. So raising questions is important but it is also important to raise the questions about the subjects that do not have a universally-agreed upon answer. That seems to be the objective of Drs. John Ambrose and Alfredo Rodríguez in crafting this volume on *Controversies in Cardiology*. Certainly there are controversies, and in this era, we are easily convinced that things are happening so fast that the controversies are multiplying exponentially. But are these questions as pertinent as they were in the 1950s, 1960s, 1970s or 1980s? One might reflect on open heart surgery, cardiac electrical pacing, defibrillation, percutaneous intervention for coronary artery disease, management of acute myocardial infarction, and a revolution of effective drugs for hypertension, congestive heart failure and atherosclerosis. Many of these issues of the prior decades may seem non-controversial now. For the patient whose heart beats too slowly to support the circulation, a pacemaker is the answer, and a 10,000 patient randomized controlled trial is clearly not necessary. Some that are not controversial now were very controversial then. In the late 1960s, coronary bypass surgery for severely symptomatic angina was an example of a highly-controversial subject that, at present, has evolved into the question of which form of revascularization should be performed. Drs. Ambrose and Rodríguez have picked 25 of their favorite controversies to explore and have recruited leading experts to probe the existing evidence, as well as current opinion, about these issues. In addition, suggestions are made for further investigations needed to bring more clarity. The editors' bias is clearly toward coronary artery disease and its diagnosis and therapy. Twenty-one chapters deal in some manner with coronary disease and its complications and treatment, while only three address the controversies surrounding structural heart disease and only one addresses a rhythm disturbance. A different look reveals that there are two chapters that address risk and prevention. Nine address coronary interventions. Another six address other issues of coronary artery disease, and three deal with access and cost benefit issues. Others might select different issues to discuss but these favorites of Ambrose and Rodríguez are ones that many of us with a focus on coronary artery disease deal with daily in our own practices. Many of these controversies will be settled within the next few years, but many of them will remain and be challenges for the judgment of physicians for years to come. Framing common clinical problems and attempting to answer them is a great contribution because that, in fact, is how we think. My former mentor, Dr. Hurst, and Dr. Eugene Stead often spoke about writing a book which would include the ten things that every cardiologist should know. That book did not materialize, but if it had it would require revisions on a frequent basis because not only the answers to our questions but the questions themselves continue to change. The controversies of today addressed in this book may not be the controversies of tomorrow but we only live in today. Drs. Ambrose and Rodríguez have helped us understand where we live today and what is needed to gain further understanding of what is needed tomorrow.

Piedmont Hospital, Atlanta, Georgia   Spencer B. King, III, M.D.

Preface

It is quite amazing to have been witnesses to the spectacular evolution of cardiology over the last 30–35 years. Just consider two achievements – the management of acute myocardial infarction and the entire discipline of interventional cardiology. In the 1970s, patients presenting with an acute myocardial infarction with ST elevation and/or pathologic Q waves on ECG (then designated as transmural infarctions) were put to bed rest for about 3 weeks to "recover." Medications were crude and morbidity and mortality were high. Now, the average length of stay for a patient with a STEMI is about 2 days, and in most we aggressively insert metal tubes in their thrombosed arteries that remain open with the appropriate technique and medications. Complications have been drastically reduced and long-term survival and quality of life have improved. Likewise, the entire field of interventional cardiology was no more than a dream in the early 1970s until the pioneering work of Gruntzig and others made it a reality. We have evolved from crude balloons to atherectomy, then to scaffolds, followed by medicated scaffolds and now disappearing scaffolds. Obviously, over these decades, there have been several other examples of these paradigm shifts in how our patients are now managed.

What has been responsible for these changes? In some, it has been in the development of new uses for old medications such as aspirin in ACS, streptokinase for STEMI and colchicine in pericarditis. However, the driving force behind most of these changes that have revolutionized our approaches has been discovery, invention and innovation with the development of new medications and technologies. And the testing ground for these innovations has been, for the most part, randomized clinical trials. Furthermore, 35 years ago there were few standardized approaches to management and national guidelines were non-existent. Clearly, several organizations, based on various trial data and expert opinion, now provide direction and options for therapy in several different patient scenarios.

However, with such rapid change comes controversy, and not all situations that a cardiologist encounters in caring for patients can always be resolved based on the conventional wisdom of the day. Furthermore, the enthusiasm for a new drug or procedure frequently leads initially to much "off-label" overuse when the new therapy is introduced to the general patient population. Additional studies in the form of registries, meta-analyses or new randomized trials attempt to focus the therapy by identifying those most likely to benefit from the new discovery. Yet, as evolution continues to occur with the development of even newer therapies, technologies and approaches, not all situations can be identified in which guidelines or studies provide an appropriate solution.

This is where the editors began a discussion about *Controversies in Cardiology*. We attempted to identify different topics that had unresolved or controversial data. Some of these subjects did not have specific recommendations from the guidelines. We also considered an approach whereby for each topic there would be a pro and con discussion, but rejected this in most chapters as the data might be too repetitive and it might also confuse the reader. Nevertheless, we have been able to recruit several internationally recognized experts in the field to contribute to the book.

Each chapter begins with an introduction that presents the subject matter to be considered and outlines where the controversies or unresolved issues exist. It is then followed by a balanced and scholarly discussion of the subject. The conclusions attempt to suggest possible solutions if they exist or provide the authors' learned opinion on the subject. The book is broadly divided into three sections: cardiovascular risk assessment/pathophysiology, cardiovascular diagnosis and cardiovascular management. You will see that for multi-vessel disease and optimal stent design, we have requested two separate and different opinions. Also, some might argue that we have omitted key topics from the book that are unresolved. While we agree that there are other topics that might have been included, we were limited in some cases by failure in engaging the appropriate author for the topic and also by space. Finally, we are deeply grateful to all of the authors for their hard work in preparing their chapters and for Springer Publishing who has been our enthusiastic partner since the inception of this project.

Fresno, CA, USA   John A. Ambrose, MD, FACC
Buenos Aires, Argentina   Alfredo E. Rodríguez, MD, PhD, FACC, FSCAI

Contents

Contributors

Tushar Acharya, MD Department of Cardiology, University of California, San Francisco, Fresno, CA, USA

Dimitrios Alexopoulos, MD, FACC, FESC Department of Cardiology, Patras University Hospital, Rion, Patras, Greece

John A. Ambrose, MD Chief of Cardiology, UCSF Fresno, Fresno, CA, USA

Department of Medicine, UCSF Community Regional Medical Center, Fresno, CA, USA

David Antoniucci, MD Division of Cardiology, Department of Cardiology, Careggi Hospital, Florence, Italy

Usman Baber, MD, MS The Icahn School of Medicine at Mount Sinai, The Zena and Michael A. Wiener Cardiovascular Institute, New York, NY, USA

Ryan Berg, MD UCSF Fresno Department of Cardiology, Community Regional Medical Center, Fresno, CA, USA

William E. Boden, MD, FACC, FAHA Department of Medicine, Albany Medical College, Samuel S. Stratton VA Medical Center and Albany Medical Center, Albany, NY, USA

Patricia Carrascosa, MD, PhD Department of Cardiovascular Imaging, Diagnostico Maipu, Vicente Lopez, Buenos Aires, Argentina

Consejo Nacional de Investigaciones Científi cas y Técnicas (CONICET), Vicente Lopez, Buenos Aires, Argentina

Alaide Chieffo, MD Department of Invasive Cardiology, San Raffaele Scientific Institute, Milan, Lombardy, Italy

Antonio Colombo, MD Department of Invasive Cardiology, San Raffaele Scientific Institute, Milan, Lombardy, Italy

EMO-GV Centro Cuore Columbus, Milan, Italy

Francesco Costa, MD Erasmus MC, Department of Interventional Cardiology, Thoraxcenter, Rotterdam, The Netherlands

Department of Clinical and Experimental Medicine, Policlinico "G. Martino", University of Messina, Messina, Italy

Prakash C. Deedwania, MD, FACC, FAHA Department of Cardiology, University of California, San Francisco, Fresno, CA, USA

Michael E. Farkouh, MD, MSc Department of Medicine, University of Toronto, Toronto, ON, Canada

Division of Cardiology, The Peter Munk Cardiac Centre and the Heart and Stroke Richard Lewar Centre of Excellence, Toronto, ON, Canada

Carlos Fernández-Pereira, MD, PhD Department of Interventional Cardiology, Otamendi Hospital, Buenos Aires, Argentina

Aloke V. Finn, MD Department of Internal Medicine, Emory University School of Medicine, Atlanta, GA, USA

Eduardo D. Gabe, MD, PhD, FACC Department of Cardiology, Otamendi Hospital, Buenos Aires, Argentina

Scot Garg, MBChB, MRCP, PhD, FESC Department of Cardiology, Royal Blackburn Hospital, East Lancashire Hospitals NHS Trust, Blackburn, Lancashire, UK

Luís Henrique Wolff Gowdak, MD, PhD, FESC Laboratory of Genetics and Molecular Cardiology, Heart Institute, São Paulo, SP, Brazil

Liliana Rosa Grinfeld, MD, PhD, FACC, FSCAI Head interventinal cardiology Clinica San Camilo, Bueno Aires, Past President Argentina Society of Cardiology, New York, NY, USA

University of Buenos Aires, Cardiovascular Physiopathology Institute, Buenos Aires, Argentina

Nicolás Herscovich, MD Department of Cardiology, Otamendi Hospital, Buenos Aires, Argentina

Dominique Himbert, MD Department of Cardiology, Bichat-Claude Bernard Hospital, Paris, France

Bernard Iung, MD Department of Cardiology, Bichat Hospital, Paris, France

Michael Joner, MD, CEO CVPath Institute, Inc., Gaithersburg, MD, USA

Steven R. Jones, MD Division of Cardiology, Department of Medicine, The Ciccarone Center or Prevention of Heart Disease, The Johns Hopkins Hospital, Baltimore, MD, USA

Pranav Kansara, MD, MS Department of Cardiology, Christiana Care Health System, Newark, DE, USA

Richard George Kiel, MD Medical Education Program, Cardiology Division, Department of Internal Medicine, University of California San Francisco-Fresno, Fresno, CA, USA

Konstantinos Kossidas, MD Department of Cardiology, Christiana Care Health System, Newark, DE, USA

Eulógio E. Martinez, MD Federal University of São Paulo Medical School, São Paulo, SP, Brazil

Catheterization and Interventional Cardiology, Heart Institute (InCor), São Paulo, SP, Brazil

Department of Cardiac Catheterization and Interventional Cardiology, Hospital do Coração (HCor), São Paulo, SP, Brazil

University of São Paulo, São Paulo, SP, Brazil

Roxana Mehran, MD Mount Sinai Medical Center, New York, NY, USA

The Icahn School of Medicine at Mount Sinai, The Zena and Michael A. Wiener Cardiovascular Institute, New York, NY, USA

Juan Mieres, MD Department of Interventional Cardiology, Otamendi Hospital and Sanatorio Las Lomas, Buenos Aires, Argentina

Hiroyoshi Mori, MD CVPath Institute, Inc., Gaithersburg, MD, USA

Shady Nakhla, MD School of Medicine, Johns Hopkins Hospital, Baltimore, MD, USA

Igor F. Palacios, MD Department of Medicine, Harvard Medical School, Boston, MA, USA

Cardiac Unit, Massachusetts General Hospital, Boston, MA, USA

Pablo Rengifo-Moreno, MD Department of Medicine, University of Miami Hospital, Miami, FL, USA

Alfredo E. Rodríguez, MD, PhD, FACC, FSCAI Cardiac Unit, Department of Interventional Cardiology, Revista Argentina de Cardioagiologia Intervencionista (RACI), Otamendi Hospital, Buenos Aires, Argentina

Interventional Cardiology Unit, Department of Interventional Cardiology, Otamendi Hospital, Buenos Aires, Argentina

Otamendi Hospital, Post Graduate Buenos Aires School of Medicine, Buenos Aires, Argentina

Director, Cardiovascular Research Center (CECI), Buenos Aires, Argentina

A. Matías Rodríguez-Granillo, MD Cardiovascular Research Center (CECI), Capital Federal, Ciudad de Buenos Aires, Argentina

Gaston A. Rodriguez-Granillo, MD, PhD Department of Cardiovascular Imaging, Diagnostico Maipu, Vicente Lopez, Buenos Aires, Argentina

Consejo Nacional de Investigaciones Científicas y Técnicas (CONICET), Buenos Aires, Argentina

Department of Cardiovascular Imaging, ENERI-Clinica La Sagrada Familia, Vicente Lopez, Buenos Aires, Argentina

Neil Ruparelia, BSc, MBBS, DPhil, MRCP Department of Invasive Cardiology, San Raffaele Scientific Institute, Milan, Lombardy, Italy

Imperial College, London, UK

Arang Samim, MD UCSF-Fresno Medical Education Program, Department of Cardiology, University of California, Fresno, CA, USA

Omar Santaera, MD Interventional Cardiology Department, Sanatorio Las Lomas, Buenos Aires, Argentina

Patrick W. Serruys, MD, PhD, FESC International Centre for Cardiovascular Health, Imperial College, London, UK

Department of Cardiology, Erasmus Medical Centre, Rotterdam, The Netherlands

Sanjum S. Sethi, MD, MPH Division of Cardiology, Ronald Reagan UCLA Medical Center, Los Angeles, CA, USA

Nabil Shafi, MD UCSF Fresno, Department of Cardiology, Community Regional Medical Center, Fresno, CA, USA

Alec Vahanian, MD, FESC, FRCP (Edin.) Department of Cardiology, Bichat Hospital, Paris, France

Marco Valgimigli, MD, PhD, FESC Erasmus MC, Department of Interventional Cardiology, Thoraxcenter, Rotterdam, The Netherlands

Thoraxcenter, Erasmus Medical Center, Rotterdam, The Netherlands

Renu Virmani, MD CVPath Institute, Inc., Gaithersburg, MD, USA

Josephine Warren, MBBS Mount Sinai Medical Center, New York, NY, USA

The Icahn School of Medicine at Mount Sinai, The Zena and Michael A. Wiener Cardiovascular Institute, New York, NY, USA

William S. Weintraub, MD, MACC Department of Cardiology, Christiana Care Health System, Newark, DE, USA

Sandra Weiss, MD, FACC Department of Cardiology, Christiana Care Health System, Newark, DE, USA

Ralph J. Wessel, MD, FACC Department of Cardiology, Medicine UCSF, Community Regional Medical Center—Fresno, Fresno, CA, USA

Division of Cardiology, UCSF – Fresno, Fresno, CA, USA

Kazuyuki Yahagi, MD CVPath Institute, Inc., Gaithersburg, MD, USA

Jennifer Yu, MBBS Mount Sinai Medical Center, New York, NY, USA

The Icahn School of Medicine at Mount Sinai, The Zena and Michael A. Wiener Cardiovascular Institute, New York, NY, USA

Part I
Special Situations of Controversial, Increased, or Unknown Cardiovascular Risk

Chapter 1
New Risk Factors of Cardiovascular Disease

Tushar Acharya and Prakash C. Deedwania

Abstract Cardiovascular (CV) disease is the leading cause of death in the US and worldwide. Primary prevention of CV disease requires identification and treatment of risk factors. Since multiple risk factors coexist and interact leading to overt CVD, use of global risk assessment scores like Framingham risk score is recommended to identify and target high risk individuals. However, scores incorporating traditional risk factors like hypertension, diabetes, dyslipidemia and smoking are imperfect as the majority of cardiac events in the general population occur in low and intermediate risk individuals. This has led to the search for novel risk factors that may provide incremental value over and above the traditional risk models in predicting adverse CV events and reclassify patients to widen the scope of primary prevention. The following chapter aims to provide a comprehensive review of the major emerging risk factors by highlighting their background, evaluating supportive evidence and providing insight into their potential clinical utility. Unresolved or controversial issues will also be addressed.

Keywords Cardiovascular disease • Primary prevention • Risk factors • Risk assessment • Reclassification • Framingham score • hsCRP • Coronary artery calcium • Ankle brachial index

In the United States, 1 in every 3 deaths is attributed to CVD and more than 200 people die as a result of CVD every day [1]. Coronary heart disease (CHD) alone contributes to approximately 1 in 6 deaths per year [1]. Advancing age and male sex are known immutable risk factors. Additionally, there are several well-established modifiable risk factors, the management of which serves as the foundation for primary prevention of CHD events. These risk factors include but are not limited to hypertension, dyslipidemia, diabetes mellitus, cigarette smoking, obesity and physical inactivity (Table 1.1). Over the years, we have developed increasing understanding of their causal effect on CVD. From 1961, when the Framingham heart study first established hypertension and hypercholesterolemia in the pathogenesis of

T. Acharya, MD • P.C. Deedwania, MD, FACC, FAHA (✉)
Department of Cardiology, University of California, San Francisco, Fresno, CA, USA
e-mail: tacharya@fresno.ucsf.edu; pdeedwaia@fresno.ucsf.edu

© Springer International Publishing Switzerland 2015
J.A. Ambrose, A.E. Rodríguez (eds.), *Controversies in Cardiology*,
DOI 10.1007/978-3-319-20415-4_1

Table 1.1 Traditional risk factors for Coronary Heart Disease

Non-modifiable risk factors:
I. Advanced age
II. Male sex
III. Family history of coronary heart disease
Modifiable risk factors:
I. Hypertension: Elevated systolic and diastolic blood pressure
II. Dyslipidemia: High total cholesterol, high LDL, low HDL
III. Diabetes mellitus
IV. Cigarette smoking
V. Obesity
VI. Physical inactivity
VII. Metabolic syndrome and insulin resistance

Abbreviations: *LDL* low density lipoprotein, *HDL* high density lipoprotein

CHD [2], the field of risk assessment and primary prevention has received significant attention. The adverse cardiovascular effects of cigarette smoking have been documented in multiple studies, some predating Framingham. Diabetes mellitus has emerged as one of the most important predictors of CVD. It is considered a coronary artery disease equivalent as patients with this condition have the same risk of future myocardial infarctions as patients with prior myocardial infarction [3]. Aggregate risk scoring systems such as the Framingham risk score (FRS) [4] (and more recently the atherosclerotic cardiovascular disease [ASCVD] calculator) take into account multiple cardiac risk factors to predict the likelihood of future coronary events. The use of such global risk calculators is desirable as patients with fatal and non-fatal CVD often have one or more risk factors [5] (Table 1.2).

There is usually a latency period between exposure to risk factors and development of first CV event. This provides an opportunity to treat high risk patients with lifestyle modifications and medications. Effective evidence-based medical therapies are available to specifically address CV risk factors and various medical and governmental agencies have established therapeutic guidelines. Although implementation of such therapy(s) can reduce clinical events, adherence is generally poor. Medication compliance can be challenging in asymptomatic patients without a prior adverse CV event. Prospectively proven global lifetime risk prediction models may help impress patients and payers of the importance of therapy even in primary prevention.

There has been an emphasis on identifying high risk individuals in whom preventative therapy would be most beneficial. However, the majority of CV events actually occur in patients with low FRS. National Health and Nutrition Examination Survey showed that low risk patients comprise the bulk (85 %) of the general population; they in fact constitute 2/3 s of the overall population risk [6]. Thus, assessment based on traditional risk factors cannot accurately predict CV events in many patients, especially those deemed traditionally at low to intermediate risk. This has led to the search of novel risk factors for CVD.

A new risk factor should be associated with incident events independent of established risk factors. Additionally, it should provide incremental risk assessment. This

Table 1.2 New risk factors for Coronary Heart Disease

Biomarkers:
I. High sensitivity C-reactive protein (hsCRP)
II. Albuminuria
III. Lipoprotein Associated Phospholipase A2 (LP-PLA2)
IV. Lipid sub-particles: Lipoprotein (a), Apolipoprotein B
V. Natriuretic peptides (ANP, BNP, NT-proANP, NT-proBNP)
VI. Cardiac troponin
Subclinical atherosclerosis imaging techniques and vascular markers:
I. Coronary artery calcium
II. Ankle brachial index
III. Carotid Intima Media Thickness
IV. Endothelial Dysfunction and peripheral flow mediated dilatation
V. Measures of arterial stiffness

Abbreviations: *ANP* atrial natriuretic peptide, *BNP* B-type natriuretic peptide, *NT* N terminal

incremental risk prediction is often documented using Receiver-Operator curve analysis showing the improvement in sensitivity and specificity of a risk prediction model above that achieved using traditional risk factors (Fig. 1.1). This improvement is expressed as an increase in area under the curve (AUC) or the C-statistic. Another measure is its ability to reclassify low to intermediate risk patients to high risk so as to influence aggressiveness of therapy and follow up. In this chapter, we will review some of the new and emerging risk factors and evaluate their association with incident CV disease, scrutinize their discriminatory power and reclassification potential. Unresolved or controversial issues will also be addressed.

Biomarkers

Biomarkers can be objectively measured in the body and serve as indicators of normal biological function or pathological processes. A number of biomarkers are associated with CVD. The following is a description of the most prominent CV biomarkers.

High-Sensitivity C-Reactive Protein (hsCRP)

Inflammation is an important player in plaque formation and progression. Chronic inflammatory conditions accelerate atherosclerosis. Inflammatory biomarkers have been evaluated for CV risk prediction with specific attention to their additive value. hsCRP has probably been most widely studied. CRP is an acute phase reactant

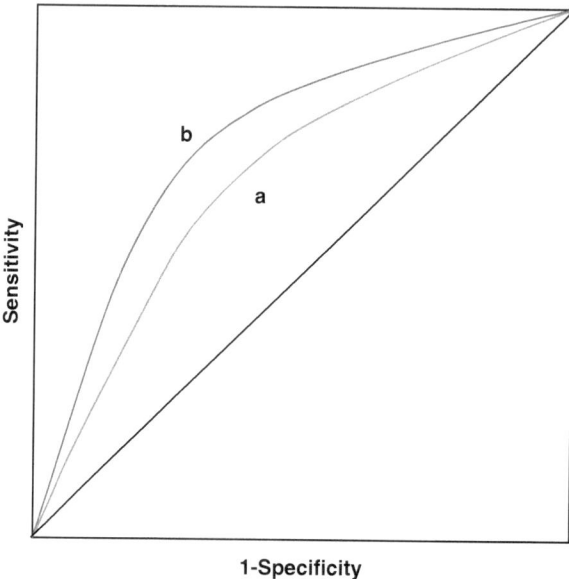

Fig. 1.1 Receiver Operator characteristic curves demonstrating the principle of incremental risk prediction. Area under the curve (*a*) represents the cardiovascular risk as predicted by established model like Framingham risk score (FRS) that incorporates traditional risk factors. Area under the curve (*b*) represents risk as predicted by FRS + novel risk factor. Addition of novel risk factor, in this example, moves the curve up and towards the left increasing the sensitivity and specificity of the new model

produced by the liver in response to Interleukin-6 and Interleukin-1 release as a result of infection, trauma or stress. It is a sensitive but non-specific marker of inflammation. CRP is also released at low levels in individuals with atherosclerosis and this can be detected accurately in the circulation. Only hsCRP should be used as a biomarker for use in predicting coronary events.

The role of CRP in atherosclerosis is complex and there is ongoing controversy regarding its mantle as a causative agent versus a marker of vascular inflammation [7]. High levels of CRP are associated with endothelial dysfunction, monocyte chemotaxis and platelet mediated pro-atherogenic effects. CRP attached to oxidized LDL particles can be found in lipid rich plaques. However, this does not establish a cause and effect relationship, particularly since animal and some human research data have failed to establish a crucial role of CRP in the causation of atherosclerosis. Genetic over expression and extraneous injection of CRP in animal models have failed to show increased atherosclerosis. Additionally, gene variants associated with high CRP expression in humans have not shown any significant association with adverse CV events. Thus, CRP might just be a marker for inflammatory changes related to atherosclerosis rather than a key player in the process itself.

Even though causality is contentious, there is substantial evidence that increased CRP is associated with poorer CV outcomes. An analysis of the Multiple Risk Factor Intervention Trial (MRFIT) showed a significant correlation between high hsCRP levels and subsequent CV mortality in healthy but high risk middle age men [8]. The Physicians' Health Study showed high levels of hsCRP can predict future MI and stroke [9]. The Women's Health Study found hsCRP to strongly predict CV events compared to LDL [10]. A meta-analysis of 22 studies found levels >3 mg/l were associated with a 60 % increased risk of coronary events versus levels <1 mg/l independent of established risk factors [11].

Does hsCRP add to CV risk prediction over and above traditional risk factors? Studies adding hsCRP to a CV risk prediction model have shown only moderate improvement of AUC. In MESA, coronary calcium score, carotid intima-media thickness, brachial flow-mediated dilatation and ankle brachial index performed better than hsCRP in improving AUC [12]. Other studies failed to show any improvement in risk prediction model at all [13]. The Reynolds risk model incorporates hsCRP and family history to the traditional Framingham risk factors and has shown to add incremental value [14]. However, most of this increment is derived from recalibration of known risk factors with minimal contribution from CRP. HsCRP does reclassify intermediate FRS patients and a low hsCRP value downgrades them to low risk. This reclassification, however, is not as robust as that derived from other testing like coronary calcium scoring.

CRP levels vary among population subgroups. BMI, diet, exercise, infection, smoking and alcohol consumption also influence levels. Interval measurements in the same individual may be significantly different making risk stratification based on a single measurement difficult. Another issue is the threshold of hsCRP to be used in clinical practice. JUPITER (Justification for the Use of Statins in Prevention: An Interventional Trial Evaluating Rosuvastatin) used a cut-off of 2 mg/l for comparing groups [15]. This value is not universally acceptable. In MESA, 3 mg/l performed better than 2 mg/l in predicting events. More importantly, based on representative samples, over 1/2 of the United States population has a CRP level >2 mg/l [16].

HsCRP has increasingly been used to guide statin therapy after JUPITER. JUPITER was a large multi-center trial that randomized 17,802 healthy low to intermediate risk men and women with LDLs <130 mg/dl and hsCRP level >2 mg/l to Rosuvastatin 20 mg daily versus placebo. The trial was stopped early after a median follow up of 1.9 years after a significant reduction (44 %) in combined primary outcome (MI, stroke, revascularization, hospitalization for unstable angina or CV death) was seen in the Rosuvastatin group. Rosuvastatin reduced LDL by 50 % and CRP by 37 %. The greatest reduction in the primary outcome was in patients with a reduction in both LDL and CRP. Some argue that the positive results could be explained by LDL reduction alone. Even in the absence of LDL reduction, the pleiotropic effects of statins with normal or low LDL levels are well established. Thus, while statins lowered CRP, there is no evidence to suggest that their benefits were attributable to their CRP lowering effect. Additionally, JUPITER did not have a low LDL (<130 mg/dl) and CRP (<2 mg/l) arm making it impossible to demonstrate the lack of statin benefit with low CRP. Lastly, some believe that the anti-inflammatory properties of statins are due to their LDL lowering effect. Ongoing trials using anti-inflammatory agents like Methotrexate and Interleukin-1 antagonists in patients with chronic inflammation might shed some light on the specific role of inflammation suppression without lipid lowering.

Due to significant controversy, the enthusiasm for hsCRP in the guidelines has decreased. The 2010 ACCF/AHA guidelines for CV risk assessment in asymptomatic adults gave hsCRP measurement a level IIA recommendation for deciding statin therapy in patients meeting JUPITER criteria [17]. A IIB recommendation was given for men >50 and women >60 years at intermediate CV risk. The 2013 guidelines have lowered all hsCRP recommendations to no higher than IIB [18].

Albuminuria

Microalbuminuria is often considered as poor man's marker of endothelial dysfunction. Microalbuminuria is generally seen in patients with diabetes mellitus and hypertension. The American Diabetes Association recommends a yearly urinalysis for all diabetic patients. Since 24 h urine collection is cumbersome, early morning samples for albumin-creatinine ratio have been used for diagnosis. Microalbuminuria is a ratio of 30–300 mg/g and macroalbuminuria as >300 mg/g. Multiple cohort studies have linked urinary albumin excretion to CVD risk. A meta-analysis of 26 studies (n = 169,949) showed a positive correlation between albuminuria and incidence of coronary disease [19]. Macroalbuminuria had twice the risk and those with microalbuminuria had a 50 % greater risk of developing CHD irrespective of coexisting hypertension, diabetes and renal function status. Urinary albumin excretion in Framingham and the Cardiovascular Health Study showed minor improvement in the C-statistic [20, 21]. The later study showed risk reclassification with the urinary albumin-creatinine ratio. Subjects with calculated Framingham risk of 5–10 % with urine albumin >30 g/mg had an observed CHD incidence of 20 % versus 6.3 % in the same risk category with lower urine albumin.

The 2010 ACCF/AHA guideline considered microalbuminuria reasonable (class IIA) for CV risk assessment in asymptomatic patients with diabetes or hypertension. For asymptomatic adults without these conditions but still at intermediate risk, the level of recommendation was IIB [17]. The 2013 ACCF/AHA guidelines, citing uncertain contribution of microalbuminuria for risk assessment, have excluded urine albumin measurement in asymptomatic adults [18].

Lipoprotein Associated Phospholipase A2 (LP-PLA2)

Lipoprotein Associated Phospholipase A2 is an enzyme produced by lymphocytes and macrophages that hydrolyzes oxidized phospholipids in LDL. Products of this degradation (lysophosphatidylcholine and oxidized nonesterified fatty acids) are pro-inflammatory and promote atherosclerosis [22]. LP-PLA2 activity is directly related to smoking and LDL and inversely related to HDL levels. Lipid lowering therapy reduces LP-PLA2 levels.

Elevated LP-PLA2 in the plasma and increased LP-PLA2 activity are associated with cardiovascular disease. Meta-analyses of 14 studies (n = 20,549) found an odds ratio of 1.60 (95 % CI 1.36–1.89) for association between LP-PLA2 and CV disease after adjusting for traditional risk factors [23]. Atherosclerosis Risk in Communities (ARIC) study and Rancho Bernardo study showed small improvements in AUC with the addition of Lp-PLA2 to CV risk prediction [24, 25]. However, two different trials evaluating LP-PLA2 inhibitors found no beneficial effect on coronary events and other outcomes [26, 27].

The 2010 ACCF/AHA guidelines thus gave measurement of LP-PLA2 a lukewarm IIb recommendation [17]. The 2013 guidelines have not recommended LP-PLA2 [18].

Lipoprotein (a) (LP [a])

Lipoprotein (a) is a lipid sub-particle synthesized in the liver that consists of apolipoprotein B100 linked to apolipoprotein (a). Its exact function in humans is unknown but it has been linked to foam cell formation, inflammation and thrombosis. LP (a) in many studies has been associated with poor CV outcomes. A recent meta-analysis of 24 prospective cohort studies, showed that in patients with 3.5-fold higher LP (a) levels, there was a small increase in CHD (risk ratio 1.13) and stroke (risk ratio 1.10) [28]. There is insufficient data to suggest any incremental risk benefit from measuring LP (a) levels beyond traditional risk factors.

Measurement of LP (a) or other lipid sub-particles for risk stratifying asymptomatic individuals was not recommended (class III) by the ACCF/AHA guideline from 2010 [17] and was not mentioned by the 2013 guidelines [18].

Natriuretic Peptides

Natriuretic peptides (Atrial natriuretic peptide, B-type natriuretic peptide, N-terminal-proatrial natriuretic peptide and N-terminal-pro B-type natriuretic peptide) are released from the myocardium in response to wall stress. Their utility in diagnosis and prognostication in heart failure is well established. Population based studies from North American (including Framingham) and Europe have found higher levels of natriuretic peptides to be associated with a higher incidence of MI, stroke, heart failure, CV death and all-cause death in asymptomatic patients [29–31]. This association may be secondary to underlying left ventricular hypertrophy and subclinical myocardial damage from hypertension or ischemia though this is speculative. The relationship between BNP and future CV events has neither been rigorously tested for incremental increase in the C-statistic when added to traditional risk factors, nor evaluated for risk reclassification.

ACCF/AHA 2010 risk assessment guidelines advised against checking them in asymptomatic patients (class III recommendation) [17]. The 2013 guidelines have not discussed their role [18].

Troponin

Cardiac troponin is the preferred biomarker to detect myocardial necrosis in acute coronary syndromes. Troponin elevation is also seen in situations of high myocardial demand and non-ischemic conditions like renal disease, heart failure, sepsis and stroke. Methods for troponin detection have become increasingly more sensitive and the new generation ultra-sensitive assays can detect troponins even in the general population. Increased troponin levels with high sensitivity assays may be associated with poor CV outcomes in asymptomatic patients. Participants (aged 54–74 years, n=9698) in ARIC with elevated cardiac troponin T ($\geq$0.003 µg/L) had a higher incidence of CAD, heart failure and all-cause mortality after adjusting for traditional risk factors, renal function, hsCRP and natriuretic peptides [32]. Younger asymptomatic individuals (aged 30–65 years, n=3546) from the Dallas Heart study had a similar increase in adjusted all-cause mortality with elevated troponin levels [33]. This raises the possibility of low level myocardial ischemia or stress in these asymptomatic patients. However, this relationship needs further evaluation and validation. It has the same limitations as natriuretic peptides and measuring troponin levels in the general population does not have a present role in clinical practice. The guidelines have not discussed it.

Subclinical Atherosclerosis Imaging Techniques and Vascular Markers

Coronary Artery Calcium

As part of atherosclerosis, calcium deposits in diseased vessel walls. Atherosclerosis progresses with age and the elderly have significantly more calcium in their arteries compared to the young. Coronary artery calcium (CAC) gives an estimate of plaque in the arterial wall. Its non-linear relationship to luminal narrowing (as seen on angiogram) is probably explained by positive remodeling of the vessel. Though calcified plaques are relatively stable, their presence indicates coexisting soft plaque responsible for most acute coronary events. CAC can be detected on 2.5–3 mm thick axial images obtained from non-contrast ECG-gated electron beam or multi detector computed tomography (CT). Based on the area and density of calcium, a calcium score (measured in Agatston units) is obtained and acts as a surrogate marker for global coronary plaque burden [34]. The test can be performed within minutes and is highly sensitive (nearly 100 % for coronary plaque) with virtually no false positive results. However, as previously mentioned, it is not very specific for 'obstructive' CAD.

CAC correlates well with future CV events. Pooled data of 27,622 asymptomatic patients from six studies showed incremental rates of MI and CV deaths with increasing CAC score. Subjects with CAC of 0 had a very low (0.4 %) 3–5 year event rate. When compared to this group, the relative risk of having an event with scores of 1–112, 100–400, 400–999 and ≥1000 were 1.9, 4.3, 7.2 and 10.8 respectively [34]. Subsequent studies have shown this relations ship to be consistent. Detrano et al. studied CAC in 6722 men and women from four major racial and ethnic groups (white, black, Hispanic and Chinese) and showed that a doubling of CAC score increased major coronary event risk by 15–35 % and risk of any coronary event by 18–39 % [35]. Predictive values of CAC scores were similar in all racial groups. Addition of CAC to traditional risk prediction models significantly improves AUC. MESA showed an AUC improvement from 0.79 to 0.83 with the addition of CAC (P=0.006) [36]. This improvement was significantly superior to that seen with hsCRP, carotid intima media thickness or ankle brachial index. CAC also has a reclassification benefit. Intermediate risk patients (with a 10 years CV event rate of 10–20 % as predicted by FRS) with scores of >300 had a 10 years event rate of approximately 28 % [37]. Thus, CAC reclassified these patients to high risk. High CAC scores in asymptomatic patients may motivate some towards healthier lifestyle changes [38, 39] and positively influence aspirin and statin use [40].

High CAC scores, especially in those reclassified to high risk, probably merit intensification of medical therapy. But there are no data to support additional testing in this patient group in the form of either stress testing or angiogram. In fact, there is no evidence that CAC testing changes CV outcomes. Thus, its utility as a screening test is not established. An important consideration and limitation with CAC imaging is radiation exposure. Although radiation from a cardiac CT for CAC is <1.5 mSv, this is not negligible and is a cause of concern especially in the young. Additionally, the diagnostic yield of CAC is men <40 and women <50 years of age is low, tilting the risk-benefit ratio towards avoiding CAC testing in this age group. Another important sub-group worthy of mention is patients with end stage renal disease on hemodialysis who, due to perturbations in calcium-phosphorus metabolism, have significantly higher calcium deposition in the coronaries. CAC testing in this population needs to be interpreted with caution due to lack of data from under-representation of these patients in trials. CAC is not recommended for follow up as there are no data to support that repeat testing influences management or outcome. In summary, among the newer risk factors of CAD, CAC has the strongest association with future CV events and its measurement adds value to traditional risk factors and helps reclassify intermediate risk patients. This may potentially be helpful in determining the aggressiveness with which to medically treat these patients.

The 2010 ACCF/AHA guidelines gave CAC testing IIA recommendation for patients at intermediate risk [17]. The 2013 guidelines suggest that CAC (level IIB) may be considered to inform decision making if treatment decisions are uncertain after quantitative risk assessment [18].

Ankle Brachial Index

The selective predilection of atherosclerosis for the lower as opposed to upper extremities has been described since the 1950s as a non-invasive marker of peripheral arterial disease (PAD). Ankle-brachial index (ABI) is the ratio of the highest blood pressure measurements from lower and upper extremities. Differential narrowing of arteries in lower extremities from the atherosclerotic disease process would cause a lower blood pressure recording when measured with a pressure cuff, leading to a lower ABI in patients with significant PAD. ABI cut-offs of ≤0.9 are significant in detecting PAD with a sensitivity and specificity of around 90 %.

CVD and PAD share similar risk factors. Low ABIs are associated with hypertension, diabetes mellitus, dyslipidemia, smoking and other CVD risk factors. In fact, peripheral atherosclerosis (as measured by ABI) is a marker for significant disease in other vascular beds including coronary and cerebrovascular circulation. Population based studies have shown strong correlations between low ABI and CAD with odds ratios ranging from 1.4 to 3 [41, 42]. This association is even stronger in diabetic patients. Similar associations are seen between low ABI and strokes. High ABIs, on the other hand, represent increased vascular stiffness secondary to calcification of blood vessels. Though not as extensively studied as low ABI, high ABI is also linked to CVD. An ABI >1.4 is associated with increased risk of stroke and heart failure [43]. MESA also found high ABIs to be associated with incident CVD [44]. Thus, the relationship between ABI and CV risk is probably best represented by a J shaped curve with increased risk in individuals with low (≤0.9) as well as high ABI (≥1.4).

Does ABI add to the predictive value of traditional risk factors in a meaningful way to reclassify patients beyond the assessment available from FRS? A meta-analysis by the ABI collaboration assessing 16 cohort studies and evaluating a total of 24,955 men and 23,339 women with a follow up of 480,325 person-years found that after adjusting for FRS, low ABI (≤0.9) remained an important predictor of 10 years cardiovascular mortality (HR 2.9 for men and 3.0 for women) [45]. Within each Framingham risk category, low ABI was associated with approximately twice the risk of all-cause mortality, CV mortality, and coronary events. The study also showed that normal ABIs could reclassify 43 % of high risk men (FRS ≥20) to intermediate risk and an abnormal ABI could reclassify 9 % of women at low (≤10) or intermediate risk [10–19] to high risk. Thus, ABI provides incremental stratification above traditional risk factors. Subsequently, MESA also found low (≤1.00) and high (≥1.40) ABI to be associated with incident CVD events independent of traditional risk factors as well as CAC scores and carotid intimal medial thickness [44].

In patients with established CAD, low ABI portends an even worse prognosis in terms of increased risk of MI, stroke, heart failure, and CV mortality independent of preexisting risk factors [46]. This is likely due to the multiplicative effects of atherosclerosis in multiple vascular beds.

Though ABI serves as a cost and time efficient non-invasive way of risk stratification, factors like patient and limb position, cuff size, Doppler vs oscillometry derived pressure measurement, inter and intra-user variability can influence accurate readings. The AHA in 2012 released a scientific statement to standardize measurement and interpretation of ABI [47].

The use of ABI was considered reasonable for CV risk assessment in asymptomatic individuals and was given IIA recommendation by the ACCF/AHA guidelines in 2010 [17]. However, the latest 2013 guideline argued that ABI (along with other newer risk factors) has not been studied prospectively as a screening tool in randomized trials to look for CV outcomes [18]. Thus, the benefit of using this tool in clinical practice is uncertain. The ACCF/AHA guidelines have subsequently watered down the strength of recommendation to a level IIB and have recommended its use specifically in patients with intermediate risk.

Carotid Intima Media Thickness

Carotid intima-media thickness (CIMT) is a non-invasive measurement of the combined thickness of intima and media layers of the carotid artery wall using ultrasound. Due to the inability of current ultrasound technology to accurately delineate these layers, they are measured in continuum from the intima-lumen interface to the media-adventitia border. Measurement made off the far wall as compared to the near wall of the vessel correlates better with actual histological wall thickness. CIMT used as a surrogate marker for atherosclerosis, is among the new risk factors to predict adverse CV events.

There are, however, several technical limitations to accurate CIMT measurement. An important conceptual caveat is that atherosclerosis and plaque formation can be focal rather than diffuse leading to significant regional variability in IMT in the same patient depending on sampling location. The angle of the probe can change the measured thickness and miniscule differences in measurement (less than 1 mm) can lead to significant variability in interpretation [48]. CIMT measurement, thus, requires high levels of precision on the part of the operator and standardization in the lab is difficult to achieve in real world practice. This also makes serial scanning to evaluate progression a problem.

Multiple large clinical studies have shown the predictive value of CIMT in the risk of future CV events like MI, stroke and death [49]. Relative risk of MI increases by 10–15 % for every 0.1 mm increase in CIMT [49]. MESA showed CIMT to be a stronger predictor of stroke than CAC score [50]. However, the heterogeneity of methods used to assess CIMT in these studies has been a source of confusion. Studies have used different segments of the carotid tree (common carotid artery, carotid bulb or internal carotid artery); unilateral vs bilateral neck imaging; single vs multiple segment sampling; inclusion or exclusion of plaque; far wall vs near wall measurements; and mean or maximum thickness for defining CIMT. Additionally, different cut offs of significance for CIMT to predict CV risk make it nearly impossible to compare or combine study results. To alleviate uncertainty, ASE in 2008 defined CIMT to be significant if it was in excess of the 75th percentile of the reference population [51].

Clinical importance of any novel risk factor relates to its ability to reclassify intermediate risk patients into high or low risk. Studies evaluating CIMT failed to show significant discrimination above traditional risk factors. A recent meta-analysis comparing 14 studies using common carotid IMT to predict 10 years risk of new MI or strokes showed only a small and clinically insignificant net reclassification benefit over FRS [52].

CIMT was initially given a class IIa recommendation in the 2010 ACCF/AHA guideline statement for CV risk assessment is asymptomatic individuals [17]. However, due to the above mentioned pitfalls and dubious clinical utility, the use of CIMT in asymptomatic adults has been downgraded to Class III (no benefit) in the most recent guideline from 2013 [18].

Endothelial Dysfunction and Peripheral Flow Mediated Dilatation

The endothelium forms the largest organ of the body and it is essential for normal coronary blood flow. The entire vascular tree is lined with endothelial cells that modulate vascular tone. Endothelial dysfunction precedes angiographically apparent coronary obstruction. Endothelial dysfunction can be elicited invasively by paradoxical vasoconstriction seen on intracoronary infusion of acetylcholine. Since endothelial dysfunction is considered the initial step in the pathogenesis of atherosclerosis, non-invasive methods for its evaluation have been developed. Peripheral arterial flow-mediated dilatation (FMD) is one such non-invasive method. A blood pressure cuff is inflated over the forearm for 4–5 min followed by release of pressure. The pressure release leads to increased blood flow that stimulates nitric oxide release, which in turn causes brachial artery vasodilatation. This vasodilation can be quantified by using an ultrasound machine or by measuring pulse wave volumes using finger cuffs (called peripheral arterial tonometry). Individuals with endothelial dysfunction (with faulty nitric oxide production) demonstrate poor or no vasodilation.

Hypertension, diabetes, hyperlipidemia and cigarette smoking cause endothelial dysfunction. In fact, addition of risk factors as demonstrated by percentage increase in FRS has been shown to be linked with decreasing FMD. However, this relationship is only seen in low risk individuals [53] suggesting that endothelial function becomes impaired early on and the addition of more risk factors does not impair it further. The Cardiovascular Health Study showed that FMD was predictive of CV events in the elderly at a 5 years follow up but its addition to the predictive model containing traditional risk factors only minimally increased the AUC [54]. A study of asymptomatic postmenopausal women showed similar correlation [55]. There are no data available on the reclassification value of FMD.

Due to the absence of robust evidence of clinical utility and significant technical limitations (variability in duration of forearm occlusion, location of cuff, inter-user variability, lack of standardized conditions), use of FMD as a marker of endothelial dysfunction to predict CV events has not gained wide application. The 2010 ACCF/AHA guidelines have recommended against FMD studies for cardiac risk assessment in asymptomatic adults [17].

Arterial Stiffness

Arterial walls stiffen and lose elasticity with increasing age and atherosclerosis. Pulse waves produced by the pumping heart propagate through vessel walls. This propagation is influenced by mechanical properties of the vessel and stiff arteries cause pulse waves to move more rapidly. Arterial pulse wave velocity (PWV) and pulse wave analysis (PWA) can thus be used as measures of arterial stiffness. Applanation tonometry is the most commonly used method to measure PWV and PWA, (though Doppler ultrasound or magnetic resonance imaging can also be used for PWV). These parameters are measured using commercial devices that use pre-specified analytic algorithms [56].

There are some studies reporting measures of arterial stiffness (PWV, ambulatory arterial stiffness index, and carotid pulse pressure versus brachial pulse pressure) in predicting CV outcomes in asymptomatic adults [57, 58]. Most have shown a positive correlation after adjusting for traditional risk factors and in some cases for blood pressure and ABI. However, the strength of association is only moderate. No studies have compared measures of arterial stiffness with other novel risk predictors like hsCRP, CIMT or CAC score. There are no data on its value in improving ROC or net reclassification.

Measures of arterial stiffness need standardization, personnel training and quality control to make them reliably reproducible. Thresholds for test positivity need to be established. ACCF/AHA 2010 guidelines for risk assessment in asymptomatic individuals recommended against measuring arterial stiffness for risk stratification (class III) and deemed them to be, at best, only a research tool [17].

Conclusions

1. Effort towards improving CV risk prediction with the aim of implementing primary prevention in appropriate group of patients has led to the search for new risk factors.
2. The last two decades have seen the emergence of numerous biomarkers, vascular markers and subclinical atherosclerosis imaging techniques, some of which are still undergoing clinical validation. Most of these have shown independent association with incident CVD. Others have shown the ability to provide incremental risk assessment above the traditional risk factors and provide reclassification advantage.

3. Among the risk factors discussed above, hsCRP, CAC and ankle brachial index have shown the most promise. But their utility in clinical practice for screening asymptomatic population remains controversial since they have not been evaluated prospectively in randomized control trials to show a difference in clinical outcomes. The issues of availability, cost effectiveness, reproducibility and risks of downstream testing are other factors limiting their widespread use.

4. The 2013 ACCF/AHA guidelines have suggested that hsCRP, CAC and ABI may be optional screening tools if the decision to initiate pharmacological therapy(s) remains uncertain after quantitative CV risk assessment using traditional risk factor model (Class IIb). An hsCRP ≥2 mg/L, CAC ≥300 Agatston units or ≥75th percentile for age, sex, and ethnicity and ABI <0.9 are suggested thresholds to support revising risk assessment upward [18]. The clinical advantage of using other novel risk factors presently remains uncertain.

5. Large scale randomized control trials are needed to validate the clinical utility of testing asymptomatic individuals for novel risk factors in reducing CV outcomes. Their universal application with special emphasis on safety, cost effectiveness and reliability needs to be established. Until such time, it is up to the clinician to continue aggressive treatment of established CV risk factors and to individualize patients based on global risk score and identify those that may benefit from additional testing with one of the newer CV risk markers.

References

1. Go AS, Mozaffarian D, Roger VL, et al.; American Heart Association Statistics Committee and Stroke Statistics Subcommittee. Heart disease and stroke statistics – 2013 update: a report from the American Heart Association. Circulation. 2013;127(1):e6–e245.
2. Kannel WB, Dawber TR, Kagan A, Revotskie N, Stokes 3rd J. Factors of risk in the development of coronary heart disease – six year follow-up experience. The Framingham Study. Ann Intern Med. 1961;55:33–50.
3. Anderson KM, Wilson PW, Odell PM, Kannel WB. An updated coronary risk profile. A statement for health professionals. Circulation. 1991;83(1):356–62.
4. Haffner SM, Lehto S, Ronnemaa T, Pyorala K, Laakso M. Mortality from coronary heart disease in subjects with type 2 diabetes and in non-diabetic subjects with and without prior myocardial infarction. N Engl J Med. 1998;339:229–34.
5. Greenland P, Knoll MD, Stamler J, et al. Major risk factors as antecedents of fatal and nonfatal coronary heart disease events. JAMA. 2003;290:891–7.
6. Ajani UA, Ford ES. Has the risk for coronary heart disease changed among U.S. adults? J Am Coll Cardiol. 2006;48:1177–82.
7. Yousuf O, Mohanty BD, Martin SS, et al. High-sensitivity C-reactive protein and cardiovascular disease: a resolute belief or an elusive link? J Am Coll Cardiol. 2013;62(5):397–408.
8. Kuller LH, Tracy RP, Shaten J, Meilahn EN. Relation of C-reactive protein and coronary heart disease in the MRFIT nested case–control study. Multiple Risk Factor Intervention Trial. Am J Epidemiol. 1996;144:537–47.
9. Ridker PM, Cushman M, Stampfer MJ, Tracy RP, Hennekens CH. Inflammation, aspirin, and the risk of cardiovascular disease in apparently healthy men. N Engl J Med. 1997;336:973–9.
10. Ridker PM, Rifai N, Rose L, Buring JE, Cook NR. Comparison of C-reactive protein and low-density lipoprotein cholesterol levels in the prediction of first cardiovascular events. N Engl J Med. 2002;347:1557–65.

11. Buckley DI, Fu R, Freeman M, Rogers K, Helfand M. C-reactive protein as a risk factor for coronary heart disease: a systematic review and meta-analyses for the U.S. Preventive Services Task Force. Ann Intern Med. 2009;151:483–95.
12. Yeboah J, McClelland RL, Polonsky TS, et al. Comparison of novel risk markers for improvement in cardiovascular risk assessment in intermediate-risk individuals. JAMA. 2012;308:788–95.
13. Melander O, Newton-Cheh C, Almgren P, et al. Novel and conventional biomarkers for prediction of incident cardiovascular events in the community. JAMA. 2009;302:49–57.
14. Ridker PM, Buring JE, Rifai N, Cook NR. Development and validation of improved algorithms for the assessment of global cardiovascular risk in women: the Reynolds Risk Score. JAMA. 2007;297(6):611–9.
15. Ridker PM, Danielson E, Fonseca FA, et al.; JUPITER Study Group. Rosuvastatin to prevent vascular events in men and women with elevated C-reactive protein. N Engl J Med. 2008;359(21):2195–207.
16. Woloshin S, Schwartz LM. Distribution of C-reactive protein values in the United States. N Engl J Med. 2005;352:1611–3.
17. Greenland P, Alpert JS, Beller GA, et al. 2010 ACCF/AHA guideline for assessment of cardiovascular risk in asymptomatic adults: a report of the American College of Cardiology Foundation/American Heart Association Task Force on Practice Guidelines. J Am Coll Cardiol. 2010;56:e50–103.
18. Goff Jr DC, Lloyd-Jones DM, Bennett G, et al. 2013 ACC/AHA guideline on the assessment of cardiovascular risk: a report of the American College of Cardiology/American Heart Association task force on practice guidelines. J Am Coll Cardiol. 2014;63(25 PtB):2935–59.
19. Perkovic V, Verdon C, Ninomiya T, et al. The relationship between proteinuria and coronary risk: a systematic review and meta-analysis. PLoS Med. 2008;5, e207.
20. Cao JJ, Biggs ML, Barzilay J, et al. Cardiovascular and mortality risk prediction and stratification using urinary albumin excretion in older adults ages 68–102: the Cardiovascular Health Study. Atherosclerosis. 2008;197:806–13.
21. Wang TJ, Gona P, Larson MG, et al. Multiple biomarkers for the prediction of first major cardiovascular events and death. N Engl J Med. 2006;355:2631–9.
22. Zalewski A, Macphee C. Role of lipoprotein-associated phospholipase A2 in atherosclerosis: biology, epidemiology, and possible therapeutic target. Arterioscler Thromb Vasc Biol. 2005;25(5):923–31.
23. Garza CA, Montori VM, McConnell JP, Somers VK, Kullo IJ, Lopez-Jimenez F. Association between lipoprotein-associated phospholipase A2 and cardiovascular disease: a systematic review. Mayo Clin Proc. 2007;82(2):159–65.
24. Folsom AR, Chambless LE, Ballantyne CM, et al. An assessment of incremental coronary risk prediction using C-reactive protein and other novel risk markers: the atherosclerosis risk in communities study. Arch Intern Med. 2006;166:1368–73.
25. Daniels LB, Laughlin GA, Sarno MJ, et al. Lipoprotein-associated phospholipase A2 is an independent predictor of incident coronary heart disease in an apparently healthy older population: the Rancho Bernardo Study. J Am Coll Cardiol. 2008;51:913–9.
26. STABILITY Investigators, White HD, Held C, Stewart R, et al. Darapladib for preventing ischemic events in stable coronary heart disease. N Engl J Med. 2014;370(18):1702–11.
27. O'Donoghue ML, Braunwald E, White HD, et al.; SOLID-TIMI 52 Investigators. Effect of darapladib on major coronary events after an acute coronary syndrome: the SOLID-TIMI 52 randomized clinical trial. JAMA. 2014;312(10):1006–15.
28. Emerging Risk Factors Collaboration, Erqou S, Kaptoge S, Perry PL, et al. Lipoprotein(a) concentration and the risk of coronary heart disease, stroke, and nonvascular mortality. JAMA. 2009;302(4):412–23.
29. Wang TJ, Larson MG, Levy D, et al. Plasma natriuretic peptide levels and the risk of cardiovascular events and death. N Engl J Med. 2004;350:655–63.
30. Kistorp C, Raymond I, Pedersen F, et al. N-terminal pro-brain natriuretic peptide, C-reactive protein, and urinary albumin levels as predictors of mortality and cardiovascular events in older adults. JAMA. 2005;293:1609–16.

31. Daniels LB, Laughlin GA, Clopton P, et al. Minimally elevated cardiac troponin T and elevated N-terminal pro-B-type natriuretic peptide predict mortality in older adults: results from the Rancho Bernardo Study. J Am Coll Cardiol. 2008;52:450–9.

32. Saunders JT, Nambi V, de Lemos JA, et al. Cardiac troponin T measured by a highly sensitive assay predicts coronary heart disease, heart failure, and mortality in the Atherosclerosis Risk in Communities Study. Circulation. 2011;123(13):1367–76.

33. de Lemos JA, Drazner MH, Omland T, et al. Association of troponin T detected with a highly sensitive assay and cardiac structure and mortality risk in the general population. JAMA. 2010;304(22):2503–12.

34. Greenland P, Bonow RO, Brundage BH, et al. ACCF/AHA 2007 clinical expert consensus document on coronary artery calcium scoring by computed tomography in global cardiovascular risk assessment and in evaluation of patients with chest pain: a report of the American College of Cardiology Foundation Clinical Expert Consensus Task Force (ACCF/AHA Writing Committee to Update the 2000 Expert Consensus Document on Electron Beam Computed Tomography). J Am Coll Cardiol. 2007;49:378–402.

35. Detrano R, Guerci AD, Carr JJ, et al. Coronary calcium as a predictor of coronary events in four racial or ethnic groups. N Engl J Med. 2008;358:1336–45.

36. Budoff MJ, Nasir K, McClelland RL, et al. Coronary calcium predicts events better with absolute calcium scores than age-sex-race/ethnicity percentiles: MESA (Multi-Ethnic Study of Atherosclerosis). J Am Coll Cardiol. 2009;53:345–52.

37. Nasir K, Budoff MJ, Post WS, et al. Electron beam CT versus helical CT scans for assessing coronary calcification: current utility and future directions. Am Heart J. 2003;146:969–77.

38. Orakzai RH, Nasir K, Orakzai SH, et al. Effect of patient visualization of coronary calcium by electron beam computed tomography on changes in beneficial lifestyle behaviors. Am J Cardiol. 2008;101:999–1002.

39. O'Malley PG, Feuerstein IM, Taylor AJ. Impact of electron beam tomography, with or without case management, on motivation, behavioral change, and cardiovascular risk profile: a randomized controlled trial. JAMA. 2003;289:2215–23.

40. Taylor AJ, Bindeman J, Feuerstein I, et al. Community-based provision of statin and aspirin after the detection of coronary artery calcium within a community-based screening cohort. J Am Coll Cardiol. 2008;51:1337–41.

41. Selvin E, Erlinger TP. Prevalence of and risk factors for peripheral arterial disease in the United States: results from the National Health and Nutrition Examination Survey, 1999–2000. Circulation. 2004;110:738–43.

42. Murabito JM, Evans JC, Nieto K, Larson MG, Levy D, Wilson PW. Prevalence and clinical correlates of peripheral arterial disease in the Framingham Offspring Study. Am Heart J. 2002;143:961–5.

43. Allison MA, Hiatt WR, Hirsch AT, Coll JR, Criqui MH. A high anklebrachial index is associated with increased cardiovascular disease morbidity and lower quality of life. J Am Coll Cardiol. 2008;51:1292–8.

44. Criqui MH, McClelland RL, McDermott MM, Allison MA, Blumenthal RS, Aboyans V, Ix JH, Burke GL, Liu K, Shea S. The ankle-brachial index and incident cardiovascular events in the MESA (Multi-Ethnic Study of Atherosclerosis). J Am Coll Cardiol. 2010;56:1506–12.

45. Fowkes FG, Murray GD, Butcher I, et al. Ankle brachial index combined with Framingham Risk Score to predict cardiovascular events and mortality: a meta-analysis. JAMA. 2008;300:197–208.

46. Agnelli G, Cimminiello C, Meneghetti G, Urbinati S; Polyvascular Atherothrombosis Observational Survey (PATHOS) Investigators. Low ankle-brachial index predicts an adverse 1-year outcome after acute coronary and cerebrovascular events. J Thromb Haemost. 2006;4:2599–606.

47. Aboyans V, Criqui MH, Abraham P, et al.; American Heart Association Council on Peripheral Vascular Disease; Council on Epidemiology and Prevention; Council on Clinical Cardiology; Council on Cardiovascular Nursing; Council on Cardiovascular Radiology and Intervention, and Council on Cardiovascular Surgery and Anesthesia. Measurement and interpretation of the

ankle-brachial index: a scientific statement from the American Heart Association. Circulation. 2012;126(24):2890–909.

48. Naqvi TZ, Lee MS. Carotid intima-media thickness and plaque in cardiovascular risk assessment. JACC Cardiovasc Imaging. 2014;7(10):1025–38.

49. Lorenz MW, Markus HS, Bots ML, Rosvall M, Sitzer M. Prediction of clinical cardiovascular events with carotid intima-media thickness: a systematic review and meta-analysis. Circulation. 2007;115:459–67.

50. Folsom AR, Kronmal RA, Detrano RC, et al. Coronary artery calcification compared with carotid intima-media thickness in the prediction of cardiovascular disease incidence: the Multi-Ethnic Study of Atherosclerosis (MESA). Arch Intern Med. 2008;168:1333–9.

51. Stein JH, Korcarz CE, Hurst RT, et al. Use of carotid ultrasound to identify subclinical vascular disease and evaluate cardiovascular disease risk: a consensus statement from the American Society of Echocardiography Carotid Intima-Media Thickness Task Force. Endorsed by the Society for Vascular Medicine. J Am Soc Echocardiogr. 2008;21:93–111.

52. Den Ruijter HM, Peters SA, Anderson TJ, et al. Common carotid intima-media thickness measurements in cardiovascular risk prediction: a meta-analysis. JAMA. 2012;308:796–803.

53. Witte DR, Westerink J, de Koning EJ, et al. Is the association between flow-mediated dilation and cardiovascular risk limited to low-risk populations? J Am Coll Cardiol. 2005;45: 1987–93.

54. Yeboah J, Crouse JR, Hsu FC, et al. Brachial flow-mediated dilation predicts incident cardiovascular events in older adults: the Cardiovascular Health Study. Circulation. 2007;115:2390–7.

55. Rossi R, Nuzzo A, Origliani G, Modena MG. Prognostic role of flow-mediated dilation and cardiac risk factors in post-menopausal women. J Am Coll Cardiol. 2008;51:997–1002.

56. Laurent S, Cockcroft J, Van Bortel L, et al. for European Network for Non-invasive Investigation of Large Arteries. Expert consensus document on arterial stiffness: methodological issues and clinical applications. Eur Heart J. 2006;27(21):2588–605.

57. Sutton-Tyrrell K, Najjar SS, Boudreau RM, et al. Elevated aortic pulse wave velocity, a marker of arterial stiffness, predicts cardiovascular events in well-functioning older adults. Circulation. 2005;111:3384–90.

58. Dolan E, Thijs L, Li Y, et al. Ambulatory arterial stiffness index as a predictor of cardiovascular mortality in the Dublin Outcome Study. Hypertension. 2006;47:365–70.

Chapter 2
Angiographic Narrowing Prior to ST Elevation MI. Are the Lesions Non Obstructive?

John A. Ambrose and Ryan Berg

Abstract In the 1980s, our group and others published studies that showed that myocardial infarction frequently arose from plaques that on angiograms prior to the event were not significantly stenotic. Over the years, this became an accepted tenet of cardiology and was even incorporated into the definition of the vulnerable plaque. However, more recently, other angiographic data performed either just before or immediately after infarction as well as intravascular data at the time of infarction assessing lesion severity have challenged this paradigm showing that the lesions were, in fact, severely stenotic. This chapter reviews these data and indicates how these two possibilities are actually not mutually exclusive.

Keywords Angiographic lesion severity • Coronary thrombus • Myocardial infarction • Sudden coronary death

Introduction

Total coronary occlusion of an epicardial coronary artery is the usual cause of acute myocardial infarction in patients presenting with ST segment elevation. Acute coronary thrombosis on a disrupted or eroded atherosclerotic plaque is the proven pathological process responsible for infarction in nearly all cases of Type 1 infarction by the Universal definition of myocardial infarction [1]. In the 1980s and early 1990s, several small, retrospective angiographic studies in selected patients

J.A. Ambrose, MD
Chief of Cardiology, UCSF Fresno, Fresno, CA, USA

Department of Medicine, UCSF Community Regional Medical Center, Fresno, CA, USA
e-mail: jamambrose@yahoo.com

R. Berg, MD (✉)
UCSF Fresno Department of Cardiology, Community Regional Medical Center, Fresno, CA, USA
e-mail: medrberg@hotmail.com

© Springer International Publishing Switzerland 2015
J.A. Ambrose, A.E. Rodríguez (eds.), *Controversies in Cardiology*,
DOI 10.1007/978-3-319-20415-4_2

presenting with an acute MI or unstable angina in whom a prior angiogram was available for analysis made a surprising finding. In a majority of cases, the culprit site was not significantly narrowed on the first angiogram and it had usually a <50 % diameter stenosis. In many cases, the site of the subsequent event on the second angiogram even appeared normal on the first angiogram [2–6]. While initially met with skepticism, additional data from other angiographic studies, intravascular ultrasound (IVUS) analyses and pathologic studies in pressure fixed coronary arteries at the time of autopsy supported the concept that the angiogram underestimated plaque size, might appear normal even in the presence of a large plaque burden related to positive or Glagovian remodeling [7] and was often non obstructive prior to an acute coronary event. Over time, this concept that the less than severe angiographic lesion preceded a majority of acute coronary events became accepted by the cardiology community and was even incorporated into the usual characteristics of the vulnerable plaque(the plaque responsible for subsequent myocardial infarction) [8].

Nevertheless, if in the pathogenesis of acute myocardial infarction (AMI), the preceding plaque did not appear angiographically severe, yet the angiogram at the onset of infarction showed total or near total coronary occlusion, how could this occur? A contrary opinion to the concept that the mild angiographic lesion usually preceded MI suggested that the lesion preceding MI was not mild but usually severe. This was based on several different studies suggesting either, (1) severe stenoses and not mild stenoses usually preceded the event, either months or just days to weeks prior to MI or (2) analysis of the angiogram during the acute event but immediately after thrombolytic therapy or mechanical thrombectomy had reopened the infarct-related lesion indicating that the residual narrowing was nearly always >70 % obstructed. This chapter revisits the controversy surrounding "mild diameter stenoses" prior to myocardial infarction and indicates, based on several sources of data, that the contrary opinion does not contradict the mild lesion concept.

A Time Line of Angiographic Narrowing to Acute Myocardial Infarction

To properly examine the relationship between angiographic narrowing and the pathogenesis of acute myocardial infarction, it would be useful to assess 3 time intervals: (1) remote from infarction when the plaque ultimately responsible for the event is quiescent, (2) in the days or weeks prior to infarction and (3) immediately after successful thrombolytic therapy or thrombectomy (see Fig. 2.1). This discussion will be limited for the most part, to patients presenting with ST elevation MI (STEMI) previously defined as transmural or Q wave myocardial infarction.

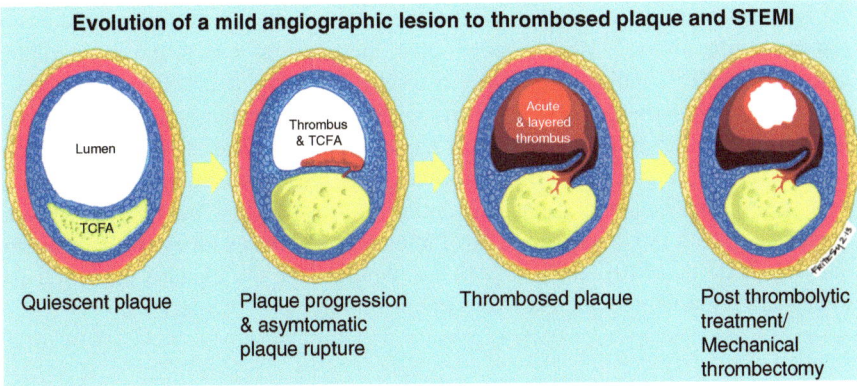

Fig. 2.1 Theoretic cross sections of a coronary artery at different stages in the evolution to STEMI. The *left panel* demonstrates a TCFA with positive remodeling and only mild luminal narrowing. The *second panel* from the left depicts an artery with some progression and an asymptomatic plaque rupture with intraluminal thrombus formation. The lumen begins to narrow. This asymptomatic progression to STEMI is accelerated in the days to weeks prior to the event. The *third panel* depicts the thrombosed plaque of an acute STEMI that has completely obliterated the lumen with acute thrombus over layered thrombus. Following thrombolytic therapy or mechanical thrombectomy, the *last panel* depicts an open but still significantly narrowed arterial cross section with both plaque and residual thrombus occluding the lumen (Reproduced from Giampaolo et al. [43], with permission of Elsevier)

Angiographic Narrowing Remote from AMI

In addition to the early retrospective angiographic studies alluded to above indicating that about 70 % had <50 % diameter stenosis and only 13 % were >70 % stenosed, other more recent studies have supported this concept although in some cases, the diagnosis was not STEMI but other acute syndromes. These data are presented to indicate a pattern seen in many but not all studies related to the pathogenesis of ACS and AMI.

In 2005, Glaser et al. reported on 216 patients from the NHLBI Dynamic PCI Registry who required an additional angiogram for clinical progression at 1 year of a non target lesion [9]. Fifty nine percent presented with unstable angina and 9 % presented with non fatal MI. Of the 216, 157 were available for independent evaluation. The mean stenosis of the progressed lesion was 41.8±20.8 % at the initial angiogram. A majority of lesions (60.5–95/157) were <50 % in severity at the time of the initial angiogram and only 13 % were >70 %. While studied at a different time and in a different population, these percentages were similar to the data reported in the 1980s.

Furthermore, in the PROSPECT (Providing Regional Observations to Study Predictors of Events in the Coronary Tree) study, non culprit events (not the culprit lesion treated during the first angiogram) represented nearly 50 % of all repeat cardiovascular events at 3 years. While these new ischemic events included very few acute infarctions, IVUS in a sub group of these lesions with visual angiographic narrowing >30 % indicated that the responsible lesion at baseline was often a thin-capped fibroatheroma (TCFA) with a large plaque volume and a small cross sectional area. Nevertheless, the mean angiographic diameter stenosis at baseline was 32.3±20.6 % and 59 % of lesions had a <50 % diameter stenosis. Thirty percent were <30 % stenotic at baseline and it is uncertain how many of these were interrogated with IVUS as only 52 % of non culprit lesions with events had accompanying IVUS data [10]. Thus, large plaques may not be significantly narrowed due to positive remodeling which is found in most infarct and ACS lesions.

Differences in Measuring Stenoses Between Technologies

Pathologic studies in patients dying after AMI or with sudden coronary death indicate that plaque rupture of a TCFA is seen in **2/3 to 3/4** of culprit thrombosed plaques [11]. Kolodgie et al. found in pressure fixed coronary arteries at autopsy, that asymptomatic TCFAs in general are not severely narrowed. Eighty percent occur in vessels with <75 % area stenosis which corresponds to <50 % diameter stenosis [12]. It should also be noted that pathology and IVUS measure narrowing differently than coronary angiography. The angiogram compares a narrowing to a proximal reference segment while area stenosis is measured by calculating the change in area at the site of narrowing to the external elastic membrane area. As lesions responsible for acute syndromes are usually positively remodeled [7] but not the proximal reference segment, area narrowing may overestimate stenosis severity relative to angiographic diameter stenosis. Thus, prior to MI or in patients with unstable symptoms, the plaque responsible for the subsequent event may be large but often exhibits <50 % diameter narrowing on angiography. These plaques are bulky but quiescent; most are TCFAs and positive remodeling usually preserves lumen diameter and luminal area.

Not all studies indicate that mild lesions precede ACS and even transmural MI. The angiographic study of Alderman et al. in 1993 appears to be contrary to the mild concept [13]. Five year angiographic follow up from participants in CASS (Coronary Artery Surgical Study) indicated that severe lesions (>80 % diameter narrowing on the first angiogram) were more likely to totally occlude on follow up study compared to less severe lesions. However, no clinical data were available to assess symptoms at the time of follow up. Furthermore, there were many more lesions that were milder or <80 % narrowed that occluded on the repeat study (71 % or 52 of 73) while only 29 % were >80 % initially (their qualitative analysis only categorized lesions into no narrowing, 5–49 %, 50–80 % and >80 % narrowed). In a subsequent publication from CASS, Ellis et al. found that the highest risk for subsequent anterior infarction (either transmural or non-transmural) was a severe stenosis (90–98 %) in the left anterior descending. However, angiographic follow up after the infarction was not available to confirm the severe stenosis as the culprit lesion [14]. Similarly, in the Program on the Surgical Control of the Hyperlipidemias

(POSCH), Buchwald et al. concluded that severe lesions preceded most transmural or Q wave infarcts. Again, no follow up angiography was available to identify the culprit [15].

The last study of import comes from the Patients in the Clinical Outcomes Utilizing Revascularization and Aggressive Drug Evaluation (COURAGE) trial. Mancini et al. analyzed 61 of 119 (56 %) of patients in the optimal medical therapy arm who subsequently had an infarct and a subsequent angiogram as well as other patients who had an ACS without infarction or just more angina requiring subsequent angiography[16]. These authors found for the entire group that lesions originally with <50 % diameter stenosis at baseline were responsible for only one third of events while the rest occurred in lesions with >50 % diameter stenosis at baseline. Yet, patients with MI were not analyzed separately and particularly in those with STEMI, baseline angiographic data were not reported. Thus, in the three studies mentioned above, 2 (Ellis and Buchwald) did not have follow up angiograms and 2 (Ellis and Mancini) included both STEMI and non STEMI cases in their analyses. We believe that because of these discrepancies, these data do not undermine the mild lesion argument.

Any follow up data that includes ACS patients that are not STEMI are also contaminated by the possible presence of supply/demand mismatch (Type 2 MI) as the mechanism for AMI [1]. Type 2 MI can occur in the presence of severe coronary disease although culprit lesions are not identified angiographically in nearly all of these patients. On the other hand, in Type I MI, single angiographic culprits were identified in 95 and 56 % of STEMI and NSTEMI patients, respectively [17].

Angiographic Narrowing in the Days to Weeks Prior to AMI and AMI Pathogenesis

Two studies have assessed angiographic narrowing in the days to weeks before STE MI. The earlier studies quoted above [2–6] did not compute angiographic stenosis data related to the timing of the baseline study prior to AMI. The largest of these two newer studies by Ojio et al. retrospectively assessed 40 patients with 2 angiograms before and after AMI onset similar to the analyses reported above [18]. However, when they analyzed the angiographic narrowing in 20 patients in whom the angiogram was obtained 3 ± 3 days before Q (n=12) or non Q AMI (n=8), the angiographic narrowing averaged 71 ± 12 % at the culprit site while it was 30 ± 18 % in the 20 control patients with a first angiogram that was 6–18 months before the subsequent AMI (see Fig. 2.2). They concluded that the lesion immediately before AMI is often severe. Likewise, in another small retrospective study, Zaman et al. found that lesions leading to STEMI were more often narrowed on the first angiogram if the clinical event was ≤3 months after the initial angiogram (n=7) compared to >3 months (n=34), 59 ± 31 % vs 36 ± 21 %, diameter stenosis respectively, p=0.02 [19].

However, the question that must be asked in both of these studies is why were these patients studied right before the MI? The likely answer was that they were either symptomatic with new onset unstable angina and/ or a lesion had asymptomatically

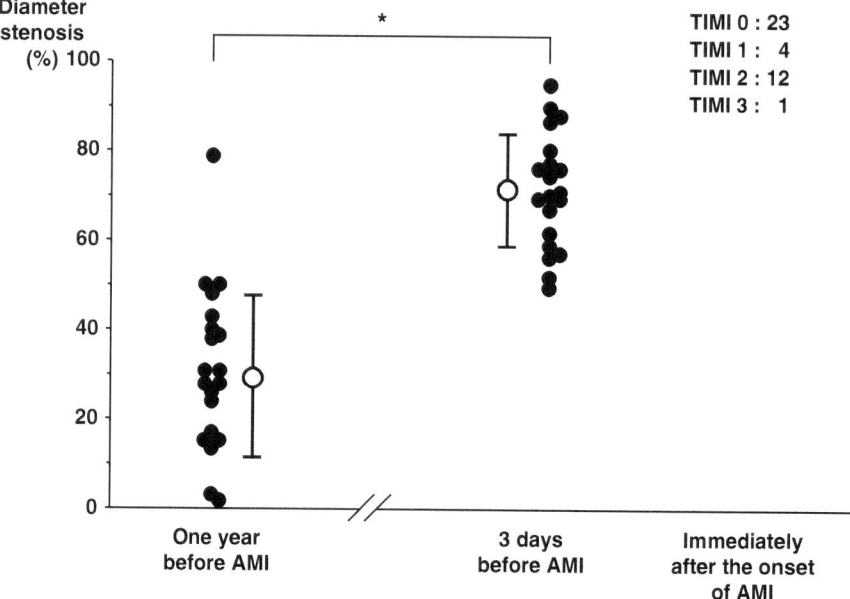

Fig. 2.2 Percent diameter stenosis of infarct related coronary stenosis 1 year before AMI, 3 days before onset, and immediately after onset of AMI (Reproduced from Ojio et al. [18], with permission of Wolters Kluwer health)

destabilized yet had not totally occluded prior to the acute clinical event. In support of that hypothesis was the fact that 70 % of patients in the group with an angiogram 3 days before AMI in the Ojio et al. study had angiographic evidence of an acute, complex culprit lesion as described originally by Ambrose et al. while these lesions were infrequent in the control group (10 %). These complex lesions indicate plaque disruption and/or intracoronary thrombus [20]. Thus, this group just happened to be studied immediately prior to the onset of either Q or non Q MI.

Growth of the plaque and narrowing of the lumen must occur at some point prior to the onset of AMI as the lesion progresses to total or near total occlusion at the time of the clinical event. Pathologically, autopsy studies indicate that the thrombosed lesion responsible for fatal MI or sudden coronary death contains both acute and healed thrombus [21, 22]. Multiple episodes of asymptomatic thrombus formation related to plaque disruptions or plaque hemorrhage usually precede the fatal event. These are the processes responsible for rapid progression of atherosclerotic lesions. Pathologic analysis of thrombectomy specimens at the time of primary PCI in ST elevation MI patients have also indicated that organized thrombus can be extracted in over 50 % of cases [23]. This also suggests some chronicity to the process. i.e. intracoronary thrombus formation does not automatically or immediately lead to a clinical event and the thrombus forms before the onset of symptoms in most patients with STEMI.

Thus, plaque instability and intraluminal thrombus formation must commonly precede the onset of infarction and total or near total coronary occlusion. This process is seen in both asymptomatic and symptomatic patients before infarction. If one considers unstable angina to be the forerunner to AMI particularly if untreated, plaque disruption and/or thrombus (a complex plaque) will be seen in >70 % of cases in the culprit vessel on coronary angiography [20]. Total occlusion in this setting is unusual but the culprit lesion has a severe diameter stenosis (>70 %) in nearly all cases [24]. These processes, we believe help to explain the findings of Ojio et al. and Zaman et al.

Angiographic Narrowing Immediately After Lysis or Thrombectomy

As mentioned earlier, ST elevation MI presents with total or near total coronary occlusion caused by intracoronary thrombus formation on a disrupted or eroded atherosclerotic plaque. Following successful opening of a totally occluded vessel with thrombolytic therapy or after mechanical thrombectomy, the culprit lesion is severely narrowed in nearly all vessels. This has been utilized as an argument favoring the concept that a severe lesion usually precedes MI. Thus, in 2007, Frobert et al. reported on 151 STEMI patients with spontaneous reflow or with immediate reflow after uncomplicated wiring of the lesion but before primary PCI. In 96 %, the underlying diameter stenosis was >50 % and in 66 %, it was >70 % [25]. Similar findings were also reported in 2009 by Manoharan et al. after mechanical thrombectomy in 102 STEMI patients. The underlying culprit lesion was severe in nearly all and was <50 % in only 11 % [26].

However, in the two studies mentioned above, did the residual stenosis represent only plaque in the culprit lesion? In an elegant angiographic study by Brown et al. in 1986, these investigators showed that residual thrombus is present following thrombolytic reopening of a vessel and that the underlying plaque was only moderate [27]. In 21 of 32 cases, the original lesion was <60 and <50 % in 31 %. Follow up angiography in three different studies performed hours to days or weeks after thrombolytic therapy to allow for endogenous thrombolysis have demonstrated that the residual diameter narrowing was moderate averaging 50–57 % on the follow up angiogram [27–29]. Pathologic studies after fatal MI or sudden death also support the concept that the underlying culprit plaque (excluding acute thrombus) may not be severely narrowed. However, unless post mortem preparations utilize pressure fixed arteries, the degree of stenosis will be overestimated as the lumen will be collapsed. Such was the case in the study of Qiao et al. who found thrombosis on plaques that had a mean stenosis of 91 % [30]. With pressure fixation, Davies and Thomas showed in thrombotic lesions responsible for sudden cardiac ischemic death that the average area stenosis was 79 % corresponding to a diameter stenosis of 52 % [31].

The presence of residual thrombus following mechanical thrombectomy at the time of primary PCI can also be inferred from the data of Rittersma et al. Organized thrombus was found on pathologic analysis of thrombectomy specimens in over 50 % of cases suggesting that some thrombotic material was left behind [22]. Furthermore, heightened vasomotion in epicardial arteries and in the microvasculature is common in acute MI which also would increase residual diameter narrowing in the acute setting [32].

Optical coherence tomography (OCT) and IVUS studies after coronary thrombectomy are flawed and have added little concerning the degree of underlying area stenosis. IVUS uses ultrasound to generate gray scale images of the vessel wall and luminal components including plaque and thrombus. While there can be subtle changes in gray scale, IVUS cannot reliably distinguish between plaque and thrombus [33]. Therefore, unless complete thrombectomy is done, the measured IVUS stenosis area is prone to significant over estimation. Hong et al. assessed IVUS images in 125 patients with STEMI [34]. However, not all patients had manual aspiration thrombectomy prior to imaging. Furthermore, the authors stated even in those who underwent aspiration, that thrombus at the culprit lesion was not completely removed. Therefore, the quantitative coronary angiography measurements and IVUS measurements indicated significant vessel narrowing of the culprit lesion which represented a combination of plaque and residual thrombus.

While OCT has better resolution than IVUS (15 μm versus about 120 μm), and can more easily identify thrombus [35], the yellow/orange color scale typically used in current Fourier transformation OCT may not easily distinguish it from surrounding plaque, as they are both seen as signal-rich objects [36]. Furthermore, lipid rich plaque or coronary thrombus causes OCT signal attenuation, which makes it difficult to observe deep layers of the coronary artery wall behind this plaque and thrombus. Thus, OCT is not optimum for the quantification of lipid core size and the evaluation of arterial remodeling [37]. Other OCT studies in AMI [38, 39] are also flawed in quantifying lumen narrowing by the lack of complete thrombus aspiration and therefore are unable to accurately characterize area stenosis. What is clear from these IVUS and OCT studies [34, 38, 39] is that the culprit lesions in STEMI are large, positively remodeled and usually contain a TCFA.

Conclusions

1. In a majority but not in all cases, severe diameter narrowings do not usually precede STEMI in the weeks to months before the event. These lesions that ultimately result in STEMI are quiescent and usually are TCFAs on pathologic or intravascular analysis in which positive remodeling has maintained lumen area in spite of being large plaques.
2. In the days to weeks prior to an acute event, some of these lesions are transformed through rapid progression from intraluminal thrombus formation or intraplaque hemorrhage into truly vulnerable plaques that subsequently progress to symptomatic, total coronary occlusion. Most patients who subsequently develop STEMI are not fortunate enough to undergo angiography in time to detect this degree of rapid progression and eventual occlusion as they are either asymptomatic beforehand or they misinterpret their symptomatology.

3. That a TCFA must expand or grow larger (i.e. become more stenotic) prior to plaque rupture and the acute event has also been recently suggested by Narula et al. [40]. Their post mortem study indicated that percent area narrowing was greater in the presence of rupture and thrombosis but was usually <75 % (<50 % diameter stenosis) in the rupture-prone TCFA.
4. Angiographic narrowing is measured differently than at pathology or with intravascular techniques likely explaining much of the discrepancy among the techniques.
5. Finally, this concept of whether or not the lesion preceding MI is mild or severe should not be considered semantics or just an idle exercise. Myocardial infarction and sudden death still account yearly for hundreds of thousands of events. Demonstrating coronary atherosclerosis either through an invasive angiogram or otherwise is a premonitory sign that can occasionally progress to an acute and/or sometimes a fatal event. Obviously, the invasive angiogram is insensitive to plaque size and not the most appropriate for defining atherosclerotic plaque burden. While some suggest that we should evaluate most moderately stenosed lesions with intravascular techniques such as IVUS or FFR, this is not always practical in our opinion and infrequently utilized [41]. Nevertheless, with so many invasive angiograms still being performed annually, the demonstration of atherosclerosis without severe diameter narrowing on invasive angiography or by other techniques such as CT angiography must be treated as aggressively medically as when severe disease is demonstrated. Otherwise, we perform a great disservice to our patients from reinventing the past.

However, we also don't want to disservice our patients by assuming that *only* mild stenoses have vulnerable potential and to not worry about fixing severe lesions. As mentioned previously, while the majority of lesions leading to STEMI have less than severe diameter stenosis, there are still some as noted even in the angiographic studies from the 1980s that had moderate or severe stenosis prior to the event. Furthermore, as mentioned in section 2 of this article, some severe stenoses are in the active process of transformation from a prior mildly stenotic vulnerable plaque. Finally, it is known from FAME 2 that intervening on a physiologic significant stenosis leads to a reduction in subsequent adverse outcomes [42].

References

1. Thygesen K, Alpert JS, White HD, et al. Universal definition of myocardial infarction. Circulation. 2007;116:2634–53.
2. Ambrose JA, Winters SL, Arora RR, et al. Angiographic evolution of coronary morphology in unstable angina. J Am Coll Cardiol. 1986;7:472–7.
3. Ambrose JA, Tannenbaum MA, Alexopoulos D, et al. Angiographic progression of coronary artery disease and the development of myocardial infarction. J Am Coll Cardiol. 1988;12:56–62.
4. Little WC, Constantinescu M, Applegate RJ, et al. Can coronary angiography predict the site of a subsequent myocardial infarction in patients with mild-to-moderate coronary artery disease? Circulation. 1988;78:1157–66.

5. Hackett D, Verwilghen J, Davies G, Maseri A. Coronary stenoses before and after acute myo-cardial infarction. Am J Cardiol. 1989;63:1517–8.

6. Giroud D, Li JM, Urban P, Meier B, Rutishauer W. Relation of the site of acute myocardial infarction to the most severe coronary serial stenosis at prior angiography. Am J Cardiol. 1992;69:729–32.

7. Glagov S, Weisenberg E, Zarins CK, Stankunavicius R, Kolettis GJ. Compensatory enlarge-ment of human atherosclerotic coronary arteries. N Engl J Med. 1987;316:1371–5.

8. Naghavi M, Libby P, Falk E, et al. From vulnerable plaque to vulnerable patient. Circulation. 2003;108:1664–72.

9. Glaser R, Selzer F, Faxon DP, et al. Clinical progression of incidental, asymptomatic lesions discovered during culprit vessel coronary intervention. Circulation. 2005;111:143–9.

10. Stone GW, Maehara A, Lansky AJ, et al. A prospective natural-history study of coronary ath-erosclerosis. N Engl J Med. 2011;364:226–35.

11. Falk E, Nakano M, Benton JF, Finn AV, Virmani R. Update on acute coronary syndromes: the pathologists' view. Eur Heart J. 2013;34:719–28.

12. Kolodgie FD, Virmani R, Burke AP, et al. Pathologic assessment of the vulnerable human coronary plaque. Heart. 2004;90:1385–91.

13. Alderman EL, Corley SD, Fisher LD, et al. Five-year angiographic follow-up of factors associ-ated with progression of coronary artery disease in the Coronary Artery Surgery Study (CASS). CASS participating Investigators and Staff. J Am Coll Cardiol. 1993;22:1141–54.

14. Ellis S, Alderman E, Cain K, et al. Prediction of risk of anterior myocardial infarction by lesion severity and measurement method of stenoses in the left anterior descending coronary distribu-tion: a CASS Registry Study. J Am Coll Cardiol. 1988;5:908–16.

15. Buchwald H, Hunter DW, Tuna N, et al. Myocardial infarction and percent arteriographic stenosis of culprit lesion. Report from the Program on the Surgical Control of the Hyperlipidemias (POSCH). Atherosclerosis. 1998;138:391–401.

16. Mancini GB, Hartigan PM, Bates ER, et al. Angiographic disease progression and residual risk of cardiovascular events while on optimal medical therapy: observations from the COURAGE Trial. Circ Cardiovasc Interv. 2011;4:545–52.

17. Ambrose JA, Loures-Vale A, Javed U, et al. Angiographic correlates in type 1 and 2 MI by the universal definition. J Am Coll Cardiol Img. 2012;5:463–4.

18. Ojio S, Takatsu H, Tanaka T, et al. Considerable time from the onset of plaque rupture and/or thrombi until the onset of acute myocardial infarction in humans: coronary angiographic find-ings within 1 week before the onset of infarction. Circulation. 2000;102:2063–9.

19. Zaman T, Agarwal S, Anabtwai AG, et al. Angiographic lesion severity and subsequent myo-cardial infarction. Am J Cardiol. 2012;110:167–72.

20. Ambrose JA, Winters SL, Stern A, et al. Angiographic morphology and the pathogenesis of unstable angina pectoris. J Am Coll Cardiol. 1985;5:609–16.

21. Mann J, Davies MJ. Mechanisms of progression in native coronary artery disease: role of healed plaque disruption. Heart. 1999;82:265–8.

22. Burke AP, Kolodgie FD, Farb A, et al. Healed plaque ruptures and sudden coronary death: evidence that subclinical rupture has a role in plaque progression. Circulation. 2001;103:934–40.

23. Rittersma SZ, van der Wal AC, Koch KT, et al. Plaque instability frequently occurs days or weeks before occlusive coronary thrombosis: a pathological thrombectomy study in primary percutaneous coronary intervention. Circulation. 2005;111:1160–5.

24. Ambrose JA, Dangas G. On the pathogenesis of unstable angina. ACC Curr J Rev. 1997;6:17–9.

25. Frobert O, van't Veer M, Aarnoudse W, Simonsen U, Koolen JJ, Pijls NH. Acute myocardial infarction and underlying stenosis severity. Catheter Cardiovasc Interv. 2007;70:958–65.

26. Manoharan G, Ntalianis A, Muller O, et al. Severity of coronary arterial stenoses responsible for acute coronary syndromes. Am J Cardiol. 2009;103:1183–8.

27. Brown BG, Gallery BA, Kennedy WA, et al. Incomplete lysis of thrombus in the moderate atherosclerotic lesion during intracoronary infusion of streptokinase for acute myocardial infarction. Quantitative angiographic conversations. Circulation. 1986;73:654–61.
28. Serruys PW, Arnold AE, Brower RW, et al. Effect of continued rt-PA administration on the residual stenosis after initially successful recanalization in acute myocardial infarction—a quantitative coronary angiography study of a randomized trial. Eur Heart J. 1987;8:1172–81.
29. Van Lierde J, De Geest H, Verstraete M, Van de Werf F. Angiographic assessment of the infarct-related residual coronary stenosis after spontaneous or therapeutic thrombolysis. J Am Coll Cardiol. 1990;16:1545–9.
30. Qiao JH, Fishbein MC. The severity of coronary atherosclerosis at sites of plaque rupture with occlusive thrombosis. J Am Coll Cardiol. 1991;17:1138–42.
31. Davies MJ, Thomas A. Thrombosis and acute coronary artery lesions in sudden cardiac ischemic death. N Engl J Med. 1984;310:1137–40.
32. Fearon WF. Is a myocardial infarction more likely to result from a mild coronary lesion or an ischemia-producing one? Circ Cardiovasc Interv. 2011;4:539–41.
33. Wu X, Mintz G, Xu K, et al. The relationship between attenuated plaque indentified by intravascular ultrasound and no-reflow after stenting in acute myocardial infarction. J Am Coll Cardiol Intv. 2011;4:495–502.
34. Hong Y, Jeong M, Choi Y, et al. Differences in intravascular ultrasound findings in culprit lesions in infarct-related arteries between ST segment elevation myocardial infarction and non-ST segment elevation myocardial infarction. J Cardiol. 2010;56:15–22.
35. Regar E, Van Soest G, Bruining N, et al. Optical coherence tomography in patients with acute coronary syndrome. EuroIntervention. 2010;6 Suppl G:G154–60.
36. Kubo T, Xu C, Wang Z, et al. Plaque and thrombus evaluation by optical coherence tomography. Int J Cardiovasc Imaging. 2011;27:289–98.
37. Kubo T, Ino Y, Tanimoto T, et al. Optical coherence tomography imaging in acute coronary syndromes. Cardiol Res Pract. 2011;2011:1–7.
38. Toutouzas K, Karanasos A, Tsiamis E, et al. New insights by optical coherence tomography into the differences and similarities of culprit ruptured plaque morphology in non-ST-elevation myocardial infarction and ST-elevation myocardial infarction. Am Heart J. 2011;161:1192–9.
39. Ino Y, Kubo T, Tanaka A, et al. Difference of culprit lesion morphologies between ST- segment elevation myocardial infarction and non-ST- segment elevation acute coronary syndrome. J Am Coll Cardiol Intv. 2011;4:76–82.
40. Narula J, Nakano M, Virmani R, et al. Histopathologic characteristics of atherosclerotic coronary disease and implications of the findings for the invasive and noninvasive detection of vulnerable plaques. J Am Coll Cardiol. 2013;61:1041–51.
41. Dattilo PB, Prasad A, Honeycutt E, Wang TY, Messenger JC. Contemporary patterns of fractional flow reserve and intravascular ultrasound use among patients undergoing PCI in the United States. Insights from the National Cardiovascular Data Registry. J Am Coll Cardiol. 2012;60:2337–9.
42. De Bruyne B, Pijls N, Kalesan B, et al. Fractional flow reserve-guided PCI versus medical therapy in stable coronary disease. N Engl J Med. 2012;367:991–1001.
43. Giampaolo N, Stafanini GG, Caopdanno D, Crea F, Ambrose JA, Berg R. Are the culprit lesions severely stenotic? JACC Cardiovasc Imaging. 2013;10:1108–14.

Chapter 3
Vulnerable Plaques Versus Patients-How to Reduce Acute Coronary Events in the Future

Richard George Kiel and John A. Ambrose

Abstract Cardiovascular disease including acute myocardial infarction and sudden death is the leading cause of death in the United States and worldwide. Important advances in prevention and therapy have been able to recently reduce their prevalence and improve therapeutic outcomes. However, much more work needs to be done. While standard risk factors can identify those most likely to succumb from these conditions, most of these events unfortunately occur in the low to intermediate risk populations.

This chapter considers the two main approaches for reducing subsequent events: (1) identifying and treating the vulnerable plaque versus (2) identification and treating the vulnerable or high risk patient. Which approach will be the most efficacious in reducing subsequent hard cardiovascular events.

Keywords Vulnerable plaque • Thin-capped fibroatheroma • Plaque rupture • Plaque erosion • Vulnerable patient

Introduction

Cardiovascular disease (CVD) including acute myocardial infarction (AMI) and sudden cardiac death (SCD) are the leading cause of mortality for adults in the United States surpassing deaths related to cancer. Through advances in medical

R.G. Kiel, MD
Medical Education Program, Cardiology Division, Department of Internal Medicine, University of California San Francisco-Fresno, Fresno, CA, USA
e-mail: rkiel@fresno.ucsf.edu

J.A. Ambrose, MD (✉)
Chief of Cardiology, UCSF Fresno, Fresno, CA, USA

Department of Medicine, UCSF Community Regional Medical Center, Fresno, CA, USA
e-mail: jamambrose@yahoo.com

© Springer International Publishing Switzerland 2015   33
J.A. Ambrose, A.E. Rodríguez (eds.), *Controversies in Cardiology*,
DOI 10.1007/978-3-319-20415-4_3

care, event rates have decreased but in 2010, according to the AHA, there were an estimated 915,000 new or recurrent AMIs and 278,000 SCDs [1].

The primary method for reducing AMI and SCD has been to identify those at risk or with the acute presentation and to then treat appropriately with guideline-directed medical, interventional and/or surgical therapies. Identifying appropriate patients at risk is relatively easy in those with established disease or in those with coronary disease equivalents such as diabetes, peripheral vascular disease or significant renal insufficiency. The difficulty is in identifying those patients without a prior history i.e. those in primary prevention. Those at highest risk according to Framingham have a 10 year event rate ≥20 % but most initial adverse CV events including AMI and SCD occur in the intermediate and low risk populations which include a larger population although at a lower event rate (percentage) than in the high risk population [2].

As an alternative to the high risk patient is the concept of identifying and treating the vulnerable or high risk plaque. This is the plaque prone to intracoronary thrombus formation and responsible for nearly all ST elevation MI, and a majority of non STEMI and SCDs. Pathologists have identified disruption of a thin-capped fibroatheroma (TCFA) as the primary cause of fatal AMI or SCD in about 2/3 s to 3/4 s of cases [3]. In the remaining cases, particularly in women <50 years of age or in cigarette smokers, the acute event appears related to plaque erosion and intracoronary thrombus formation. The controversies that form the basis of this chapter revolve around the question as to the best methods for reducing future acute coronary events? Will we be able to better identify and treat the high risk patient and prevent the initial or subsequent events? Will identification and local therapy of a vulnerable plaque ever be an evidenced-based strategy for selected patients?

The Vulnerable or High Risk Plaque Concept

If the thrombosed plaque is the immediate cause of most acute coronary events, can one find the so-called vulnerable plaque, that is likely to progress in the future and cause the acute event? The post mortem data referred to in the introduction concerning the histopathology of thrombosed plaque responsible for acute syndromes, have been supported by angiography and intravascular techniques such as intravascular ultrasound, ocular coherence tomography or infrared spectroscopy which can be performed at the time of percutaneous coronary intervention [4]. Table 3.1 highlights the most commonly used modalities for imaging the vulnerable plaque. As most vulnerable plaques are angiographically non-obstructive in the weeks to months prior to the event [5–8], relying on symptomatology alone prior to the event is usually not useful. For vulnerable plaque detection, one would need to find a device either invasive or preferably noninvasive that could detect the vulnerable plaque. For the vulnerable plaque strategy to be evidenced-based would necessitate knowing the natural history of such plaques and being able to show that intervening on a presumed vulnerable plaque by some approach such as a stent was safer and more cost effective in reducing future events than the best medical therapy alone [9].

Table 3.1 Commonly used imaging techniques for identifying the vulnerable plaque

Technique	Imaging benefit
Intravascular ultrasound (IVUS)	Quantify plaque burden, identify positive remodeling, calculate area stenosis, calcification
IVUS + virtual histology	Better define plaque characteristics; identify pathological intimal thickening, thick and thin capped fibroatheromas, degree of calcification
Optical coherence tomography (OCT)	Quantify fibrous cap thickness, identify plaque rupture, erosion, calcification
Infrared spectroscopy (LipiScan)	Quantify plaque lipid content
CT coronary angiography	Identify low attenuation plaques, determine presence of positive remodeling, identify ruptured plaque, punctate calfication

The first study to attempt to define invasively the natural history of vulnerable plaque was the landmark PROSPECT (Providing Regional Observations to Study Predictors of Events in the Coronary Tree) trial [10]. Patients undergoing percutaneous intervention for an acute coronary syndrome were evaluated. After all culprit and other severe lesions were intervened upon, based on the decision of the angiographer, the remaining non culprit arteries were evaluated with angiography, intravascular ultrasound and virtual histology. Patients were followed for 3 years and those with another event- either a myocardial infarction, need for another angiogram because of increasing or unstable angina or aborted sudden death were restudied to assess the cause (culprit lesion) for the syndrome. At 3 years follow up, 23 % had an event and this was nearly equally distributed between the prior culprit lesion/lesions that had been intervened upon or a different lesion in a non culprit vessel. While Stone et al. found that the presence of a TCFA identified by VH technology, with a large plaque burden on IVUS (>70 %) and a plaque area <4 mm^2 had an 18 % incidence of a non culprit event at 3 years, there were only 6 non culprit myocardial infarctions and no documented sudden deaths at follow up. Most non culprit events were increasing or unstable angina. Furthermore, identification of a TCFA was a non specific finding as there were nearly 600 TCFA's at baseline but so few acute events at follow up.

Thus, more date on plaques responsible for subsequent acute events are required. We still do not know the natural history of presumed vulnerable plaques and a plaque that looks vulnerable on an initial evaluation may change at some later point and appear stabilized [11]. Additional studies are required if the local approach to reducing subsequent acute events will become a viable option. There are additional studies, some on-going that are trying to address the natural history question. Utilizing IVUS, angiography and infrared spectroscopy to identify lipid core, PROSPECT 2 (Prospective natural history of coronary atherosclerosis – NCT02171065). will try to further characterize this plaque. Furthermore, a subset with lipid-rich plaques will be randomized to a bio-absorbable stent and optimal medical therapy versus optimal medical therapy alone to test whether this local approach can reduce subsequent events on follow up.

One concern with an invasive methodology is the fact that all of the detectors are concentrating on finding the responsible TCFA and not considering plaque erosion which is not an infrequent cause of STEMI, NSTEMI or SCD. Several studies have suggested that acute myocardial infarctions secondary to plaque erosion may constitute more than 30 % of all acute coronary syndromes [12, 13]. Furthermore, if the detector is invasive, what about individuals in whom the first presentation of symptomatic coronary disease is AMI or SCD. In the Framingham study, 53 % of men and 36 % of women respectively, presented with either AMI or SCD [14]. While a non invasive detector of a vulnerable plaque would be preferable to an invasive detector, there is no consensus, at present, as to the appropriate technique/s and additional prospectively evaluation is required.

The Vulnerable or High Risk Patient

While there are established therapies to reduce subsequent events for patients with known cardiovascular disease manifestations or coronary disease equivalents, can one identify the vulnerable or high risk patient particularly in primary prevention? This is the most difficult challenge to prevent the initial acute event. Nearly half of all patients who die from cardiovascular disease will do so as a result of sudden cardiac death, and this is often the initial presenting symptom of coronary artery disease [15]. Table 3.2 lists common tools used to assess patient risk.

In an effort to better characterize and treat these lower risk populations that might be at risk for AMI or SCD (most events not in the high risk population by Framingham), the new cholesterol guidelines have broadened their recommendations for statin therapy to include individuals 40–75 years of age with a 10 years risk of ≥ 7.5 % [16]. Other markers of atherosclerosis have been studied to enhance risk prediction. These include calcium scoring, carotid intima-medial thickness measurements, hsCRP and several others. On-going studies such as the High Risk Plaque initiative and the Progression and Early detection of Subclinical Atherosclerosis (PESA) study are assessing the additive benefit of some of these non invasive imaging markers above standard risk factors in predicting first adverse cardiac events [17, 18].

Serum markers of inflammation have been predictive of plaque vulnerability in multiple studies. Paul Ridker and collegues have demonstrated that high sensitivity CRP is predictive of the development of cardiovascular events, and that the use of potent statins in patients with elevated hsCRP reduces the incidence of cardiac events [19, 20]. The JUPITER study randomized 17,802 low to medium risk patients with normal levels of LDL cholesterol and an elevated HsCRP to either 20 mg of rosuvastatin or placebo. The group receiving statin therapy had a 53 % relative risk reduction in the composite endpoint of myocardial infarction, stroke, or cardiovascular death. However, the event rates at follow up were low. Several other potential markers of plaque vulnerability including lipoprotein phospholipase A2, osteoglycan and NGAL/MMP9 have also demonstrated the ability to predict some coronary

Table 3.2 Common tools for estimating patient risk of atherosclerotic cardiovascular disease

Traditional scoring systems	Imaging techniques
Pooled Cohort Risk Equation	Magnetic Resonance Imaging Coronary Angiography (MRA)
Framingham Risk Core	Positron Emesion Tomography/Computed Tomography (PET-CT, SPECT)
European Society Risk Score	Coronary calcium scoring
PROCAM Study Risk Score	Molecular Imaging
Reynolds Risk Score	Ankle brachial index (ABI)
	Carotid intimal medial thickness
	Iliac-femoral imaging
Non-traditional markers of CV risk	**Biomarkers**
Left ventricular Hypertrophy	High sensitivity C-reactive protein (hsCRP)
Triglycerides	Homosystine
Small dense Low density lipoprotein (LDL)	Fibrinogen
Apo-lipoprotein B	Lipoprotein associated phospholipas A_2 (LP-PLA$_2$)
Microalbuminuria	Myeloperoxidase
Abdominal obesity	Oxidized LDL
Physical inactivity	Fractalkine
Poor socioeconomic status (QRISK, ASSIGN)	CD36
Erectile dysfunction	
Physiologic assessment of atherosclerosis	**Genetic markers**
Stress testing	Single nucleotide polymorphism (Microarray)
Endothelial dysfunction techniques	
Arterial compliance	

events but have yet to be demonstrated to be effective reducing cardiovascular events in primary prevention trials [21, 22].

The High-Risk Plaque Initiative as previously mentioned, is an ongoing research and development effort designed to evaluate the role of a variety of biomarkers and advanced imaging techniques in providing a more accurate assessment of cardiovascular risk [17]. This ambitious effort should shed some light regarding the role of genetic analysis, coronary calcium scoring, ankle-brachial index, carotid intimal thickness, iliofemoral ultrasound and other emerging technologies on estimating the risk of silent atherosclerotic cardiovascular disease. The 2013 ACC/AHA joint guidelines on the assessment of cardiovascular risk suggest that all patients be screened for traditional atherosclerotic cardiovascular disease risk factors every 4–6 years in adults 20–79 years of age and to estimate a 10 years risk of an acute event [23]. The ACC/AHA has also endorsed a race and sex specific pooled cohort equation which was derived from the Atherosclerosis Risk in Communities (ARIC), Cardiovascular Health Study, Coronary Artery Risk Development in Young Adults

(CARDIA) Study, and the original Framingham study as well as its offspring cohorts. These studies are well validated to provide a reasonable assessment of both 10 year and lifetime risk of ASCVD in non-hispanic whites and African Americans. In addition, the guidelines suggest that the same Pooled Cohort Equation may be used in populations other than non-hispanic African Americans and whites. Table 3.3 lists the properties of this risk stratification tool. When compared to the more traditional method of utilizing the Framingham data base to estimate risk, the Pooled Cohort Equations tend to encourage broader use of risk factor modification, particularly in terms of statin use, as mentioned previously. The guidelines go on to suggest that if, after undergoing risk assessment using the Pooled Cohort Equation, a therapeutic decision hasn't been reached then it is reasonable to utilize either a hs CRP level, coronary artery calcium score, or ankle-brachial index for treatment making decisions. Citing the lack of outcomes data, the ACC/AHA joint guideline committee currently recommends against the use of carotid intima medial thickness, apolipoprotein B, albuminuria and cardiorespiratory fitness as part of a risk assessment for atherosclerotic cardiovascular disease [23].

As the initial manifestation of atherosclerotic cardiovascular disease is often an acute coronary syndrome or sudden cardiac death, it is important to focus on primary prevention in patients at increased risk. Our current treatment strategies for primary prevention has primarily included risk factor identification and modification targeting blood pressure, serum LDL cholesterol, lifestyle modification and weight loss. Given that atherosclerosis is primarily a disease of chronic inflammation, therapies which reduce inflammation have also been targeted as a mechanism

Table 3.3 Components of the ACC/AHA pooled cohort equation

Registries/databases incorporated	Validation study
Cardia	REGARDS
Framingham	
ARIC	
CHS	
Risk factors/covariates included	
Age	
Sex	
Total cholesterol	
HDL-cholesterol	
Systolic blood pressure	
Use of antihypertensives	
Diabetes mellitus	
Smoking	
Cardiovascular disease events utilized	
Myocardial infarction	
CHD death	
Stroke	
Stroke death	

Online risk calculator available at http://tools.cardiosource.org/ASCVD-Risk-Estimator/

for reducing cardiovascular events. The Cardiovascular Inflammation Reduction Trial (CIRT) is an ongoing, large scale, multicenter randomized, double blinded, placebo-controlled trial of low dose methotrexate for the primary prevention of major cardiovascular events in subjects with either diabetes mellitus or the metabolic syndrome [24]. It will be evaluating the effects of chronic immunosuppression in this moderate to high risk population, which, if positive, should then prompt additional studies to look into lower risk populations.

The use of the polypill has been another strategy that has been proposed to reduce patient non-compliance and insure that those at risk receive appropriate therapies in a single pill. The polypill is a single tablet which typically combines low dose aspirin with an antihypertensive and statin. With up to 50 % of patients demonstrating non-compliance with medical therapy, the polypill could improve adherence [25]. There have been numerous phase II clinical trials which have demonstrated the efficacy of the polypill in reducing both blood pressure and cholesterol at the expense of mildly increased side effects [26–29]. The Indian Poly Pill (TIPS) study was a multicenter, double blinded, randomized control trial of 2053 subjects in India between the ages of 45 and 80 years with one cardiovascular risk factor [26]. This polypill contained low doses of a thiazide diuretic, beta blocker, ACE inhibitor, statin and aspirin. Patients were randomized to receive the polypill or a treatment group with various combinations of the above medications. The polypill was found to show a similar reduction in blood pressure when compared to groups receiving three blood pressure lowering drugs. When compared to statin therapy alone, the polypill group had less of a reduction of LDL cholesterol. There was no significant difference in tolerance between the different groups. While the study demonstrated that the polypill could be safely tolerated, the study wasn't designed to look at long term reduction in major adverse cardiovascular events.

The UMPIRE (Use of a Multidrug Pill In Reducing cardiovascular Events) trial was the first study to demonstrate an improvement in medication adherence when compared to standard therapy. This European and Indian study was a randomized, open labeled, single blinded trial of 2000 subjects who received either a fixed dose combination polypill or standard care [29]. At the conclusion of the study, 73 % of subjects were adherent to the medication protocol versus 23 % in the control group. Rates of adverse events and reductions in blood pressure and serum cholesterol were similar between the two arms. There are several ongoing studies looking to compare the efficacy of fixed dose combination polypills versus standard therapy on reducing cardiovascular events, and the adoption of this strategy will be dependent upon those outcomes.

One of the most effective strategies to decrease the rates of acute cardiac events may not require direct medical intervention. Cigarette smoking is the second most significant population attributable risk factor for cardiovascular disease after hypertension [1]. In 2005, smoking was responsible for an estimated 467,000 adult deaths, with approximately 1/3rd of these occurring from cardiovascular complications. Despite the well established and irrefutable link to acute coronary events as well as cancer, more than 20 % of males and 15 % of females continue to actively smoke cigarettes [1]. In contrast, nearly 45 % of STEMI patients in the NCDR database of primary PCI were active or recent smokers [30]. The effect of cigarette smoke on mortality is not limited to active smokers. It is estimated that 11 % of smoking-related deaths were the result of passive (second-hand) smoke exposure [31]. Smoking cessation has been proven to decrease all cause mortality within 2 years of quitting, with an effect which increases exponentially over time [31]. Public bans on smoking have been shown to significantly decrease AMI incidence [32]. One relatively simple, albeit politically unpopular, way to significantly reduce cardiovascular mortality and myocardial infarctions within two years would be to simply make the cost of cigarettes so prohibitive that it encourages non use [33]. Given the enormous financial burden of added health care expenses caused by tobacco consumption, such measures to encourage cessation should be strongly considered.

As mentioned previously, though the patient with multiple cardiovascular risk factors is at the highest risk of experiencing an acute cardiovascular event in primary prevention, the majority of patients who have an acute event are at moderate or low risk. From an epidemiologic perspective, our efforts might be better spent on primary prevention and control of standard risk factors for atherosclerotic disease before the patient becomes vulnerable or high risk. Donald Lloyd-Jones and colleagues looked at patients in the Framingham Heart Study who, at the age of 50, were free of all cardiovascular disease (including coronary artery disease, stroke, and peripheral arterial disease). Subjects who, at the age of 50, had zero Framingham cardiovascular risk factors (non smoker, no diabetes, total cholesterol <180 and blood pressure <120/80) had markedly reduced lifetime rates of major adverse cardiovascular events compared to similar groups with two or more risk factors (5.2 % versus 68.9 % in men, 8.2 % versus 50.2 % in women) and significantly longer median survivals (39 versus 28 years in men, 39 versus 31 years in women [34]).

Conclusions

1. While the vulnerable plaque is a concept supported by several lines of evidence, it is too premature to suggest that intervention on these lesion/lesions, if they could be identified, can prevent hard cardiovascular events such as AMI or SCD in the future. It is possible that this strategy might be applicable to a subset in secondary prevention if ongoing natural history and therapeutic trials turn out positive. However, to be an effective large scale strategy, we believe the detector of a true vulnerable plaque should be non invasive. Such a detector is not presently available.
2. Thus, the vulnerable or high risk patient is the appropriate target. The usual therapies are capable of reducing events in secondary prevention although these therapies are not completely effective. However, detection of the higher risk patient in primary prevention is challenging. Standard risk assessment will not identify most patients, so other strategies are needed. The ideal tool/tools remain to be determined.

3. Identification of at risk patients with newer or established markers might allow for a more comprehensive management strategy that could be applied early and thus reduce events over one's entire life time. However, identification does not necessarily ensure that an event can be prevented. Better medications/strategies are required. An easy solution to reduce acute events would be to eliminate cigarette exposure although logistically this would be challenging.

References

1. Go AS, Mozaffarian D, Roger VL, et al. Heart disease and stroke statistics – 2014 update: a report from the American Heart Association. Circulation. 2014;129(3):e28–292.
2. Vasas RS, Sullivan LM, Wilson PWF, et al. Relative importance of borderline and elevated levels of coronary heart disease risk factors. Ann Intern Med. 2005;142(6):393–402.
3. Bentzon JF, Otsuka R, Virmani R, Falk E. Mechanisms of plaque formation and rupture. Circ Res. 2014;114(12):1852–66.
4. Fujii K, Mintz GS, Carlier SG, Costa Jr JD, et al. Intravascular ultrasound profile analysis of ruptured coronary plaques. Am J Cardiol. 2006;98:429–35.
5. Ambrose JA, Tannenbaum MA, Alexopoulos D, et al. Angiographic progression of coronary artery disease and the development of myocardial infarction. J Am Coll Cardiol. 1988;12:56–62.
6. Litttle WC, Constantinescu M, Applegate RJ, et al. Can coronary angiography predict the site of a subsequent myocardial infarction in patients with mild to moderate coronary artery disease? Circulation. 1988;78:1157–66.
7. Yamagishi M, Terashima M, Awano K, et al. Morphology of vulnerable coronary plaque: insights from follow-up of patients examined by intravascular ultrasound before an acute coronary syndrome. J Am Coll Cardiol. 2000;35:106–11.
8. Giroud D, Li JM, Urban P, Meier B, Rutishauser W. Relation of the site of acute myocardial infarction to the most severe coronary arterial stenosis at prior angiography. Am J Cardiol. 1992;69:729–32.
9. Ambrose JA. In search of the "vulnerable plaque": can it be localzied and will focal regional therapy ever be an option for cardiac prevention? J Am Coll Cardiol. 2008;51(16):1539–42.
10. Stone GW, Maehara A, Lansky AJ, et al. A prospective natural-history study of coronary atherosclerosis. N Engl J Med. 2011;364:226–35.
11. Kubo T, Imanishi T, Takarada S, et al. Assessment of culprit lesion morphology in acute myocardial infarction. Ability of ocular coherence tomography compared with intravascular ultrasound and coronary angioscopy. J Am Coll Cardiol. 2007;50:933–9.
12. Jia H, Abtahian F, Aguirre AD, Lee S, et al. In vivo diagnosis of plaque erosion and calcified nodule in patients with acute coronary syndrome by intravascular optical coherence tomography. J Am Coll Cardiol. 2013;62(19):1748–58.
13. Virmani R, Burke AP, Farb A, Kolodgie FD. Pathology of the vulnerable plaque. J Am Coll Cardiol. 2006;47:C13–8.
14. Lerner DJ, Kannel WB. Patterns of coronary heart disease morbidity and mortality in the sexes: a 26 year follow-up of the Framingham population. Am Heart J. 1986;111:383–90.
15. Zipes DP, Wellens HJJ. Sudden cardiac death. Circulation. 1998;98:2334–51.
16. Stone NJ, Robinson J, Lichtenstein AH, et al. 2013 ACC/AHA guidelines on the treatment of blood cholesterol to reduce atherosclerotic cardiovascular risk in adults: a report of the American College of Cardiology/American Heart Association Task Force on Practice Guidelines. Circulation. 2014;129(25 Suppl 2):S1–45.

17. Falk F, Sillesen H, Fuster V. The high-risk plaque initiative: primary prevention of athero-thrombotic events in the asymptomatic population. Curr Atheroscler Rep. 2011;13:359–66.
18. Fernández-Ortiz A, Jiménez-Borrequero LJ, Peñalvo JL, et al. The progression and early detection of subclinical atherosclerosis (PESA) study: rational and design. Am Heart J. 2013;166(6):990–8.
19. Ridker PM, Rifai N, Rose L, Burning JE, Cook NR. Comparison of C-reactive protein and low-density lipoprotein cholesterol levels in the prediction of first cardiovascular events. N Engl J Med. 2002;347:1557–65.
20. Ridker PM, Danielson E, Fonseca FAH, et al. Rosuvastatin to prevent vascular events in men and women with elevated c-reactive protein. N Engl J Med. 2008;359:2195–207.
21. Cheng JM, Akkerhuis KM, Meilhac O, et al. Circulating osteoglycin and NGAL/MMP9 complex concentrations predict 1-year major adverse cardiovascular events after coronary angiography. Arterioscler Thromb Vasc Biol. 2014;34:1078–84.
22. Liu CF, Qin L, Ren JY, Chen H, Wang WM, Liu J, Song JX, Li LJ. Elevated plasma lipoprotein-associated phospholipase A2 activity is associated with plaque rupture in patients with coronary artery disease. Chin Med J. 2011;124(16):2469–73.
23. Goff DC, Loyd-Jones DM, Bennett G, Coady MS, et al. 2013 ACC/AHA guideline on the assessment of cardiolovascular risk. Circulation. 2014;129:S49–73.
24. Clinical trials.gov. Cardiovascular Inflammation Reduction Trial (CIRT). www.clinicaltrials.gov/show/NCT0159433.
25. Catellano JM, Sanz G, Fernandez OA, Garrido E, Bansilal S, Fuster V. A polypill strategy to improve global secondary cardiovascular prevention: from concept to reality. J Am Coll Cardiol. 2014;64:613–21.
26. The Indian Polycaps Study (TIPS) Investigators. Effects of a polypill (Polycap) on risk factors in middle-aged individuals without cardiovascular disease (TIPS): a phase II, double-blind randomized trial. Lancet. 2009;373:1341–3151.
27. Rodgers A, Patel A, Berwanger O, et al.; The PILL Collaborative Group. An international randomized placebo-controlled trial of a four-component combination pill ("polypill") in people with raised cardiovascular risk. PLoS One. 2011;6(5):e19857.
28. Wald DS, Morris JK, Wald NJ. Randomized Polypill crossover trial in people aged 50 and over. PLoS One. 2012;7, e41297.
29. Malekzadeh F, Marshall T, Pourshams A, et al. A pilot double-blind randomised placebo-controlled trial of the effects of fixed-dose combination therapy ('polypill') on cardiovascular risk factors. Int J Clin Pract. 2010;64:1220–7.
30. Akhter N, Milford-Beland S, Roe MT, Piana RN, Kao J, Shroff A. Gender difference among patients with acute coronary syndromes undergoing percutaneous coronary intervention in the American College of Cardiology-National Cardiovascular Data Registry (ACC-NCDR). Am Heart J. 2009;157:141–8.
31. Centers for Disease Control and Prevention (CDC). Smoking-attributable mortality, years of potential life lost, and productivity losses: United States, 2000–2004. MMWR Morb Mortal Wkly Rep. 2008;57:1226–8.
32. Mackay DF, Irfan MO, Haw S, Pell JP. Meta-analysis of the effect of comprehensive smoke-free legislation on acute coronary events. Heart. 2010;96:1525–30.
33. Ambrose JA, Acharya T. Reducing acute coronary events- the solution is not so difficult. Am J Med. 2015;128:105–6.
34. Lloyd-Jones DM, Leip EP, Larson MG, et al. Prediction of lifetime risk for cardiovascular disease by risk factor burden at 50 years of age. Circulation. 2006;113:791–8.

Chapter 4
Diabetes and Coronary Artery Disease

Sanjum S. Sethi and Michael E. Farkouh

Abstract Diabetes is a major risk factor for developing aggressive coronary artery disease. Since lifestyle modification and glycemic control efforts have not proven to reduce long term mortality, management still hinges on medical therapy and invasive revascularization. Guideline recommended medical therapy targeting secondary prevention efforts is warranted in all patients with diabetes and coronary artery disease. Higher risk populations benefit from revascularization, with coronary artery bypass grafting providing durable reductions in myocardial infarction and mortality relative to contemporary percutaneous coronary revascularization. However, coronary artery bypass grafting is not the appropriate approach in all patients, given elevated risk of short term stroke and equivalent long term symptom relief. Thus, controversy exists as to the appropriate management strategy in different sub groups. We advocate for an interdisciplinary heart team approach to provide a balanced perspective on the various options and a thoughtful discussion of the risks and benefits for each patient.

Keywords Diabetes • CAD • Coronary artery disease • Revascularization • Percutaneous coronary intervention • PCI • Coronary artery bypass grafting • CABG

Introduction

Over 25 million people (8.3 % of the population) in the United States are affected with diabetes [1]. Compared with their non diabetic peers of similar age, sex, and ethnicity, diabetic individuals have a well-established twofold to fourfold relative risk increase for the development of coronary artery disease (CAD) [2, 3]. This

S.S. Sethi, MD, MPH
Division of Cardiology, Ronald Reagan UCLA Medical Center, Los Angeles, CA, USA
e-mail: ssethi@mednet.ucla.edu

M.E. Farkouh, MD, MSc (✉)
Division of Cardiology, The Peter Munk Cardiac Centre and the Heart and Stroke
Richard Lewar Centre of Excellence, Toronto, ON, Canada

Department of Medicine, University of Toronto, Toronto, ON, Canada

© Springer International Publishing Switzerland 2015
J.A. Ambrose, A.E. Rodríguez (eds.), *Controversies in Cardiology*,
DOI 10.1007/978-3-319-20415-4_4

43

increased risk in the development of CAD translates into an elevated risk of mortality of about two–four times compared to those without diabetes [1]. Part of this elevated mortality is derived from the fact that diabetic patients with CAD develop acute coronary syndromes (ACS) with a 7 year incidence of 20 % [4]. Furthermore, diabetic patients are at increased risk for more extensive CAD [5, 6], heart failure, renal failure, and cardiogenic shock [7].

Given the elevated risk of CAD conferred by diabetes, early research postulated that optimal treatment of the underlying hyperglycemia would reduce CAD and the downstream incidence of ACS or heart failure [8, 9]. However recent data from the ACCORD (The Action to Control Cardiovascular Risk in Diabetes) study indicated that strict glycemic control did not significantly influence the composite macrovascular outcome of nonfatal myocardial infarction, nonfatal stroke, or death [10]. Interestingly, there were fewer nonfatal MI (hazard ratio 0.79, 95 % confidence interval [CI] 0.66–0.95), but death from any cause was increased (hazard ratio 1.21, 95 % CI 1.02–1.44). These data confirm that the benefit for glycemic control rests solely on microvascular outcomes such as nephropathy.

As a result, the basic treatment of CAD in diabetic patients does not differ from nondiabetic persons and hinges on optimal management of the atherosclerosis process to prevent long-term death, stroke and myocardial infarction. Given the propensity for developing ACS and the aggressive nature of CAD in the diabetic population, careful management is prudent to prevent long-term complications. However controversy exists as to the appropriate management strategy in different subsets with diabetes. The foundation of managing of coronary artery disease can be divided into three basic strategies: lifestyle modification, aggressive medical therapy, and coronary revascularization.

Lifestyle Modification

Lifestyle modification is a mainstay of any treatment program beginning before the diagnosis of diabetes is even made. One randomized trial of 3234 high-risk nondiabetic individuals found that a lifestyle intervention of 7 % weight loss and 150 min of physical activity per week decreased the incidence of diabetes by 58 % [11]. Similarly in the CAD population, many studies have confirmed long term mortality benefits for participation in cardiac rehabilitation programs that focus on increasing physical activity and promoting optimal dietary habits [12, 13]. Therefore, diabetic CAD patients have multiple reasons to develop healthy lifestyle habits. However, an analysis from the 2008 National Health and Nutrition Examination Survey found that less than 1 % of US adults exhibited ideal cardiovascular health for seven predefined metrics (diet, physical activity, body mass index, smoking, blood pressure, total cholesterol, and fasting blood glucose) [14].

Aside from the difficulty in achieving optimal control of health behaviors, recent trial data do not support reduction in hard cardiovascular outcomes with successful lifestyle interventions. The multicenter Look AHEAD (Action for Health in

Diabetes) trial randomly assigned 5145 diabetes patients between the ages of 45 and 75 with a body mass index of 25 or greater to lifestyle modification with decreased caloric intake and increased physical activity designed to promote weight loss versus control (diabetes support and education) [15]. At a median follow up of 9.6 years, the investigators found no difference between groups in the composite outcomes of cardiac death, nonfatal MI, nonfatal stroke, or hospitalization for angina (403 intervention vs. 418 control; hazard ratio in the intervention group, 0.95; 95 % CI, 0.83–1.09; p=0.51). This was despite greater weight loss in the intervention group compared to control (8.6 % vs. 0.7 % at 1 year; 6.0 % vs. 3.5 % at study end). With difficulties in adherence and unclear long-term efficacy, lifestyle modification remains only an adjunct strategy in diabetic patients with CAD. Further management relies on medical therapy and/or invasive revascularization.

Medical Therapy

Primary and secondary prevention efforts for CAD have evolved quite considerably over the last 25–30 years. The first therapy proven to reduce long-term mortality post acute coronary syndrome (ACS) was aspirin. In the early 1980s, a randomized controlled trial of 1266 patients diagnosed with unstable angina or non ST elevation myocardial infarction (NSTEMI) were enrolled to aspirin versus placebo on hospital discharge. They found a 51 % mortality reduction in the aspirin group compared to placebo [16]. Since this landmark study, multiple medications have been approved for the secondary prevention of coronary artery disease. Aside from aspirin, angiotensin converting enzyme inhibitors, beta blockers, and statins have all subsequently become guideline-recommended approved therapies for secondary prevention in diabetic patients with coronary artery disease [17].

As diabetic patients tend to have a more aggressive form of CAD, they particularly benefit from adherence to established medical therapies aimed at the secondary prevention of CAD [18, 19]. However, adherence that translates into obtaining objective measurements of risk factor control is difficult even under the most rigorous of circumstances. An analysis of three large randomized controlled trials that promoted strict risk factor control pooling data from over 5000 diabetic patients found that reaching optimal target levels of 4 important risk factors: glycemic control, systolic blood pressure, low density lipoprotein cholesterol, and smoking cessation ranged from only 8–23 % across the studies [20] (Fig. 4.1).

Medical Therapy vs. Revascularization

It has been well established that revascularization improves mortality and reduced the incidence of subsequent myocardial infarction in all subsets of patients presenting with acute coronary syndromes [21]. Furthermore, early data from the Coronary

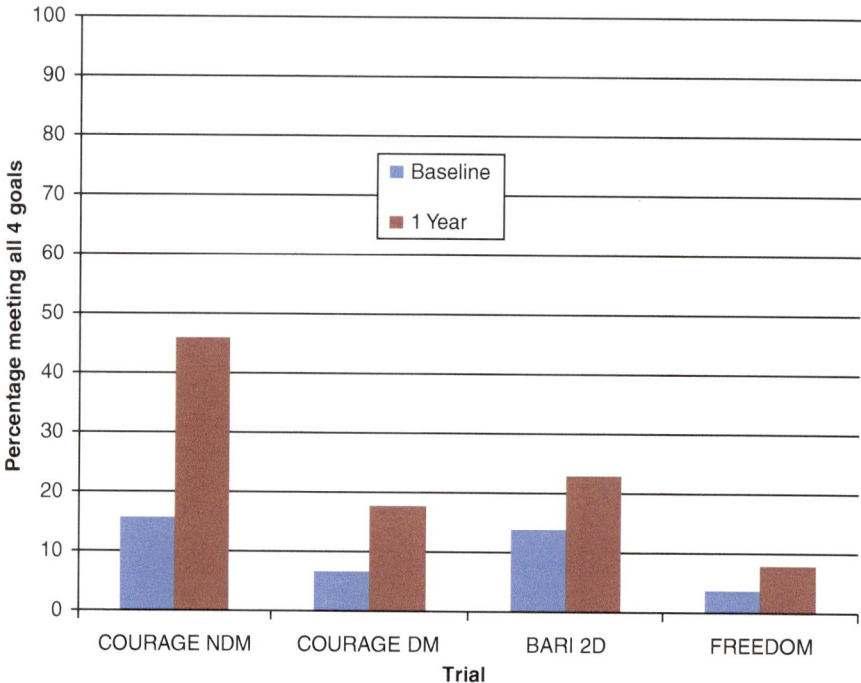

Fig. 4.1 Percentage of Patients Meeting All 4 Targets (LDL-C, SBP, HbA1c, and Smoking Cessation) Among the 3 Trials From Baseline to 1 Year of Follow-Up. The COURAGE trial was divided into DM and NDM cohorts. Targets were pre-specified by trial and included 4 items: LDL-C, SBP, HbA1c, and smoking cessation. *LDL – C* low density lipoprotein cholesterol, *SBP* systolic blood pressure, *HBA1c* hemoglobin A1c, *DM* diabetes mellitus, *NDM* non diabetes mellitus (Reproduced from Farkouh ME, et al. [20]) with permission of Elsevier

Artery Surgery Study (CASS) study revealed that stable CAD that includes left main and proximal left anterior descending stenosis also benefited from revascularization [22–24]. The issue that was less clear was whether significant stenoses ($\geq 70\%$) in patients with stable CAD benefited from revascularization compared to medical management.

The pivotal trial examining the comparative effectiveness of medical therapy versus percutaneous coronary intervention (PCI) for the management of stable coronary artery disease is the Clinical Outcomes Utilizing Revascularization and Aggressive Drug Evaluation (COURAGE) trial released in 2007 [25]. In this trial 2287 patients with stable CAD were randomized to a strategy of optimal medical therapy versus optimal medical therapy plus PCI. They included patients with stable ischemic heart disease and stenosis in one or more epicardial vessel of $\geq 70\%$. After excluding high-risk patients, including those with persistent angina, depressed ejection fraction, and markedly positive stress tests; almost one half of patients were asymptomatic or Canadian Cardiovascular Society (CCS) I. Over a median follow up of 4.6 years, the primary outcome, a composite of nonfatal myocardial infarction

(MI) and all-cause mortality, occurred in 211 (19 %) patients in the PCI arm versus 202 (18.5 %) patients in the optimal medical therapy group (P=0.62). Although there was a statistically significant improvement in rates of freedom from angina in the PCI group relative to the medical therapy group, this trial demonstrated no benefit for stenting with regards to MI or death.

Approximately 34 % percentage of patients in COURAGE had diabetes. Subgroup analyses did not demonstrate any appreciable difference in this subset [26]. Expanding on these results by focusing solely on diabetic patients, the multinational Bypass Angioplasty Revascularization Investigation 2 Diabetes (BARI 2D) study investigated the questions of medical management versus revascularization for diabetic patient with stable CAD [27]. The investigators randomized a total of 2368 patients from almost 50 sites to elective revascularization (PCI or coronary artery bypass grafting (CABG) at the discretion of the treating physician) plus aggressive medical therapy versus medical therapy alone. Mortality was similar between the two groups (11.7 % vs. 12.2 % p=0.97) as well the composite outcome of death, stroke, or myocardial infarction (MACE) (22.8 % vs. 24.1 % p=0.70). Interestingly, those who underwent CABG had a lower major cardiovascular event (MACE) rate compared to the medical therapy group (22.4 % vs. 30.5 % p=0.01). Since this group was naturally higher risk with more extensive underlying disease compared to those selected for the PCI group, there appeared to be a signal indicating beneficial effects of surgical revascularization in high-risk diabetic patients. Of note, less than half the patients received contemporary drug eluting stents (DES) and there was significant crossover of the patients in the medical therapy arm to revascularization.

PCI vs. CABG

Whereas medical therapy has not proven inferior in low risk patients, those with aggressive multivessel CAD benefit from revascularization. The first large trial to look at this question in diabetic patients was the Bypass Angioplasty Revascularization Investigation (BARI) trial which looked at 1928 patients with multivessel CAD randomizing them to PCI with percutaneous coronary angioplasty (PTCA) or CABG [28]. Between group 5-year survival rates were similar (86.3 % PTCA vs. 89.3 % CABG, p=0.019), despite significantly higher rates of revascularization in the PTCA arm (54 % vs. 8 %). In a subgroup analysis looking only at diabetic patients, CABG offered a substantial mortality benefit with survival rates of 80.6 % versus 65.5 % in the PTCA group (p=0.03). This dramatic reduction in mortality led to a National Heart Lung and Blood institute alert recommending CABG for as the preferred method for revascularization in diabetic patient with multivessel disease [29].

Since this was a post-hoc subgroup analysis, confirmation was needed in a larger prospectively enrolled randomized control trial of only diabetic patients to conclusively answer this question. The first attempt was the Coronary Artery Revascularization in Diabetes (CARDia) trial, which was underpowered and terminated early only enrolling 510 patients [30]. Although they did not find a difference between CABG and PCI for major cardiovascular endpoints, consensus remains that the trial was not adequately powered to answer the initial hypothesis.

With this context, the Future REvascularization Evaluation in patients with Diabetes mellitus: Optimal management of Multivessel disease (FREEDOM) trial sought to compare PCI vs. CABG in the contemporary era of medical therapy [31]. A total of 1900 patients were enrolled at over 130 international sites that randomized patients to PCI with DES versus CABG for diabetic patients with multivessel CAD. Similar to COURAGE and BARI 2D, aggressive risk factor modification and medical therapy was used in both groups. While COURAGE and BARI 2D used nurse practitioners or study coordinators to coach their participants, the protocol used in FREEDOM relied on site supervision. This less intensive approach was favored by the NHLBI to mimic real world conditions.

Despite the difference in medical therapy protocols amongst the trials, in FREEDOM, 93 % were receiving antiplatelet therapy; 88 %, antianginal agents; 86 %, lipid-lowering agents; and 78 %, a renin-angiotensin system inhibiting agents. These rates were similar compared to COURAGE and BARI 2D [20]. Along with appropriate and high utilization of guideline directed medical therapies, both PCI and CABG were performed using established and contemporary approaches. In the PCI arm, DES was used in 94 % of patients. These were first generation DES (sirolimus and paclitaxel eluting). Acknowledging the advances in DES stent design and drug delivery versus bare metal stents, a meta analysis of data from over 100,000 patients does not suggest any large-scale efficacy differences that would impact the results of the trial [32]. In the CABG arm, the left internal mammary artery (LIMA) graft was also used in 94 % of patients.

The primary outcome consisted of a composite of all-cause mortality, nonfatal MI, and nonfatal stroke. Follow up was 5 years with a median follow up of 3.8 years. The primary outcome occurred more often in the PCI group vs. CABG group (26.6 % vs. 18.7 %, $p = 0.005$) (Fig. 4.2). The statistically significant composite outcome was primarily driven by higher rates of MI (13.9 % vs. 6.0 %; $P < 0.001$) and all-cause mortality (16.3 % vs. 10.9 %; $P = 0.049$) in the PCI group vs. the CABG group. On the other hand, stroke occurred more often in the CABG patients (5.2 % vs. 2.4 %; $p = 0.03$) [31]. These events were mostly periprocedural occurring within the first 30 days of randomization. Interestingly, a prespecified sub group analysis dividing the participants into tertiles by The SYNergy between percutaneous coronary intervention with TAXus and cardiac surgery (SYNTAX) score did not find any between group differences. This finding indicated that unlike nondiabetic patients, diabetic patients preferentially benefited from CABG regardless of anatomic complexity of disease.

The mortality benefit described in the FREEDOM study was confirmed by a recent meta-analysis of 8 trials that included 3612 diabetic participants. At 5-year follow up, diabetic individuals with multivessel CAD who underwent CABG had lower all-cause mortality as compared to those undergoing PCI (RR 0.67, 95 % CI 0.52–0.86; $p = 0.0002$) [33]. This analysis evaluated over 7000 patients across the 8 trials including 4 trials using bare metal stents and 4 trials utilizing DES. There was no difference in outcome based on stent type indicating that same mortality benefit with CABG was present regardless of advances in stent technology.

a **Primary outcome**

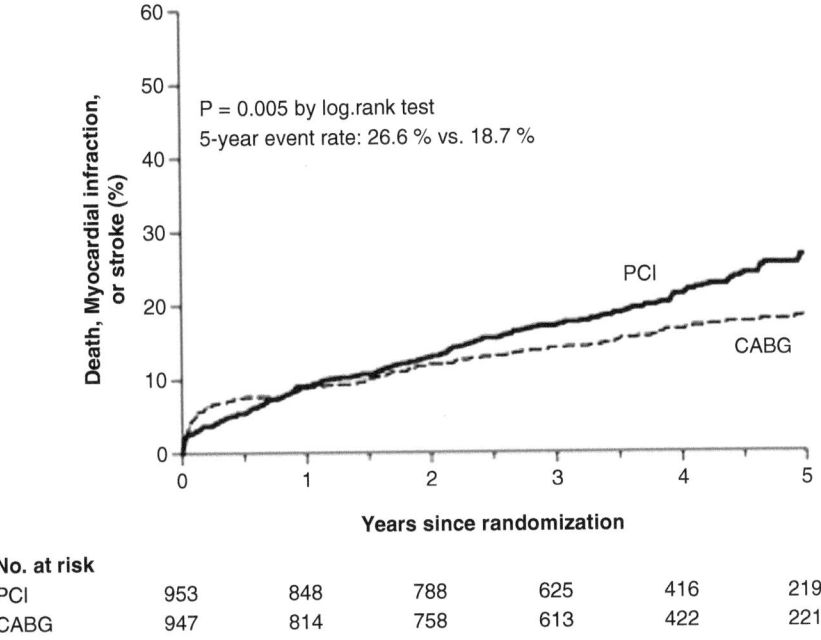

b **Death**

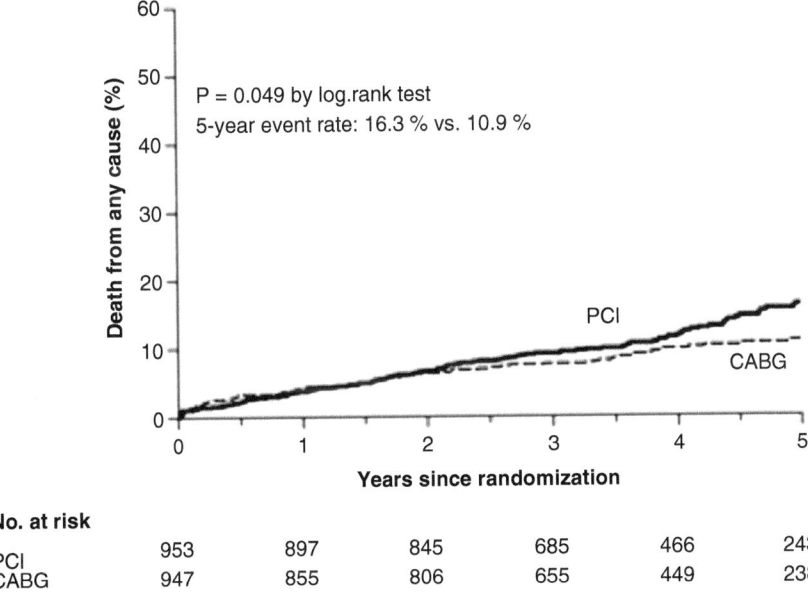

Fig. 4.2 Kaplan–Meier Estimates of the Composite Primary Outcome and Death. Shown are rates of the composite primary outcome of death, myocardial infarction, or stroke (Panel **a**) and death from any cause (Panel **b**) truncated at 5 years after randomization. The P value was calculated by means of the log-rank test on the basis of all available follow-up data (Reproduced from Farkouh ME, et al. [31]), with permission from the Massachusetts Medical Society

Although we know that strict glycemic control does not improve long-term mortality rates, accruing data suggest that the degree of insulin resistance may have an impact on cardiovascular outcome post revascularization. In the FREEDOM trial, all pre specified subgroups appeared to have outcomes congruent with the main trial (Fig. 4.3). One of these subgroups was stratified based on a glycated hemoglobin A1c of greater than or less than 7 %. There was no difference in the primary outcome based on this stratification with both groups favoring CABG (<7 % 23 % PCI vs. 16 % CABG, ≥7 % 28 % PCI vs. 20 % CABG; p value for interaction=0.99). However, a subsequent analysis stratified the groups based on insulin usage [34]. Insulin treated patients (n=602) had a significantly higher rate of stroke/death/MI as opposed to non insulin treated patients (28.7 % vs. 19.5 %, p<0.001) despite adjustment for potential confounders including baseline factors, angiographic complexity, and treatment group. There was no difference in the degree of PCI versus CABG treatment effect. CABG was superior to PCI in both diabetes subtypes (p value interaction=0.40). These data were similar to a subgroup analysis from the SYNTAX trial [35]. Out of

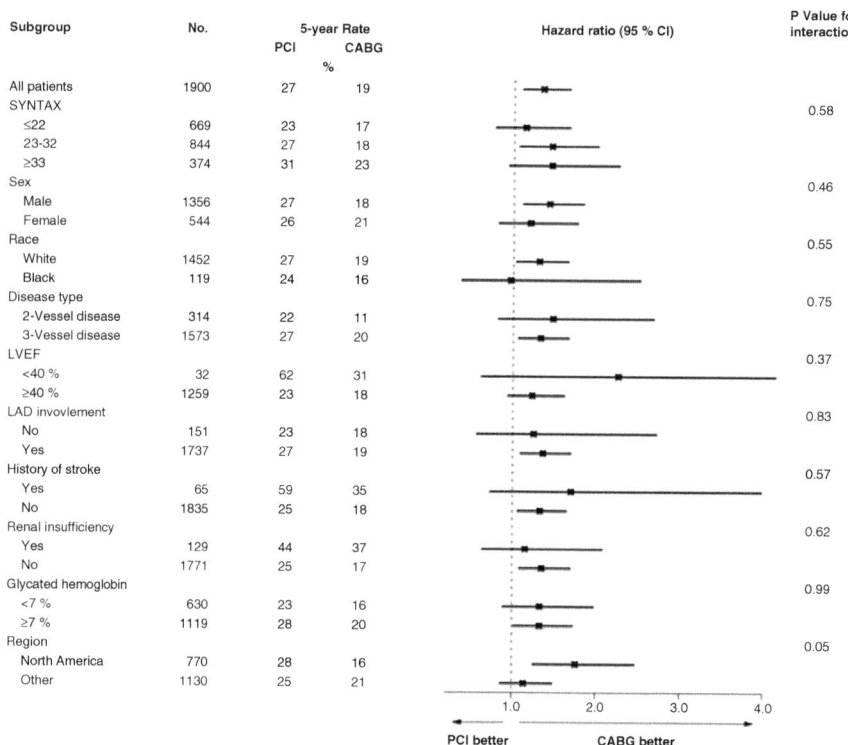

Fig. 4.3 Primary Composite Outcome, According to Subgroup. Subgroup analyses were performed with the use of Cox proportional-hazards regression. Five-year composite event rates for death, myocardial infarction, or stroke are shown. LAD denotes left anterior descending artery, and LVEF left ventricular ejection fraction (Reproduced from Farkouh ME, et al. [31]), with permission of the Massachusetts Medical Society

the 1800 patients enrolled in the SYNTAX trial, 452 had diabetes. While there was no difference in all cause mortality/stroke/MI between PCI and CABG based on diabetes, the investigators found worsened rates of the composite outcome in the diabetes patients undergoing PCI who were treated with insulin versus those who were not (32.1 % vs. 18.8 %; p=0.018). The sum of these data suggest that the degree of insulin resistance may have an impact on long-term revascularization outcomes.

Data to date do not suggest the utilization of CABG as the revascularization strategy for every patient with diabetes. As noted, the vast majority of patients in FREEDOM had triple-vessel disease (over 80 %) and over 90 % received a left internal mammary artery graft. Applying these data to populations that do not fit the underlying criteria would not be appropriate. Furthermore, the benefit for CABG relative to PCI with regards to nonfatal MI and death must be weighed against the increased risk of stroke. At 5 years, there were 37 strokes in the CABG group (5.2 %) versus 20 in the PCI group (2.4 %) [31]. This difference was statistically significant with a p=0.03. This difference is largely driven by outcomes during the during the periprocedural period (first 30 days) with 16 strokes in the CABG group and three in the PCI group. Careful evaluation for stroke risk in potential revascularization patients would be prudent given this short-term risk of cerebrovascular event.

Aside from objective clinical outcomes, consideration must also be given to quality of life factors. Quality of life measures were integrated into the FREEDOM trial with participants answering the Seattle Angina Questionnaire (SAQ) at regular intervals throughout the trial. Domains included angina frequency, physical limitations, and quality-of-life subscales. While long-term scores did not differ between the groups, there was significantly less angina in the CABG group during the first 2 years (p=0.03) [36]. The lack of durable benefit in the CABG group may have been confounded by higher rates of repeat revascularization in the PCI group. Regardless, despite the increased risk of MI, patients in the PCI group had equal quality of life. Given multiple options and complex decision making, a heart team approach incorporating risk of MI, mortality, or stroke along with quality of life factors is warranted for all stable diabetic CAD patients. With such an approach, it can be ensured that the patients are provided with balanced explanations of the various therapy options including lifestyle modification, medical therapy, and invasive revascularization [37].

Conclusion

1. The treatment of CAD in diabetic patients hinges on the fundamental approaches of lifestyle modification, medical therapy, and invasive revascularization including PCI and CABG. Data clearly support a combination of these approaches depending on the risk profile of the patient. Aggressive medical therapy is recommended for all patients given proven benefits regardless of long-term management strategy chosen. Adherence to therapy must be pursued earnestly by both patients and clinicians, as achieving optimal risk factor targets can be challenging even under the most rigorous of circumstances.

2. For the higher risk diabetic patients with multivessel disease that require invasive revascularization, CABG provides durable long-term reduction in MI and mortality relative to PCI.
3. However, we do not advocate subjecting all diabetic patients to CABG. Careful patient selection is warranted using a heart team approach in which the long term benefit of mortality and MI reduction is weighed against the short-term stroke risk and equivalent long-term quality of life. Using this method, evidence based trial data can be successfully applied to individual patients to improve long-term cardiovascular outcomes.
4. At the same time, there is no justification for further PCI versus CABG trials. We need to spend resources to optimize outcomes for CABG by limiting perioperative stroke and for PCI by limiting nontarget lesion progression.

References

1. Centers for Disease Control and Prevention. National diabetes fact sheet: national estimates and general information on diabetes and prediabetes in the United States, 2011. Atlanta: U.S. Department of Health and Human Services, Centers for Disease Control and Prevention; 2011.
2. Kannel WB, McGee DL. Diabetes and cardiovascular disease. The Framingham study. JAMA. 1979;241:2035–8.
3. Howard BV, Rodriguez BL, Bennett PH, et al. Prevention conference VI: diabetes and cardiovascular disease: writing group I: epidemiology. Circulation. 2002;105:e132–7.
4. Haffner SM, Lehto S, Rönnemaa T, et al. Mortality from coronary heart disease in subjects with type 2 diabetes and in nondiabetic subjects with and without prior myocardial infarction. N Engl J Med. 1998;339:229–34.
5. Norhammar A, Malmberg K, Diderholm E, et al. Diabetes mellitus: the major risk factor in unstable coronary artery disease even after consideration of the extent of coronary artery disease and benefits of revascularization. J Am Coll Cardiol. 2004;43:585–91.
6. Granger CB, Califf RM, Young S, et al. Outcome of patients with diabetes mellitus and acute myocardial infarction treated with thrombolytic agents. The thrombolysis and angioplasty in myocardial infarction (TAMI) study group. J Am Coll Cardiol. 1993;21:920–5.
7. Franklin K, Goldberg RJ, Spencer F, et al.; GRACE Investigators. Implications of diabetes in patients with acute coronary syndromes. The global registry of acute coronary events. Arch Intern Med. 2004;164:1457–63.
8. Gerstein HC, Swedberg K, Carlsson J, et al.; CHARM Program Investigators. The hemoglobin A1c level as a progressive risk factor for cardiovascular death, hospitalization for heart failure, or death in patients with chronic heart failure: an analysis of the Candesartan in Heart failure: Assessment of Reduction in Mortality and Morbidity (CHARM) program. Arch Intern Med. 2008;168(15):1699–704.
9. Selvin E, Steffes MW, Zhu H, et al. Glycated hemoglobin, diabetes, and cardiovascular risk in nondiabetic adults. N Engl J Med. 2010;362:800–11.
10. ACCORD Study Group, Gerstein HC, Miller ME, Genuth S, Ismail-Beigi F, Buse JB, Goff Jr DC, Probstfield JL, Cushman WC, Ginsberg HN, Bigger JT, Grimm Jr RH, Byington RP, Rosenberg YD, Friedewald WT. Long-term effects of intensive glucose lowering on cardiovascular outcomes. N Engl J Med. 2011;364(9):818–28.
11. Knowler WC, Barrett-Connor E, Fowler SE, et al.; Diabetes Prevention Program Research Group. Reduction in the incidence of type 2 diabetes with lifestyle intervention or metformin. N Engl J Med. 2002;346(6):393–403.

12. Hammill BG, Curtis LH, Schulman KA, Whellan DJ. Relationship between cardiac rehabilitation and long-term risks of death and myocardial infarction among elderly Medicare beneficiaries. Circulation. 2010;121:63–70.

13. Goel K, Lennon RJ, Tilbury RT, Squires RW, Thomas RJ. Impact of cardiac rehabilitation on mortality and cardiovascular events after percutaneous coronary intervention in the community. Circulation. 2011;123:2344–52.

14. Shay CM, Ning H, Allen NB, Carnethon MR, Chiuve SE, Greenlund KJ, Daviglus ML, Lloyd-Jones DM. Status of cardiovascular health in US adults. Circulation. 2012;125:45–56.

15. Look AHEAD Research Group, Wing RR, Bolin P, Brancati FL, et al. Cardiovascular effects of intensive lifestyle intervention in type 2 diabetes. N Engl J Med. 2013;369(2):145–54.

16. Lewis Jr HD, Davis JW, Archibald DG, et al. Protective effects of aspirin against acute myocardial infarction and death in men with unstable angina. Results of a veterans administration cooperative study. N Engl J Med. 1983;309(7):396–403.

17. Smith Jr SC, Benjamin EJ, Bonow RO, et al. AHA/ACCF secondary prevention and risk reduction therapy for patients with coronary and other atherosclerotic vascular disease: 2011 update: a guideline from the American Heart Association and American College of Cardiology Foundation endorsed by the World Heart Federation and the Preventive Cardiovascular Nurses Association. J Am Coll Cardiol. 2011;58(23):2432–46.

18. Brown LC, Johnson JA, Majumdar SR, Tsuyuki RT, McAlister FA. Evidence of suboptimal management of cardiovascular risk in patients with type 2 diabetes mellitus and symptomatic atherosclerosis. CMAJ. 2004;171(10):1189–92.

19. Delcré S, Anselmino M, Moretti C, Biondi-Zoccai G, Sheiban I. Clinical and pharmacological management of a high risk diabetic population undergoing percutaneous coronary interventions. Minerva Cardioangiol. 2008;56(3):267–75.

20. Farkouh ME, Boden WE, Bittner V, et al. Risk factor control for coronary artery disease secondary prevention in large randomized trials. J Am Coll Cardiol. 2013;61(15):1607–15.

21. Amsterdam EA, Wenger NK, Brindis RG, et al. 2014 AHA/ACC Guideline for the Management of Patients with Non-ST-Elevation Acute Coronary Syndromes: a report of the American College of Cardiology/American Heart Association Task Force on Practice Guidelines. J Am Coll Cardiol. 2014;64(24):e139–228.

22. Yusuf S, Zucker D, Peduzzi P, et al. Effect of coronary artery bypass graft surgery on survival: overview of 10-year results from randomised trials by the Coronary Artery Bypass Graft Surgery Trialists Collaboration. Lancet. 1994;344:563–70.

23. Caracciolo EA, Davis KB, Sopko G, et al. Comparison of surgical and medical group survival in patients with left main coronary artery disease. Long-term CASS experience. Circulation. 1995;91:2325–34.

24. Fihn SD, Gardin JM, Abrams J, et al.; American College of Cardiology Foundation; American Heart Association Task Force on Practice Guidelines; American College of Physicians; American Association for Thoracic Surgery; Preventive Cardiovascular Nurses Association; Society for Cardiovascular Angiography and Interventions; Society of Thoracic Surgeons. 2012 ACCF/AHA/ACP/AATS/PCNA/SCAI/STS Guideline for the diagnosis and management of patients with stable ischemic heart disease: a report of the American College of Cardiology Foundation/American Heart Association Task Force on Practice Guidelines, and the American College of Physicians, American Association for Thoracic Surgery, Preventive Cardiovascular Nurses Association, Society for Cardiovascular Angiography and Interventions, and Society of Thoracic Surgeons. J Am Coll Cardiol. 2012;60(24):e44–164.

25. Boden WE, O'Rourke RA, Teo KK, et al; COURAGE Trial Research Group. Optimal medical therapy with or without PCI for stable coronary disease. N Engl J Med. 2007;356:1503–16.

26. Maron DJ, Boden WE, Spertus JA, et al.; COURAGE Trial Research Group. Impact of metabolic syndrome and diabetes on prognosis and outcomes with early percutaneous coronary intervention in the COURAGE (Clinical Outcomes Utilizing Revascularization and Aggressive Drug Evaluation) trial. J Am Coll Cardiol. 2011;58(2):131–7.

27. BARI 2D Study Group, Frye RL, August P, Brooks MM, et al. A randomized trial of therapies for type 2 diabetes and coronary artery disease. N Engl J Med. 2009;360(24):2503–15.

28. The Bypass Angioplasty Revascularization Investigation (BARI) Investigators. Comparison of coronary bypass surgery with angioplasty in patients with multivessel disease. N Engl J Med. 1996;335:217–25.
29. Ferguson JJ. NHLI BARI clinical alert on diabetics treated with angioplasty. Circulation. 1995;92(12):3371.
30. Kapur A, Hall RJ, Malik IS, et al. Randomized comparison of percutaneous coronary intervention with coronary artery bypass grafting in diabetic patients. 1-year results of the CARDia (Coronary Artery Revascularization in Diabetes) trial. J Am Coll Cardiol. 2010;55:432–40.
31. Farkouh ME, Domanski M, Sleeper LA, et al; FREEDOM Trial Investigators. Strategies for multivessel revascularization in patients with diabetes. N Engl J Med. 2012;367:2375–84.
32. Bangalore S, Kumar S, Fusaro M, et al. Short- and long-term outcomes with drug-eluting and bare-metal coronary stents: a mixed-treatment comparison analysis of 117 762 patient-years of follow-up from randomized trials. Circulation. 2012;125(23):2873–91.
33. Verma S, Farkouh ME, Yanagawa B, Fitchett DH, Ahsan MR, Ruel M, Sud S, Gupta M, Singh S, Gupta N, Cheema AN, Leiter LA, Fedak PW, Teoh H, Latter DA, Fuster V, Friedrich JO. Comparison of coronary artery bypass surgery and percutaneous coronary intervention in patients with diabetes: a meta-analysis of randomised controlled trials. Lancet Diabetes Endocrinol. 2013;1(4):317–28.
34. Dangas GD, Farkouh ME, Sleeper LA, et al.; FREEDOM Investigators. Long-term outcome of PCI versus CABG in insulin and non-insulin-treated diabetic patients: results from the FREEDOM trial. J Am Coll Cardiol. 2014;64(12):1189–97.
35. Kappetein AP, Head SJ, Morice MC, et al.; SYNTAX Investigators. Treatment of complex coronary artery disease in patients with diabetes: 5-year results comparing outcomes of bypass surgery and percutaneous coronary intervention in the SYNTAX trial. Eur J Cardiothorac Surg. 2013;43(5):1006–13.
36. Abdallah MS, Wang K, Magnuson EA, et al.; FREEDOM Trial Investigators. Quality of life after PCI vs CABG among patients with diabetes and multivessel coronary artery disease: a randomized clinical trial. JAMA. 2013;310(15):1581–90.
37. Head SJ, Kaul S, Mack MJ, et al. The rationale for heart team decision-making for patients with stable, complex coronary artery disease. Eur Heart J. 2013;34(32):2510–8.

Chapter 5
Elevated Triglycerides, Atherosclerosis and Adverse Clinical Events

Steven R. Jones and Shady Nakhla

Abstract Mendelian randomization studies have confirmed the causal relationship of triglycerides and triglyceride-rich remnant lipoprotein cholesterol with ischemic heart disease. The mechanism of atherogenicity is complex involving elevated levels of chylomicron and very low density lipoprotein remnants, generation of small dense low density lipoprotein particles frequently in the setting of obesity, insulin resistance or genetic disorders of lipoprotein metabolism. Management remains controversial but centers on reduction of overall atherogenic lipoprotein particle burden and use of triglyceride-rich lipoprotein lowering therapies such as fibrates and niacin in selected patients with elevated triglycerides, especially when accompanied by reduced levels of high density lipoprotein cholesterol.

Keywords Triglycerides • Lipoproteins • Very low density lipoprotein (VLDL) • Low density lipoprotein (LDL) • Chylomicrons • Hepatic lipase • Lipoprotein lipase (LPL) • Atherosclerosis

Introduction

Decades of research have revealed an association between elevated triglyceride (TG) levels, TG rich lipoproteins and cardiovascular disease (CVD) [1]. Through various population based studies and clinical trials, these associations have been somewhat weakened after adjustment for other markers of dyslipidemia. While it is generally accepted that elevated TG levels are found in patients with established CVD, it remains unclear whether they play a causal role in atherosclerosis or present as a biomarker of

S.R. Jones, MD (✉)
Division of Cardiology, Department of Medicine, The Ciccarone Center or Prevention of Heart Disease, The Johns Hopkins Hospital, Zayed 7125U, Baltimore, MD 21287, USA
e-mail: sjones64@jhmi.edu

S. Nakhla, MD
School of Medicine, Johns Hopkins Hospital, 733 N Broadway, Baltimore, MD 21205, USA
e-mail: snakhla1@jhmi.edu

© Springer International Publishing Switzerland 2015   55
J.A. Ambrose, A.E. Rodríguez (eds.), *Controversies in Cardiology*,
DOI 10.1007/978-3-319-20415-4_5

disease. Given this dilemma, the role of TGs in risk prediction models as well as the management of hypertriglyceridemia remains blurred and controversial.

This chapter aims to review the lack of uniformity in epidemiologic evidence linking hypertriglyceridemia to atherosclerosis. Furthermore, a review of TG and TG rich lipoprotein metabolism is described to potentially shed light on why such discordance in the literature exists.

TG Biology and Role in Atherosclerosis

TGs are mainly derived from dietary and hepatic sources. In the exogenous, dietary form, TGs are broken down and absorbed in the intestines, forming Apolipoprotein B48 (ApoB48) tagged chylomicrons that are released into the lymphatics and ultimately into the venous system. In the endogenous pathway, Very Low Density Lipoprotein (VLDL) is assembled in hepatocytes, associated with ApoB100 and then released into the circulation [2].

Hypertriglyceridemia occurs secondary to the combination of genetic predispositions as well as other metabolic (e.g., insulin resistance) or environmental effects (high fat, carbohydrate and alcohol diet). This ultimately increases the TG content of the main Triglyceride Rich Lipoproteins (TRLs): VLDL and chylomicrons [3].

Remnant Atherogenicity

At the level of the vascular endothelium, VLDL cholesterol and chylomicrons undergo partial hydrolysis by Lipoprotein Lipase (LPL). This results in the release of triglyceride rich Remnant Lipoprotein Particles (denser subfractions of VLDL and chylomicrons, as well as IDL; collectively, RLP) and Free Fatty Acids (FFA) [2]. It is indeed the former that is potentially the cause of atherosclerosis and CVD in hypertriglyceridemic states [3].

Several mechanisms of atherogenicity due to RLPs have been proposed. Notably, studies have shown that cholesterol rich remnants are taken up by the vascular subendothelium in a manner similar to Low Density Lipoprotein (LDL) resulting in leukocyte adhesion molecule expression. This in turn leads to endothelial uptake of monocytes, conversion to macrophages and the initiation of a local inflammatory cytokine mediated response, resulting in apoptosis, oxidation, foam cell formation as well as smooth muscle cell proliferation and eventual plaque formation [4].

TGs and Small, Dense LDL in Atherosclerosis

In humans with normal TG levels, about 50 % of VLDL molecules undergo hepatic uptake from plasma, and the remaining molecules are hydrolyzed by LPL to form RLP, as described above. The VLDL derived RLPs undergo further hydrolysis by Hepatic Lipase (HL) to form mainly LDL.

In the setting of hypertriglyceridemia (particularly associated with Insulin Resistance – IR), marked by the prominence of VLDL and VLDL derived RLPs, Cholesteryl Ester Transfer Protein (CETP) catalyzes the transfer of Cholesteryl Esters (CE) from LDL to remnant protein and VLDL in exchange for TGs from the highly enriched remnants (Fig. 5.1). This process results in cholesterol deplete, small, dense LDL particles [5]. The significance of this process is highlighted through decades of population-based studies that showed an association between small, dense LDL and CVD beyond measured LDL cholesterol, particularly in patients with Familial Combined Hypertriglyceridemia (discussed below, Type IIb phenotype). It is thought that the smaller and denser LDL particles are more susceptible to oxidation and can easily penetrate the arterial intima compared to normal LDL [6]. Hence, one can infer that patients with equal LDL cholesterol may not necessarily have comparable LDL Particle concentrations (LDL-P) and consequently, non-comparable risk for CVD (Fig. 5.2).

Epidemiologic Background

Data from the National Health and Nutrition Examination Survey (NHANES) shows that 31 % of the US population has a TG level of >150 mg/dL, commonly considered "borderline high". Further, about 16 % of the US population has a TG

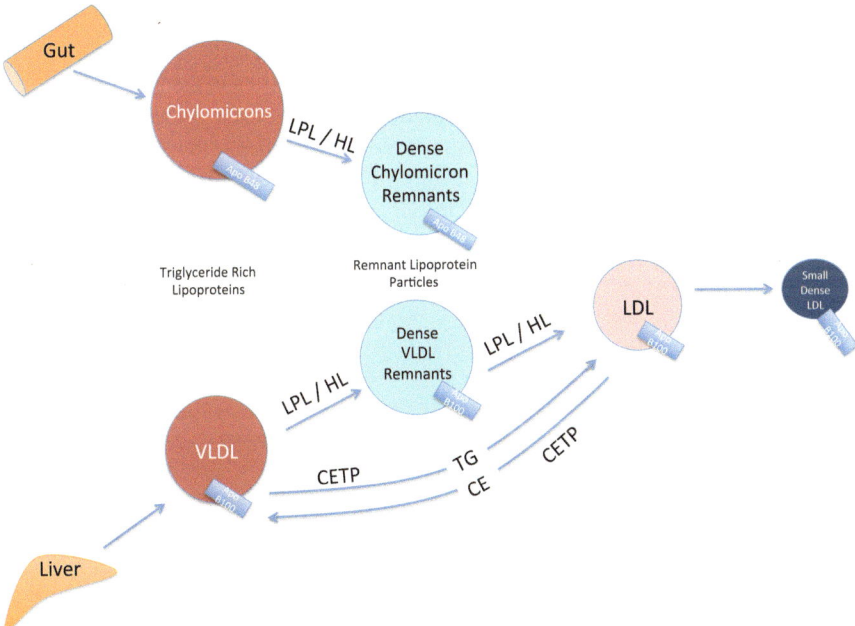

Fig. 5.1 Triglycerides are incorporated into lipoproteins via the exogenous and endogenous pathways to form chylomicrons and VLDL, the TRLs. Activity by LPL and HL results in partial hydrolysis and the formation of RLPs. VLDL remnants, including IDL, undergo further hydrolysis to form LDL-C. CEPT activity results in the formation of cholesterol deplete, small, dense LDL

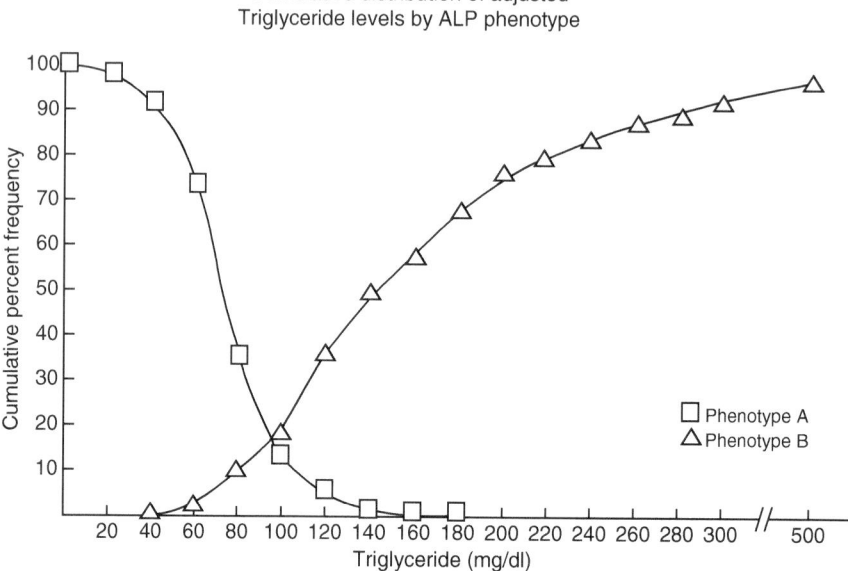

Fig. 5.2 Distribution of the small dense LDL atherogenic lipoprotein (ALP) phenotype demarcated as phenotype B across a continuum of triglyceride values shown compared to phenotype A: large buoyant LDL (Reproduced from Austin MA, et al. [6] with permission from Wolters-Kluwer Health)

level of >200 mg/dL, designated as "high". While there has only been a mild increase in median TG levels across genders and ethnicities in the past two decades, these increases were primarily encountered in younger age groups compared to prior [2]. In fact, some argue that this increased prevalence of hypertriglyceridemia is a reflection of the Type 2 Diabetes and Metabolic Syndrome epidemic. Despite such a large-scale problem, years of research have only fueled the controversy in implicating elevated TG's as causal in atherosclerotic CVD.

Familial Dyslipidemias

A reason for the initial dismissal of TGs as a potential marker for CVD was the finding that some subgroups of patients with familial genetic dyslipidemias (mainly Fredrickson-Levy classification type I and V), and severely elevated TGs (>1000 mg/dL), did not seem especially prone to developing atherosclerosis but rather were at high risk for chylomycronemia and pancreatitis [7]. Further research has shown that the genetic dyslipidemias with TGs in the 200–800 mg/dL range accompanied by the presence of TG rich lipoproteins (Fredrickson-Levy classification type IIb, III and IV) were inversely associated with premature atherosclerosis and CVD [8]. This paradox was accounted for by the thought that when TGs are >1000 mg/dL, remnants are too large to incorporate into the arterial intima and participate in the development of atherosclerosis.

Recent Epidemiologic Studies

In 2008, the INTERHEART study investigated apolipoproteins and conventional lipids as indices of risk for a first acute myocardial infarction (MI) [9]. This was an international, multi ethnic case control study with 12,461 cases and 14,637 age and sex matched controls in 52 countries. The investigators found that a high ApoB: ApoAI ratio had the highest population attributable risk for acute MI at 54 % which was statistically significant compared to conventional lipid ratios (p<0.0001). Given the distribution of ApoB across all non-HDL lipoproteins, these results highlight the notion that lipid atherogenicity goes beyond LDL cholesterol, to include the variety of TRL's and their downstream remnants: VLDL, IDL and chylomicron remnants.

The Emerging Risk Factors Collaboration released a 2009 meta-analysis (with data from 68 long term prospective studies analyzing 302,430 individuals) showing that raised TG levels regardless of fasting status were associated with an increased risk of Coronary Heart Disease (CHD) after adjustment for non-lipid risk factors [10]. However, this association was completely attenuated after adjustment for High Density Lipoprotein Cholesterol (HDL-C) and non-HDL-C (HR 0.99, 95 % CI, 0.94–1.05), suggesting that there was no added benefit of using TGs for CHD risk prediction beyond standard lipoprotein measurements. However, the latest guidelines recommend that risk prediction focuses on the combined endpoint of CHD and stroke, not just CHD. In addition, the usefulness by sex and in different ethnicities should also be considered.

Drawing on the previously mentioned role of small, dense LDL, a population based cohort study using the Multi-Ethnic Study of Atherosclerosis (MESA) database examined the discordance between LDL-C and LDL Particle concentration (LDL-P) [11]. This study examined 6814 subjects free of clinical CVD at baseline and followed up participants for 5.5 years during which time 319 incident CVD events occurred. The study showed that for patients with discordant LDL-C and LDL-P levels, only LDL-P was associated with incident CVD. Further, in patients with LDL-P greater than LDL-C, there was an increased incidence of hypertriglyceridemia and insulin resistance, with 54 % of those patients meeting criteria for metabolic syndrome. Finally, this study also showed that carotid intima-media thickness, a marker for subclinical atherosclerosis had a stronger correlation with LDL-P levels than LDL-C.

A subsequent Mendelian randomization study investigated the notion that if TG levels remained genetically low lifelong, there would be an expected decrease in all-cause mortality [12]. The study showed that genetically reduced nonfasting plasma TG levels due to allelic variants in LPL gene loci, resulted in lower levels of plasma TGs, inversely proportional to the number of alleles present (more alleles corresponded to lower TG levels and survival benefit). Further, the study did indeed find that genetically low concentrations of nonfasting TGs are associated with reduced all-cause mortality. The authors felt that TGs per se were not necessarily causal, but rather, RLPs were the more likely causal factor, based on other similar studies by the same group [13, 14].

The aforementioned select studies, with clear discordance in establishing a relationship between CVD and hypertriglyceridemia, highlight the extent of the controversy in the field. Despite this discordance, several conclusions can potentially be extrapolated: (i) there is some evidence for an association between hypertriglyceridemia and atherosclerosis in epidemiologic studies, (ii) Mendelian randomization studies do indeed provide relatively concrete evidence to establish causality, and (iii) elevated TG clearly alters the atherogenicity of lipoproteins, particularly remnant particles and small, dense LDL.

Controversy in Clinical Trial Data

While focus over the past decade in the clinical trial realm has been on LDL lowering medications, several clinical trials have looked at TG lowering agents. In addition to the prospective cohort and case control studies discussed previously, the following representative primary and secondary prevention studies further illustrate mixed results.

Primary Prevention Trials

One of the earlier trials to examine TG lowering and CVD was the Helsinki Heart Study (HHS). This was a primary prevention trial examining 4081 dyslipidemic men without CVD who were randomized to gemfibrozil vs placebo [15]. While there was a 34 % reduction in CVD incidence in the gemfibrozil group, there was no difference in all cause mortality between the two groups. Further, despite reduction in TG levels in HHS patients, this was not associated with the observed reduction in CVD events.

Another study examining fibrate therapy was the Fenofibrate Intervention and Event Lowering in Diabetes trial (FIELD). Patients with Type 2 Diabetes, regardless of their lipid profile, were randomized to fenofibrate vs placebo [16]. While there were significant reductions in non-fatal MI, microvascular disease, total CVD events, coronary and non-coronary revascularization in the fibrate group, unfortunately – likely secondary to higher crossover to statins in the placebo treated patients - FIELD failed to show a difference in all-cause mortality. In fact, there was a trend toward increased mortality, pulmonary embolus and pancreatitis in the treated patients. Notably, post-hoc analysis of FIELD did show that fenofibrate was most beneficial in patients with metabolic syndrome and marked dyslipidemia (high TG, low HDL).

The most recent fibrate based trial was the Action to Control Cardiovascular Risk in Diabetes (ACCORD). This study was designed to investigate whether fibrate therapy provided mortality benefit in addition to statin therapy in patients with type

2 diabetes [17]. In this study, 10,251 patients were randomized to fenofibrate plus simvastatin vs placebo plus simvastatin. While there was significant, albeit modest, lowering in TG levels (186–170 mg/dL), there was no primary outcome reduction in the study group (fatal CVD, non fatal MI or non fatal stroke). However, further subgroup analysis showed that in patients with marked dyslipidemia (TG > 204 mg/dL and HDL < 34 mg/dL), there was a trend towards benefit.

Another trial investigating combination therapy was the Japan Eicosapentaenoic Acid Lipid Intervention Study (JELIS). Here, patients were randomized to pravastatin or simvastatin in addition to the fish oil eicosapentaenoic acid vs. a statin alone [18]. In follow-up, patients in the study group had about a 20 % reduction in primary and recurrent CVD events but no difference was seen in sudden cardiac death or overall mortality. Notably, here as well, the improved effects were likely not related to TG lowering over and above statins.

Secondary Prevention

A landmark secondary prevention trial was the Veterans Affairs High-Density Lipoprotein Intervention Trial (VA-HIT). In this study, men with known CVD and HDL-C <40 mg/dL, LDL-C <140 mg/dL and TG <300 mg/dL were randomized to gemfibrozil vs placebo [19]. With mean follow up of about 5 years, patients who were treated with fibrate therapy had a significant 22 % reduction in the primary endpoint of nonfatal MI or death due to CVD. While there was a 31 % reduction in mean TG levels in the treated group, this was not associated with the reduction in primary endpoints. Initial statistical analysis pointed towards increased HDL levels as what may have accounted for the positive result given that LDL-C levels in both treatment groups were equivalent and not changed with gemfibrozil. However, further analysis with Nuclear Magnetic Resonance spectroscopy did show that treatment with gemfibrozil increased LDL size and decreased LDL-P, likely explaining the observed reduction in endpoints with therapy concomitant with TG lowering [20]. As with the primary prevention trials noted above, there was a further significant reduction in overall death and CVD-related death in patients with diabetes at baseline.

Another secondary prevention trial of fibrate therapy was Bezafibrate Infarction Prevention (BIP). Here 3090 patients with known prior MI and dyslipidemia were randomized to bezafibrate vs placebo. While there was no difference in the primary endpoint of fatal, nonfatal MI and sudden death in either group, patients with TG >200 mg/dL at baseline had a significant reduction in the primary endpoint [21].

While the PROVE-IT TIMI 22 trial successfully established that reduction in LDL-C to <70 mg/dL was superior to previous more conservative cutoffs in patients with Acute Coronary Syndromes (ACS), a subgroup analysis explored the impact of on-treatment TG levels on CHD. There was a reduced risk of the incidence of death, MI and recurrent ACS associated with low on-treatment TG levels (<150 mg/dL) even after adjustment for other covariates [22]. While only a post-hoc analysis, these results are consistent with evidence that hypertriglyceridemia may be associated with hypercoagulability, worsened in post-MI states.

Lastly, the most recent trial to examine the effects of niacin in secondary prevention was the Atherothrombosis Intervention in Metabolic Syndrome With Low HDL/High Triglycerides and Impact on Global Health Outcomes (AIM-HIGH) study [23]. Here, 3414 patients with known CVD and low HDL-C were randomized to high dose niacin versus placebo, with both arms receiving varying doses of simvastatin and ezetimibe to maintain LDL-C of 40–80 mg/dL. The study was halted early given no significant differences in primary outcomes. Further post-hoc analysis of a pre-specified subgroup with HDL-C <32 mg/dL and TG of >200 mg/dL showed that niacin decreased the primary endpoint by 37 % [24].

The results of the primary and secondary prevention trials discussed here are clearly not consistent with one another in terms of the potential efficacy of TG targeted therapy or TG lowering in reducing the risk of CVD. Altogether, these trials make it quite difficult to extrapolate treatment strategies to clinical practice. In an attempt to consolidate the evidence above, it seems plausible that the groups of patients that benefit the most from targeted TG lowering agents are those with insulin resistance and marked dyslipidemia. While TG lowering was not consistently and independently associated with benefit in most of these studies, it is somewhat clear that the downstream effects of TG lowering, namely, decreased non-HDL-C levels, remnants and LDL-P are likely responsible for the observed changes, potentially of greatest benefit in those with characteristic lipid phenotype characterized by concurrently high TG and low HDL-C.

Highlights of Management

Fasting vs. Non-fasting Evaluation

While it has been traditional that an overnight fast preceded lipid testing, a growing body of evidence seems to support non-fasting measurements, particularly of TG. Several large population-based prospective cohort studies over the past decade have found that postprandial TG levels better predicted the risk of CVD than post-fast levels of TG. The thought here is that in the hypertriglyceridemic, insulin resistant, obese individual, a postprandial elevation in TG may persist, resulting in the remnant and small, dense, LDL cascade [25]. Fasting TGs has been required for usage in the estimation of LDL-C by the Friedwald equation [26]. Further, fasting measurement TGs allow for a standard, predictable state allowing temporal tracking of TG response to therapy

Current Management Strategies and Their Pitfalls

The National Cholesterol Education Program (NCEP), Adult Treatment Panel III provided insights about management of patients with hypertriglyceridemia [27]. The definitions of optimum, elevated and very high TG established in this landmark guideline are widely accepted and represent the current consensus across major dyslipidemia guidelines worldwide (Table 5.1).

The NCEP outlined that the primary goal of therapy in patients with borderline-high and high TG levels is to achieve LDL-C goals. Once LDL-C goals are achieved, non-HDL-C (defined as TC – HDL-C) becomes a secondary target of therapy.

Using the Very Large Database of Lipids (VLDL) of more than 1.3 million adult patients, two recent studies have reinforced the complementary nature of using LDL-C and Non-HDL-C in these patients. The first study compared the Friedwald estimated and directly measured LDL-C values. It found that the Friedwald equation generated LDL-C measurement underestimated directly assessed LDL-C particularly in patients with TG >150 mg/dL [28, 29]. Further, an additional study using the same database showed that a significant degree of patient level discordance between LDL-C and non-HDL-C percentiles for risk stratification resulted in a significant degree of patient reclassification based on non-HDL-C (a potentially more accurate reflection of true atherogenicity than LDL-C) [30]. This discordance was again most notable in patients with low LDL-C and high TG (>150 mg/dL).

Dietary and Lifestyle Modification

In patients such as those with the Type I and V distribution, where TG levels are well above 500 mg/dL, the aim of therapy is to bring down TG to <500. This recommendation is included in prior guidelines as well as the latest 2013 ACC/AHA cholesterol treatment guideline. Typically, a low-fat diet is recommended given their chylomicron predominant phenotype. Further, the addition of unsaturated, medium chain fats and proteins in their diet could further contribute to TG lowering in severe cases with inadequate response to dietary fat restriction [31].

In patients with borderline-high and high levels of TGs accompanied by the typical obesity-insulin resistance dyslipidemia, metabolic syndrome phenotype, data have been considerably more uniform. Beyond doubt, the combination of weight loss, exercise, low carbohydrate and low alcohol consumption has shown significant benefit in TG lowering particularly in those patients with the highest levels of TG at baseline [32]. Weight loss is essential in these patients given the well known contribution of metabolically active visceral fat stores in the dyslipidemia of obesity [33]. This is exemplified in Fig. 5.3, which describes beneficial changes in metabolic syndrome hallmarks in obese patients who have undergone bariatric surgery.

Table 5.1 Therapeutic targets based on severity of TG elevation, from the NCEP ATP-III guideline

TG level	Severity designation	Target of therapy
TG < 150	Normal	None
TG 150–200	Borderline high	LDL-C
TG 200–500	High	LDL-C then Non-HDL-C
TG > 500	Very high	TG

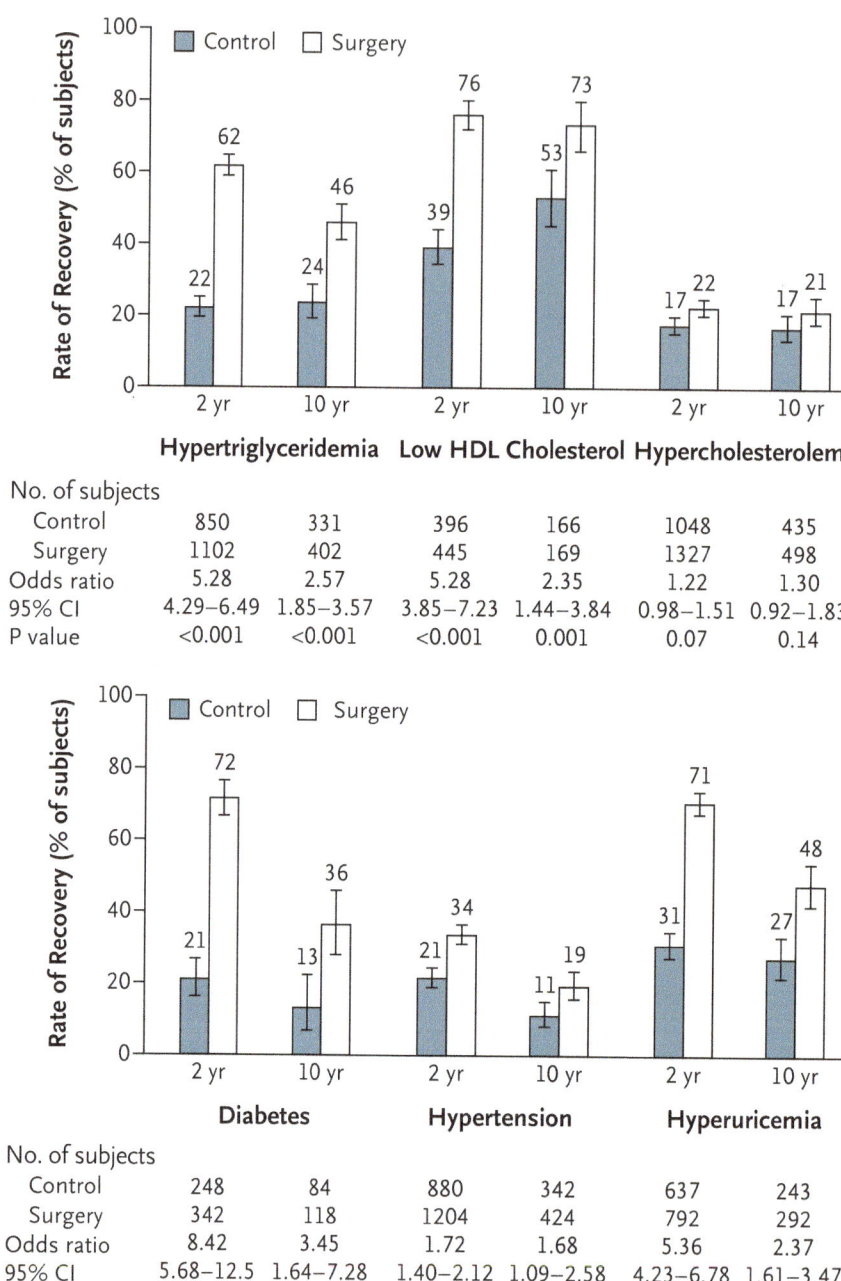

Fig. 5.3 Two and ten year recovery rates for post bariatric surgery patients compared to controls in hypertriglyceridemia and other markers of the metabolic syndrome (Reproduced from: Sjostrom L, et al.[32], with permission off the Massachusetts Medical Society)

Conclusion

1. Over the past several decades, an association between hypertriglyceridemia and incident CVD has resulted in extensive research with mixed results.
2. Population based studies as well as clinical trials have failed to consistently link elevated TGs with CVD though recent Mendelian randomization studies do support the potential causal nature of RLPs.
3. Insight into the TG induced mechanisms of atherogenesis through remnant particles and small, dense LDL may potentially consolidate the perceived, controversially mixed, clinical trial and population based study outcomes.
4. Extrapolating information from trial data and guidelines to appropriately target lipoprotein levels in the treatment of elevated TGs is further complicated by poor reliability of lipoprotein measurements in hypertriglyceridemic states.
5. The best evidence from **post hoc** subgroup analyses of randomized trials would suggest a significant reduction in clinical events by addition of a fibrate in secondary prevention with TG >200 mg/dL or in combination with a statin in diabetic patients with concurrent elevations in TG >204 mg/dL and low HDL-C <34 mg/dL. Similarly, the addition of niacin to statins may be of benefit in secondary prevention in those with concurrent TG >200 mg/dL and HDL-C <32 mg/dL.

References

1. Austin MA, Hokanson JE, Edwards KL. Hypertriglyceridemia as a cardiovascular risk factor. Am J Cardiol. 1998;81(4A):7B–12.
2. Miller M, Stone NJ, Ballantyne C, Bittner V, Criqui MH, Ginsberg HN, et al. Triglycerides and cardiovascular disease: a scientific statement from the American Heart Association. Circulation. 2011;123(20):2292–333.
3. Ginsberg HN. New perspectives on atherogenesis: role of abnormal triglyceride-rich lipoprotein metabolism. Circulation. 2002;106(16):2137–42.
4. Liu L, Wen T, Zheng XY, Yang DG, Zhao SP, Xu DY, et al. Remnant-like particles accelerate endothelial progenitor cells senescence and induce cellular dysfunction via an oxidative mechanism. Atherosclerosis. 2009;202(2):405–14.
5. Austin MA. Triglyceride, small, dense low-density lipoprotein, and the atherogenic lipoprotein phenotype. Curr Atheroscler Rep. 2000;2(3):200–7.
6. Austin MA, King MC, Vranizan KM, Krauss RM. Atherogenic lipoprotein phenotype. A proposed genetic marker for coronary heart disease risk. Circulation. 1990;82(2):495–506.
7. Leaf DA. Chylomicronemia and the chylomicronemia syndrome: a practical approach to management. Am J Med. 2008;121(1):10–2.
8. Hopkins PN, Heiss G, Ellison RC, Province MA, Pankow JS, Eckfeldt JH, et al. Coronary artery disease risk in familial combined hyperlipidemia and familial hypertriglyceridemia: a case–control comparison from the national heart, lung, and blood institute family heart study. Circulation. 2003;108(5):519–23.
9. McQueen MJ, Hawken S, Wang X, Ounpuu S, Sniderman A, Probstfield J, et al. Lipids, lipoproteins, and apolipoproteins as risk markers of myocardial infarction in 52 countries (the INTERHEART study): a case–control study. Lancet. 2008;372(9634):224–33.

10. Emerging Risk Factors Collaboration, Di Angelantonio E, Sarwar N, Perry P, Kaptoge S, Ray KK, et al. Major lipids, apolipoproteins, and risk of vascular disease. JAMA. 2009;302(18):1993–2000.
11. Mora S, Szklo M, Otvos JD, Greenland P, Psaty BM, Goff Jr DC, et al. LDL particle subclasses, LDL particle size, and carotid atherosclerosis in the multi-ethnic study of atherosclerosis (MESA). Atherosclerosis. 2007;192(1):211–7.
12. Thomsen M, Varbo A, Tybjaerg-Hansen A, Nordestgaard BG. Low nonfasting triglycerides and reduced all-cause mortality: a mendelian randomization study. Clin Chem. 2014;60(5):737–46.
13. Varbo A, Benn M, Tybjaerg-Hansen A, Nordestgaard BG. Elevated remnant cholesterol causes both low-grade inflammation and ischemic heart disease, whereas elevated low-density lipoprotein cholesterol causes ischemic heart disease without inflammation. Circulation. 2013;128(12):1298–309.
14. Varbo A, Benn M, Tybjaerg-Hansen A, Jorgensen AB, Frikke-Schmidt R, Nordestgaard BG. Remnant cholesterol as a causal risk factor for ischemic heart disease. J Am Coll Cardiol. 2013;61(4):427–36.
15. Frick MH, Elo O, Haapa K, Heinonen OP, Heinsalmi P, Helo P, et al. Helsinki heart study: primary-prevention trial with gemfibrozil in middle-aged men with dyslipidemia. Safety of treatment, changes in risk factors, and incidence of coronary heart disease. N Engl J Med. 1987;317(20):1237–45.
16. Keech A, Simes RJ, Barter P, Best J, Scott R, Taskinen MR, et al. Effects of long-term fenofibrate therapy on cardiovascular events in 9795 people with type 2 diabetes mellitus (the FIELD study): randomised controlled trial. Lancet. 2005;366(9500):1849–61.
17. ACCORD Study Group, Ginsberg HN, Elam MB, Lovato LC, Crouse 3rd JR, Leiter LA, et al. Effects of combination lipid therapy in type 2 diabetes mellitus. N Engl J Med. 2010;362(17):1563–74.
18. Yokoyama M, Origasa H, Matsuzaki M, Matsuzawa Y, Saito Y, Ishikawa Y, et al. Effects of eicosapentaenoic acid on major coronary events in hypercholesterolaemic patients (JELIS): a randomised open-label, blinded endpoint analysis. Lancet. 2007;369(9567):1090–8.
19. Rubins HB, Robins SJ, Collins D, Fye CL, Anderson JW, Elam MB, et al. Gemfibrozil for the secondary prevention of coronary heart disease in men with low levels of high-density lipoprotein cholesterol veterans affairs high-density lipoprotein cholesterol intervention trial study group. N Engl J Med. 1999;341(6):410–8.
20. Otvos JD, Collins D, Freedman DS, Shalaurova I, Schaefer EJ, McNamara JR, et al. Low-density lipoprotein and high-density lipoprotein particle subclasses predict coronary events and are favorably changed by gemfibrozil therapy in the veterans affairs high-density lipoprotein intervention trial. Circulation. 2006;113(12):1556–63.
21. Bezafibrate Infarction Prevention (BIP) Study. Secondary prevention by raising HDL cholesterol and reducing triglycerides in patients with coronary artery disease. Circulation. 2000;102(1):21–7.
22. Miller M, Cannon CP, Murphy SA, Qin J, Ray KK, Braunwald E, et al. Impact of triglyceride levels beyond low-density lipoprotein cholesterol after acute coronary syndrome in the PROVE IT-TIMI 22 trial. J Am Coll Cardiol. 2008;51(7):724–30.
23. Guyton JR, Slee AE, Anderson T, Fleg JL, Goldberg RB, Kashyap ML, et al. Relationship of lipoproteins to cardiovascular events: the AIM-HIGH trial (atherothrombosis intervention in metabolic syndrome with low HDL/high triglycerides and impact on global health outcomes). J Am Coll Cardiol. 2013;62(17):1580–4.
24. Al-Hijji M, Martin SS, Joshi PH, Jones SR. Effect of equivalent on-treatment apolipoprotein levels on outcomes (from the AIM-HIGH and HPS2-THRIVE). Am J Cardiol. 2013;112(10):1697–700.
25. Bansal S, Buring JE, Rifai N, Mora S, Sacks FM, Ridker PM. Fasting compared with nonfasting triglycerides and risk of cardiovascular events in women. JAMA. 2007;298(3):309–16.

26. Mora S, Rifai N, Buring JE, Ridker PM. Comparison of LDL cholesterol concentrations by friedewald calculation and direct measurement in relation to cardiovascular events in 27,331 women. Clin Chem. 2009;55(5):888–94.
27. National Cholesterol Education Program (NCEP) Expert Panel on Detection, Evaluation, and Treatment of High Blood Cholesterol in Adults (Adult Treatment Panel III). Third report of the national cholesterol education program (NCEP) expert panel on detection, evaluation, and treatment of high blood cholesterol in adults (adult treatment panel III) final report. Circulation. 2002;106(25):3143–421.
28. Martin SS, Blaha MJ, Elshazly MB, Brinton EA, Toth PP, McEvoy JW, et al. Friedewald-estimated versus directly measured low-density lipoprotein cholesterol and treatment implications. J Am Coll Cardiol. 2013;62(8):732–9.
29. Martin SS, Blaha MJ, Elshazly MB, Toth PP, Kwiterovich PO, Blumenthal RS, et al. Comparison of a novel method vs the friedewald equation for estimating low-density lipoprotein cholesterol levels from the standard lipid profile. JAMA. 2013;310(19):2061–8.
30. Elshazly MB, Martin SS, Blaha MJ, Joshi PH, Toth PP, McEvoy JW, et al. Non-high-density lipoprotein cholesterol, guideline targets, and population percentiles for secondary prevention in 1.3 million adults: the VLDL-2 study (very large database of lipids). J Am Coll Cardiol. 2013;62(21):1960–5.
31. Jacobson TA, Ito MK, Maki KC, Orringer CE, Bays HE, Jones PH, et al. National lipid association recommendations for patient-centered management of dyslipidemia: part 1 - executive summary. J Clin Lipidol. 2014;8(5):473–88.
32. Sjostrom L, Lindroos AK, Peltonen M, Torgerson J, Bouchard C, Carlsson B, et al. Lifestyle, diabetes, and cardiovascular risk factors 10 years after bariatric surgery. N Engl J Med. 2004;351(26):2683–93.
33. Bays HE, Toth PP, Kris-Etherton PM, et al. Obesity, adiposity, and dyslipidemia: a consensus statement from the national lipid association. J Clin Lipidol. 2013;7:304–83.

Chapter 6
Patent Foramen Ovale Closure and Stroke

Pablo Rengifo-Moreno and Igor F. Palacios

Abstract A patent foramen ovale (PFO) is highly prevalent among the adult population and has been associated to cryptogenic strokes. The diagnosis of PFO is done through echocardiographic studies. Due to the high prevalence of PFO, the identification of "high risk" features such as atrial septal aneurysm (ASA) becomes extremely important in the management of these patients. Currently, the major controversy regarding the treatment and secondary prevention of patients with cryptogenic stroke and PFO is based on the fact that most of the studies investigating medical and interventional based therapies, failed to include patients with "high risk" features.

Keywords Patent foramen ovale • Atrial septal aneurysm • Transcatheter PFO closure devices • Eustachian valves

Introduction

A patent foramen ovale (PFO) is highly prevalent among the adult population. It allows shunting of blood through the inter-atrial septum and has been associated with cryptogenic stroke and migraines with aura. Currently, echocardiography is the most important diagnostic tool, and, the sensitivity and specificity of the study depends on the modalities available: transthoracic (TTE), transesophageal (TEE) and transcranial Doppler (TCD), as well as the use of agitated saline and the site of injection.

It has been over 140 years since the controversy regarding the potential cause-effect relationship between a PFO and cryptogenic strokes was originally proposed

P. Rengifo-Moreno, MD
Department of Medicine, University of Miami Hospital, Miami, FL, USA
e-mail: Pablo.rengifo@gmail.com

I.F. Palacios, MD (✉)
Cardiac Unit, Department of Medicine, Massachusetts General Hospital,
Harvard Medical School, Boston, MA, USA

© Springer International Publishing Switzerland 2015
J.A. Ambrose, A.E. Rodríguez (eds.), *Controversies in Cardiology*,
DOI 10.1007/978-3-319-20415-4_6

69

by Dr. Julius Cohnheim [1]. Since then, multiple attempts have tried to prove that closure of PFO could be an effective therapy to prevent subsequent neurological events. Medical therapy alone seems to be appropriate for patients with "low risk anatomy" but those with "high risk" features might not obtain sufficient protection. Transcatheter (TC) PFO closure has been shown in observational and prospective studies to be a safe and efficient therapy. However, the results of multiple randomized clinical trials (RCT) have failed to show significant benefits from catheter closure, mostly due to the fact that each study was underpowered. Thus, meta-analysis of the combined studies is important. The fact that there are no randomized clinical trials studying the impact of TC-PFO closure versus standardized medical therapy in patients with "high risk" anatomy PFO, contributes to the controversy surrounding secondary prevention in patients with cryptogenic stroke and PFO.

The purpose of this chapter is to provide a review of different aspects regarding PFO and neurological syndromes, including anatomy, diagnosis and therapeutic options, as well as the data supporting these different strategies.

Embryology and Anatomy

The development of the foramen ovale is critical in the embryological development of the heart. Approximately at the 5th week of development, a very thin septum primum begins to migrate downwards towards the endocardial cushion. The hiatus in between both structures forms the foramen primum. As the migration of the septum primum continues, apoptotic changes within the septum will originate the foramen secundum. On the right atrial surface of the foramen secundum a more muscular and thicker septum secundum migrates downwards covering the foramen secundum and leaving a small foramen on the bottom of the atrium, the foramen ovale. This structure will provide a right to left shunt necessary for fetal circulation. After birth, this communication will spontaneously close in approximately 75 % of the population [2].

The anatomy of the PFO is highly variable and may be associated with a long tunnel of >10 mm, an atrial septal aneurysm which is a redundancy of the atrial septum of over 15 mm, a hypermobile septum or a persistent Eustachian valve.

Prevalence

In multiple autopsy reports, the prevalence of PFO in the adult population is approximately 26 % [3]. The prevalence of PFO is similar by non-invasive methods with TEE [4]. However, the incidence of PFO in young patients presenting with cryptogenic stroke can reach up to 50 % [5].

Factors Associated with Paradoxical Embolization

The PFO in Cryptogenic Stroke Study (PICSS) was a multicenter study that evaluated TEE findings in patients randomly assigned to warfarin or aspirin in the Warfarin-Aspirin Recurrent Stroke Study (WARSS). PICSS found that patients with cryptogenic stroke had a significantly higher incidence of a large PFO when compared to those patients having a stroke of known cause (20 % vs. 9.7 % p<0.001) [6]. Moreover, Steiner et al. performed TEE in 95 patients with a first ischemic stroke over 39 years of age [7]. The stroke subtype and MRI/CT imaging data were evaluated blinded to the presence of a PFO. These findings were compared between two groups: patients with a medium to large PFO (>2 mm) and small (<2 mm) or no PFO. Stroke patients with larger PFOs showed more brain imaging features of embolic infarcts than those with small PFOs.

The presence of a prominent Eustachian valve (EV) has been proposed as responsible for re-directing blood flow towards the septum, potentially allowing emboli to travel through the inter-atrial septum into the left atrium. This hypothesis was evaluated with TEE by Schuchlenz et al. by comparing patients who had cryptogenic strokes to healthy volunteers and found a significantly higher incidence of PFO and EV in those patients with cryptogenic stroke [8].

The PFO and ASA study group followed 581 ischemic stroke patients under the age of 55 years of age. The patients were started on aspirin within 3 months of their neurological event, and followed up for a period of 4 years. The patients were divided into groups depending of the characteristics of the inter-atrial septum. Mas et al. found that the presence of both atrial septal abnormalities (PFO and ASA) was a significant predictor of increased risk of recurrent cerebrovascular events, whereas the presence of a PFO alone or an ASA alone was not [9]. Moreover, their finding suggested that aspirin as secondary prevention for recurrent events may not be enough for this subgroup of patients. These findings are in agreement with findings of other studies, especially in patients with right-to-left shunting at rest [10]. Stone et al. followed prospectively a group of stroke patients found to have a PFO during TEE and divided them into "large" degree shunting (≥20 microbubbles) and "small" degree shunting (≥3 but <20 microbubbles). Patients with "large" shunts had a 31 % incidence of a recurrent event versus none in the "small" shunt group despite the use of antiplatelet and/or anticoagulation. Therefore, patients with "large" shunts, should be considered at a significantly higher risk for subsequent adverse neurologic events [11]. It has also been proposed that "long-tunnel" PFO anatomy represents an environment fertile for clot formation, with subsequent embolization. However, there is no clear evidence supporting this hypothesis [12].

In a venography study, Stollberger et al. presented evidence that patients with ischemic stroke due to suspected paradoxical embolization have a higher incidence of deep venous thrombosis [13]. Therefore, conditions that facilitate the formation of deep venous thrombosis deserve special attention when evaluating patients with PFO and cryptogenic stroke. The May-Thurner syndrome, in which the right common iliac artery compresses the overlying left common iliac vein has been found to have a higher incidence in patients with PFO-related stroke [14, 15]. In a prospective study of patients with large pulmonary embolism, it was found that those patients with PFO had a sixfold higher risk of stroke when compared to those without PFO [16] Table. 6.1.

PFO Diagnosis

It is very important to remember when evaluating a patient for the presence of a PFO, that a PFO is present in approximately 25 % of the general healthy population [3]. Thus, it is important to be mindfull of the clinical presentation of every particular case. Moreover, the clinician should be able to identify particular "high risk" features that might make the presence of a PFO more relevant (Table. 6.1).

There are different modalities available for the diagnosis of PFO. The most commonly used are TTE, TEE and TCD coupled with agitated saline injection in association with the Valsalva manuever. The most common initial modality is TTE for evaluation of cardiac sources of emboli. Agitated saline contrast increases the diagnostic sensitivity by enhancing echocardiographic detection of the trivial intermittent right-to-left shunting across the PFO. However, the sensitivity of TEE is higher than TTE despite the use of agitated saline [3]. Hamman et al. [17] demonstrated increased sensitivity when the injection of agitated saline was performed from the femoral vein versus the traditional antecubital vein. This is probably due to the fact that the bubbles ascending through the inferior vena cava will encounter the EV and flow preferentially towards the septum. These findings were more evident when using TEE and TCD versus TTE.

Medical Therapy for Secondary Prevention of Cryptogenics Strokes

Medical therapy for secondary prevention in cryptogenic strokes continues to be the most common initial approach for patients after the initial neurological event. However, the type of medical therapy has been loosely defined in different studies and there is no consensus regarding the use of either antiplatelet agents or anticoagulation. Furthermore, there is no agreement regarding an escalation in therapy for patients with "high risk" PFO anatomical features.

Table. 6.1 "High risk" features of a PFO increasing stroke risk

PFO associated with an ASA
Large size of the PFO
PFO associated with a prominent EV
PFO associated with a large degree of shunt

WARSS, was the first randomized controlled study to compare the effect of warfarin and aspirin after prior non-cardioembolic ischemic stroke. WARSS showed that aspirin was as effective as warfarin in prevention of stroke recurrence, but the presence of a PFO was not specifically systematically evaluated [18]. Moreover, WARSS showed that the incidence of death and recurrent ischemic strokes was similar in both groups of patients (Warfarin vs. Aspirin). However, the incidence of recurrent ischemic strokes was equally high (17.8 % vs. 16.0 % for the Warfarin and the Aspirin groups respectively, $p=0.2$). Of interest that same year in the same journal, the report from the PFO and ASA study group [9] was published. In their prospective study of cryptogenic stroke patients treated with aspirin, when the PFO was associated with an ASA, aspirin was not as effective for secondary prevention. A year later, a substudy of WARSS, the PICCS trial compared secondary prevention with aspirin versus warfarin. In the cohort of patients with cryptogenic stroke, there was a trend towards fewer neurological events in the arm treated with warfarin when a PFO was present [6]. The evidence seems to indicate that warfarin might be more appropriate for secondary prevention in patients with "high risk" PFO. However, this was associated with an increase in bleeding complications. New anticoagulation agents are now available, and it will be interesting to see how the use of this new medication class will impact the secondary prevention of cryptogenic strokes in patients with a PFO, especially those with "high risk" features. Studies are on going.

Surgical Therapy for Secondary Prevention of Cryptogenic Strokes

Surgical closure of PFO has shown good results, with a low incidence of recurrent events [3]. However, due to the invasive nature of the intervention, it is not a commonly used therapy. Currently, it is reserved for cases that will require surgical intervention for another condition or in those in whom percutaneous closure can not be performed related to the inter-atrial septal anatomy.

PFO-TC Closure for Secondary Prevention of Cryptogenic Strokes

Although there are no FDA approved devices for TC-PFO closure in the United States, there is a vast experience using off-label devices for secondary prevention. Reports have shown that TC-PFO closure is a safe intervention that is associated with favorable short- and intermediate-term outcomes [19]. Moreover, studies show excellent long-term outcomes when used for secondary prevention in patients with cryptogenic stroke (Fig. 6.1) [20]. A systematic review and meta-analysis of observational studies showed the annual rate of strokes after PFO-closure is

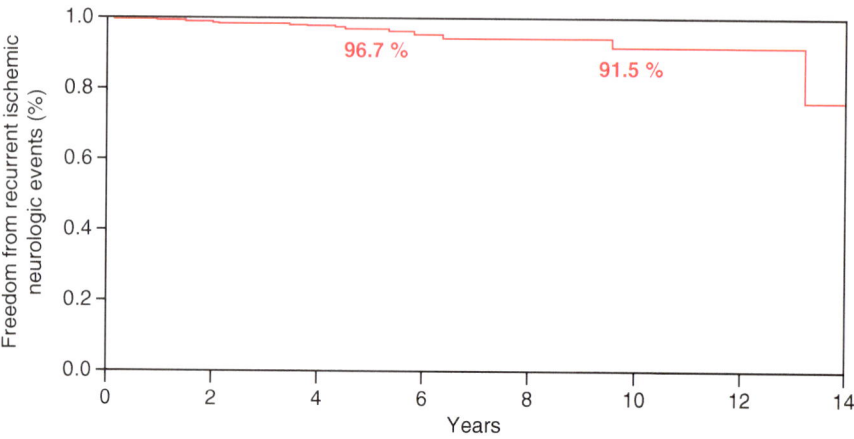

Fig. 6.1 Kaplan-Mayer recurrent neurological event after TC-PFO closure

approximately 0.3–0.8 %, lower than the 1.98–5.0 % in the medical group [3, 21]. This translates into an 84 % reduction in the rate of recurrent neurological events when compared to medical management alone.

A prospective study with long term follow-up showed that the presence of a substantial residual shunt after TC-PFO closure was an important predictor of recurrent neurological events with a relative risk of 4.2 [22]. Therefore, the use of a second device for secondary prevention of recurrent neurological events has been an important clinical question. In a retrospective study by Diaz et al., 424 patients with at least a 5 % substantial residual shunt found that the placement of a second device was safe and effective in treating the residual shunt. Moreover, there were no neurological events at a mean follow-up of 3 years. However, the clinical significance of treating residual shunts with a second device would be at least difficult to prove, since the event rate is low even with untreated PFOs [23].

However, results from three recently published RCTs failed to show a significant benefit of TC PFO closure over medical therapy [24–26]. One trial utilized the StarFlex device [24], the other two studied the Amplatzer device [25, 26]. The main limitation of all three RCTs was the small number of events during follow-up, raising the possibility of a "type 2 error" (failure to detect a true difference between treatments due to lack of power). This lack of power can be explained by the difficulties in enrolling patients in a trial, while the study device was available as an off-label therapy. Another important observation about the three RCTs was the inclusión of relatively "low risk" PFOs into their analysis [24–26]. The presence of an ASA in patients included in the RCTs, a feature that has been associated with a higher incidence of recurrent neurological events, ranged from only 23–26 %.

A recent meta-analysis of the three RCTs that attempted to overcome the lack of power of the individual studies found that in the intention-to-treat analyses, there was a statistically significant 41 % risk reduction in stroke and/or transient ischemic attack in the TC PFO closure group when compared to medical treatment

Review: PFO closure and adverse CV events
Comparison: 01 PFO closure Vs medical treatment
Outcome: 09 PFO closure and TLA/stroke

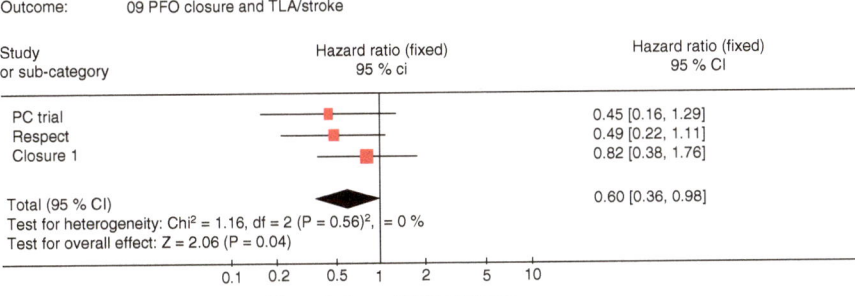

Fig. 6.2 Medical therapy versus TC-PFO closure for prevention of TIA/Stroke

(Fig. 6.2) [27]. Device implantation was successful in 93.8 % on average, being lowest with the STARFlex device in the CLOSURE I trial (89.4 %). Moreover, the meta-analysis showed that the development of new-onset atrial fibrillation was significantly higher in the TC PFO group when compared to medical therapy. However, when stratified by type of device (excluding the STARFlex device), the Amplatzer device had a non-significant increased risk for developing new-onset atrial fibrillation. This analysis was consistent with a recently reported meta-analysis of observational studies showing that STARFlex or CardiolSEAL, but not the Amplatzer device was associated with an increased risk of developing new-onset atrial fibrillation [28].

Rengifo-Moreno et al. also showed that subjects with a significant shunt (substantial vs. trace, none, or moderate) had a tendency towards decreased vascular events in patients when randomized to the TC PFO closure compared to medical therapy [27]. A recent subgroup analysis of the patients enrolled in the CLOSURE I trial identified diabetes and atrial fibrillation as independent predictors of recurrent stroke. Therefore, a substantial proportion of recurrent events within the CLOSURE I trial was probably not due to paradoxical embolization [29], but was, in fact, likely related to atrial fibrillation developing post-randomization and to the presence of diabetes.

Until further analyses with individual-level data are available or new on-going RCTs with similar outcomes and appropriate follow-up are published, TC PFO closure continues to be an individualized decision. A multi-disciplinary approach with input from the cardiologist, neurologist, hematologist and interventional cardiologist provides the best therapeutic plan for each patient taking into account the available data, but also, medical, social and occupational considerations.

PFO and Migraines

The association between migraines with aura and the presence of a PFO remains controversial and small non-randomized studies assessing the response to PFO closure provided inconsistent results [30–40]. Two major mechanisms have being proposed to explain the putative association of PFO and migraine: 1- vasoactive substances from the general circulation may bypass the metabolic filters of the lung thereby altering the natural equilibrium. Substance P and serotonin have been suggested as possible culprit agents. Furthermore, it has being suggested that patients with migraine have a high rate of abnormal pulmonary function that could result in decreased metabolism of vasoactive amines [41]. 2- PFO may result in the passage of microemboli resulting in hypoxia and ischemia into the occipital cortex [42–44].

The MIST trial [45], evaluated the Starflex device versus a sham procedure in a randomized fashion. The primary end point was cessation of migraine headache. The primary end-point was not significantly different between both arms. However, the exploratory analysis supported further investigation. The PRIMA trial was presented at TCT 2014 [46]. In PRIMA, 107 patients with migraines were randomized to either PFO closure or medical therapy. Only 45 of 53 randomized to the device actually agreed to undergo the procedure. Of these, only 41 actually underwent PFO closure. At 1 year, the primary end-point of mean reduction in headache days from baseline was 2.9 in the closure group and 1.7 in the medical-treatment group, a nonsignificant difference. However, for the secondary end point of reduction in migraine-with-aura days, closure patients saw reductions significantly greater than in the control group. These results highlight the need for additional RCTs with enough power and the appropriate primary end-points to investigate the impact of TC PFO closure in patients with migraine and aura.

Conclusions

1. PFO is highly prevalent in the general population approaching 25 %. However, the incidence doubles in young patients presenting with cryptogenic stroke.
2. Currently, there are no RCTs comparing different medical therapy strategies for secondary prevention in patients with cryptogenic strokes. However, aspirin is not as efficient in preventing recurrent strokes in patients with "high risk" PFO.
3. RCTs have not systematically studied the population at highest risk for recurrent stroke after a cryptogenic event. Thus, RCTs enrolling exclusively patients with cryptogenic stroke and "high risk" PFO should be conducted.
4. Systematic reviews, meta-analysis of RCTs and observational studies suggest a possible benefit of TC-PFO closure for secondary prevention in patients with cryptogenic stroke associated with PFO but more data are needed. The recently published ASA/AHA guidelines for stroke prevention, give a class III recommendation for PFO closure in patients with a cryptogenic ischemic stroke or TIA and a PFO without evidence for DVT. The new guidelines give a IIb recommendation for consideration of TC-PFO closure, in the setting of a cryptogenic stroke associated to DVT [47].
5. Until further studies are available with emphasis on patients with "high risk" anatomy, TC PFO closure continues to be an individualized decision.

References

1. Cohnheim J. Untersuchungen uber die embolischen processe. Berlin: August Hirschwald; 1872.
2. Moore KL, Persaud TVN. The developing human: clinical oriented embryology. 5th ed. Philadelphia: Saunders; 1994.
3. Homma S, Sacco RL. Patent foramen ovale and stroke. Circulation. 2005;112:1063–72.
4. Lechat P, Mas JL, Lascault G, Loron PH, Theard M, Klimczac M, Drobinski G, Thomas D, Grosgogeat Y. Prevalence of patent foramen ovale in patients with stroke. N Engl J Med. 1988;318:1148–52.
5. Webster MWI, Smith HJ, Sharpe DN, Chancellor AM, Swift DL, Bass NM, Glasgow GL. Patent foramen ovale in young stroke patients. Lancet. 1988;332:11–2.
6. Homma S, Sacco RL, Di Tullio MR, Sciacca RR, Mohr JP. Effect of medical treatment in stroke patients with patent foramen ovale: patent foramen ovale in cryptogenic stroke study. Circulation. 2002;105:2625–31.
7. Steiner MM, Di Tullio MR, Rundek T, Gan R, Chen X, Liguori C, Brainin M, Homma S, Sacco RL. Patent foramen ovale size and embolic brain imaging findings among patients with ischemic stroke. Stroke. 1998;29:944–8.
8. Schuchlenz HW, Saurer G, Weihs W, Rehak P. Persisting eustachian valve in adults: relation to patent foramen ovale and cerebrovascular events. J Am Soc Echocardiogr. 2004;17:231–3.
9. Mas JL, Arquizan C, Lamy C, Zuber M, Cabanes L, Derumeaux G, COSTE J. Recurrent cerebrovascular events associated with patent foramen ovale, atrial septal aneurysm, or both. N Engl J Med. 2001;345:1740–6.
10. De Castro S, Cartoni D, Fiorelli M, Rasura M, Anzini A, Zanette EM, Beccia M, Colonnese C, Fedele F, Fieschi C, Pandian NG. Morphological and functional characteristics of patent foramen ovale and their embolic implications. Stroke. 2000;31:2407–13.
11. Stone DA, Godard J, Corretti MC, Kittner SJ, Sample C, Price TR, Plotnick GD. Patent foramen ovale: association between the degree of shunt by contrast transesophageal echocardiography and the risk of future ischemic neurologic events. Am Heart J. 1996;131:158–61.
12. Landzberg MJ, Khairy P. Indications for the closure of patent foramen ovale. Heart. 2004;90:219–24.
13. Stollberger C, Slany J, Schuster I, Leitner H, Winkler WB, Karnik R. The prevalence of deep venous thrombosis in patients with suspected paradoxical embolism. Ann Intern Med. 1993;119:461–5.
14. Greer DM, Buonanno FS. Cerebral infarction in conjunction with patent foramen ovale and May-Thurner syndrome. J Neuroimaging. 2001;11(4):432–4.
15. Kiernan TJ, Yan BP, Cubeddu RJ, Rengifo-Moreno P, Gupta V, Inglessis I, Ning M, Demirjian ZN, Jaff MR, Buonanno FS, Schainfeld RM, Palacios IF. May-Thurner syndrome in patients with cryptogenic stroke and patent foramen ovale: an important clinical association. Stroke. 2009;40:1502–4.
16. Konstantinides S, Geibel A, Kasper W, Olschewski M, Blumel L, Just H. Patent foramen ovale is an important predictor of adverse outcomes in patients with major pulmonary embolism. Circulation. 1998;97:1946–51.
17. Hamman GF, Schatzer-Klotz D, Frohlig G, Strittmatter M, Jost V, Berg G, Stopp M, Schimrigk K, Schieffer H. Femoral injection of echo contrast medium may increase the sensitivity of testing for a patent foramen ovale. Neurology. 1998;50:1423–8.
18. Mohr JP, Thompson JLP, Lazar RM, Levin B, Sacco RL, Furie KL, Kistler JP JP, Albers GW, Pettigrew LC, Adams HP, Jackson CM, Pullicino P. A comparison of warfarin and aspirin for the prevention of recurrent ischemic stroke. N Engl J Med. 2001;345:1444–51.
19. Martin F, Sánchez PL, Doherty E, et al. Percutaneous transcatheter closure of patent foramen ovale in patients with paradoxical embolism. Circulation. 2002;106:1121–6.
20. Inglessis I, Elmariah S, Rengifo-Moreno P, Margey R, O'Callaghan C, Cruz-Gonzalez I, Baron S, Mehrotra P, Tan TC, Hung J, Demirjian Z, Buonanno F, Ning MM, Silverman SB,

Cubeddu RJ, Pomerantsev E, Schainfeld RM, Dec GW, Palacios IF. Long-term experience and outcomes with transcatheter closure of patent foramen ovale. J Am Coll Cardiol Intv. 2013;6:1176–83.

21. Agarwal S, Bajaj NS, Kumbhani DJ, Tuzcu EM, Kapadia SR. Meta-analysis of transcatheter closure versus medical therapy for patent foramen ovale in prevention of recurrent neurological events after presumed paradoxical embolism. J Am Coll Cardiol Intv. 2012;5:777–89.

22. Windecker S, Wahl A, Chatterjee T, Garachemani A, Eberli FR, Seiler C, Meier B. Percutaneous closure of patent foramen ovale in patients with paradoxical embolism: long-term risk of recurrent thromboembolic events. Circulation. 2000;101(8):893–8.

23. Diaz T, Cubeddu RJ, Rengifo-Moreno PA, Cruz-Gonzalez I, Solis-Martin J, Buonanno FS, Inglessis I, Palacios IF. Management of residual shunts after initial percutaneous patent foramen ovale closure: a single center experience with immediate and long-term follow-up. Catheter Cardiovasc Interv. 2010;76(1):145–50.

24. Furlan AJ, Reisman M, Massaro J, Mauri L, Adams H, Albers GW, Felberg R, Herrmann H, Kar S, Landzberg M, Raizner A. Closure or medical therapy for cryptogenic stroke with patent foramen ovale. N Engl J Med. 2012;366:991–9.

25. Carroll JD, Saver JL, Thaler DE, Smalling RW, Berry S, MacDonald LA, Marks DS, Tirschwell DL. Closure of patent foramen ovale versus medical therapy after crypto-genic stroke. N Engl J Med. 2013;368:1092–100.

26. Meier B, Kalesan B, Mattle HP, Khattab AA, Hildick-Smith D, Dudek D, Andersen G, Ibrahim R, Schuler G, Walton AS, Wahl A, Windecker S, Juni P. Percutaneous closure of patent foramen ovale in cryptogenic embolism. N Engl J Med. 2013;368:1083–91.

27. Rengifo-Moreno P, Palacios IF, Junpaparp P, Witzke CF, Morris LD, Romero-Corral A. Patent foramen ovale transcatheter closure vs. medical therapy on recurrent vascular events: a systematic review and meta-analysis of randomized controlled trials. Eur Heart J. 2013;34(43):3342–52.

28. Li Y, Zhou K, Hua Y, Wang C, Xie L, Fang J, Rong X, Shen J. Amplatzer occluder versus CardioSEAL/STARFlex occluder: a meta-analysis of the efficacy and safety of transcatheter occlusion for patent foramen ovale and atrial septal defect. Cardiol Young. 2013;23:582–96.

29. Elmariah S, Furlan AJ, Reisman M, Burke D, Vardi M, Wimmer NJ, Ling S, Chen X, Kent DM, Massaro J, Mauri L. Predictors of recurrent events in patients with cryptogenic stroke and patent foramen ovale within the Closure I (Evaluation of the Starflex Septal Closure System in Patients with a Stroke and/or Transient Ischemic Attack due to Presumed Paradoxical Embolism Through a Patent Foramen Ovale) trial. J Am Coll Cardiol Intv. 2014;7:913–20.

30. Wilmshurst PT, Nightingale S, Walsh KP, Morrison WL. Effect on migraine of closure of cardiac right-to-left shunts to prevent recurrence of decompression illness or stroke or for haemodynamic reasons. Lancet. 2000;356:1648–51.

31. Morandi E, Anzola GP, Angeli S, Melzi G, Onorato E. Transcatheter closure of patent foramen ovale: a new migraine treatment? J Interv Cardiol. 2003;16:39–42.

32. Schwerzmann M, Wiher S, Nedeltchev K, Mattle HP, Wahl A, Seiler C, Meier B, Windecker S. Percutaneous closure of patent foramen ovale reduces the frequency of migraine attacks. Neurology. 2004;62:1399–401.

33. Post MC, Thijs V, Herroelen L, Budts WI. Closure of patent foramen ovale is associated with a decrease in prevalence of migraine. Neurology. 2004;62:1439–40.

34. Azarbal B, Tobis J, Suh W, Chan V, Dao V, Gaster R. Association of interatrial shunts and migraine headaches: impact of transcatheter closure. J Am Coll Cardiol. 2005;45:489–92.

35. Reisman M, Christofferson RD, Jesurum J, Olsen JV, Spencer MP, Krabill KA, Diehl L, Aurora S, Gray WA. Migraine headache relief after transcatheter closure of patent foramen ovale. J Am Coll Cardiol. 2005;45:493–5.

36. Giardini A, Donti A, Formigari R, Salomone L, Prandstraller D, Bonvicini M, Palareti G, Guidetti D, Gaddi O, Picchio FM. Transcatheter patent foramen ovale closure mitigates aura migraine headaches abolishing spontaneous right-to-left shunting. Am Heart J. 2006;151:922-e1–5.

37. Anzola G, Frisoni GB, Morandi E, Casilli F, Onorato E. Shunt-associated migraine responds favorably to atrial septal repair: a case control study. Stroke. 2006;37:430–4.
38. Anzola GP, Magoni M, Guindani M, Rozzini L, Dalla Volta G. Potential source of cerebral embolism in migraine with aura: a trans-cranial Doppler study. Neurology. 1999;52:1622–5.
39. Domitrz I, Mieszkowshi J, Kwiecinski H. The Prevalence of patent foramen ovale in patients with migraines. Neurol Neurochir Pol. 2004;38:89–92.
40. Schwedt TJ, Demaerschalk BM, Dodick DW. Patent foramen ovale and migraine: a quantitative systematic review. Cephalalgia. 2008;28:531–40.
41. Ozge A, Ozge C, Oztürk C, Kaleagasi H, Ozcan M, Yalçinkaya DE, Ozveren N, Yalçin F. The relationship between migraine and atopic disorders—the contribution of pulmonary function tests and immunological screening. Cephalalgia. 2005;26:172–9.
42. Gorji A. Spreading depression: a review of the clinical relevance. Brain Res Brain Res Rev. 2001;38:33–60.
43. Olesen J, Friberg L, Olsen TS, Andersen AR, Lassen NA, Hansen PE, Karle A. Ischaemia-induced (symptomatic) migraine attacks may be more frequent than migraine induced ischaemic insults. Brain. 1993;116:187–202.
44. Venketasubramanian N, Sacco RL, Di Tullio M, Sherman D, Homma S, Mohr JP. Vascular distribution of paradoxical emboli by transcranial Doppler. Neurology. 1993;43:1533–5.
45. Dowson A, Mullen MJ, Peatfield R, Muir K, Khan AA, Wells C, Lipscombe SL, Rees T, De Giovanni JV, Morrison WL, Hildick-Smith D, Elrington G, Hillis WS, Malik IS, Rickards A. Migraine intervention with STARFlex technology (MIST) trial: a prospective, multicenter, double-blind, sham-controlled trial to evaluate the effectiveness of patent foramen ovale closure with STARFlex septal repair implant to resolve refractory migraine headache. Circulation. 2008;117(11):1397–404.
46. Wood S. PFO closure fails anew in migraine: PRIMA. Kansas: Heartwire; 2014.
47. Kernan WN, Ovbiagele B, Black HR, Bravata DM, Chimowitz MI, Ezekowitz MD, Fang MC, Fisher M, Furie KL, Heck DV, Johnston SC, Kasner SE, Kittner SJ, Mitchell PH, Rich M, Richardson D, Schwamm LH, Wilson JA. Guidelines for the prevention of stroke in patients with stroke and transient ischemic attack. Stroke. 2014;45:2160–236.

Part II
Cardiovascular Diagnosis

Chapter 7
CT Angiography Versus Routine Stress Testing for Patients with Chest Pain Seen in the Emergency Room to Exclude Significant Coronary Artery Disease

Gaston A. Rodriguez-Granillo and Patricia Carrascosa

Abstract The triage of low-to-intermediate risk patients presenting at the emergency department (ED) with acute chest pain based on symptoms, initial 12-lead ECG, and a single set of biomarkers of myocardial necrosis usually fails to provide a fast and safe discharge without further diagnostic testing. Among low risk patients with normal or non-diagnostic ECG and negative initial cardiac enzymes, stress imaging (particularly stress-only SPECT) is an effective strategy to safely discharge patients; with a very high negative predictive value to predict myocardial infarction or future adverse cardiac events. Computed tomography coronary angiography (CTCA) has emerged as a fast, safe, and possibly cost effective means to exclude coronary artery disease (CAD) as the cause of an acute coronary syndrome in the ED in patients at low-to-intermediate risk of CAD; and provides a long-term event-free safety window with zero events after a mean 52-month follow-up. CTCA is associated with a mild (2 %) but significant difference in the rates of invasive angiography and coronary revascularization, but with a higher diagnostic yield. Further studies are warranted to define whether CTCA plus confirmatory stress imaging for indeterminate results might be the most cost effective strategy.

G.A. Rodriguez-Granillo, MD, PhD (✉)
Department of Cardiovascular Imaging, Diagnostico Maipu,
Vicente Lopez, Buenos Aires, Argentina

Consejo Nacional de Investigaciones Científicas y Técnicas (CONICET),
Buenos Aires, Argentina
e-mail: grodriguezgranillo@gmail.com

P. Carrascosa, MD, PhD
Department of Cardiovascular Imaging, Diagnostico Maipu,
Vicente Lopez, Buenos Aires, Argentina

© Springer International Publishing Switzerland 2015
J.A. Ambrose, A.E. Rodríguez (eds.), *Controversies in Cardiology*,
DOI 10.1007/978-3-319-20415-4_7

Keywords Computed tomography • Emergency department • Perfusion • Functional • Outcome • Cost • Invasive coronary angiography • Negative predictive value • Revascularization

Introduction

Timely and accurate triage of patients presenting at the emergency department (ED) with acute chest pain remains challenging. Identification of acute coronary syndromes (ACS) is relatively simple and straightforward in intermediate to high risk patients, particularly in the presence of typical symptoms. Notwithstanding, the triage of low to intermediate risk patients based on symptoms, initial 12-lead ECG, and a single set of biomarkers of myocardial necrosis usually fails to provide a fast and safe discharge without further diagnostic testing [1, 2]. Consequently, more than 60 % of patients with chest pain admitted to the hospital ultimately do not end up having an ACS [3–5]. This over triage has a huge economical impact to health care systems, estimated at an annual cost of U$D 8 billion [6]. Indeed, only in the United States, more than seven million patients are admitted every year with acute chest pain suspected of ACS, and are evaluated for approximately 24 h including serial ECGs, enzyme level assessment, and eventually the performance of functional tests [2]. Furthermore, while most turn out not to have underlying coronary artery disease (CAD), about 5 % of patients with ACS are not recognized by standard diagnostic algorithms, potentially leading to serious legal implications [2]. Given this scenario, it is therefore imperative to develop tools that enable a faster discharge of patients with acute chest pain from the ED.

The field of cardiovascular imaging provides different diagnostic tools to evaluate patients with suspected CAD. These can be discriminated into two major groups relevant to this chapter: anatomical (computed tomography coronary angiography, CTCA), and functional (stress-echocardiography, nuclear medicine, stress-magnetic resonance). Moreover, an additional discrimination should be made between methods that evaluate coronary artery atherosclerosis, and those that evaluate CAD. This small distinction might conceal sizeable diagnostic and prognostic implications.

Diagnostic methods that assess the presence of CAD, either by means of functional tests or by invasive coronary angiography (ICA), target the evaluation of the luminal impact of the disease. On the contrary, CTCA has the ability to characterize not only the lumen (Fig. 7.1), but the vessel wall as well, being able to identify features associated with potential plaque instability such as low density (<30 HU), spotty calcification, napkin-ring sign, and large plaque volume that are associated with potential plaque instability (Figs. 7.2 and 7.3) [7–15].

In the past decade, the safety, promptness, and high negative predictive value of CTCA has driven its incorporation as an alternative for the triage of patients with acute chest pain at low to intermediate risk of CAD. Notwithstanding, several controversies persist, particularly concerns regarding whether this technique might lead to an increase in downstream costs and in revascularization rates.

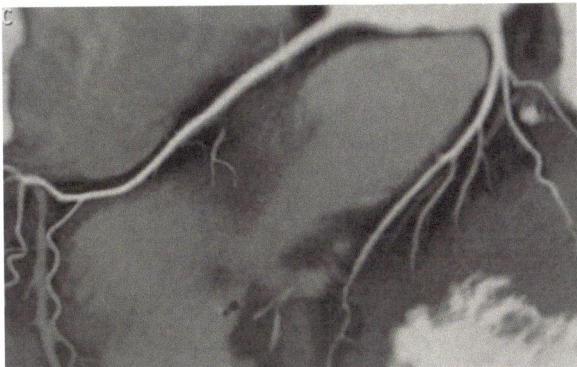

Fig. 7.1 Acute chest pain with normal ECG in a 55 year old female with hypertension and hyper-cholesterolemia as coronary risk factors. The patient is rapidly discharged after computed tomography coronary angiography shows absence of coronary atherosclerosis in the early triage

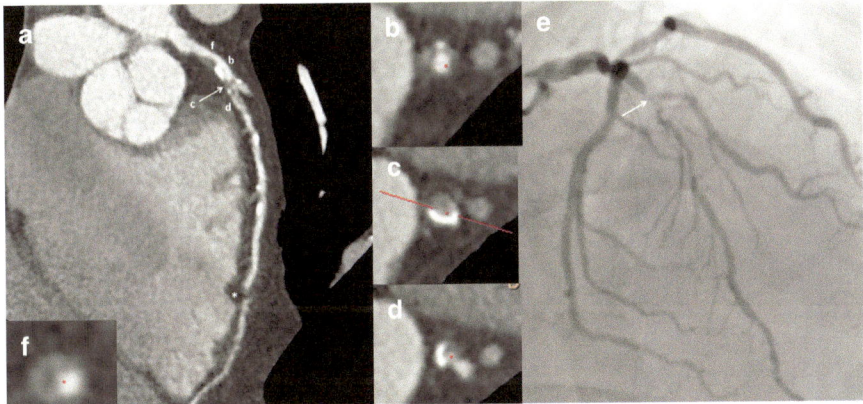

Fig. 7.2 Atypical acute chest pain in a 58 year old male with hypercholesterolemia and smoking as coronary risk factors, and non-specific repolarization abnormalities. Computed tomography coronary angiography is performed as part of the early triage (curved multiplanar reconstructions), showing a critical lesion at the mid left anterior descending (LAD) artery, with compromise of a large diagonal branch (panel **a**, *arrow*). The asterisk refers to a motion artifact attributed to prospective ECG-gating (effective dose 4.1 mSv in a patient with a body mass index of 29 kg/m^2). An orthogonal view of the lesion depicts the subtotal occlusion, with mild eccentric calcification (**c**), whereas panels (**b, d**) show the immediately proximal and distal reference sites with extensive disease. Invasive angiography confirms the findings (panel **e**). Of note, a large eccentric non-calcified plaque with positive remodeling, low attenuation, and napkin-ring sign (panel **f**); all characteristics of plaque vulnerability, is observed at the proximal LAD

Computed Tomography Coronary Angiography (CTCA)

CTCA is more closely related to intravascular ultrasound than to ICA [16]. Based on that principle, CTCA has significantly contributed to visualize atherosclerosis in the earlier phases and has therefore contributed to a better understanding of the

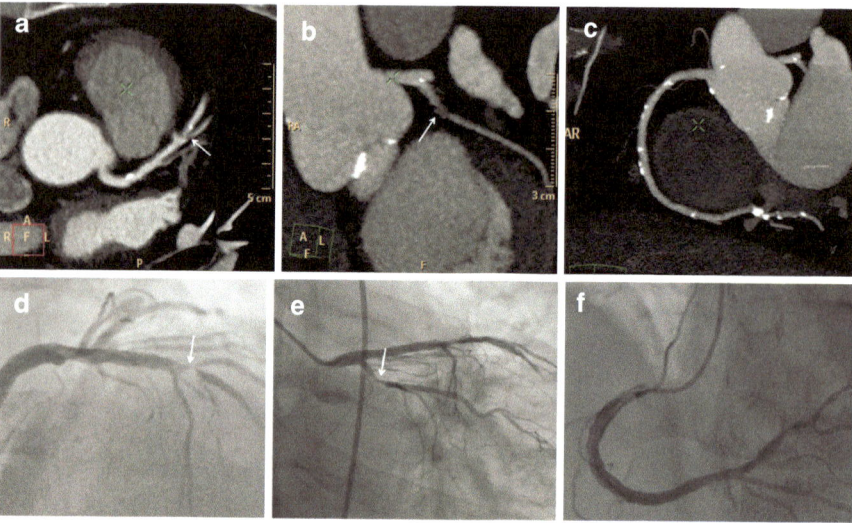

Fig. 7.3 Sixty eight year old male with hypertension and hypercholesterolemia as coronary risk factors. Typical rest angina with normal ECG and normal first set of cardiac enzyme levels. Computed tomography coronary angiography is performed as part of the early triage (maximum intensity projections area shown), demonstrating a critical lesion at the mid left anterior descending artery (panel **a**, *arrow*), and a severe lesion at the proximal left circumflex (panel **b**, *arrow*); whereas mild calcifications are seen at the right coronary artery (panel **c**). Invasive angiography confirmed the findings (panels **d–f**)

blind gap between the onset of coronary atherosclerosis and the development of obstructive CAD [10–15]. This feature of CTCA has potential important clinical implications since most acute thrombotic coronary events arise from angiographically non significant lesions [17–19]. As a matter of fact, until recently, only ex vivo and catheter-based diagnostic tools enabled the assessment of the anatomic substrate of presumed high risk plaques [20–25].

During the past decade, CTCA has earned a more active role in different diagnostic algorithms of patients suspected of CAD. Several studies have explored the role of CTCA for the detection of obstructive *de novo* lesions [26–28]. These studies have demonstrated that CTCA has a high diagnostic accuracy to detect obstructive CAD in diverse populations, although patients at intermediate risk appear as the best scenario. A number of multicenter studies have confirmed these earlier findings, with sensitivities ranging between 85 and 95 %, specificities between 83 and 90 %, and similar diagnostic accuracy compared to ICA regarding the ability to predict short term revascularization. Despite slight differences in study design and populations, there is robust evidence that positions CTCA as the non invasive diagnostic tool with the highest negative predictive value (Fig. 7.1) [26–28].

In the past decade, great technical advances in the field of CTCA have been witnessed, that have a major effect in effective dose radiation (EDR), image quality, scan duration, physiological assessment, iodine volume load, and myocardial perfusion imaging. Numerous tools have been successfully elaborated in order to reduce radiation dose associated with CTCA, such as iterative reconstruction, tube modulation, prospective ECG-gating, and high-pitch spiral acquisitions [29–31]. Using a combination of these techniques enable high quality acquisitions with radiation dose levels lower than 3 mSv for CTCA with prospective triggering and below 1 mSv for high-pitch helical mode studies using dual source scanners [29, 30, 32]. For instance, high pitch scans can be performed in 258 ms with a mean EDR of barely 0.87 msV [31]. Nevertheless, the Prospective Multicenter Study on Radiation Dose Estimates of Cardiac CT Angiography I and II (PROTECTION I and II) reported a wide range of effective radiation doses according to the acquisition technique. Therefore, the use of one or more of the aforementioned dose reduction techniques should be encouraged [33, 34].It should be noted that prospective ECG triggering should not be considered as a first choice in obese patients, and if heart rate is high (≥ 70 bpm) or irregular.

Despite the considerable technical developments of the past decades, the high sensitivity and negative predictive value of CTCA has remained consistently over 90 % and relatively unaffected since the 16-row CTCA generation. On the contrary, the specificity and the positive value has significantly improved with the incorporation of newer generations of scanners [35]. From a clinical standpoint, this has been translated into a reduced number of normal downstream invasive diagnostic procedures (~14 % to ~4 %) [26, 27].

Role of CTCA in Patients with Acute Chest Pain

Recently, CTCA has emerged as an alternative for patient triage with acute chest pain and low to intermediate probability of CAD. Three large randomized multicenter studies (CT-STAT, ACRIN-PA, and ROMICAT II) have shown that CTCA is a safe strategy that allows a significant reduction in diagnostic time, thereby leading to a larger percentage of patients with discharge from the emergency department (ED). Importantly, this benefit derived a significant reduction in costs [36–38].

The CT-STAT trial randomized 749 patients with low-risk acute chest pain to CTCA or standard of care (SOC). Despite a similar diagnostic performance between the two strategies, patients assigned to CTCA had a significant reduction in diagnostic time (54 %; 2.9 h vs. 6.2 h; $p < 0.001$) as well as in total cost (38 %; USD $2137 vs. USD $3458, $p < 0.001$) [36]. The ACRIN-PA trial randomized 1370 patients with low to intermediate risk to CTCA or SOC. In this study, CTCA had significantly higher rates of discharge from the ED (50 % vs. 23 %, $p < 0.001$), and a significantly lower number of unnecessary (false positive) invasive angiograms (p < 0.05). Moreover, it is worth mentioning that of the 640 patients with a negative CTCA, none had an adverse event at 30 days follow-up [37]. Finally, the ROMICAT II trial randomized 1000 patients with acute chest pain and no ischemic ECG changes to CTCA or SOC. Patients assigned to CTCA showed a significant reduction in diagnostic time (5.8 h vs. 21.0 h; p < 0.001), and a significantly higher rates of discharge from the ED (47 % vs. 12 %, p < 0.001). In addition, no differences were observed regarding costs, even though it was pre-specified in the protocol that diagnostic tools within the control group were used at the treating physician's discretion [38]. Hulten et al. recently published a meta-analysis of studies that explored the role of CTCA for the triage of patients with acute chest pain and concluded that CTCA is a safe strategy, improving patient management in the ED, reducing costs and hospital admission rates [39]. In addition, patients with acute chest pain with negative or mild CT findings can be safely and rapidly discharged without further testing, with excellent 30 day event-free survival [40]. The aforementioned evidence has lead to the integration of CTCA in a number of guidelines of clinical practice for acute chest pain management [41–44].

The potential role of cardiac CT in the triage of acute chest pain is not only related to the ability of CTCA to identify obstructive CAD. During the past decade, major technological advances in the field of CT have enabled a comprehensive assessment of both CTCA and stress myocardial perfusion during a single procedure [45]. Several clinical studies have validated this application using different scanners, pharmacological agents, and acquisition protocols [46, 47]. A recent prospective study compared two strategies to evaluate myocardial perfusion by CT (CTP) for the assessment of acute chest pain in patients who were clinically referred to stress/rest SPECT and cardiac MRI: real-time adenosine stress CTP using second generation dual-source CT (group A), and adenosine-stress first-pass dual energy CTP (group B). Compared to stress cardiac magnetic resonance, real-time CTP (versus SPECT) had a 86 % sensitivity, 98 % specificity, 94 % positive predictive value, and 96 % negative predictive value for the detection of myocardial perfusion defects. Furthermore, dual energy CTP had 93 % sensitivity, 99 % specificity, 92 % positive predictive value, and 96 % negative predictive value for detecting perfusion defects [48].

The incremental value of dual-energy CTP over CTCA for the detection of obstructive CAD has recently been considered. Wang et al. reported that the combination of dual energy CTP and CTCA may improve diagnostic performance compared to CTA alone for the diagnosis of significant coronary stenosis [49]. Furthermore, Bettencourt et al. showed that an integrated protocol including CTCA and CTP has an excellent sensitivity and very good specificity for detecting obstructive CAD (assessed by invasive fractional flow reserve), and that CTP provides a significant incremental value over CTCA in patients with intermediate to high pretest probability [50]. Finally, rest CTP simultaneously evaluated during routine CTCA might aid the identification of perfusion defects in the presence of acute coronary occlusion [51]. Indeed, in a recent study that included patients presenting with chest pain to the ED, the evaluation of rest myocardial CTP showed a high diagnostic performance as compared with SPECT-MPI, and improved the accuracy of CTCA mainly by reducing rates of false-positive findings [52]. It should be stressed that most patients with acute chest pain arrive at the CT scanner with an IV line in and heart rate control medications already administrated. Therefore, the exam is usually fast and straightforward. Patients with high or irregular heart rates, pregnant woman, and those with renal failure should avoid this strategy.

Stress Myocardial Perfusion Imaging for the Triage of Acute Chest Pain

Low-risk patients for ACS (negative or unremarkable ECG, and negative initial troponin levels) require confirmatory functional tests including exercise treadmill testing or cardiac imaging evaluation. Early exercise testing in patients who present with chest pain in the ED has been shown to provide limited prognostic information over established clinical scores [53]. Furthermore, exercise testing is precluded in patients with uninterpretable ECG and in patients unable to exercise [54]. Stress imaging such as myocardial perfusion scintigraphy or dobutamine stress echocardiography (DSE) have been positioned in the past two decades as valuable tools with improved prognostic value [55, 56]. Among low risk patients with normal or non-diagnostic ECG and negative initial cardiac enzymes, stress myocardial perfusion imaging (MPI) by means of single photon emission CT (SPECT) has been convincingly established as an effective strategy to safely discharge patients; with a very high negative predictive value to predict myocardial infarction (99 %) or future adverse cardiac events (97 %) [57]. Furthermore, patients with a normal stress-only SPECT have similar mortality rates than those with normal rest-stress studies. Accordingly, rest imaging can be avoided in patients with normal stress, resulting in a significant reduction in radiation exposure [58].

Rest myocardial perfusion imaging in these patients has shown to improve ED triage decision making, with a high negative predictive value that results in reducing unnecessary hospitalizations [59, 60]. Nevertheless, the specificity and positive predictive value of rest MPI is fairly low, because perfusion defects at rest cannot discriminate between acute or chronic ischemia, and can also be due to attenuation artifacts. Accordingly, the strength of rest MPI is mainly its very high negative predictive value, with a 30-day rate of adverse cardiac events <1 %.

Several studies have demonstrated that adding stress myocardial perfusion imaging to conventional SOC strategy (clinical evaluation, serial ECGs, and cardiac markers) for patients presenting with acute chest pain improves clinical decision making by significantly reducing the need for hospitalization, without an increment in adverse event rates at 30 days or 1 year [61].

However, there is evidence suggesting that clinical risk scores (GRACE and TIMI risk scores) but not stress imaging predict long-term cardiovascular mortality in patients with normal or non-diagnostic electrocardiogram after ruling out ACS [62].

It could be hypothesized that aside from the ischemic burden, the anatomic burden of CAD might play an important role in these patients. A recent subanalysis of the COURAGE (Clinical Outcomes Utilizing Revascularization and Aggressive Drug Evaluation) trial showed that when both anatomic burden and ischemic burden of disease at baseline are considered concomitantly, the anatomic burden and the left ventricular ejection fraction, but not the ischemic burden were independent predictors of death, myocardial infarction, or non-ST elevation myocardial infarction [63]. These results are in line with recently published data both from COURAGE indicating that the extent of site-defined ischemia did not predict events and did not modify treatment effectiveness [64]; and from the STICH (Comparison of Surgical and Medical Treatment of Congestive Heart Failure and Coronary artery Disease) trial, showing that in patients with severely reduced systolic function, inducible ischemia did not identify those with worse prognosis or those whom would have obtained greater benefit from revascularization over optimal medical treatment [65].

In the near future, these novel diagnostic methods might lead to identification of three different groups of patients, possibly with dissimilar prognoses: (1) patients with CAD (obstructive disease); (2) patients with coronary atherosclerosis but normal stress tests; and (3) patients without epicardial coronary atherosclerosis but with microvascular disease. Indeed, a recent analysis of the CONFIRM registry (COronary CT Angiography EvaluatioN For Clinical Outcomes: An InteRnational Multicenter Registry) validated previous data showing that the extent of plaque burden, regardless of stenosis severity, has an independent prognostic value [66].

Does CTCA Lead to an Increment in Downstream Costs and More Revascularizations?

As discussed above, the use of CTCA for the triage of patients with acute chest pain is safe, reduces the time to diagnosis and the admission rates, and does not lead to an increment in costs. Nevertheless, there is concern that CTCA might lead to an increment in downstream costs mainly related to an increase in the rates of ICA and revascularization [39]. These have been raised mainly by the aforementioned meta-analysis of Hulten et al., although several issues should be addressed in this regard. This meta-analysis included 3266 patients, 1869 undergoing CTCA and 1397 undergoing SOC. The authors concluded that the use of CTCA for the triage of low-to intermediate risk patients in the ED is safe and reduces the length of stay. However, they found a mild (2 %) but significant differences in the rates of invasive angiography and coronary revascularization [39]. None of the individual studies found significant differences in this regard. Furthermore, the pooled rate of ICA was 8.4 % versus 6.3 % [OR 1.36 (CI 95 % 1.03–1.80)], and of revascularization, 4.6 % versus 2.6 % [OR 1.81 (CI 95 % 1.20–2.72)] for CTCA and SOC, respectively.

The clinical significance of such small difference is uncertain. The diagnostic yield of coronary angiograms induced by CTCA (54 %) was higher than those induced by SOC (41 %). Accordingly, is the question that CTCA leads to increased rate of revascularizations, or does SOC lead to fewer revascularizations? Furthermore, are patients with obstructive disease discharged without a diagnosis?

It might be believed that CTCA could eventually lead to an increment in downstream costs driven by the higher rates of ICA and revascularization. Nevertheless, since more than 90 % of patients did not undergo ICA, the major source of cost is the diagnostic workup per se. Moreover, the decision to revascularize depends on the interventional cardiologist, not on the CTCA that leads to it. Finally, it is noteworthy that two of the studies included in the meta-analysis performed SPECT in all patients with stenoses >25 % or calcium score (Agatston) >100. This very conservative strategy has probably leaded to increased rates of ICA in the CTCA group [36, 67].

The CT-STAT trial provided a head-to-head comparison of CTCA versus stress-rest SPECT in patients with acute chest pain presenting at the ED, and thus deserves a comment. In this study, the rates of ICA during the index visit (CTCA 6.7 %, SPECT 6.2 %, p = 0.80) and the total revascularization rates (CTCA 3.6 %, SPECT 2.4 %, p = 0.34) were similar between groups. Furthermore, the cumulative event rates were comparable (CTCA 5.2 %, SPECT 3.7 %, p = 0.36) [36].Clinical outcome studies in this population are warranted, although they would require very large sample sizes given the low event rate.

Further data regarding downstream cost utilization arises from a recent large multicenter registry (CONFIRM) that included 155,207 CTCA patients at intermediate risk of CAD and demonstrated that patients without CAD and those with only mild disease had low rates of ICA (2.5 % vs. 8.3 %, respectively), and very low revascularization rates (0.3 % vs. 2.5 %, respectively), after a 2.3 year follow-up [68].

Most of the aforementioned favorable evidence of CTCA is related to its unsurpassed negative predictive value, positioning the technique as a fast, safe, and possibly cost effective means to exclude CAD as the cause of an ACS in the ED. Such negative predictive value provides an unparalleled long-term event-free safety window, with zero events in a large cohort of patients with normal coronary arteries after a mean 52-month follow-up [69].

A recent decision analytic model possibly summarizes the concept of this chapter that one method is not meant to exclude the other. In this study that included patients with acute chest pain at low risk of CAD, CTCA plus confirmatory SPECT for indeterminate results might be the most cost effective strategy compared to stress ECG, echocardiography, and SPECT. This combination also reduced hospitalization of patients with an initially false-positive CTA [70]. Furthermore, two recently published meta-analyses indicate that the utilization of CTCA is a cost- and time-effective strategy for evaluation of low and intermediate risk acute chest pain patients in ED and can be used for safe exclusion of acute coronary syndrome (ACS) [39, 71].

Nevertheless, it should be stressed that results from these trials cannot be directly applied to the real world. Only highly trained physicians should read CTCA scans and patients presenting to the ED during evening or weekends were excluded. An attempt to incorporate CTCA in patients with acute chest pain and TIMI risk score ≤2 in a large urban health care system yielded promising results, analogous to the findings from randomized studies. Cury et al. proposed to risk stratification based on the following groups of risk of ACS: 0, low (negative CTA findings); 1, mild (1–49 % stenosis); 2, moderate (50–69 % stenosis); or 3, severe (≥70 % stenosis). Patients with negative CTCA were discharged, those with mild disease were discharged but followed up at the outpatient clinic, those with moderate stenosis underwent further stress testing, and patients with severe stenosis underwent ICA. The rate of MACEs in patients with stenosis ≥70 % (8.3 %) was significantly higher than in patients with negative CTA findings (0 %) or those with mild stenosis (0.2 %). Moreover, a 51 % decreased length of stay from 28.8 to 14.0 h (p < 0.0001) was observed after implementation of the dedicated chest pain protocol [40].

Limitations of CTCA

Aside from the evaluation of CTP that has been discussed above, CTCA does not provide a significant incremental value over functional tests in patients with high pretest probability [72]. This limitation is partially related to the fact that high risk patients usually have diffusely calcified coronary arteries. Furthermore, although the incorporation of significant technical developments in the field has greatly improved temporal and spatial resolution, diffuse calcification remains the only variable with a major impact on diagnostic accuracy [73]. A number of studies have reported a significant decline in diagnostic accuracy with calcium scores (Agatston) >400 related mainly to blooming artifacts that commonly lead to overestimation stenosis severity [27, 74]. A post-hoc analysis of the CORE-64 study disclosed this limitation. Non-calcified segments yielded a positive likelihood ratio (LR +) of 34.4 (95 % CI 23.1, 51.2), compared to a LR+ of 9.9 (95 % CI 7.5, 13.1) among mildly calcified segments, a LR+ of 4.3 (95 % CI 3.3, 5.5) among segments with moderate calcification, and a LR+ of 2.8 (95 % CI 2.2, 3.5) among severely calcified segments, respectively; exposing the negative impact of calcification in the diagnostic accuracy of CTCA. Furthermore, 16 % of segments with mild calcification had poor image quality versus 43 % of segments with severe calcification [75].

Dual energy CT imaging shows promise to overcome some of these limitations, by the ability to attenuate the adverse effect of beam hardening and blooming artifacts, thereby potentially aiding in the assessment of severely calcified vessels [45, 76, 77]. Future studies using dual energy imaging are warranted to explore whether this technique might lead to the inclusion of patients with intermediate to high probability of CAD, usually excluded from any analysis with conventional single energy scanners. Furthermore, dual energy imaging might also have improved diagnostic performance compared to conventional CT for the assessment of myocardial perfusion, preserving image quality without increasing effective radiation dose levels [45]. This might be of interest in the further functional assessment of patients with intermediate to high probability of CAD with stress myocardial perfusion CT.

Conclusions

1. Among low risk patients with chest pain presenting at the ED with normal or non-diagnostic ECG and negative initial cardiac enzymes, stress imaging (particularly stress-only SPECT) is an effective strategy to safely discharge patients; with a very high negative predictive value to predict myocardial infarction or future adverse cardiac events.

2. CTCA has emerged as a fast, safe, and possibly cost effective means to exclude CAD as the cause of an ACS in the ED in patients at low-to-intermediate risk of CAD.
3. CTCA is associated with a mild (2 %) but significant difference in rates of invasive angiography and coronary revascularization, but with a higher diagnostic yield.
4. A normal CTCA provides a long-term event-free safety window, with zero events after a mean 52-month follow-up.
5. Further studies might define whether CTCA plus confirmatory stress imaging for indeterminate results might be the most cost effective strategy.
6. The potential prognostic value of CTCA regarding plaque burden in comparison to stenosis severity and myocardial ischemia warrants further investigation.

References

1. Pope JH, Aufderheide TP, Ruthazer R, Woolard RH, Feldman JA, Beshansky JR, Griffith JL, Selker HP. Missed diagnoses of acute cardiac ischemia in the emergency department. N Engl J Med. 2000;342:1163–70.
2. Christenson J, Innes G, McKnight D, Boychuk B, Grafstein E, Thompson CR, Rosenberg F, Anis AH, Gin K, Tilley J, Wong H, Singer J. Safety and efficiency of emergency department assessment of chest discomfort. CMAJ Can Med Assoc J J Assoc Med Can. 2004;170: 1803–7.
3. Hollander JE, Sease KL, Sparano DM, Sites FD, Shofer FS, Baxt WG. Effects of neural network feedback to physicians on admit/discharge decision for emergency department patients with chest pain. Ann Emerg Med. 2004;44:199–205.
4. McCaig LF, Nawar EW. National hospital ambulatory medical care survey: 2004 emergency department summary. Adv Data. 2006:1–29.
5. Kohn MA, Kwan E, Gupta M, Tabas JA. Prevalence of acute myocardial infarction and other serious diagnoses in patients presenting to an urban emergency department with chest pain. J Emerg Med. 2005;29:383–90.
6. Tosteson AN, Goldman L, Udvarhelyi IS, Lee TH. Cost-effectiveness of a coronary care unit versus an intermediate care unit for emergency department patients with chest pain. Circulation. 1996;94:143–50.
7. Carrascosa PM, Capunay CM, Garcia-Merletti P, Carrascosa J, Garcia MF. Characterization of coronary atherosclerotic plaques by multidetector computed tomography. Am J Cardiol. 2006;97:598–602.
8. Rodriguez-Granillo GA, Rosales MA, Degrossi E, Durbano I, Rodriguez AE. Multislice ct coronary angiography for the detection of burden, morphology and distribution of atherosclerotic plaques in the left main bifurcation. Int J Cardiovasc Imaging. 2007;23:389–92.
9. Rodriguez Granillo GA. Non-invasive assessment of vulnerable plaque. Expert Opin Med Diagn. 2009;3:53–66.
10. Motoyama S, Sarai M, Harigaya H, Anno H, Inoue K, Hara T, Naruse H, Ishii J, Hishida H, Wong ND, Virmani R, Kondo T, Ozaki Y, Narula J. Computed tomographic angiography characteristics of atherosclerotic plaques subsequently resulting in acute coronary syndrome. J Am Coll Cardiol. 2009;54:49–57.
11. Voros S, Rinehart S, Qian Z, Joshi P, Vazquez G, Fischer C, Belur P, Hulten E, Villines TC. Coronary atherosclerosis imaging by coronary ct angiography: current status, correlation with intravascular interrogation and meta-analysis. JACC Cardiovasc Imaging. 2011;4:537–48.
12. Hoffmann U, Moselewski F, Nieman K, Jang IK, Ferencik M, Rahman AM, Cury RC, Abbara S, Joneidi-Jafari H, Achenbach S, Brady TJ. Noninvasive assessment of plaque morphology and composition in culprit and stable lesions in acute coronary syndrome and stable lesions in stable angina by multidetector computed tomography. J Am Coll Cardiol. 2006;47:1655–62.

13. Motoyama S, Kondo T, Sarai M, Sugiura A, Harigaya H, Sato T, Inoue K, Okumura M, Ishii J, Anno H, Virmani R, Ozaki Y, Hishida H, Narula J. Multislice computed tomographic characteristics of coronary lesions in acute coronary syndromes. J Am Coll Cardiol. 2007;50: 319–26.

14. Kashiwagi M, Tanaka A, Kitabata H, Tsujioka H, Kataiwa H, Komukai K, Tanimoto T, Takemoto K, Takarada S, Kubo T, Hirata K, Nakamura N, Mizukoshi M, Imanishi T, Akasaka T. Feasibility of noninvasive assessment of thin-cap fibroatheroma by multidetector computed tomography. JACC Cardiovasc Imaging. 2009;2:1412–9.

15. Kruk M, Wardziak L, Mintz GS, Achenbach S, Pregowski J, Ruzyllo W, Dzielinska Z, Demkow M, Witkowski A, Kepka C. Accuracy of coronary computed tomography angiography vs intravascular ultrasound for evaluation of vessel area. J Cardiovasc Comput Tomogr. 2014;8:141–8.

16. Fischer C, Hulten E, Belur P, Smith R, Voros S, Villines TC. Coronary ct angiography versus intravascular ultrasound for estimation of coronary stenosis and atherosclerotic plaque burden: a meta-analysis. J Cardiovasc Comput Tomogr. 2013;7:256–66.

17. Stone GW, Maehara A, Lansky AJ, de Bruyne B, Cristea E, Mintz GS, Mehran R, McPherson J, Farhat N, Marso SP, Parise H, Templin B, White R, Zhang Z, Serruys PW, Investigators P. A prospective natural-history study of coronary atherosclerosis. N Engl J Med. 2011;364: 226–35.

18. Little WC, Constantinescu M, Applegate RJ, Kutcher MA, Burrows MT, Kahl FR, Santamore WP. Can coronary angiography predict the site of a subsequent myocardial infarction in patients with mild-to-moderate coronary artery disease? Circulation. 1988;78:1157–66.

19. Ambrose JA, Tannenbaum MA, Alexopoulos D, Hjemdahl-Monsen CE, Leavy J, Weiss M, Borrico S, Gorlin R, Fuster V. Angiographic progression of coronary artery disease and the development of myocardial infarction. J Am Coll Cardiol. 1988;12:56–62.

20. Glaser R, Selzer F, Faxon DP, Laskey WK, Cohen HA, Slater J, Detre KM, Wilensky RL. Clinical progression of incidental, asymptomatic lesions discovered during culprit vessel coronary intervention. Circulation. 2005;111:143–9.

21. Virmani R, Kolodgie FD, Burke AP, Farb A, Schwartz SM. Lessons from sudden coronary death: a comprehensive morphological classification scheme for atherosclerotic lesions. Arterioscler Thromb Vasc Biol. 2000;20:1262–75.

22. Rodriguez-Granillo GA, Regar E, Schaar JA, Serruys PW. New insights towards catheter-based identification of vulnerable plaque. Rev Esp Cardiol (Engl Ed). 2005;58:1197–206.

23. Rodriguez-Granillo GA, Agostoni P, Garcia-Garcia HM, de Feyter P, Serruys PW. In-vivo, cardiac-cycle related intimal displacement of coronary plaques assessed by 3-d ECG-gated intravascular ultrasound: exploring its correlate with tissue deformability identified by palpography. Int J Cardiovasc Imaging. 2006;22:147–52.

24. Rodriguez-Granillo GA, Garcia-Garcia HM, Valgimigli M, Vaina S, van Mieghem C, van Geuns RJ, van der Ent M, Regar E, de Jaegere P, van der Giessen W, de Feyter P, Serruys PW. Global characterization of coronary plaque rupture phenotype using three-vessel intravascular ultrasound radiofrequency data analysis. Eur Heart J. 2006;27:1921–7.

25. Asakura M, Ueda Y, Yamaguchi O, Adachi T, Hirayama A, Hori M, Kodama K. Extensive development of vulnerable plaques as a pan-coronary process in patients with myocardial infarction: an angioscopic study. J Am Coll Cardiol. 2001;37:1284–8.

26. Miller JM, Rochitte CE, Dewey M, Arbab-Zadeh A, Niinuma H, Gottlieb I, Paul N, Clouse ME, Shapiro EP, Hoe J, Lardo AC, Bush DE, de Roos A, Cox C, Brinker J, Lima JA. Diagnostic performance of coronary angiography by 64-row CT. N Engl J Med. 2008;359:2324–36.

27. Raff GL, Gallagher MJ, O'Neill WW, Goldstein JA. Diagnostic accuracy of noninvasive coronary angiography using 64-slice spiral computed tomography. J Am Coll Cardiol. 2005;46:552–7.

28. Meijboom WB, Meijs MF, Schuijf JD, Cramer MJ, Mollet NR, van Mieghem CA, Nieman K, van Werkhoven JM, Pundziute G, Weustink AC, de Vos AM, Pugliese F, Rensing B, Jukema JW, Bax JJ, Prokop M, Doevendans PA, Hunink MG, Krestin GP, de Feyter PJ. Diagnostic accuracy of 64-slice computed tomography coronary angiography: a prospective, multicenter, multivendor study. J Am Coll Cardiol. 2008;52:2135–44.

29. Carrascosa P, Rodriguez-Granillo GA, Capunay C, Deviggiano A. Low-dose CT coronary angiography using iterative reconstruction with a 256-slice CT scanner. World J Cardiol. 2013;5:382–6.
30. Hausleiter J, Meyer T, Hadamitzky M, Huber E, Zankl M, Martinoff S, Kastrati A, Schomig A. Radiation dose estimates from cardiac multislice computed tomography in daily practice: impact of different scanning protocols on effective dose estimates. Circulation. 2006;113:1305–10.
31. Achenbach S, Marwan M, Schepis T, Pflederer T, Bruder H, Allmendinger T, Petersilka M, Anders K, Lell M, Kuettner A, Ropers D, Daniel WG, Flohr T. High-pitch spiral acquisition: a new scan mode for coronary ct angiography. J Cardiovasc Comput Tomogr. 2009;3:117–21.
32. Sabarudin A, Sun Z, Ng KH. A systematic review of radiation dose associated with different generations of multidetector ct coronary angiography. J Med Imaging Radiat Oncol. 2012; 56:5–17.
33. Bischoff B, Hein F, Meyer T, Krebs M, Hadamitzky M, Martinoff S, Schomig A, Hausleiter J. Comparison of sequential and helical scanning for radiation dose and image quality: results of the prospective multicenter study on radiation dose estimates of cardiac ct angiography (protection) I study. AJR Am J Roentgenol. 2010;194:1495–9.
34. Hausleiter J, Meyer TS, Martuscelli E, Spagnolo P, Yamamoto H, Carrascosa P, Anger T, Lehmkuhl L, Alkadhi H, Martinoff S, Hadamitzky M, Hein F, Bischoff B, Kuse M, Schomig A, Achenbach S. Image quality and radiation exposure with prospectively ecg-triggered axial scanning for coronary ct angiography: the multicenter, multivendor, randomized protection-III study. JACC Cardiovasc Imaging. 2012;5:484–93.
35. Hamon M, Morello R, Riddell JW, Hamon M. Coronary arteries: diagnostic performance of 16- versus 64-section spiral CT compared with invasive coronary angiography–meta-analysis. Radiology. 2007;245:720–31.
36. Goldstein JA, Chinnaiyan KM, Abidov A, Achenbach S, Berman DS, Hayes SW, Hoffmann U, Lesser JR, Mikati IA, O'Neil BJ, Shaw LJ, Shen MY, Valeti US, Raff GL, Investigators C-S. The CI-stat (coronary computed tomographic angiography for systematic triage of acute chest pain patients to treatment) trial. J Am Coll Cardiol. 2011;58:1414–22.
37. Litt HI, Gatsonis C, Snyder B, Singh H, Miller CD, Entrikin DW, Leaming JM, Gavin LJ, Pacella CB, Hollander JE. Ct angiography for safe discharge of patients with possible acute coronary syndromes. N Engl J Med. 2012;366:1393–403.
38. Hoffmann U, Truong QA, Schoenfeld DA, Chou ET, Woodard PK, Nagurney JT, Pope JH, Hauser TH, White CS, Weiner SG, Kalanjian S, Mullins ME, Mikati I, Peacock WF, Zakroysky P, Hayden D, Goehler A, Lee H, Gazelle GS, Wiviott SD, Fleg JL, Udelson JE, Investigators R-I. Coronary CT angiography versus standard evaluation in acute chest pain. N Engl J Med. 2012;367:299–308.
39. Hulten E, Pickett C, Bittencourt MS, Villines TC, Petrillo S, Di Carli MF, Blankstein R. Outcomes after coronary computed tomography angiography in the emergency department: a systematic review and meta-analysis of randomized, controlled trials. J Am Coll Cardiol. 2013;61:880–92.
40. Cury RC, Feuchtner GM, Batlle JC, Pena CS, Janowitz W, Katzen BT, Ziffer JA. Triage of patients presenting with chest pain to the emergency department: implementation of coronary CT angiography in a large urban health care system. AJR Am J Roentgenol. 2013;200:57–65.
41. Taylor AJ, Cerqueira M, Hodgson JM, Mark D, Min J, O'Gara P, Rubin GD; American College of Cardiology Foundation Appropriate Use Criteria Task F, Society of Cardiovascular Computed T, American College of R, American Heart A, American Society of E, American Society of Nuclear C, North American Society for Cardiovascular I, Society for Cardiovascular A, Interventions, Society for Cardiovascular Magnetic R, Kramer CM, Berman D, Brown A, Chaudhry FA, Cury RC, Desai MY, Einstein AJ, Gomes AS, Harrington R, Hoffmann U, Khare R, Lesser J, McGann C, Rosenberg A, Schwartz R, Shelton M, Smetana GW, Smith Jr SC. ACCF/SCCT/ACR/AHA/ASE/ASNC/NASCI/SCAI/SCMR 2010 appropriate use criteria for cardiac computed tomography. A report of the american college of cardiology foundation appropriate use criteria task force, the society of cardiovascular computed tomography, the american college of radiology, the american heart association, the american society of echocardiography, the american society of nuclear cardiology, the north american society for

cardiovascular imaging, the society for cardiovascular angiography and interventions, and the society for cardiovascular magnetic resonance. J Am Coll Cardiol. 2010;56:1864–94.

42. Hamm CW, Bassand JP, Agewall S, Bax J, Boersma E, Bueno H, Caso P, Dudek D, Gielen S, Huber K, Ohman M, Petrie MC, Sonntag F, Uva MS, Storey RF, Wijns W, Zahger D; ESC Committee for Practice Guidelines. ESC guidelines for the management of acute coronary syndromes in patients presenting without persistent st-segment elevation: The task force for the management of acute coronary syndromes (ACS) in patients presenting without persistent st-segment elevation of the european society of cardiology (ESC). Eur Heart J. 2011;32:2999–3054.

43. Wright RS, Anderson JL, Adams CD, Bridges CR, Casey Jr DE, Ettinger SM, Fesmire FM, Ganiats TG, Jneid H, Lincoff AM, Peterson ED, Philippides GJ, Theroux P, Wenger NK, Zidar JP, Anderson JL, Adams CD, Antman EM, Bridges CR, Califf RM, Casey Jr DE, Chavey 2nd WE, Fesmire FM, Hochman JS, Levin TN, Lincoff AM, Peterson ED, Theroux P, Wenger NK, Zidar JP, American College of Cardiology Foundation/American Heart Association Task Force on Practice Guidelines. 2011 ACCF/AHA focused update incorporated into the ACC/AHA 2007 guidelines for the management of patients with unstable angina/non-ST-elevation myocardial infarction: a report of the American College of Cardiology Foundation/American Heart Association Task Force on Practice Guidelines Developed in Collaboration with the American Academy of Family Physicians, Society for Cardiovascular Angiography and Interventions, and the Society of Thoracic Surgeons. J Am Coll Cardiol. 2011;57:e215–367.

44. Raff GL, Chinnaiyan KM, Cury RC, Garcia MT, Hecht HS, Hollander JE, O'Neil B, Taylor AJ, Hoffmann U. Scct guidelines on the use of coronary computed tomographic angiography for patients presenting with acute chest pain to the emergency department: a report of the society of cardiovascular computed tomography guidelines committee. J Cardiovasc Comput Tomogr. 2014;8:254–71.

45. Carrascosa P, Deviggiano A, Capunay C, Campisi R, Lopez de Munin M, Vallejos J, Tajer C, Rodriguez-Granillo G. Incremental value of myocardial perfusion over coronary angiography by spectral computed tomography in patients with intermediate to high likelihood of coronary artery disease. Eur J Radiol. 2015;84(4):637–42.

46. Rossi A, Merkus D, Klotz E, Mollet N, de Feyter PJ, Krestin GP. Stress myocardial perfusion: imaging with multidetector CT. Radiology. 2014;270:25–46.

47. Kurata A, Kawaguchi N, Kido T, Inoue K, Suzuki J, Ogimoto A, Funada J, Higaki J, Miyagawa M, Vembar M, Mochizuki T. Qualitative and quantitative assessment of adenosine triphosphate stress whole-heart dynamic myocardial perfusion imaging using 256-slice computed tomography. PLoS One. 2013;8, e83950.

48. Weininger M, Schoepf UJ, Ramachandra A, Fink C, Rowe GW, Costello P, Henzler T. Adenosine-stress dynamic real-time myocardial perfusion CT and adenosine-stress first-pass dual-energy myocardial perfusion CT for the assessment of acute chest pain: initial results. Eur J Radiol. 2012;81:3703–10.

49. Wang R, Yu W, Wang Y, He Y, Yang L, Bi T, Jiao J, Wang Q, Chi L, Yu Y, Zhang Z. Incremental value of dual-energy ct to coronary CT angiography for the detection of significant coronary stenosis: comparison with quantitative coronary angiography and single photon emission computed tomography. Int J Cardiovasc Imaging. 2011;27:647–56.

50. Bettencourt N, Chiribiri A, Schuster A, Ferreira N, Sampaio F, Pires-Morais G, Santos L, Melica B, Rodrigues A, Braga P, Azevedo L, Teixeira M, Leite-Moreira A, Silva-Cardoso J, Nagel E, Gama V. Direct comparison of cardiac magnetic resonance and multidetector computed tomography stress-rest perfusion imaging for detection of coronary artery disease. J Am Coll Cardiol. 2013;61:1099–107.

51. Ichinose T, Yamase M, Yokomatsu Y, Kawano Y, Konishi H, Tanimoto K, Oigawa T, Katoh Y, Nakazato Y, Suwa S, Sakurai H, Sumiyoshi M. Acute myocardial infarction with myocardial perfusion defect detected by contrast-enhanced computed tomography. Intern Med. 2009;48: 1235–8.

52. Feuchtner GM, Plank F, Pena C, Battle J, Min J, Leipsic J, Labounty T, Janowitz W, Katzen B, Ziffer J, Cury RC. Evaluation of myocardial CT perfusion in patients presenting with acute chest pain to the emergency department: comparison with SPECT-myocardial perfusion imaging. Heart. 2012;98:1510–7.

53. Sanchis J, Bodi V, Nunez J, Bertomeu-Gonzalez V, Gomez C, Consuegra L, Bosch MJ, Bosch X, Chorro FJ, Llacer A. Usefulness of early exercise testing and clinical risk score for prognostic evaluation in chest pain units without preexisting evidence of myocardial ischemia. Am J Cardiol. 2006;97:633–5.
54. Rodgers GP, Ayanian JZ, Balady G, Beasley JW, Brown KA, Gervino EV, Paridon S, Quinones M, Schlant RC, Winters Jr WL, Achord JL, Boone AW, Hirshfeld Jr JW, Lorell BH, Rodgers GP, Tracy CM, Weitz HH. American College of Cardiology/American Heart Association clinical competence statement on stress testing: a report of the American College of Cardiology/American Heart Association/American College of Physicians – American Society of Internal Medicine Task Force on Clinical Competence. J Am Coll Cardiol. 2000;36: 1441–53.
55. Travin MI, Heller GV, Johnson LL, Katten D, Ahlberg AW, Isasi CR, Kaplan RC, Taub CC, Demus D. The prognostic value of ECG-gated SPECT imaging in patients undergoing stress TC-99m sestamibi myocardial perfusion imaging. J Nucl Cardiol Off Publ Am Soc Nucl Cardiol. 2004;11:253–62.
56. Biagini E, Elhendy A, Bax JJ, Rizzello V, Schinkel AF, van Domburg RT, Kertai MD, Krenning BJ, Bountioukos M, Rapezzi C, Branzi A, Simoons ML, Poldermans D. Seven-year follow-up after dobutamine stress echocardiography: impact of gender on prognosis. J Am Coll Cardiol. 2005;45:93–7.
57. Vesely MR, Dilsizian V. Nuclear cardiac stress testing in the era of molecular medicine. J Nucl Med Off Publ Soc Nucl Med. 2008;49:399–413.
58. Chang SM, Nabi F, Xu J, Raza U, Mahmarian JJ. Normal stress-only versus standard stress/ rest myocardial perfusion imaging: similar patient mortality with reduced radiation exposure. J Am Coll Cardiol. 2010;55:221–30.
59. Udelson JE, Beshansky JR, Ballin DS, Feldman JA, Griffith JL, Handler J, Heller GV, Hendel RC, Pope JH, Ruthazer R, Spiegler EJ, Woolard RH, Selker HP. Myocardial perfusion imaging for evaluation and triage of patients with suspected acute cardiac ischemia: a randomized controlled trial. JAMA. 2002;288:2693–700.
60. Better N, Karthikeyan G, Vitola J, Fatima A, Peix A, Novak MD, Soares Jr J, Bien VD, Briones PO, Vangu M, Soni N, Nguyen A, Dondi M. Performance of rest myocardial perfusion imaging in the management of acute chest pain in the emergency room in developing nations (premier trial). J Nucl Cardiol Off Publ Am Soc Nucl Cardiol. 2012;19:1146–53.
61. Lim SH, Anantharaman V, Sundram F, Chan ES, Ang ES, Yo SL, Jacob E, Goh A, Tan SB, Chua T. Stress myocardial perfusion imaging for the evaluation and triage of chest pain in the emergency department: a randomized controlled trial. J Nucl Cardiol Off Publ Am Soc Nucl Cardiol. 2013;20:1002–12.
62. van der Zee PM, Verberne HJ, Cornel JH, Kamp O, van der Zant FM, Bholasingh R, De Winter RJ. GRACE and TIMI risk scores but not stress imaging predict long-term cardiovascular follow-up in patients with chest pain after a rule-out protocol. Neth Heart J Mon J Neth Soc Cardiol Neth Heart Found. 2011;19:324–30.
63. Mancini GB, Hartigan PM, Shaw LJ, Berman DS, Hayes SW, Bates ER, Maron DJ, Teo K, Sedlis SP, Chaitman BR, Weintraub WS, Spertus JA, Kostuk WJ, Dada M, Booth DC, Boden WE. Predicting outcome in the courage trial (clinical outcomes utilizing revascularization and aggressive drug evaluation): coronary anatomy versus ischemia. JACC Cardiovasc Interv. 2014;7:195–201.
64. Shaw LJ, Weintraub WS, Maron DJ, Hartigan PM, Hachamovitch R, Min JK, Dada M, Mancini GB, Hayes SW, O'Rourke RA, Spertus JA, Kostuk W, Gosselin G, Chaitman BR, Knudtson M, Friedman J, Slomka P, Germano G, Bates ER, Teo KK, Boden WE, Berman DS. Baseline stress myocardial perfusion imaging results and outcomes in patients with stable ischemic heart disease randomized to optimal medical therapy with or without percutaneous coronary intervention. Am Heart J. 2012;164:243–50.
65. Panza JA, Holly TA, Asch FM, She L, Pellikka PA, Velazquez EJ, Lee KL, Borges-Neto S, Farsky PS, Jones RH, Berman DS, Bonow RO. Inducible myocardial ischemia and outcomes in patients with coronary artery disease and left ventricular dysfunction. J Am Coll Cardiol. 2013;61:1860–70.

66. Hadamitzky M, Achenbach S, Al-Mallah M, Berman D, Budoff M, Cademartiri F, Callister T, Chang HJ, Cheng V, Chinnaiyan K, Chow BJ, Cury R, Delago A, Dunning A, Feuchtner G, Gomez M, Kaufmann P, Kim YJ, Leipsic J, Lin FY, Maffei E, Min JK, Raff G, Shaw LJ, Villines TC, Hausleiter J, Investigators C. Optimized prognostic score for coronary computed tomographic angiography: results from the confirm registry (coronary ct angiography evaluation for clinical outcomes: an international multicenter registry). J Am Coll Cardiol. 2013;62: 468–76.

67. Goldstein JA, Gallagher MJ, O'Neill WW, Ross MA, O'Neil BJ, Raff GL. A randomized controlled trial of multi-slice coronary computed tomography for evaluation of acute chest pain. J Am Coll Cardiol. 2007;49:863–71.

68. Shaw LJ, Hausleiter J, Achenbach S, Al-Mallah M, Berman DS, Budoff MJ, Cademartiri F, Callister TQ, Chang HJ, Kim YJ, Cheng VY, Chow BJ, Cury RC, Delago AJ, Dunning AL, Feuchtner GM, Hadamitzky M, Karlsberg RP, Kaufmann PA, Leipsic J, Lin FY, Chinnaiyan KM, Maffei E, Raff GL, Villines TC, Labounty T, Gomez MJ, Min JK, Investigators CR. Coronary computed tomographic angiography as a gatekeeper to invasive diagnostic and surgical procedures: results from the multicenter confirm (coronary CT angiography evaluation for clinical outcomes: an international multicenter) registry. J Am Coll Cardiol. 2012;60:2103–14.

69. Andreini D, Pontone G, Mushtaq S, Bartorelli AL, Bertella E, Antonioli L, Formenti A, Cortinovis S, Veglia F, Annoni A, Agostoni P, Montorsi P, Ballerini G, Fiorentini C, Pepi M. A long-term prognostic value of coronary CT angiography in suspected coronary artery disease. JACC Cardiovasc Imaging. 2012;5:690–701.

70. Priest VL, Scuffham PA, Hachamovitch R, Marwick TH. Cost-effectiveness of coronary computed tomography and cardiac stress imaging in the emergency department: a decision analytic model comparing diagnostic strategies for chest pain in patients at low risk of acute coronary syndromes. JACC Cardiovasc Imaging. 2011;4:549–56.

71. D'Ascenzo F, Cerrato E, Biondi-Zoccai G, Omede P, Sciuto F, Presutti DG, Quadri G, Raff GL, Goldstein JA, Litt H, Frati G, Reed MJ, Moretti C, Gaita F. Coronary computed tomographic angiography for detection of coronary artery disease in patients presenting to the emergency department with chest pain: a meta-analysis of randomized clinical trials. Eur Heart J Cardiovasc Imaging. 2013;14:782–9.

72. Meijboom WB, van Mieghem CA, Mollet NR, Pugliese F, Weustink AC, van Pelt N, Cademartiri F, Nieman K, Boersma E, de Jaegere P, Krestin GP, de Feyter PJ. 64-slice computed tomography coronary angiography in patients with high, intermediate, or low pretest probability of significant coronary artery disease. J Am Coll Cardiol. 2007;50:1469–75.

73. Brodoefel H, Burgstahler C, Tsiflikas I, Reimann A, Schroeder S, Claussen CD, Heuschmid M, Kopp AF. Dual-source CT: effect of heart rate, heart rate variability, and calcification on image quality and diagnostic accuracy. Radiology. 2008;247:346–55.

74. Ong TK, Chin SP, Liew CK, Chan WL, Seyfarth MT, Liew HB, Rapaee A, Fong YY, Ang CK, Sim KH. Accuracy of 64-row multidetector computed tomography in detecting coronary artery disease in 134 symptomatic patients: influence of calcification. Am Heart J. 2006;151:1323. e1321–6.

75. Vavere AL, Arbab-Zadeh A, Rochitte CE, Dewey M, Niinuma H, Gottlieb I, Clouse ME, Bush DE, Hoe JW, de Roos A, Cox C, Lima JA, Miller JM. Coronary artery stenoses: accuracy of 64-detector row ct angiography in segments with mild, moderate, or severe calcification–a subanalysis of the core-64 trial. Radiology. 2011;261:100–8.

76. Scheske JA, O'Brien JM, Earls JP, Min JK, LaBounty TM, Cury RC, Lee TY, So A, Hague CJ, Al-Hassan D, Kuriyabashi S, Dowe DA, Leipsic JA. Coronary artery imaging with single-source rapid kilovolt peak-switching dual-energy CT. Radiology. 2013;268:702–9.

77. Rodriguez-Granillo GA, Rosales MA, Degrossi E, Rodriguez AE. Signal density of left ventricular myocardial segments and impact of beam hardening artifact: Implications for myocardial perfusion assessment by multidetector CT coronary angiography. Int J Cardiovasc Imaging. 2010;26:345–54.

Chapter 8
Takotsubo Cardiomyopathy – An Interesting and Somewhat Unexplained Clinical Entity

Eduardo D. Gabe and John A. Ambrose

Abstract Takotsubo cardiomyopathy is a curious, underreported syndrome of transient left ventricular dysfunction unrelated to coronary artery disease, often presenting as an ACS in postmenopausal women usually following a significant mental or physical stress. Since its initial description nearly 25 years ago, it has been reported under various scenarios. While criteria for diagnosis have been proposed, there remain several unresolved issues pertaining to its incidence, pathophysiology and treatment. This chapters reviews these unresolved issues.

Keywords Takotsubo • "Broken Heart" syndrome

Introduction

Takotsubo cardiomyopathy (TCM) is a curious clinical entity characterized by transient left ventricular dysfunction usually involving the antero apical and infero apical regions of the myocardium in the absence of significant coronary artery disease (Fig. 8.1). The syndrome often presents with chest pain and/or dyspnea, dynamic reversible ST-T segment abnormalities, and mildly increased cardiac enzymes disproportionate to the extent of wall motion abnormalities. Most patients are usually elderly women and there is often a significant mental or physical stress preceding the appearance of symptoms. Common triggers that have been identified which include the death of a loved one, becoming a victim of theft, the experience of a great loss such as with gambling, a surprise party or severe illness (hospitalization in an intensive care unit), etc. [1]. In others, an acute neurologic event, most commonly a subarachnoid hemorrhage is the precipitating event. While elevated catecholamine

E.D. Gabe, MD, PhD, FACC (✉)
Department of Cardiology, Otamendi Hospital, Buenos Aires, Argentina
e-mail: edudagabe@gmail.com

J.A. Ambrose, MD
Chief of Cardiology, UCSF Fresno, Fresno, CA, USA

Department of Medicine, UCSF Community Regional Medical Center, Fresno, CA, USA

© Springer International Publishing Switzerland 2015
J.A. Ambrose, A.E. Rodríguez (eds.), *Controversies in Cardiology*,
DOI 10.1007/978-3-319-20415-4_8

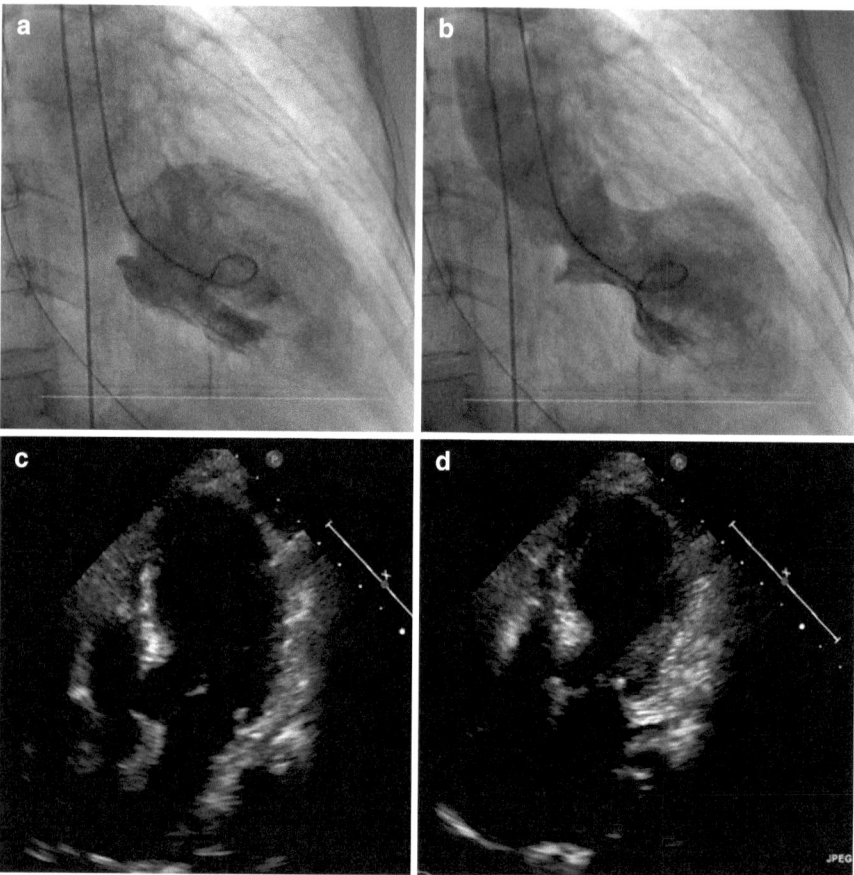

Fig. 8.1 The typical end diastolic (**a**) and end systolic (**c**) left ventricular angiographic frames from a 72 year old female who presented with an ACS after the death of her sister. Similar findings are also seen on a four chamber echocardiogram-End diastole (**b**) and end systole (**d**)

levels have been suggested as a significant pathophysiologic mechanism in most patients, in others, the pathophysiology is unknown as well as how elevated catecholamines alter left ventricular function. Since it was first described in 1991, multiple articles have been published on this subject. However, several aspects of the disease remain unresolved. These revolve around its incidence, pathophysiology, the diagnostic criteria used to define it and its appropriate management [2–5].

Incidence

Since it was first recognized, it has been reported in most studies that about 1–2 % of patients diagnosed as an ACS could suffer from TCM. However, its true incidence is largely unknown. Possible reasons that contribute to this include the fact that there is often a low index of clinical suspicion for TCM and TCM can often masquerade as other syndromes. While diagnostic criteria have been proposed, these criteria are very specific although probably relatively insensitive leading to under diagnosis. Since the presence of severe coronary artery disease is an exclusion according to the Mayo criteria, a typical presentation in an elderly female may be misdiagnosed as related to coronary disease [6]. The prevalence estimate of TCM comes from small series of consecutive patients with suspected ACS [7–10]. While each of these series included a small number of patients with TCM, they represented approximately 1.7–2.2 % of the cases admitted to the coronary care unit with suspected ACS. In a preliminary investigation, researchers at the University of Arkansas identified 21,748 patients diagnosed with TCM in 2011 using a database of national hospital discharge in the USA [11]. In an analysis of cases by state, it was observed that Vermont and Missouri had the highest rate, with 380 per million population in Vermont and 169 per million in Missouri. The rate of patients with TCM in Vermont in 2011 was more than double that in the other states. This was the same year that Tropical Storm Irene hit the state with heavy rains and wind. Similarly, the researchers found a rate of 169 cases per million in Missouri in 2011, the same year that a massive tornado devastated Joplin, Mo. Most states had fewer than 150 cases per million inhabitants [11].

There are other data suggesting that the incidence may be more common than previously published particularly if one examines post menopausal women presenting with ACS. Sy et al. prospectively evaluated 1297 consecutive postmenopausal women with a positive troponin, 323 (24.9 %) of whom met criteria for acute myocardial infarction according to the Universal Definition. Of these, 19 (5.9 %) met criteria for definite or probable TCM [12]. We also believe that TCM can pose as other syndromes previously reported in the literature. Other than the cerebral T waves associated with subarachnoid hemorrhage, LV dysfunction associated with sepsis [13], the occasional patient with normal appearing coronary arteries on angiography after thrombolytic therapy and viral myocarditis masquerading as acute myocardial infarction may represent, in many cases, TCM. In the later report, most patients were elderly women with transient LV dysfunction and no coronary obstruction [14]. Their biopsies were not inconsistent with that seen in TCM.

Pathophysiology

Several theories have been proposed to explain the pathophysiology of TCM. These include catecholamine excess, multiple epicardial coronary artery spasm, microvascular dysfunction and acute outflow tract obstruction in the presence of low estrogen levels. These theories are not mutually exclusive.

In general, the LV dysfunction of TCM whether it is the apical variant or the other less frequent presentations (mid ventricular or basal) does not correspond to a single coronary artery territory. In the usual apical variant, the akinesis is more extensive than the territory supplied by the left anterior descending artery. While Migliore et al. [15] found that myocardial bridging of the left anterior descending on angiography or CT imaging was a common finding in patients with TCM, it is highly unlikely that this is causative. Likewise, Ibanez et al. suggested that TCM could be an aborted myocardial infarction with spontaneous lysis of the thrombus [16]. Again, the overall evidence is not supportive.

What has been suggested is that reversible dysfunction of the coronary microcirculation might be an important pathophysiologic mechanism. Utilizing myocardial contrast echocardiography and infusions of adenosine, Galiuto et al. showed that adenosine transiently improved microvascular perfusion and wall motion in TCM but not in acute anterior STEMI [17]. The cause of this intense microvascular constriction and the predilection for this region of the myocardium is still largely unknown, although the effect of sympathetic stimulation on the vasculature is probably an important mechanism. Supraphysiologic levels of catecholamines have been described in most but not all patients with TCM and it has been suggested that this leads to myocardial stunning. Catecholamine and dopamine plasma levels during the acute presentation of TCM are significantly higher than those found in individuals with acute myocardial infarction and Killip class III/IV and remain very high even a week after the onset of symptoms [18]. Cardiac biopsy specimens when performed acutely in some patients with TCM have shown monocyte infiltration and contraction band necrosis consistent with catecholamine excess [18]. Excessive catecholamine release might generate microvascular spasm and endothelial dysfunction leading to myocardial stunning [19–21]. Transient LV dysfunction similar to TCM could be induced in rats exposed to physical stress with elevated levels of catecholamines [22]. It has also been suggested that increased catecholamines generate increases in reactive oxygen species that directly injure vascular cells and cardiac myocytes [18].

Why is the apex of the left ventricle usually involved in TCM? Ballooning of the apical region might be related to the predominance of sympathetic receptor density in the apical portion of the left ventricle. Sympathetic receptor density is not uniformly distributed in the heart with the greatest density at the distal LV segment and apex providing a possible explanation for the classic LV apical ballooning seen in TCM. High levels of catecholamines may be negatively ionotropic when the $\beta1$ receptor is over stimulated leading to transient myocardial stunning [23]. Supporting this hypothesis is the high frequency of antecedent mental or physical stress and the similarity of the wall motion abnormalities in TCM to those with the cardiomyopathy of pheochromocytoma or catecholamine excess [24, 25]. Unfortunately, elevated catecholamine levels have not been found in all patients with TCM.

Another hypothesis that has been proposed is multivessel spasm of epicardial coronary arteries. It seems unlikely that the left ventricular dysfunction occurring in this syndrome could be due only to spasm of a single coronary artery as mentioned above. No conclusive evidence of multivessel spasm has been found to explain most cases of TCM, although it is suggested that transient spasm might explain a minority particularly in Japan. In a study in which spasm was evaluated, multivessel spasm was demonstrated in a few patients [2]. However, persistent ST elevation without coronary stenosis on angiography could not be related to epicardial spasm as the primary pathophysiology of TCM [2].

Another possibility regarding the pathophysiology of TCM has been the demonstration of acute outflow tract obstruction in some patients with TCM [20].

Hypercontractility of the basal segments in the usual apical variant may lead to outflow tract obstruction in the small left ventricles of postmenopausal women. The acute pressure overload at the thinned out apex related to obstruction could lead to transient apical akinesis. However, if this mechanism is causative, it is involved in only the minority of cases.

Metabolic abnormalities have also been described in TCM, including a reduction in fatty acid metabolism similar to what occurs under conditions of ischemia. This has been documented through SPECT imaging with I-123 BMIPP [26]. On PET imaging, reduced perfusion with N-13 ammonia and decreased metabolism with F-18 FDG imaging have also been described. The radio-iodinated analog for norepinephrine, I-123 MIBG has also been used to demonstrate a suppression of myocardial sympathetic nerve function in response to myocardial ischemia in TCM. These findings of transient decreased perfusion with reduction in metabolism and sympathetic nerve function are characteristic of myocardial stunning. These findings are likely secondary to TCM rather than primary mechanisms.

All authors agree that the vast majority of patients (typically ≥90 %) diagnosed with TCM are postmenopausal women. How does estrogen and specifically the estrogen deficiency following menopause contribute to TCM? The answer is not clear. There could be a complex interaction between neuro-hormonal factors, the genetic profile, anatomical abnormalities and other factors that jointly contribute to the cardiac dysfunction. Stress-mediated vasoconstriction may be enhanced in the presence of estrogen deficiency [27]. Estrogen deficiency promotes vasomotor instability prone to vasoconstriction, endothelial dysfunction and thus microvascular dysfunction. Lower estrogen levels may explain the gender disparity in the expression of this cardiac entity [27–29].

In summary, there are probably multiple interrelated pathophysiologic mechanisms in TCM. Most revolve around the effects of a transient increase in catecholamine levels in the presence of estrogen deficiency. Transient left ventricular dysfunction results, possibly related to catecholamine effects on β receptors upregulated at the apex and transient microvascular dysfunction. In a few patients, basal hypercontractility leads to outflow tract obstruction or multi vessel epicardial spasm is present. Both of these later conditions might be causative of TCM or just epi phenomena. Of course, these mechanisms might not apply to the occasional man or younger woman with TCM. One wonders whether or not there is a genetic component that predisposes some individuals to this condition. We believe that the molecular mechanisms underlying this syndrome also require further study.

Making the Diagnosis of TCM

Diagnostic criteria have been proposed by various authors (Tables 8.1, 8.2, 8.3, and 8.4) [30–33]. The Mayo Clinic (Table 8.5) [34, 35] criteria are the most widely accepted. Most criteria exclude patients with head trauma, intracranial or subarachnoid hemorrhage which does not seem logical since these patients often develop the typical signs of TCM on ECG and non invasive imaging. Significant epicardial

Table 8.1 Abe and Kondo criteria

Major criteria:
Reversible left ventricular ballooning with abnormalities of apical motility and hypercontractility of the basal segments.
Abnormalities of the ST segment/T wave on the ECG, simulating acute myocardial infarction.
Minor criteria:
Physical or emotional stress as triggering factors.
Limited elevation of the cardiac enzymes.
Precordial pain.
Exclusion criteria:
Ischaemic myocardial stunning.
Subarachnoid haemorrhage.
Pheochromocytoma crisis.
Acute myocarditis.
Tachycardia-induced cardiomyopathy.

Table 8.2 Prasad criteria

Transient hypokinesia, akinesia, or dyskinesia of the middle segments of the LV, with or without alterations at the apex.
Regional abnormalities of wall motion extend beyond the area of distribution of a single epicardial vessel.
Absence of an obstructed coronary artery or angiographic evidence of acute rupture of a plaque.
New ECG abnormalities (ST elevation and/or T-wave inversion) or elevation of cardiac troponin.
Absence of:
Recent head injury
Intracranial haemorrhage
Pheochromocytoma
Myocarditis
Hypertrophic cardiomyopathy

coronary artery disease is a natural exclusion although, as mentioned earlier, this probably leads to under diagnosis since TCM is not ordinarily diagnosed in the presence of severe CAD even when the acute signs are otherwise classic and the recovery of function is typical. Given the advanced age of most patients, concomitant coronary artery disease probably excludes many potential patients. Other situations may also preclude diagnosis such as not performing an angiogram to exclude CAD because the patient is too sick, i.e. ICU patients with trauma or sepsis etc. Occasionally, potential patients die before a diagnosis can be confirmed by a repeat imaging study showing improvement in regional wall motion.

After initial reports of TCM as the typical apical left ventricular dysfunction, new variants of altered ventricular geometry were reported. The dysfunction can preserve the apex and affect different segments of the left ventricle and right ventricle as well. Akinesia of the middle ventricular segment with normal or increased apical and basal contraction is termed the mid ventricular variant. Basal akinesia

Table 8.3 Segovia Cubero criteria

Previous conditions (both obligatory):

1. Evidence of a transient apical dysfunction of the LV with the typical form in systole (rounded apex with narrow neck due to hypercontractility of the basal segments), diagnosed by angiography, echocardiography, isotope scans, or cardiac magnetic resonance imaging. The disturbance typically reverts in 2–3 weeks, although it can persist for up to 2 months.

2. Absence of other conditions associated with regional transient systolic dysfunction of the LV: subarachnoid hemorrhage, pheochromocytoma, ischemic myocardial stunning, drugs (cocaine), myocarditis, etc.

Diagnostic criteria:

1. Major: Early coronary angiography (within the first 24 h) showing no anatomical lesions.

2. Minor:

| Early coronary angiography showing non-significant lesions (less than 50 % without characteristics of a complicated plaque or intraluminal thrombus). |
| Late coronary angiography (from the second to the seventh day after the onset of the syndrome) showing no significant lesions. |
| Physical or psychological stress as the trigger of the disorder. |
| Typical ECG changes: |
| ST segment elevation in the acute phase, more marked in V4–V6 than in V1–V3. |
| Appearance of Q waves that disappear after the acute phase. |
| Very prominent negative T waves in V1–V6. |
| QTc prolongation. |
| Woman over 50 years of age. |

Confirmed TADS: 1 major criterion or 2 or more minor criteria, including an angiographic criterion.

Probable TADS: 2 or more minor criteria, with no angiographic criterion.

TADS: transient apical dysfunction syndrome.

with preserved apical contractility is referred to as "inverted Takotsubo". The typical apical variant is observed in over 2/3 s of patients [8, 36].

Eitel et al. [37] have examined the role of MRI in 59 patients with clinical manifestations of TCM (patients with an ACS without significant obstructive coronary disease and characteristic wall motion abnormalities). Based on magnetic resonance imaging only, a diagnosis of MCT was established in 68 % of patients. Typically, there is no late enhancement of gadolinium with TCM in comparison to LV dysfunction related to infarction. Presumably, this technique might be used in some patients with CAD and otherwise a typical TCM presentation to suggest the diagnosis.

Acute and Chronic Management of TCM

There is no specific treatment and the same supportive therapy used in any cardiomyopathy is employed. The optimal treatment has not been established. Most would use beta blockers given the presumed role of excessive catecholamines but it is

Table 8.4 Kawai criteria

Exclusion criteria:

1. Significant organic stenosis or spasm of a coronary artery. In particular, AMI due to a lesion of the anterior descending artery of the left coronary artery, which irrigates a large territory including the apex of the LV (urgent coronary angiography is desirable in order to view the image in the acute phase; during the chronic phase, coronary angiography is necessary to confirm the presence or absence of significant stenotic lesions or abnormal lesions that could explain the ventricular contraction).

2. Cerebrovascular disturbances.

3. Pheochromocytoma.

4. Viral or idiopathic myocarditis.

(Note: Coronary angiography is required for the exclusion of coronary artery lesions. Takotsubo-like myocardial dysfunction can occur in conditions such as cerebrovascular disorders or phaeochromocytoma).

Diagnostic references:

1. Symptoms: Precordial pain and dyspnoea similar to the findings in the acute coronary syndrome. Takotsubo cardiomyopathy can also occur without symptoms.

2. Triggers: Emotional or physical stress, although it can also occur without any obvious trigger.

3. Age and gender: There is a recognized tendency to a higher frequency in elderly individuals, principally women.

4. Ventricular morphology: Apical ballooning with rapid recovery on ventriculography and echocardiography.

5. ECG: ST elevation may be observed immediately after the event. T waves progressively become negative in various leads and the QT interval progressively lengthens. These changes gradually improve, but the T waves may remain negative for months. Pathological Q waves and alterations of the QRS voltage may be observed in the acute phase.

6. Cardiac biomarkers: There is only a slight rise in the cardiac enzymes and troponin.

7. Nuclear medicine scan of the heart: Abnormalities may be detected on myocardial gamma scan in some cases.

8. Prognosis: Recovery is rapid in most cases, but some patients develop acute pulmonary edema and other sequelae, even death.

Table 8.5 Diagnostic criteria of the Mayo Clinic

Suspicion of AMI based on precordial pain and ST elevation observed on the acute-phase ECG.

Transient hypokinesia or akinesia of the middle and apical regions of the LV and functional hyperkinesia of the basal region, observed on ventriculography or echocardiography.

Normal coronary arteries confirmed by arteriography (luminal narrowing of less than 50 % in all the coronary arteries) in the first 24 h after the onset of symptoms.

Absence of recent significant head injury, intracranial hemorrhage, suspicion of pheochromocytoma, myocarditis, or hypertrophic cardiomyopathy

unknown whether these hasten recovery. Furthermore, it is unclear whether selective beta blockers such as metoprolol (a selective β1 blocker) versus carvedilol (both a non selective β and α blocker) are the preferred agent. While most would continue beta blockers chronically, there are also no data supporting the fact that these agents reduce recurrences. Fortunately, the recurrence rate is ≤10 %.

If there is adequate blood pressure, medical therapy usually includes not only a beta-blocker but also an angiotensin converting enzyme inhibitor, or angiotensin II receptor blocker. Systemic anticoagulation should be considered if a left ventricular thrombus is identified or the wall motion abnormalities are slow to recover. Inotropic support may be necessary if the blood pressure is low but should not be used in patients with outflow tract obstruction. Thus, this indicates the importance of a complete echocardiographic study or hemodynamic measurements at the time of angiography. A definitive diagnosis of TCM requires that the coronary arteries are visualized and are normal or non obstructive. An intra-aortic balloon pump or other methods of circulatory support is indicated with marked left ventricular dysfunction associated with severe hypotension or shock in the absence of outflow tract obstruction. Hospital mortality in most of the published series is <3 %. These patients should also be monitored carefully after admission to prevent significant arrhythmias.

If an elderly female is admitted with a STEMI- like presentation particularly involving the anterior wall and is not at or near a hospital with primary PCI capability, should she receive thrombolytic therapy? One must always individualize therapy but, unless she is at high risk of bleeding, the answer is yes as the therapy could be life saving. However, angiography is always preferable to exclude the occasional TCM and provide the appropriate interventional therapy. This is particularly suggested if the index of suspicion for TCM is high such as when there is a preceding great emotional stress and a large apical wall motion abnormality is seen on echocardiography or angiography.

Conclusion

In spite of being a reversible, mostly benign form of cardiomyopathy, there must always be a high index of suspicion for this diagnosis particularly in post menopausal women presenting with an ACS or unexplained LV dysfunction. Although there are controversial data regarding the incidence, pathophysiologic mechanisms, diagnostic criteria, therapeutic strategies and perhaps even the name of the syndrome, always consider TCM as a possibility particularly in this population. You might be surprised how often you will find it!

References

1. Sharkey SW, Lesser JR, Zenovich AG, et al. Acute and reversible cardiomyopathy provoked by stress in women from the United States. Circulation. 2005;111:472–9.
2. Tsuchihashi K, Ueshima K, Uchida T, et al. Transient left ventricular apical ballooning without coronary artery stenosis: a novel heart syndrome mimicking acute myocardial infarction: Angina Pectoris–Myocardial Infarction Investigations in Japan. J Am Coll Cardiol. 2001;38:11–8.

3. Kurisu S, Sato H, Kawagoe T, et al. Tako-tsubo-like left ventricular dysfunction with ST-segment elevation: a novel cardiac syndrome mimicking acute myocardial infarction. Am Heart J. 2002;143:448–55.
4. Akashi YJ, Musha H, Kida K, et al. Reversible ventricular dysfunction takotsubo cardiomyopathy. Eur J Heart Fail. 2005;7:1171–6.
5. Eitel I, von Knobelsdorff-Brenkenhoff F, Bernhardt P, et al. Clinical characteristics and cardiovascular magnetic resonance findings in stress (takotsubo) cardiomyopathy. JAMA. 2011;306:277–86.
6. Gaibazzi N, Ugo F, Vignali L, Zoni A, Reverberi C, Gherli T. Tako-Tsubo cardiomyopathy with coronary artery stenosis: a case-series challenging the original definition. Int J Cardiol. 2009;133:205–12.
7. Akashi YJ, Goldstein DS, Goldstein DS, Barbaro G, Ueyama T. Takotsubo cardiomyopathy: a new form of acute, reversible heart failure. Circulation. 2008;118:2754–62.
8. Kurowski V, Kaiser A, von Hof K, et al. Apical and midventricular transient left ventricular dysfunction syndrome (tako-tsubo cardiomyopathy): frequency, mechanisms, and prognosis. Chest. 2007;132:809–16.
9. Bybee KA, Kara T, Prasad A, et al. Transient left ventricular apical ballooning syndrome: a mimic of ST-segment elevation myocardial infarction. Ann Intern Med. 2004;141:858–65.
10. Gianni M, Dentali F, Grandi AM, et al. Apical ballooning syndrome or takotsubo cardiomyopathy: a systematic review. Eur Heart J. 2006;27:1523–9.
11. Pant S, Deshmukh A, Mehta K, et al. Clustering of takotsubo cardiomyopathy cases in United States in 2011. J Am Coll Cardiol. 2014;63(12):A828.
12. Sy F, Basroan J, Zheng H, et al. Frequency of takotsubo cardiomyopathy in postmenopausal women presenting with an acute coronary syndrome. Am J Cardiol. 2013;112:479–82.
13. Cunnion RE, Parrillo JE. Myocardial dysfunction in sepsis: recent insights. Chest. 1989;95:941–5.
14. Narula J, Khaw BA, Dec GW, et al. Brief report: recognition of acute myocarditis masquerading as acute myocardial infarction. N Engl J Med. 1993;328:100–4.
15. Migliore F, Maffei E, Perazzolo MM, et al. LAD coronary artery myocardial bridging and apical ballooning syndrome. JACC Cardiovasc Imaging. 2013;6(1):32–41.
16. Ibanez B, Navarro F, Cordoba M, Alberca PM, Farre J. Tako-tsubo transient left ventricular apical ballooning: is intravascular ultrasound the key to resolve the enigma? Heart. 2005;91:102–4.
17. Galiuto L, De Caterina AR, Porfidia A, et al. Reversible coronary microvascular dysfunction: a common pathogenetic mechanism in apical ballooning or Tako-Tsubo syndrome. Eur Heart J. 2010;31:1319–27.
18. Wittstein IS, Thiemann DR, Lima JA, et al. Neurohumoral features of myocardial stunning due to sudden emotional stress. N Engl J Med. 2005;352(6):539–48.
19. Bielecka-Dabrowa A, Mikhailidis DP, Hannam S, et al. Takotsubo cardiomyopathy-the current state of knowledge. Int J Cardiol. 2010;142:120–5.
20. Merli E, Sutcliffe S, Gori M, Sutherland GG. Tako-Tsubo cardiomyopathy: new insights into the possible underlying pathophysiology. Eur J Echocardiogr. 2006;7:53–61.
21. Goldstein DS, Eisenhofer G, Kopin IJ. Sources and significance of plasma levels of catechols and their metabolites in humans. J Pharmacol Exp Ther. 2003;305:800–11.
22. Ueyama T, Kawabe T, Hano T, et al. Upregulation of heme oxygenase-1 in an animal model of Takotsubo cardiomyopathy. Circ J. 2009;73:1141–6.
23. Lyon AR, Rees PSC, Prasad S, Poole-Wilson PA, Harding SE. Stress (Takotsubo) cardiomyopathy—a novel pathophysiological hypothesis to explain catecholamine-induced acute myocardial stunning. Nat Clin Pract Cardiovasc Med. 2008;5, E2. doi:10.1038/ncpcardio1236.
24. Shaw T, Rafferty P, Tait GW. Transient shock and myocardial impairment caused by phaeochromocytoma crisis. Br Heart J. 1987;57:194–8.
25. Yamanaka O, Fujiwara Y, Takamura T, et al. 'Myocardial stunning'-like phenomenon during a crisis of pheochromocytoma. Jpn Circ J. 1994;58:737–42.

26. Alexanderson E, Cruz P, Talayero JA, Damas F, Zeron J, Meave A. Transient perfusion and motion abnormalities in takotsubo cardiomyopathy. J Nucl Cardiol. 2007;14(1):129–33.

27. Kaski JC. Cardiac syndrome X in women: the role of oestrogen deficiency. Heart. 2006;92 Suppl 3:iii5–9.

28. Johnson BD, Shaw LJ, Buchthal SD, et al. Prognosis in women with myocardial ischemia in the absence of obstructive coronary disease: results from the National Institutes of Health-National Heart, Lung, and Blood Institute-Sponsored Women's Ischemia Syndrome Evaluation (WISE). Circulation. 2004;109:2993–9.

29. Demir H, Kahraman G, Isgoren S, et al. Evaluation of post-stress left ventricular dysfunction and its relationship with perfusion abnormalities using gated SPECT in patients with cardiac syndrome X. Nucl Med Commun. 2008;29:208–14.

30. Abe Y, Kondo M, Matsuoka R, et al. Assessment of clinical features in transient left ventricular apical ballooning. J Am Coll Cardiol. 2003;41:737–42.

31. Prasad A. Apical ballooning syndrome. An important differential diagnosis of acute myocardial infarction. Circulation. 2007;115:e56–9.

32. Segovia Cubero J, Peraira Moral R. Transient apical ballooning syndrome: a transition towards adulthood. Rev Esp Cardiol. 2004;57:194–7 [in Spanish with English abstract].

33. Kawai S, Kitabatake A, Tomoike H, et al. Guidelines for diagnosis of takotsubo (ampulla) cardiomyopathy. Circ J. 2007;71:990–2.

34. Prasad A, Lerman A, Rihal CS. Apical ballooning syndrome (Tako-Tsubo or stress cardiomyopathy): a mimic of acute myocardial infarction. Am Heart J. 2008;155:408–17.

35. Madhavan M, Prasad A. Proposed Mayo Clinic criteria for the diagnosis of Tako-Tsubo cardiomyopathy and long-term prognosis. Herz. 2010;35(4):240–3. doi:10.1007/s00059-010-3339-x.

36. Cortese B, Robotti S, Puggioni E, et al. Transient left ventricular apical ballooning syndrome: all that glitters is not apical. J Cardiovasc Med (Hagerstown). 2007;8:934–6.

37. Eitel I, Behrendt F, Schindler K, Kivelitz D, Gutberlet M, Schuler G, et al. Differential diagnosis of suspected apical ballooning syndrome using contrast-enhanced magnetic resonance imaging. Eur Heart J. 2008;29:2651–9.

Chapter 9
Chest Pain in Women: Evaluation and Management

Josephine Warren, Jennifer Yu, Liliana Rosa Grinfeld, and Roxana Mehran

Abstract Despite the significant burden of ischemic heart disease (IHD) in women, the optimal evaluation and management of chest pain in this population is unclear, complicated by gender differences in presentation, etiology and disease perception as well as a relative paucity of specific, well-powered studies in this field. In contrast to male IHD, which is typically characterized by classical symptomology and demonstrable obstruction on angiography, chest pain in women is often more vague and more likely caused by an atypical etiology such as microvascular disease or endothelial dysfunction. The absence of macroscopic coronary obstruction presents a management challenge to physicians, and a large proportion of index cardiac events in women result in fatality. Evaluating chest pain is further complicated by gender discrepancies in the accuracy of diagnostic testing due to anatomical and physical variation. Furthermore, there is a distinct lack of awareness of disease severity among women and treating physicians, placing the imperative on the need for improving public education. This chapter will analyze current controversies pertaining to the evaluation and management of chest pain in women.

Keywords Chest pain • Ischemic heart disease • Women • Gender • Coronary artery disease

J. Warren, MBBS • J. Yu, MBBS • R. Mehran, MD (✉)
Mount Sinai Medical Center, New York, NY, USA

The Icahn School of Medicine at Mount Sinai, The Zena and Michael A. Wiener
Cardiovascular Institute, New York, NY, USA
e-mail: roxana.mehran@mountsinai.org

L.R. Grinfeld, MD, PhD, FACC, FSCAI
Head Interventinal Cardiology Clinica San Camilo, Bueno Aires,
Past President Argentina Society of Cardiology, New York, NY, USA

University of Buenos Aires, Cardiovascular Physiopathology Institute,
Buenos Aires, Argentina

© Springer International Publishing Switzerland 2015
J.A. Ambrose, A.E. Rodríguez (eds.), *Controversies in Cardiology*,
DOI 10.1007/978-3-319-20415-4_9

Introduction

Cardiovascular disease represents the leading cause of mortality in women, claiming more lives annually than it does men [1]. Despite this, the evaluation and management of women presenting with chest pain remains suboptimal, and there is underutilization of invasive and medical management in women versus men. Not surprisingly, this has translated into worse outcomes and greater healthcare costs. With almost 40 % of index cardiac events in women resulting in fatality, the need for an effective diagnostic strategy for those at risk is clear [2, 3]. The clinical assessment of women presenting with chest pain is complicated by the prevalence of atypical symptomology, lack of awareness of risk, higher burden of symptoms, lower functional capacity and atypical etiology [4]. Controversy lies in defining an investigative and management strategy that best reflects the pathophysiological differences between genders. Recently, it has been proposed that coronary disease in women should be considered a different entity to that in men, and that management should be modified accordingly to challenge the current paradigm that chiefly revolves around the identification and revascularization of large vessel coronary obstruction [5]. This chapter will outline the available evidence regarding the optimal evaluation and treatment of woman presenting with chest pain.

Clinical Assessment

Clinical Presentation

Several key features differentiate the clinical presentation of chest pain between men and women. Women present on average 10 years older than men, and experience significantly greater delay from symptom onset to diagnosis, with a more extensive risk factor profile [6–8]. The primary priority in the assessment of chest pain in women is to establish the nature of the presenting complaint, which mandates establishing a history of duration, onset, distribution, intensity, character and aggravating or alleviating factors associated with the pain. Importantly, women are more likely to underestimate the severity of their presentation and to attribute their pain to a non-cardiac cause [9], necessitating perseverance from the physician.

In women, an atypical pattern of chest pain is not the rule, but occurs more frequently than in men. Features are described in Table 9.1 [10]. Though the mechanism is poorly understood, it is thought that this is due to higher frequency

Table 9.1 Atypical chest pain

Distribution: jaw, neck, back, arm, abdomen, left chest
Onset: at rest, during sleep, post-prandial, during mental stress
Character: sharp, stabbing, fleeting
Associated symptoms: nausea, vomiting, fatigue, dyspnea, palpitations, indigestion, sweating, syncope

Table 9.2 Red flag diagnoses

Diagnosis	Differentiating signs and symptoms	Investigations
Acute coronary syndrome (ACS)	Acute chest pain	Elevated biomarkers
	± dyspnea, fatigue, nausea, syncope	Ischemic ECG changes
Takotsubo cardiomyopathy[a]	Acute chest pain	Mild biomarker elevation
	± dyspnea, shock	No obstruction on angiography
	Precipitated by emotional stress	Circumferential ballooning on echo (apex, mid or base).
Aortic dissection	Tearing chest pain, radiation to the back	Widened mediastinum on CXR
	± aortic regurgitation, neurological deficits	Echocardiography
	Pulse deficits	CT scan
Pulmonary embolism	Chest pain, may be pleuritic	V:Q scan
	± dyspnea, tachycardia, fever	CT pulmonary angiography
Cardiac tamponade	Chest pain	Pericardial effusion on echocardiography
	Tachycardia, hypotension, muffled heart sounds	
	Pulsus paradoxus	
Tension pneumothorax	Acute dyspnea, pleuritic chest pain	Pneumothorax ± displaced mediastinum on CXR
	Reduced breath sounds, resonance to percussion, tracheal deviation	
Spontaneous coronary artery dissection[a]	Symptoms of ACS, recent child birth	Angiography or intravascular ultrasound demonstrating true and false lumen
Coronary vasospasm[a]	Chest pain at rest, sometimes during sleep	ST-changes on EKG
	Younger women	

[a]More common in women

of atypical ischemic etiology in women, such as microvascular angina, endothelial dysfunction, and vasospasm [11, 12]. Therefore, a lowered index of suspicion for a cardiac etiology is required for women, particularly if the presentation is atypical. Indeed, while women are more likely to present with non-cardiac chest pain than men, their angina is still associated with an increased risk of mortality [13].

Typical chest pain still occurs more frequently in women. A history of typical angina confers a predictive value of greater than 60 % for coronary artery disease (CAD) on the coronary angiogram [14]. Common atypical triggers for women include stress, rest and sleep [15]. An effective history also screens for non-cardiac causes and prevents the need for further invasive testing. Red flag diagnoses are presented in Table 9.2.

Systems Review

Women are significantly more likely than men to report multiple symptoms [16] in the setting of chest pain so it is important to conduct a thorough cardiovascular systems review, with particular emphasis on the presence of palpitations, dyspnea and fatigue. In addition, a brief screening of other systems assists both in ruling out common differentials in women, such as esophageal spasm, anxiety and pleurisy, and in as identifying further risk factors for coronary vascular disease (Table 9.3).

Gender-Specific Assessment

The assessment of chest pain is incomplete without a thorough obstetric and gynecological history (Table 9.4) as many of these conditions may mask or exacerbate cardiovascular disease.

Risk Factor Assessment and Risk Stratification

Women present with a more extensive risk factor profile at their index event than men, due in part to an older age at presentation, but are less likely to have prior history of IHD or revascularization [30]. Table 9.5 shows the risk factors for CAD in women. The presence of cardiovascular risk factors is a stronger predictor of CAD in women than in men [12].

The Framingham risk estimation score, which is the current standard of risk stratification, is a poor predictor of subclinical disease in women, and has the tendency to misclassify those who would benefit from investigation as low risk. As a result, these women potentially evade adequate assessment and thus the threshold for investigation should be lower [33]. Accuracy may be improved with the use of imaging assessment, such as the coronary artery calcium score, which is discussed later in this chapter.

Diabetes mellitus is the strongest independent predictor of CAD in women, to a much greater extent than in men. The presence of DM increases the chance of developing CAD three-fold [34, 35]. Similarly, the presence of concurrent peripheral vascular disease is equivalent to an existing diagnosis of CAD. The presence of one or more major risk factor should warrant consideration of further investigation.

Investigations

Despite best practice guidelines, women are significantly less likely to undergo exercise ECG stress testing and coronary angiography than their male counterparts [36]. Not surprisingly, women presenting with stable angina have an increased risk of 1-year mortality, which highlights the need for a shift in the paradigm in the assessment and treatment of women with chest pain. Female gender, coupled with age <55, functions as an independent risk factor for missed myocardial infarction [37].

Several factors complicate the investigation of chest pain in women [38]. Anatomically, women have smaller body surface area, narrower coronary arteries

Table 9.3 Systems review

Systems: [17]
Cardiovascular
Dyspnea[a]
Palpitations[a]
Peripheral edema
Cyanosis
Syncope[a]
Diaphoresis[a]
Gastroenterological
Reflux, indigestion, esophageal spasm[b]
Nausea and vomiting[a]
Abdominal pain or discomfort
Psychosocial
Depression[b]
Anxiety[b]
Somatoform disorders
Respiratory
Pleuritic chest pain
Musculoskeletal
History of trauma[b]
Neuropathic pain
Swelling, deformity
Rheumatological
Rheumatoid arthritis, systemic lupus erythematosus, psoriatic arthritis[c]

[a]Red flags
[b]Differential diagnoses
[c]Increase risk for CAD

and a higher frequency of abnormal plaque morphology, rendering invasive procedures and assessment more difficult [39]. Risk stratification standards in women
remain suboptimal, as evidenced by the higher incidence of women undergoing
angiography only to find normal coronary anatomy, highlighting the need for
improvement in triage and investigation [11]. Figure 9.1 shows investigations for
women presenting with chest pain.

Acute Chest Pain

ECG

The standard 12-lead ECG is integral to the initial evaluation and triage of patients
with suspected ACS. Ideally, this needs to be performed within 10 min of presentation, but this occurs less frequently in women [40, 41]. Discrepancies in the ECG
seen in women include a prolonged QT interval, reduced QRS amplitude and

Table 9.4 Obstetric/gynecological review

Menopausal status
Risk factor for CAD, compounded by effects of ageing
Loss of protective effects of oestrogen on the vasculature and cholesterol profile [18–20]
Hormone replacement therapy (HRT) as a cardiovascular protection agent in post-menopausal women is controversial, with the HERS trial finding no benefit to this regime, with an increased rate of venous thromboembolic events (VTE) and MI in the early stages of therapy.
Pre-eclampsia
Pregnancy is often seen as a physiological stress test for cardiovascular disease, and is also a time when women first undergo blood pressure and blood glucose monitoring, thus making it an essential part of a cardiovascular risk assessment in women [21].
There is a link between hypertensive disorders of pregnancy (HDP) and development of coronary vascular disease, as well as stroke, and hypertension [22, 23].
Pre-eclampsia is a marker of maternal predisposition to vascular disease, particularly at a younger age [24]
Gestational diabetes
Increased risk of cardiovascular disease and type 2 diabetes [25].
Polycystic Ovarian Syndrome (PCOS)
Increased cardiovascular risk, as well as increasing the risk of co-morbidities such as insulin resistance, obesity and hyperlipidemia [26].
Women with PCOS are at a higher risk than their age-matched counterparts and require earlier screening for CVD
Oral contraceptive pill (OCP)
However, the use of OCPs in women over the age of 35 who smoke is contraindicated due to the risk of venous thromboembolic events and myocardial infarction [27, 28].
While some meta-analyses have indicated a higher risk of MI attributable to increased thrombogenicity, the overall attributable risk is low, and thus considered safe [29].

Table 9.5 Risk stratification tool

Moderate risk criteria	High risk criteria
One or more of the following	Known coronary artery disease
Smoking	Other arterial disease, including
Poor diet	Cerebrovascular disease
Sedentary lifestyle	Peripheral arterial disease
Obesity (particularly central)	Abdominal aortic aneurysm
Family history of premature CVD	Chronic renal impairment
Hypertension	Diabetes mellitus
Dyslipidemia (particularly hypertriglyceridemia [31])	10-year Framingham Global Risk >20 %
Subclinical vascular disease	
Metabolic syndrome	
Poor exercise capacity on ETT	

Adapted from: Mosca et al. [32]

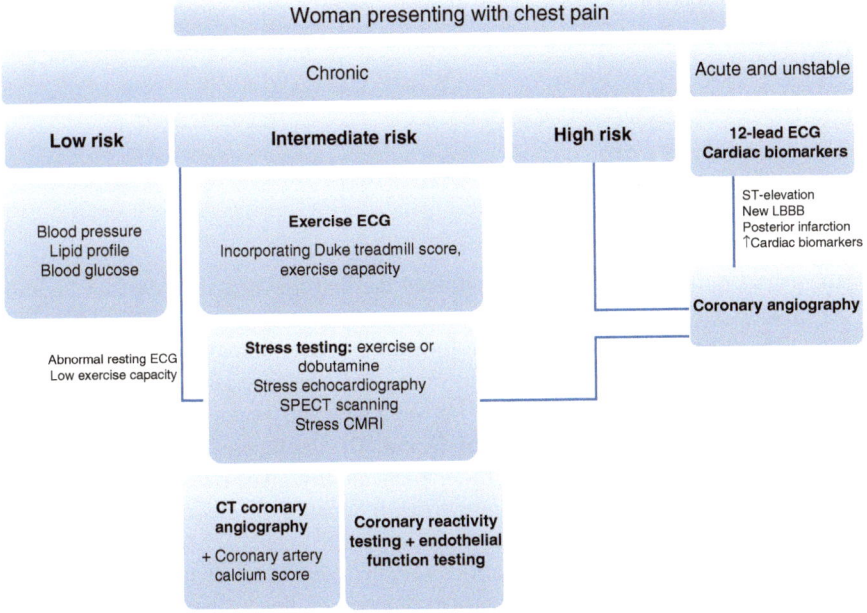

Fig. 9.1 Investigations for women presenting with chest pain

duration, and reduced baseline ST deviation. In particular, these parameters reduce the efficacy of diagnostic criteria for left ventricular hypertrophy, and despite the development of gender specific criteria, this condition continues to be under-diagnosed [42]. For STEMI, current guidelines advocate a lower threshold for diagnosis of ST elevation in women in leads V2-3, with ≥1.5 mm elevation signifying STEMI, as opposed to ≥2 mm in men [43, 44].

Potentially, there may be a role for echocardiography in women presenting with suspected IHD in the absence of diagnostic ECG changes or an atypical pattern of symptomatology.

Cardiac Biomarkers

A multi-marker approach is advocated in the assessment of women with chest pain due to gender discrepancies in reference range and specific biomarker expression, with women less likely to present with troponin elevations than men [45]. The TACTICS-TIMI 18 trial found that in women with non-ST-segment acute coronary syndromes were more likely to have elevated BNP and hs-CRP than men, who were more likely to present with elevated troponin and CK-MB [46]. In addition, CRP is related to micro-vascular coronary disease, a common but atypical cause of ischemic chest pain in women, and may be associated with the post-menopausal drop in estrogen [47]. It may also play a role as a risk marker in women [48]. Advantages and disadvantages of imaging modalities are presented in Table 9.6.

Chronic Chest Pain

Exercise ECG Stress Test

The exercise ECG test (ETT) is considered the first line non-invasive investigation for patients with a moderate risk of CAD and a normal baseline ECG [49]. ETT provides ischemic provocation in the form of exercise and allows interpretation of corresponding ECG abnormalities. However, there are clear gender discrepancies in the accuracy of exercise ECG testing between men and women. The sensitivity and specificity of ETT in women is just 61 % and 70 %, compared to 72 % and 77 % in men, respectively [50]. Critically, the low specificity gives rise to almost 30 % of women receiving a false negative diagnosis, indicating the clear need for improvement in diagnostic strategy. Gender variation in the accuracy of ETT is thought to be due to the baseline ST abnormalities seen in women, lower functional capacity, lower voltage and the impact of fluctuating estrogen levels on electrical recording [51, 52].

The ETT can be of value in symptomatic women when interpreted in conjunction with the Duke treadmill score [53], shown below (see Table 9.7). Exercise time is measured in minutes and the ST deviation is the absolute distance from baseline in any lead except aVR.

Duke treadmill score = Exercise time − (5 × ST deviation) − (4 × Treadmill Angina index[1]) [53]

Also of value is the ability of the ETT to provide information on exercise capacity, which is a strong prognostic indicator in CAD. Women are considered high risk if they are incapable of performing more than five metabolic equivalents of graded exercise [54]. Heart rate recovery might also provide valuable information in women. Recovery of resting heart rate within 1–2 min post-ETT has good prognostic power [55].

Stress Echocardiography

Stress echocardiography is a highly effective non-invasive means for assessing and stratifying symptomatic women with intermediate risk of CAD. In addition, it provides the added benefit of structural assessment which allows identification of localized ventricular dysfunction, valvular disease and wall motion abnormalities when confronted with ischemic stress [56] in the form of either exercise or

---

[1]Treadmill angina index: 0 = no angina during exercise, 1 = non-limiting angina during exercise, 2 = exercise-limiting angina.

Table 9.6   Advantages and disadvantages of imaging modalities

Modality	Advantages	Disadvantages
Exercise ECG	Tests exercise capacity Prognostic information	Lower sensitivity and specificity in women due to baseline ST variation
Stress Echo	Higher sensitivity and specificity than exercise ECG Provides information on wall motion abnormality, LVEF, structural abnormalities No radiation, quick procedure Good negative predictive value	Operator variability
Coronary artery CT	Non-invasive Identifies non-obstructive and subclinical CAD (plaque burden) Prognostic indicator +++ sensitivity and specificity	Radiation exposure Good negative predictive value Limited availability
Cardiac MRI	Structural and functional assessment Sub-endocardial perfusion ++ sensitivity and specificity	Cost Patient discomfort Operator variability
SPECT	High sensitivity Risk stratification tool Less variation between operators	Radiation exposure Breast attenuation Smaller heart Poor detection of multi-vessel and micro-vascular disease
Coronary angiography	Gold standard for CAD diagnosis Assessment of structure and function Intervention can be performed simultaneously	May miss extra-luminal plaque, microvascular disease Costly Invasive procedure, patient discomfort, radiation
Coronary reactivity testing	Diagnoses endothelial dysfunction and micro-vascular disease	High rate of inconclusive results Risk of coronary artery dissection

LVEF left ventricular ejection fraction, *CAD* coronary artery disease

Table 9.7 Interpretation of Duke treadmill score

Risk	Score	Action
Low	≥5	Preventative measures only
Moderate	5 to −11	Cardiac imaging ± coronary angiography
High	≤−11	Coronary angiography

dobutamine. Wall motion abnormalities are an early indication of ischemia. Dobutamine stress echocardiography is recommended in women incapable of exercising regardless of baseline ECG. Stress echocardiography has a higher specificity and sensitivity than stress ECG, with a combined accuracy of roughly 85 % [49, 57–59]. The efficacy of stress echo is not gender specific. The higher specificity allows for lower rates of false positives and therefore reduces the rate of unnecessary angiography [60].

SPECT

Single photo-emission computed tomography (SPECT) scanning provides informa-tion on perfusion defects and left ventricular function and volume. This modality has a higher sensitivity and specificity for detecting CAD than exercise stress test-ing, particularly in conjunction with ECG. Many studies have indicated that SPECT is an accurate means of risk-stratifying women in conjunction with pre-test proba-bility calculation [61]. However, it is not without its limitations. For women, breast attenuation, whereby the artifact of overlying breast tissue mimics areas of increased activity, can lead to false positives and reduce the accuracy of assessment [62]. The relatively smaller dimensions of the left ventricle in women also reduces diagnostic accuracy [63], and there is concern that radiation exposure may be linked to certain cancers. As such, SPECT scanning should be used sparingly in pre-menopausal women, and should be reserved for symptomatic women with high pre-test likeli-hood ratio of CAD.

The introduction of technetium-99 m has reduced the impact of breast attenua-tion and the risk of radiation, rendering it the agent of choice in the evaluation of chest pain in women [60]. In conjunction with gating, which is the simultaneous assessment with echocardiography, SPECT scanning has the highest sensitivity and specificity for detecting IHD.

CT Coronary Angiography (CTCA)

CTCA is a non-invasive procedure that can provide useful information on the pres-ence and extent of both obstructive and non-obstructive CAD [51, 64]. It also func-tions as a prognostic and risk stratification tool through the identification of early markers of disease processes such as arterial remodeling, plaque development, and calcification [65]. The identification of non-obstructive CAD using CTCA is a pre-dictor of long term mortality in women [66].

CTCA also allows quantifiable assessment of calcific plaque burden with the coronary artery calcium (CAC) score, which confers high specificity for predicting disease, and is of particular use in women who have higher rates of significant sub-clinical disease [67]. When used in conjunction with the Framingham risk score, CAC assessment provides incremental value to effectively identify candidates for aggressive preventative strategies [33].

CTCA could also potentially assume a role in the triage of women presenting with non-specific chest pain, as its high negative predictive value allows avoidance of invasive assessment with coronary angiography, reducing the risk of inherent peri-procedural complications. Furthermore, CTCA affords exclusion of alternative red flag diagnoses, such as pulmonary embolism and aortic dissection, which are more common in women and present a comparable clinical picture to CAD.

Cardiac MRI (CMRI)

Stress CMRI allows assessment of perfusion defects, structural dysfunction, and ventricular function. Cardiac MRI also provides visualization of sub-endocardial perfusion, even in the absence of visible coronary obstruction, which is beneficial in women as risk is often underestimated in the absence of demonstrable coronary obstruction [68]. As such, it is useful in patients who are symptomatic but fail to manifest pathology on coronary angiography. It also has the added advantage of no radiation exposure, but is costly and uncomfortable.

Coronary Angiography

Studies have demonstrated that women are significantly less likely to undergo invasive testing than their male counterparts, even in the setting of AMI [69, 70]. However, due to the prevalence of atypical etiology and poor correlation between degree of CAD and presence of angina, more than 50 % of women undergoing angiography have no evidence of obstruction in the epicardial arteries [71]. Despite this, women with normal coronaries but symptomatic disease are at an increased risk of major adverse cardiovascular events [5, 71]. Nonetheless, coronary angiography remains the gold standard diagnostic test for CAD, but should only be performed in women with a high pre-test probability. The use of radial access will be discussed in management.

Coronary Reactivity Testing

Due to the high prevalence of non-obstructive CAD among women [3, 45, 71], coronary reactivity testing is an important test for assessing endothelial function and microvascular disease. This population is generally poorly managed, costly, and has a higher risk of mortality [72–75]. Abnormal vasomotor function is also a known predictor of atherosclerosis and adverse cardiovascular events, an association independent of the presence of obstructive CAD [73].

These tests are indicated in women with symptoms suggestive of ischemia in the absence of obstruction on angiography, and involve the administration of dilatory agents such as adenosine, acetylcholine and nitrates to assess microvascular and endothelial function in the catheterization laboratory [76]. Though these tests provide valuable prognostic and diagnostic information, there is still risk of coronary artery dissection, and so testing should be reserved for those at high risk.

Management

The management of chest pain in women spans multiple modalities, including lifestyle modification, pharmacological therapy and interventional or surgical approaches.

Invasive Management

Acute Coronary Syndrome

The optimal treatment strategy of acute coronary syndromes, including choice of revascularization therapy – invasive or conservative – remains to be defined in women, who continue to be underrepresented in large clinical trials. The current AHA/ACC guidelines advocate an invasive strategy for women who present with high risk non-ST-elevation ACS and a conservative strategy with low risk [77]. For STEMI, PCI is recommended within a target timeframe of 90 min, and the adjunctive medical regime is the same for men, but with dose adjustment for weight [78].

The indications for women undergoing elective PCI for stable angina should be the same as for men [79], using risk stratification tools and consultation with the heart team to determine the optimal method of revascularization.

Percutaneous Coronary Intervention

There is conflicting evidence on whether women have worse outcomes following percutaneous coronary intervention (PCI) due to gender alone or higher baseline risk and treatment delay. Nonetheless, women have higher rates of short-term complications but better long-term outcomes [80]. Women experience greater delays to PCI [81], often due to greater delay from symptom onset presentation, and are referred much less frequently for diagnostic catheterization [82–84]. Crude mortality and adverse outcome rates are higher in women undergoing PCI, but after adjustment for age and co-morbidities, the majority of studies have found adverse event rates comparable between genders [85]. The difference in outcomes is more likely attributable to a higher risk profile, due to a higher burden of co-morbidities, older age at presentation and confounding factors complicating the procedure, including poorer access due to smaller vessels, smaller body surface area, and higher prevalence of diabetes [86–88]. These factors also translate into higher rates of stent restenosis, a risk which appears to be at least partially mitigated with the introduction of drug eluting stents (DES). A large meta-analysis examining the effect of sex on the efficacy of newer DES determined that women experienced significant reductions in all ischemic endpoints, including mortality [89].

Women experience an increased risk of bleeding post-PCI in both the short and long-term, with female gender functioning as an independent baseline predictor of bleeding risk across several risk predictor scores [90]. An analysis of a large ACS cohort found that the risk of bleeding associated with female gender persisted at

30 day and 3 year follow up, necessitating the implementation of appropriate reduction strategies [84].

Women with positive biomarkers benefit from invasive strategy significantly more than those who do not exhibit biomarker elevation. The American College of Cardiology currently indicates that biomarker negative women should not receive a GP IIb/IIIa inhibitor due to high bleeding risk [91]. Due to a greater bleeding tendency, women have a higher rate of vascular complications. However, the risk has decreased substantially with the development of anti-bleeding regimes, including weight-determined anti-coagulation dosing, smaller sheath and stent use, and early sheath removal [92–94].

The use of a transradial approach for PCI in women has not been extensively studied, but presents an attractive alternative to transfemoral angioplasty due to the reduced risk of access site bleeding [95]. However, women have narrower arteries, thus increasing the complexity of achieving transradial access. A recent randomized controlled trial, SAFE-PCI, was designed to examine the safety and efficacy of a transradial approach in a cohort exclusively of women, but was stopped prematurely due to a small number of events [96].

Surgical

Similar to PCI, bypass surgery is complicated by the higher risk factor burden in women. CABG in women is also rendered more technically difficult by smaller coronary vessel size, smaller surface area, a greater extent of CAD and co-morbidity profile, and older age [97]. As a result, women have higher rates of procedural complications, in-hospital events and short-term mortality [98]. However, this does not translate into worse long-term outcomes, and survival rates are improving along with surgical expertise [99]. However, quality of life is impacted more significantly in women following CABG, with women experiencing greater loss of functional status, higher rates of revascularization and graft occlusion, and anxiety and depression than men [38, 100, 101]. The decision to perform CABG on or off pump has important implications, as it appears that off-pump bypass yields better survival and lower complication rates in women than in men [102]. The efficacy of CABG in women is still poorly studied, and improvement relies heavily on trials incorporating larger numbers of women.

Optimal Medical Management

Lifestyle Modification

The first line treatment for IHD is aggressive risk factor reduction through lifestyle modification, including dietary changes, exercise and elimination of risk factors such as smoking and stress. Major gender-specific barriers to guideline adherence include incompatibility with busy lifestyle and low perceived risk of cardiovascular disease – appropriate counseling and improving practicality of management strategies are paramount to assisting women in controlling risk factors.

Pharmacological Therapy

Current clinical guidelines do not recommend different pharmacological management of diagnosed IHD in women compared to men [38]. However, appropriate selection and dosage of agents is often poorly managed, as best practice is informed by large scale trials on study populations in whom the vast majority are men. Antithrombotic therapy, for example, is often associated with adverse bleeding events due to physicians' failure to adjust dosing to mitigate the increased bleeding risk seen in many women due to lower body weight, older age, and pre-existing kidney disease [103].

Medical reduction of cardiac risk factors, using anti-hypertensives and cholesterol lowering agents, is also inadequately managed in women. Women are less likely to receive evidence based secondary prevention therapy even after confirmed diagnosis of CAD, including beta-blocker and statin therapy post STEMI [36, 84]. Aspirin, for example, is of significant benefit for secondary prevention in women, but it is still widely under-prescribed [104]. Women have higher platelet reactivity, and have been shown to demonstrate a more marked response even to low-dose aspirin [105].

Due to the unique atypical etiology of many women presenting with IHD, there is emerging evidence for pharmacological therapies tailored to treat micro-vascular angina. Some examples of therapies for improving endothelial dysfunction include L-arginine and beta-blockers, while ACE inhibitors and statins have shown promising results in improving micro-vascular dysfunction [107].

Public Education

The public understanding of heart disease in women is limited. Among women, self-perception of risk is vastly underestimated, translating to a greater delay from symptom development to eventual presentation and a lower likelihood to consent to invasive procedures [84, 108]. Similarly, there is a poor understanding of risk among physicians which persists even after CAD is diagnosed [106], with women less likely to be referred to cardiac rehabilitation following myocardial infarction [109]. The deficiency in focused initiatives targeting primary prevention strategies and risk identification needs to be addressed.

Conclusion

As the incidence and impact of IHD in women continues to rise, it is increasingly apparent that further female-oriented research is required to better understand the unique etiology of chest pain in women, and the optimal methods of reducing the burden of disease in our population.

1. There are differences in the underlying pathophysiology causing chest pain in women, and so different investigative and management strategies must be explored.
2. Gender bias persists in the use of invasive treatment.
3. There is a deficiency in literature that examines pharmacological and interventional strategies in women specifically.
4. There is conflicting evidence as to whether women have worse outcomes following invasive revascularization due to gender alone or higher baseline risk and treatment delay.
5. The public understanding of heart disease in women is limited and requires targeted public awareness campaigns.

Disclosures   All authors declare no conflict of interest.

References

1. American Heart Association. Heart disease and stroke statistics: 2004 Update United States 2004. Available from: http://americanheart.org/downloadable/heart/1072969766940HSStats2 004Update.pdf.
2. Mosca L, Grundy SM, Judelson D, King K, Limacher M, Oparil S, et al. Guide to preventive cardiology for women. Circulation. 1999;99(18):2480–4.
3. Bairey Merz CN, Shaw LJ, Reis SE, Bittner V, Kelsey SF, Olson M, et al. Insights from the NHLBI-Sponsored Women's Ischemia Syndrome Evaluation (WISE) Study: part II: gender differences in presentation, diagnosis, and outcome with regard to gender-based pathophysiology of atherosclerosis and macrovascular and microvascular coronary disease. J Am Coll Cardiol. 2006;47(3 Suppl):S21–9. PubMed PMID: 16458167. Epub 2006/02/07. eng.
4. Shaw LJ, Bairey Merz CN, Pepine CJ, Reis SE, Bittner V, Kelsey SF, et al. Insights from the NHLBI-Sponsored Women's Ischemia Syndrome Evaluation (WISE) study: part I: gender differences in traditional and novel risk factors, symptom evaluation, and gender-optimized diagnostic strategies. J Am Coll Cardiol. 2006;47(3 Suppl):S4–20.
5. Gulati M, Shaw LJ, Bairey Merz CN. Myocardial ischemia in women: lessons from the NHLBI WISE study. Clin Cardiol. 2012;35(3):141–8.
6. Kannel WB, Vokonas PS. Demographics of the prevalence, incidence, and management of coronary heart disease in the elderly and in women. Ann Epidemiol. 1992;2(1–2):5–14. PubMed PMID: 1342264. Epub 1992/01/01. eng.
7. Orencia A, Bailey K, Yawn BP, Kottke TE. Effect of gender on long-term outcome of angina pectoris and myocardial infarction/sudden unexpected death. JAMA. 1993;269(18):2392–7. PubMed PMID: 8479065. Epub 1993/05/12. eng.
8. Cowley MJ, Mullin SM, Kelsey SF, Kent KM, Gruentzig AR, Detre KM, et al. Sex differences in early and long-term results of coronary angioplasty in the NHLBI PTCA Registry. Circulation. 1985;71(1):90–7. PubMed PMID: 3155449. Epub 1985/01/01. eng.
9. Philpott S, Boynton PM, Feder G, Hemingway H. Gender differences in descriptions of angina symptoms and health problems immediately prior to angiography: the ACRE study. Appropriateness of Coronary Revascularisation study. Soc Sci Med. 2001;52(10):1565–75. PubMed PMID: 11314852. Epub 2001/04/21. eng.
10. Milner KA, Funk M, Richards S, Wilmes RM, Vaccarino V, Krumholz HM. Gender differences in symptom presentation associated with coronary heart disease. Am J Cardiol. 1999;84(4):396–9. PubMed PMID: 10468075. Epub 1999/09/01. eng.

11. Sullivan AK, Holdright DR, Wright CA, Sparrow JL, Cunningham D, Fox KM. Chest pain in women: clinical, investigative, and prognostic features. BMJ (Clin Res ed). 1994;308(6933):883–6.

12. Douglas PS, Ginsburg GS. The evaluation of chest pain in women. N Engl J Med. 1996;334(20):1311–5.

13. Berecki-Gisolf J, Humphreyes-Reid L, Wilson A, Dobson A. Angina symptoms are associated with mortality in older women with ischemic heart disease. Circulation. 2009;120(23):2330–6. PubMed PMID: 19933930. Epub 2009/11/26. eng.

14. Weiner DA, Ryan TJ, McCabe CH, Kennedy JW, Schloss M, Tristani F, et al. Exercise stress testing. N Engl J Med. 1979;301(5):230–5. PubMed PMID: 449990.

15. Pepine CJ, Abrams J, Marks RG, Morris JJ, Scheidt SS, Handberg E. Characteristics of a contemporary population with angina pectoris. TIDES Investigators. Am J Cardiol. 1994;74(3):226–31. PubMed PMID: 8037126. Epub 1994/08/01. eng.

16. Khan NA, Daskalopoulou SS, Karp I, Eisenberg MJ, Pelletier R, Tsadok MA, et al. Sex differences in acute coronary syndrome symptom presentation in young patients. JAMA Intern Med. 2013;173(20):1863–71. PubMed PMID: 24043208. Epub 2013/09/18. eng.

17. Talley NJ, O'Connor S. Clinical examination: a systematic guide to physical diagnosis. Sydney: Elsevier/Churchill Livingstone; 2010.

18. Barrett-Connor E, Bush TL. Estrogen and coronary heart disease in women. JAMA. 1991;265(14):1861–7.

19. Colditz GA, Willett WC, Stampfer MJ, Rosner B, Speizer FE, Hennekens CH. Menopause and the risk of coronary heart disease in women. N Engl J Med. 1987;316(18):1105–10. PubMed PMID: 3574358.

20. van der Schouw YT, van der Graaf Y, Steyerberg EW, Eijkemans JC, Banga JD. Age at menopause as a risk factor for cardiovascular mortality. Lancet. 1996;347(9003):714–8. PubMed PMID: 8602000. Epub 1996/03/16. eng.

21. Yu J, Johnson J, Theodoropoulos K, Mungee S, Couri M, Malasky B, et al. TCT-365 pregnancy-induced disorders identify high-risk women who benefit from cardiovascular screening: results from the Women's Heart Health Initiative, an OB/GYN Screening Pilot Program. J Am Coll Cardiol. 2012;60(17_S):B104.

22. Newstead J, von Dadelszen P, Magee LA. Preeclampsia and future cardiovascular risk. Expert Rev Cardiovasc Ther. 2007;5(2):283–94.

23. Smith GC, Pell JP, Walsh D. Pregnancy complications and maternal risk of ischaemic heart disease: a retrospective cohort study of 129,290 births. Lancet. 2001;357(9273):2002–6. PubMed PMID: 11438131. Epub 2001/07/05. eng.

24. Ahmed R, Dunford J, Mehran R, Robson S, Kunadian V. Preeclampsia and future cardiovascular risk among women: a review. J Am Coll Cardiol. 2014;63(18):1815–22. PubMed PMID: 24613324. Epub 2014/03/13. Eng.

25. Archambault C, Arel R, Filion KB. Gestational diabetes and risk of cardiovascular disease: a scoping review. Open Med Peer Rev Independent Open Access J. 2014;8(1):e1–9. PubMed PMID: 25009679. Pubmed Central PMCID: PMC4085089. Epub 2014/07/11. eng.

26. Randeva HS, Tan BK, Weickert MO, Lois K, Nestler JE, Sattar N, et al. Cardiometabolic aspects of the polycystic ovary syndrome. Endocr Rev. 2012;33(5):812–41. PubMed PMID: 22829562. Pubmed Central PMCID: PMC3461136. Epub 2012/07/26. eng.

27. Chasan-Taber L, Stampfer MJ. Epidemiology of oral contraceptives and cardiovascular disease. Ann Intern Med. 1998;128(6):467–77. PubMed PMID: 9499331. Epub 1998/03/14. eng.

28. Croft P, Hannaford PC. Risk factors for acute myocardial infarction in women: evidence from the Royal College of General Practitioners' oral contraception study. BMJ (Clin Res Ed). 1989;298(6667):165–8. PubMed PMID: 2493841. Pubmed Central PMCID: PMC1835478. Epub 1989/01/21. eng.

29. Baillargeon JP, McClish DK, Essah PA, Nestler JE. Association between the current use of low-dose oral contraceptives and cardiovascular arterial disease: a meta-analysis. J Clin Endocrinol Metab. 2005;90(7):3863–70. PubMed PMID: 15814774. Epub 2005/04/09. eng.

30. O'Donoghue M, Boden WE, Braunwald E, Cannon CP, Clayton TC, de Winter RJ, et al. Early invasive vs conservative treatment strategies in women and men with unstable angina and non-ST-segment elevation myocardial infarction: a meta-analysis. JAMA. 2008;300(1):71–80. PubMed PMID: 18594042. Epub 2008/07/03. eng.

31. Lerner DJ, Kannel WB. Patterns of coronary heart disease morbidity and mortality in the sexes: a 26-year follow-up of the Framingham population. Am Heart J. 1986;111(2):383–90.

32. Mosca L, Banka CL, Benjamin EJ, Berra K, Bushnell C, Dolor RJ, et al. Evidence-based guidelines for cardiovascular disease prevention in women: 2007 update. Circulation. 2007;115(11):1481–501.

33. Michos ED, Vasamreddy CR, Becker DM, Yanek LR, Moy TF, Fishman EK, et al. Women with a low Framingham risk score and a family history of premature coronary heart disease have a high prevalence of subclinical coronary atherosclerosis. Am Heart J. 2005;150(6):1276–81. PubMed PMID: 16338271. Epub 2005/12/13. eng.

34. Spencer E, Pirie K, Stevens R, Beral V, Brown A, Liu B, et al. Diabetes and modifiable risk factors for cardiovascular disease: the prospective Million Women Study. Eur J Epidemiol. 2008;23(12):793–9. English.

35. Barrett-Connor EL, Cohn BA, Wingard DL, Edelstein SL. Why is diabetes mellitus a stronger risk factor for fatal ischemic heart disease in women than in men? The Rancho Bernardo study. JAMA. 1991;265(5):627–31.

36. Daly C, Clemens F, Lopez Sendon JL, Tavazzi L, Boersma E, Danchin N, et al. Gender differences in the management and clinical outcome of stable angina. Circulation. 2006;113(4):490–8.

37. Pope JH, Aufderheide TP, Ruthazer R, Woolard RH, Feldman JA, Beshansky JR, et al. Missed diagnoses of acute cardiac ischemia in the emergency department. N Engl J Med. 2000;342(16):1163–70. PubMed PMID: 10770981. Epub 2000/04/20. eng.

38. Varughese CJ, Pinnelas R, Yu J, Mehran R. Textbook of cardiovascular intervention. London: Springer; 2014.

39. Blum A, Blum N. Coronary artery disease: are men and women created equal? Gend Med. 2009;6(3):410–8. PubMed PMID: 19850237. Epub 2009/10/24. eng.

40. Hollander JE, Chang AM. Evaluation of chest pain in the emergency department 2013 [cited 2014 March]. Available from: http://www.uptodate.com/contents/evaluation-of-chest-pain-in-the-emergency-department?source=see_link.

41. Diercks DB, Peacock WF, Hiestand BC, Chen AY, Pollack Jr CV, Kirk JD, et al. Frequency and consequences of recording an electrocardiogram >10 minutes after arrival in an emergency room in non-ST-segment elevation acute coronary syndromes (from the CRUSADE Initiative). Am J Cardiol. 2006;97(4):437–42. PubMed PMID: 16461033. Epub 2006/02/08. eng.

42. Okin PM, Roman MJ, Devereux RB, Kligfield P. Gender differences and the electrocardiogram in left ventricular hypertrophy. Hypertension. 1995;25(2):242–9.

43. O'Gara PT, Kushner FG, Ascheim DD, Casey DE, Chung MK, de Lemos JA, et al. 2013 ACCF/AHA guideline for the management of ST-elevation myocardial infarction: a report of the American College of Cardiology Foundation/American Heart Association Task Force on Practice Guidelines. J Am Coll Cardiol. 2013;61(4):e78–140.

44. Thygesen K, Alpert JS, Jaffe AS, Simoons ML, Chaitman BR, White HD, et al. Third universal definition of myocardial infarction. Circulation. 2012;126(16):2020–35. PubMed PMID: 22923432. Epub 2012/08/28. eng.

45. Lagerqvist B, Säfström K, Ståhle E, Wallentin L, Swahn E. Is early invasive treatment of unstable coronary artery disease equally effective for both women and men? J Am Coll Cardiol. 2001;38(1):41–8.

46. Wiviott SD, Cannon CP, Morrow DA, Murphy SA, Gibson CM, McCabe CH, et al. Differential expression of cardiac biomarkers by gender in patients with unstable angina/non-ST-elevation myocardial infarction: a TACTICS-TIMI 18 (Treat Angina with Aggrastat and determine Cost of Therapy with an Invasive or Conservative Strategy-Thrombolysis in Myocardial Infarction

18) substudy. Circulation. 2004;109(5):580–6. PubMed PMID: 14769678. Epub 2004/02/11. eng.

47. Agarwal M, Mehta PK, Bairey Merz CN. Nonacute coronary syndrome anginal chest pain. Med Clin North Am. 2010;94(2):201–16. PubMed PMID: 20380951. Pubmed Central PMCID: PMC2876979. Epub 2010/04/13. eng.

48. Ridker PM, Rifai N, Rose L, Buring JE, Cook NR. Comparison of C-reactive protein and low-density lipoprotein cholesterol levels in the prediction of first cardiovascular events. N Engl J Med. 2002;347(20):1557–65. PubMed PMID: 12432042.

49. Members C, Gibbons RJ, Balady GJ, Timothy Bricker J, Chaitman BR, Fletcher GF, et al. ACC/AHA 2002 guideline update for exercise testing: summary article: a report of the American College of Cardiology/American Heart Association Task Force on Practice Guidelines (Committee to Update the 1997 Exercise Testing Guidelines). Circulation. 2002;106(14):1883–92.

50. Kwok Y, Kim C, Grady D, et al. Meta-analysis of exercise testing to detect coronary artery disease in women. Am J Cardiol. 1999;83:660–6.

51. Shaw LJTS, Rosen S, Mieres JH. Evaluation of suspected ischemic heart disease in symptomatic women. Can J Cardiol. 2014;30(7):729–37.

52. Stangl V, Witzel V, Baumann G, Stangl K. Current diagnostic concepts to detect coronary artery disease in women. Eur Heart J. 2008;29(6):707–17. PubMed PMID: 18272503. Epub 2008/02/15. eng.

53. Mark DB, Hlatky MA, Harrell Jr FE, Lee KL, Califf RM, Pryor DB. Exercise treadmill score for predicting prognosis in coronary artery disease. Ann Intern Med. 1987;106:793–800.

54. Gulati M, Black HR, Shaw LJ, Arnsdorf MF, Merz CNB, Lauer MS, Marwick TH, Pandey DK, Wicklund RH, Thisted RA. The prognostic value of a nomogram for exercise capacity in women. N Engl J Med. 2005;353(5):468–75.

55. Gibbons RJ. Abnormal heart-rate recovery after exercise. Lancet. 2002;359(9317):1536–7.

56. Mieres JH, Shaw LJ, Arai A, Budoff MJ, Flamm SD, Hundley WG, et al. Role of noninvasive testing in the clinical evaluation of women with suspected coronary artery disease: consensus statement from the Cardiac Imaging Committee, Council on Clinical Cardiology, and the Cardiovascular Imaging and Intervention Committee, Council on Cardiovascular Radiology and Intervention. Am Heart Assoc Circ. 2005;111(5):682–96. PubMed PMID: 15687114. Epub 2005/02/03. eng.

57. Williams MJ, Marwick TH, O'Gorman D, Foale RA. Comparison of exercise echocardiography with an exercise score to diagnose coronary artery disease in women. Am J Cardiol. 1994;74(5):435–8. PubMed PMID: 8059721. Epub 1994/09/01. eng.

58. Douglas PS. Is noninvasive testing for coronary artery disease accurate? Circulation. 1997;95(2):299–302.

59. Grundy SM, Pasternak R, Greenland P, Smith S, Fuster V. Assessment of cardiovascular risk by use of multiple-risk-factor assessment equations: a statement for healthcare professionals from the American Heart Association and the American College of Cardiology. Circulation. 1999;100(13):1481–92.

60. Mieres JH, Shaw LJ, Hendel RC, Miller DD, Bonow RO, Berman DS, Heller GV, Mieres JH, Bairey-Merz CN, Berman DS, Bonow RO, Cacciabaudo JM, Heller GV, Hendel RC, Kiess MC, Miller DD, Polk DM, Shaw LJ, Smanio PE, Walsh MN, Writing Group on Perfusion Imaging in Women. American Society of Nuclear Cardiology consensus statement: Task Force on Women and Coronary Artery Disease—the role of myocardial perfusion imaging in the clinical evaluation of coronary artery disease in women. J Nucl Cardiol. 2003;10:95–101.

61. Shaw LJ, Iskandrian AE. Prognostic value of gated myocardial perfusion SPECT. J Nucl Cardiol Off Publ Am Soc Nucl Cardiol. 2004;11(2):171–85. PubMed PMID: 15052249. Epub 2004/03/31. eng.

62. Nurkalem Z, Sahin S, Uslu N, Emre A, Alper AT, Gorgulu S, et al. Predicting breast attenuation in patients undergoing myocardial perfusion scintigraphy: a digital x-ray study. J Digit Imaging. 2008;21(4):446–51. PubMed PMID: 17703339. Pubmed Central PMCID: PMC3043850. Epub 2007/08/19. eng.

63. Mieres JH, Shaw LJ, Hendel RC, Miller DD, Bonow RO, Berman DS, et al. American Society of Nuclear Cardiology consensus statement: Task Force on Women and Coronary Artery Disease–the role of myocardial perfusion imaging in the clinical evaluation of coronary artery disease in women [correction]. J Nucl Cardiol Off Publ Am Soc Nucl Cardiol. 2003;10(1):95–101. PubMed PMID: 12569338. Epub 2003/02/06. eng.
64. Ajlan AM, Heilbron BG, Leipsic J. Coronary computed tomography angiography for stable angina: past, present, and future. Can J Cardiol. 2013;29(3):266–74.
65. Min JK, Shaw LJ, Berman DS. The present state of coronary computed tomography angiography. A process in evolution. J Am Coll Cardiol. 2010;55(10):957–65.
66. Min JK, Dunning A, Lin FY, Achenbach S, Al-Mallah M, Budoff MJ, et al. Age- and sex-related differences in all-cause mortality risk based on coronary computed tomography angiography findings: Results from the international multicenter CONFIRM (Coronary CT Angiography Evaluation for Clinical Outcomes: an International Multicenter Registry) of 23,854 patients without known coronary artery disease. J Am Coll Cardiol. 2011;58(8): 849–60.
67. Litwin SE, Priester TC. Diagnosing coronary artery disease in women: an update on cardiac imaging modalities. Obstet Gynecol. 2010;115(1):156–69. PubMed PMID: 20027049. Epub 2009/12/23. eng.
68. Wenger NK. Coronary heart disease in women. Springer; 2009. p. 337–69.
69. Gan SC, Beaver SK, Houck PM, MacLehose RF, Lawson HW, Chan L. Treatment of acute myocardial infarction and 30-day mortality among women and men. N Engl J Med. 2000;343(1):8–15.
70. Scirica BM, Moliterno DJ, Every NR, Anderson HV, Aguirre FV, Granger CB, et al. Differences between men and women in the management of unstable angina pectoris (The GUARANTEE Registry). The GUARANTEE Investigators. Am J Cardiol. 1999;84(10):1145–50. PubMed PMID: 10569321. Epub 1999/11/24. eng.
71. Jespersen L, Hvelplund A, Abildstrøm SZ, Pedersen F, Galatius S, Madsen JK, et al. Stable angina pectoris with no obstructive coronary artery disease is associated with increased risks of major adverse cardiovascular events. Eur Heart J. 2012;33(6):734–44.
72. Shaw LJ, Merz CNB, Pepine CJ, Reis SE, Bittner V, Kip KE, et al. The economic burden of angina in women with suspected ischemic heart disease: results from the National Institutes of Health-National Heart, Lung, and Blood Institute-sponsored Women's Ischemia Syndrome Evaluation. Circulation. 2006;114(9):894–904.
73. Von Mering GO, Arant CB, Wessel TR, McGorray SP, Bairey Merz CN, Sharaf BL, et al. Abnormal coronary vasomotion as a prognostic indicator of cardiovascular events in women: results from the National Heart, Lung, and Blood Institute-Sponsored Women's Ischemia Syndrome Evaluation (WISE). Circulation. 2004;109(6):722–5.
74. Pepine CJ, Anderson RD, Sharaf BL, Reis SE, Smith KM, Handberg EM, et al. Coronary microvascular reactivity to adenosine predicts adverse outcome in women evaluated for suspected ischemia. Results from the National Heart, Lung and Blood Institute WISE (Women's Ischemia Syndrome Evaluation) study. J Am Coll Cardiol. 2010;55(25): 2825–32.
75. Halcox JPJ, Schenke WH, Zalos G, Mincemoyer R, Prasad A, Waclawiw MA, et al. Prognostic value of coronary vascular endothelial dysfunction. Circulation. 2002;106(6):653–8.
76. Bairey Merz CN, Pepine CJ. Syndrome X and microvascular coronary dysfunction. Circulation. 2011;124(13):1477–80.
77. Anderson JL, Adams CD, Antman EM, Bridges CR, Califf RM, Casey DE, et al. ACC/AHA 2007 guidelines for the management of patients with unstable angina/non–ST-elevation myocardial infarction: executive summary: a report of the American College of Cardiology/American Heart Association Task Force on Practice Guidelines (Writing Committee to Revise the 2002 Guidelines for the Management of Patients With Unstable Angina/Non–ST-Elevation Myocardial Infarction): developed in collaboration with the American College of Emergency Physicians, the Society for Cardiovascular Angiography and Interventions, and the Society of Thoracic Surgeons: endorsed by the American Association of Cardiovascular and Pulmonary

Rehabilitation and the Society for Academic Emergency Medicine. Circulation. 2007;116(7):803–77.

78. Antman EM, Hand M, Armstrong PW, Bates ER, Green LA, Halasyamani LK, et al. 2007 focused update of the ACC/AHA 2004 guidelines for the management of patients with ST-elevation myocardial infarction. J Am Coll Cardiol. 2008;51(2):210–47.

79. Levine GN, Bates ER, Blankenship JC, Bailey SR, Bittl JA, Cercek B, et al. 2011 ACCF/AHA/SCAI guideline for percutaneous coronary intervention: executive summary: a report of the American College of Cardiology Foundation/American Heart Association Task Force on Practice Guidelines and the Society for Cardiovascular Angiography and Interventions. Circulation. 2011;124(23):2574–609.

80. Anderson ML, Peterson ED, Brennan JM, Rao SV, Dai D, Anstrom KJ, et al. Short- and long-term outcomes of coronary stenting in women versus men: results from the National Cardiovascular Data Registry Centers for Medicare & Medicaid services cohort. Circulation. 2012;126(18):2190–9. PubMed PMID: 22988009. Epub 2012/09/19. eng.

81. Angeja BG, Gibson CM, Chin R, Frederick PD, Every NR, Ross AM, et al. Predictors of door-to-balloon delay in primary angioplasty. Am J Cardiol. 2002;89(10):1156–61.

82. Ayanian JZ, Epstein AM. Differences in the use of procedures between women and men hospitalized for coronary heart disease. N Engl J Med. 1991;325(4):221–5. PubMed PMID: 2057022. Epub 1991/07/25. eng.

83. Rathore SS, Wang Y, Radford MJ, Ordin DL, Krumholz HM. Sex differences in cardiac catheterization after acute myocardial infarction: the role of procedure appropriateness. Ann Intern Med. 2002;137(6):487–93. PubMed PMID: 12230349. Epub 2002/09/17. eng.

84. Yu J, Mehran R, Grinfeld L, Xu K, Nikolsky E, Brodie BR, et al. Sex-based differences in bleeding and long term adverse events after percutaneous coronary intervention for acute myocardial infarction: three year results from the HORIZONS-AMI trial. Catheter Cardiovasc Interv Off J Soc Card Angiogr Interv. 2015;85(3):359–68. PubMed PMID: 25115966. Epub 2014/08/15. Eng.

85. Lansky AJ, Pietras C, Costa RA, Tsuchiya Y, Brodie BR, Cox DA, et al. Gender differences in outcomes after primary angioplasty versus primary stenting with and without abciximab for acute myocardial infarction: results of the Controlled Abciximab and Device Investigation to Lower Late Angioplasty Complications (CADILLAC) trial. Circulation. 2005;111(13):1611–8. PubMed PMID: 15811868. Epub 2005/04/07. eng.

86. Lansky AJ, Hochman JS, Ward PA, Mintz GS, Fabunmi R, Berger PB, et al. Percutaneous coronary intervention and adjunctive pharmacotherapy in women: a statement for healthcare professionals from the American Heart Association. Circulation. 2005;111(7):940–53.

87. Lansky AJ, Costa RA, Mooney M, Midei MG, Lui HK, Strickland W, et al. Gender-based outcomes after paclitaxel-eluting stent implantation in patients with coronary artery disease. J Am Coll Cardiol. 2005;45(8):1180–5. PubMed PMID: 15837246. Epub 2005/04/20. eng.

88. Lansky AJ. Outcomes of percutaneous and surgical revascularization in women. Prog Cardiovasc Dis. 2004;46(4):305–19.

89. Stefanini GG, Baber U, Windecker S, Morice MC, Sartori S, Leon MB, et al. Safety and efficacy of drug-eluting stents in women: a patient-level pooled analysis of randomised trials. Lancet. 2013;382(9908):1879–88. PubMed PMID: 24007976. Epub 2013/09/07. eng.

90. Mehran R, Pocock SJ, Nikolsky E, Clayton T, Dangas GD, Kirtane AJ, et al. A risk score to predict bleeding in patients with acute coronary syndromes. J Am Coll Cardiol. 2010;55(23):2556–66.

91. Boersma E, Harrington RA, Moliterno DJ, White H, Theroux P, Van de Werf F, et al. Platelet glycoprotein IIb/IIIa inhibitors in acute coronary syndromes: a meta-analysis of all major randomised clinical trials. Lancet. 2002;359(9302):189–98. PubMed PMID: 11812552. Epub 2002/01/29. eng.

92. Kelsey SF, James M, Holubkov AL, Holubkov R, Cowley MJ, Detre KM. Results of percutaneous transluminal coronary angioplasty in women. 1985–1986 National Heart, Lung, and Blood Institute's Coronary Angioplasty Registry. Circulation. 1993;87(3):720–7.

93. Lincoff AM, Tcheng JE, Califf RM, Bass T, Popma JJ, Teirstein PS, et al. Standard versus Low-dose weight-adjusted heparin in patients treated with the platelet glycoprotein IIb/IIIa receptor antibody fragment abciximab (c7E3 Fab) during percutaneous coronary revascularization. Am J Cardiol. 1997;79(3):286–91.

94. Mandak JS, Blankenship JC, Gardner LH, Berkowitz SD, Aguirre FV, Sigmon KN, et al. Modifiable risk factors for vascular access site complications in the IMPACT II trial of angioplasty with versus without eptifibatide. Integrilin to Minimize Platelet Aggregation and Coronary Thrombosis. J Am Coll Cardiol. 1998;31(7):1518–24. PubMed PMID: 9626829. Epub 1998/06/17. eng.

95. Bernat I, Horak D, Stasek J, Mates M, Pesek J, Ostadal P, et al. ST-segment elevation myocardial infarction treated by radial or femoral approach in a multicenter randomized clinical trial: the STEMI-RADIAL trial. J Am Coll Cardiol. 2014;63(10):964–72. PubMed PMID: 24211309. Epub 2013/11/12. eng.

96. Rao SV, Hess CN, Barham B, Aberle LH, Anstrom KJ, Patel TB, et al. A registry-based randomized trial comparing radial and femoral approaches in women undergoing percutaneous coronary intervention: the SAFE-PCI for Women (Study of Access Site for Enhancement of PCI for Women) trial. JACC Cardiovasc Interv. 2014;7(8):857–67. PubMed PMID: 25147030. Epub 2014/08/26. eng.

97. Brown PP, Mack MJ, Simon AW, Battaglia S, Tarkington L, Horner S, et al. Outcomes experience with off-pump coronary artery bypass surgery in women. Ann Thorac Surg. 2002;74(6):2113–9; discussion 20. PubMed PMID: 12643404. Epub 2003/03/20. eng.

98. Blankstein R, Ward RP, Arnsdorf M, Jones B, Lou Y-B, Pine M. Female gender is an independent predictor of operative mortality after coronary artery bypass graft surgery: contemporary analysis of 31 Midwestern Hospitals. Circulation. 2005;112(9 Suppl):I323–7.

99. Humphries KH, Gao M, Pu A, Lichtenstein S, Thompson CR. Significant improvement in short-term mortality in women undergoing coronary artery bypass surgery (1991 to 2004). J Am Coll Cardiol. 2007;49(14):1552–8. PubMed PMID: 17418294. Epub 2007/04/10. eng.

100. Boersma E, Harrington RA, Moliterno DJ, White H, Simoons ML. Platelet glycoprotein IIb/IIIa inhibitors in acute coronary syndromes. Lancet. 2002;360(9329):342–3. PubMed PMID: 12147403. Epub 2002/07/31. eng.

101. Fernandes LS, Tcheng JE, O'Shea JC, Weiner B, Lorenz TJ, Pacchiana C, et al. Is glycoprotein IIb/IIIa antagonism as effective in women as in men following percutaneous coronary intervention? Lessons from the ESPRIT study. J Am Coll Cardiol. 2002;40(6):1085–91. PubMed PMID: 12354432. Epub 2002/10/02. eng.

102. Ebbinghaus J, Maier B, Schoeller R, Schuhlen H, Theres H, Behrens S. Routine early invasive strategy and in-hospital mortality in women with non-ST-elevation myocardial infarction: results from the Berlin Myocardial Infarction Registry (BMIR). Int J Cardiol. 2012;158(1):78–82. PubMed PMID: 21277642. Epub 2011/02/01. eng.

103. Alexander KP, Chen AY, Roe MT, Newby LK, Gibson CM, Allen-LaPointe NM, et al. Excess dosing of antiplatelet and antithrombin agents in the treatment of non-ST-segment elevation acute coronary syndromes. JAMA. 2005;294(24):3108–16. PubMed PMID: 16380591. Epub 2005/12/29. eng.

104. Juul-Moller S, Edvardsson N, Jahnmatz B, Rosen A, Sorensen S, Omblus R. Double-blind trial of aspirin in primary prevention of myocardial infarction in patients with stable chronic angina pectoris. The Swedish Angina Pectoris Aspirin Trial (Sapat) Group. Lancet. 1992;340(8833):1421–5. PubMed PMID: 1360557. Epub 1992/12/12. eng.

105. Becker DM, Segal J, Vaidya D, Yanek LR, Herrera-Galeano JE, Bray PF, et al. Sex differences in platelet reactivity and response to low-dose aspirin therapy. JAMA. 2006;295(12):1420–7. PubMed PMID: 16551714. Epub 2006/03/23. eng.

106. Xhyheri B, Bugiardini R. Diagnosis and treatment of heart disease: are women different from men? Prog Cardiovasc Dis. 2010;53(3):227–36. PubMed PMID: 21130920. Epub 2010/12/07. eng.

107. Bugiardini R, Bairey Merz CN. Angina with "normal" coronary arteries: a changing philosophy. JAMA. 2005;293(4):477–84. PubMed PMID: 15671433. Epub 2005/01/27. eng.

108. Sadowski M, Gasior M, Gierlotka M, Janion M, Polonski L. Gender-related differences in mortality after ST-segment elevation myocardial infarction: a large multicentre national registry. EuroIntervention J EuroPCR Collaboration Working Group Interv Cardiol Eur Soc Cardiol. 2011;6(9):1068–72. PubMed PMID: 21518678. Epub 2011/04/27. eng.
109. Allen JK, Scott LB, Stewart KJ, Young DR. Disparities in women's referral to and enrollment in outpatient cardiac rehabilitation. J Gen Intern Med. 2004;19(7):747–53. PubMed PMID: 15209588. Pubmed Central PMCID: PMC1492482. Epub 2004/06/24. eng.

Part III
Cardiovascular Management

Chapter 10
Myocardial Infarction Diagnosis, Troponin Elevation and Angiographic Coronary Artery Disease

Arang Samim and John A. Ambrose

Abstract The advancements in technology and diagnostic studies in cardiology have helped the clinician but also resulted in sometimes confusing clinical pictures when attempting to diagnosis an acute MI. This chapter will review the use of cardiac biomarkers in the setting of the current universal definition of acute MI, the pitfalls in interpreting the cause of troponin elevations, and discuss controversies regarding AMI presentations when angiography reveals 'normal' coronary arteries.

Keywords Troponin • Universal Definition of Myocardial infarction • Microvascular dysfunction

Introduction

Acute myocardial infarction (AMI) has traditionally been defined as myocardial necrosis related to a supply demand mismatch which in the case of STEMI and most non STEMI is related to an acute reduction in blood supply due to a thrombotic total or near total occlusion of an epicardial artery. The terminology of AMI has changed over the last 40 years and with the routine use of sensitive biomarkers of myocardial necrosis such as high sensitivity troponins, the diagnosis of an AMI has likewise evolved. A Universal Definition of MI was introduced in 2007 in an attempt to provide some standardization to diagnosis particularly in the era of the sensitive troponin assays [1]. Of the five types of AMI included in this definition (Table 10.1), the

A. Samim, MD
UCSF-Fresno Medical Education Program, Department of Cardiology, University of California, Fresno, CA, USA
e-mail: asamim@fresno.ucsf.edu

J.A. Ambrose, MD (✉)
Chief of Cardiology, UCSF Fresno, Fresno, CA, USA

Department of Medicine, UCSF Community Regional Medical Center, Fresno, CA, USA

© Springer International Publishing Switzerland 2015
J.A. Ambrose, A.E. Rodríguez (eds.), *Controversies in Cardiology*,
DOI 10.1007/978-3-319-20415-4_10

Table 10.1 Universal classification of myocardial infarction

Type 1: Spontaneous myocardial infarction
Spontaneous myocardial infarction related to atherosclerotic plaque rupture, ulceration, erosion, or dissection with resulting intraluminal thrombus in one or more of the coronary arteries leading to decreased myocardial blood flow or distal platelet emboli with ensuing myocyte necrosis. The patient may have underlying severe CAD but on occasion non-obstructive or no CAD.

Type 2: Myocardial infarction secondary to an ischemic imbalance
In instances of myocardial injury with necrosis where a condition other than CAD contributes to an imbalance between myocardial oxygen supply and/or demand, e.g. coronary endothelial dysfunction, coronary artery spasm, coronary embolism, tachy-/brady-arrhythmias, anemia, respiratory failure, hypotension, and hypertension with or without LVH.

Type 3: Myocardial infarction resulting in death when biomarker values are unavailable
Cardiac death with symptoms suggestive of myocardial ischemia and presumed new ischemic ECG changes or new LBBB, but death occurring before blood samples could be obtained, before cardiac biomarker could rise, or in rare cases, cardiac biomarkers were not collected.

Type 4a: Myocardial infarction related to percutaneous coronary intervention (PCI)
Myocardial infarction associated with PCI is arbitrarily defined by elevation of cTn values 5×99th percentile URL in patients with normal baseline values (99th percentile URL) or a rise of cTn values 20 % if the baseline values are elevated and are stable or falling. In addition, either (i) symptoms suggestive of myocardial ischemia, or (ii) new ischemic ECG changes or new LBBB, or (iii) angiographic loss of patency of a major coronary artery or a side branch or persistent slow- or no-flow or embolization, or (iv) imaging demonstration of new loss of viable myocardium or new regional wall motion abnormality are required.

Type 4b: Myocardial infarction related to stent thrombosis
Myocardial infarction associated with stent thrombosis is detected by coronary angiography or autopsy in the setting of myocardial ischemia and with a rise and/ or fall of cardiac biomarkers values with at least one value above the 99th percentile URL.

Type 5: Myocardial infarction related to coronary artery bypass grafting (CABG)
Myocardial infarction associated with CABG is arbitrarily defined by elevation of cardiac biomarker values 10×99th percentile URL in patients with normal baseline cTn values (99th percentile URL). In addition, either (i) new pathological Q waves or new LBBB, or (ii) angiographic documented new graft or new native coronary artery occlusion, or (iii) imaging evidence of new loss of viable myocardium or new regional wall motion abnormality.

clinician if frequently confronted with the following scenario: the patient who presents to the emergency room with clinical symptoms that might be ischemic and has an elevated troponin. Is this an AMI or is the troponin increase related to another possible mechanism? Furthermore, in patients who meet criteria for AMI, angiography does not always reveal significant epicardial disease. This chapter discusses the diagnosis of AMI, troponin elevation and angiographic coronary artery disease. How often is the angiogram "normal" and what are the potential mechanisms? Also, how often does a positive troponin meet criteria for AMI?

Diagnosing an AMI in the Era of the Sensitive Troponin Assay

Prior to the era of coronary angiography and revascularization, AMI had been predominantly a clinical diagnosis based on symptoms and classic electrocardiographic changes. The pathology in non survivors showed evidence of coagulation necrosis of the myocardium corresponding to the detection of occlusive coronary thrombosis of an epicardial coronary artery, with the degree of necrosis or reparative changes correlating to the time between onset of AMI and death [2]. Clinically, chemical biomarkers were introduced and added to the accuracy of diagnosis. Initially, serum glutamic oxaloacetic transaminase (also known as aspartate transaminase) was used as a biomarker of myocardial injury [3]. However, this was neither sensitive nor specific for myocardial injury, only to be replaced by lactate dehydrogenase (LDH) or creatine kinase, both of which also lacked specificity for the myocardium [3]. The search for a more specific marker for myocardial injury lead to discovery of the creatinine kinase myocardial band (CKMB) isoenzyme and then the troponin proteins [3, 4]. Troponins have essentially replaced all other biomarkers and they have now become the standard laboratory screening test for cardiac disease. The troponin assays have improved over time and now the current fourth generation troponin assays have excellent sensitivity.

With such a sensitive test, the troponin assay has become a ubiquitous test for myocardial disease. Yet, the clinical picture of many patients with elevated serum troponin levels was not consistent with AMI. Over the years, the definition of a true AMI has been redefined to incorporate the use of these more sensitive biomarkers and reflect not simply just an elevated troponin level. The first Global MI Task Force convened in 2000 to reach a consensus on the definition of a myocardial infarction. The most recent iteration of this was the third Universal Definition of myocardial infarction, a consensus expert statement in 2012, endorsed by the ACC, ESC, AHA, and the WHF [5].

While it is understood that myocardial infarctions involved myocardial necrosis due to myocardial ischemia, the Universal Definition of myocardial infarction delineated the spectrum of etiologies. It has become apparent that elevated cardiac biomarkers were present in disease states other than classical acute coronary syndromes. This definition, as mentioned above, categorized MI into five subtypes in order to sort out all the known clinical presentations. A type I MI was a spontaneous myocardial infarction due to an acute disturbance within the coronary arterial tree [5]. This can be due to atherosclerotic plaque rupture, erosion or a calcified nodule with superimposed thrombosis. This is the usual scenario in a patient with obstructive coronary artery disease but occasionally a type 1 MI was seen with no apparent significant atherosclerotic disease on angiography as will be discussed later.

With its superior sensitivity, the preferred biomarker for diagnosing AMI, as already alluded to, is now troponin. Both troponin I and T are used and the commonly utilized assays are very sensitive for even minute quantities of myocardial necrosis. However, the more sensitive the test, the less specific they have become. While assays for CKMB have not changed appreciably over the years, the new era of troponin assays has advanced with improved detection of myocardial necrosis. Troponin assays are ever evolving in precision and biochemical research is steering to even more sophisticated laboratory testing. At our institution, the assay for troponin T was changed about 7 years ago. The new assay for high sensitivity troponin I (TnI-Ultra assay on the ADVIA Centaur XP immunoanalyzer, Siemens Healthcare Diagnostics) was about 25 times more sensitive than the prior assay with an upper reference level for the new assay of .04 ngs/ml. The ever changing spectrum of biochemical analysis of cardiac biomarkers created a need for standardization of nomenclature and interpretation of results. The International Federation of Clinical Chemistry and Laboratory Medicine (IFCC) task force on clinical applications of cardiac biomarkers standardized the nomenclature so various assays can be considered a 'high-sensitivity' troponin assay if the total imprecision (coefficient of variance) was <10 % at the 99th percentile value in the population of interest [4]. Furthermore, the assay should attain measureable concentrations for samples below the 99th percentile, above the assays limit of detection in at least 50 % of healthy individuals [4].

As such, elevated troponin I levels are sensitive to detect myocardial necrosis, but there remains controversy whether small rises in troponin signify myocyte infarction versus reversible ischemia or other mechanisms. It has been shown that troponin levels may rise above the 99th percentile in patients undergoing rigorous exercise [6]. Complimenting this idea was data that perhaps measurable troponin levels can be induced during routine stress testing. The TIMI 35 group published data demonstrating detectable levels of troponin I in patients undergoing exercise stress testing who had positive ischemic responses [7]. The proposed theory for these small elevations in troponin include changes in cell membrane permeability with release of free troponin from the cytosol, which accounts for about 5 % of the total myocyte troponin [8]. Other proposed mechanisms of troponin release in patients who do not meet clinical criteria for myocardial infarction included apoptosis, cellular release of proteolytic products, increased cell wall permeability with stress or stretch and the production of membranous blebs containing troponin [9, 10]. However, the counter argument is that this small troponin elevation still reflects minute levels of myocyte necrosis [11].

Regardless of the sensitivity of the assay, no biochemical test alone will help the clinician determine the diagnosis. While the primary concern is that of an acute coronary syndrome, there are multiple other conditions associated with (or causing) elevated troponin values (Table 10.2). Some patients will meet criteria for AMI that are not related to an acute disturbance within the epicardial coronary arterial tree, but rather due to another cause for a supply demand mismatch. This has been designated as a type 2 MI by the Universal Definition [5]. Common causes include severe anemia, a hypertensive crisis, severe aortic valve disease, tachyarrhythmias and sepsis. Still there are other causes of troponin elevation that appear in low levels and do not clinically meet the current definition of AMI (a rise and /or fall in troponin and clinical evidence of ischemia related to symptoms, ECG changes or new wall motion abnormalities). Several conditions including pulmonary embolism, congestive heart failure, acute neurological disease and renal failure can elevate troponin levels but do not meet diagnostic criteria.

As the number of positives increased with the newer assay at our institution, there was a marked increase in the number of consults to cardiology given the routine use of measuring troponin levels for patients presenting with suspected cardiac–related symptoms. We then performed a study to evaluate how often a positive troponin met criteria for AMI utilizing the Universal Definition [12]. Of the four definitions included in the Universal Definition document, the criteria utilized

Table 10.2 Causes of (or conditions associated with) elevated troponin

Coronary Plaque rupture
Intraluminal coronary artery thrombus formation
Tachy-/brady-arrhythmias
Aortic dissection or severe aortic valve disease
Hypertrophic cardiomyopathy
Cardiogenic, hypovolemic, or septic shock
Severe respiratory failure
Severe anemia
Hypertension with or without LVH
Coronary spasm
Coronary embolism or vasculitis
Coronary endothelial dysfunction without significant CAD
Cardiac contusion, surgery, ablation, pacing, or defibrillator shocks
Rhabdomyolysis with cardiac involvement
Myocarditis
Cardiotoxic agents, e.g. anthracyclines, herceptin
Heart failure
Stress (Takotsubo) cardiomyopathy
Severe pulmonary embolism or pulmonary hypertension
Sepsis and critically ill patients
Renal failure
Severe acute neurological diseases, e.g. stroke, subarachnoid
Hemorrhage
Infiltrative diseases, e.g. amyloidosis, sarcoidosis
Strenuous exercise

was a rise and/or fall in troponin related to the upper reference level along with clinical evidence of ischemia related to either typical symptoms, ECG changes, new pathologic Q waves and/or new wall motion abnormalities. All patients with troponin measurements were evaluated and those with a positive result were interviewed. Over 90 % of troponin measurements were initiated by the emergency department and this study did not routinely measure troponin after PCI or CABG. The results showed that only about 30 % of patients with a positive troponin met the universal definition of myocardial infarction and only about 2/3 s of those with an infarct could be classified as a type I MI (Fig. 10.1) Thus, approximately 70 % of positive troponins at our institution during the study period did not meet AMI criteria according to the Universal Definition [12].

Since the majority of patients found to have an elevated troponin level do not meet criteria for AMI, it is important to avoid clinically labeling these patients as such. For example, a patient admitted with severe sepsis found to have a slightly elevated troponin levels may recover from illness and may not be subsequently discharged on the standard cardiac regimen of beta blockers, statins and aspirin. In the era of electronic health records and quality of care indicators, the physician and/or hospital may be penalized if AMI is documented as a discharge diagnosis.

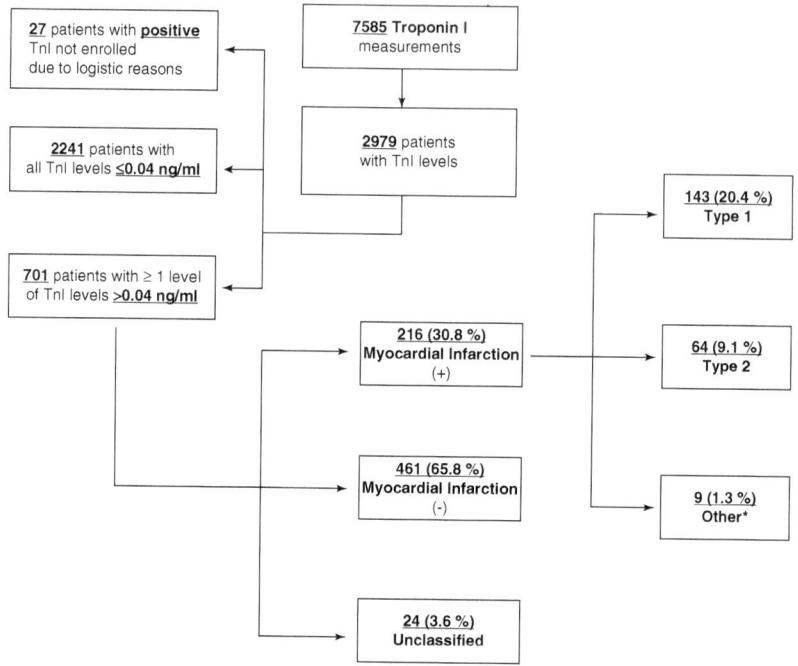

Fig. 10.1 Frequency of elevated Troponin I and diagnosis of AMI. * Includes Types 3 and 4 myocardial infarction. *TnI* Troponin I (From Javed et al. [12], with permission of Elsevier)

Furthermore, there are medical-legal implications when someone is labelled as having presumed ischemic heart disease. Thus, due to the ubiquitous use of the troponin assay in common clinical practice, we believe that this example and other such cases should be documented as a troponin elevation without AMI without ascribing a specific case.

A further unresolved issue is how does one diagnosis a type 2 MI? Sometimes the clinical situation precludes differentiation from a type I vs a type 2 MI. While it is practical in some cases to pursue noninvasive assessment with stress echocardiography or nuclear myocardial perfusion imaging, we prefer visualization of the coronary arteries for most cases to document the presence of significant coronary disease. In a subsequent study comparing the angiographic findings in type 1 versus type 2 MI, angiography in patients with a type 2 MI produced a bimodal distribution as they usually had either normal appearing coronary arteries, or severe multivessel CAD [13]. Accordingly, if normal or non-obstructive coronary arteries are visualized without an acute culprit lesion, we believe this speaks in favor of a type 2 MI. Likewise, severe CAD without a defined culprit and in the presence of an obvious supply/demand external perturbation will more likely be type 2. The treatment of such patients is open to debate, but we believe that if there is no evidence of CAD on angiography then treatment should focus on the underlying cause and acute anticoagulation is not necessary. Those with severe CAD should be treated with the appropriate guideline-based optimal medical therapies in addition to the precipitating cause. More data in the future are needed in these cases.

Of all the subtypes of myocardial infarction, the definition of a type 4a is perhaps the most widely debated. In the era of percutaneous coronary intervention, research registries and clinicians alike have noted increases in troponin levels above the 99th percentile of the upper reference limit (URL) commonly on routine measurement after uncomplicated PCI. Often, the troponin elevation will not result in clinical evidence of ischemia and is of uncertain prognostic relevance. The writing committee on the third universal definition attempted to refine this further by using the cutoff value of a fivefold increase in troponin concentration above the 99th percentile of the URL in addition to either evidence of clinical ischemia, new angiographic evidence of flow limitation or imaging evidence of a new loss of viable myocardium [5]. However, this definition was arbitrarily defined and there is no consensus that this designation affects long term prognosis. Some even argue that a much higher cut-off be established to avoid unnecessarily labeling patients as having a periprocedural complication [14]. Further discussion of this issue is beyond the scope of this chapter.

One last consideration on the Universal Definition of myocardial infarction is that the distinction between a type 1 versus a type 2 MI versus a non infarct (no clinical evidence) is not, in all situations, crystal clear. There are cases that appear to overlap and a diagnosis cannot be definitively established. The physician must then decide, on the best available evidence, how this patient is to be managed.

AMI and Angiographically Normal Coronary Arteries

There is an appreciable subset of patients who meet clinical criteria for the diagnosis of myocardial infarction yet have little or no angiographic evidence of coronary artery disease. At our institution, our prospective evaluation of 224 patients with AMI revealed that 10 % of patients with an apparent type 1 NSTEMI had non obstructive or normal coronary arteries on angiography, including 1.4 % of patients with a diagnosis of STEMI [13]. Other studies have found a similar incidence on angiography in men with NSTEMI with higher rates found in women [15–18]. How is it that with such rigorously defined criteria for AMI can the angiogram be non-diagnostic?

AMI with "normal" coronary arteries reflects a heterogeneous group of clinical syndromes, as listed in Table 10.3. As often seen clinically, a type 2 MI will occur in the setting of an imbalance of blood supply to myocardial demand precipitated by various medical illnesses. This diagnosis can occur with or without significant epicardial disease. Aside from a type 2 MI, one of the oldest appreciated causes of MI with or without angiographic coronary disease is the phenomenon of coronary vasospasm. Initially described by Myron Prinzmetal in the 1950s, coronary vasospasm is an intense vasoconstriction of the epicardial coronary arteries that can cause total or subtotal vessel occlusion. While the initial reports involved patients with severe

Table 10.3 Causes of acute myocardial infarction with normal coronary arteries

Type II myocardial infarction
Coronary artery vasospasm (Prinzmetal angina)
Embolic phenomena (paradoxical embolus, endocarditis, mural thrombus, etc.)
Spontaneous coronary artery dissection
Myocarditis
Plaque rupture in 'normal' appearing coronary arteries
Flush occlusion of a coronary side branch
Microvascular coronary dysfunction
Taokotsubo cardiomyopathy
Cardiotoxic agents, anthracyclines, herceptin, cocaine
Autoimmune vasculitis
Coronary thrombosis *in situ* with spontaneous lysis
Hypertrophic cardiomyopathy
Infiltrative disease, e.g. amyloidosis, sarcoidosis

proximal CAD, subsequent reports occurred in the absence of epicardial disease on angiography [19]. Symptoms can vary on the degree of vasoconstriction and may lead to AMI and even sudden death. However, often the vasoconstriction is transient and by the time the patient reaches angiography the vasospastic episode may have terminated. Spontaneous vasospasm alone on a coronary artery without angiographic narrowing is an uncommon cause for AMI in the United States although cocaine or methamphetamine-induced vasospasm of the epicardial or microvasculature leading to an AMI is not that uncommon.

Another uncommon cause of AMI and normal angiographic coronaries can be embolic phenomena to the coronaries. This can be seen in left sided valvular heart disease including endocarditis, left atrial or LV mural thrombus, left atrial myxoma, aortic valve fibroelastoma or with a patent foramen ovale. Of course, if the patient is studied acutely, there can be an acute cut off usually in a distal epicardial vessel without any other evidence of angiographic disease elsewhere. Angiographic misdiagnosis is another possible cause related to severe ostial stenosis or flush occlusions of an epicardial branch vessel. Takotsubo cardiomyopathy may also masquerade as AMI. If fact in one recent study, up to 6 % of post-menopausal women who presented with an AMI based on the Universal Definition, met criteria for definite or probable takotsubo cardiomyopathy [20]. Other cardiomyopathies, such as hypertrophic obstructive cardiomyopathy, cardiac amyloidosis or sarcoidosis may present with AMI. Even patients who are alcoholics, classically thought to be protective of ischemic heart disease, can present with crushing chest pain and STEMI yet have normal or non-obstructive coronary artery disease. In fact, a post mortem studies on alcoholic patients with AMI showed evidence of acute transmural infarction and regional scar formation [21]. These patients had no other systemic illness and all but one had normal complete blood counts. Evaluation of their coronary arteries showed normal or minimal obstructive coronary disease but did show evidence of periarterial fibrosis of unclear significance [21].

Years ago, patients who presented with chest pain consistent with angina pectoris yet had normal coronary arteries on angiography became a recognized entity with unclear significance. These patients were labelled as 'Cardiac Syndrome X'. As it was more prevalent in women, it was thought to pose a benign prognosis [22]. However, cardiac syndrome x represents a heterogeneous group of patients. Often times, the clinical symptoms of chest pain were later revealed to be non-cardiac in nature. These patients were found to have GI pathology, anxiety or pulmonary etiologies of their chest pain. As our understanding and definition of AMI evolved and these confounding patients were teased out, there still remained patients who had angina, objective evidence of ischemia by stress testing, yet non obstructive coronary artery disease. Data from the National Heart, Lung and Blood institute sponsored the Women's Ischemia Syndrome Evaluation (WISE) study demonstrated that patients with the triad of angina, abnormal stress testing and non-obstructive coronary artery disease on angiography had microvascular coronary dysfunction using coronary reactivity testing (CRT) [23, 24]. CRT is an invasive test during angiography, incorporating the use of vasoactive substances such as acetylcholine, adenosine and nitroglycerin to test coronary flow reserve on the microvascular level [25]. Therefore, the term cardiac syndrome x has become an out of date classification and if patients truly suffer from microvascular coronary dysfunction, then it is important to treat these patients accordingly as data show these patients have a 2.5 % annual risk of adverse cardiac events including MI, stroke, congestive heart failure or death [26].

While coronary microvascular dysfunction has become more appreciated as an etiology in patients presenting with exertional symptoms and carries an increased risk of future myocardial infarction, what about patients who present with what appears to be a typical type 1 STEMI or NSTEMI? One expects a significant obstructive lesion, whether it is either related to plaque rupture, erosion or a calcified nodule with a superimposed thrombus. However, as mentioned previously, in some studies, up to 10 % of patients and possibly up to 25 % of women who present with acute coronary syndrome have no obstructive coronary artery disease on coronary angiography [15–18]. Although this has been recognized for several years, there is little information on possible pathophysiology on how this could occur. Some have suggested these patient may have had vasospasm, while others thought it due to endothelial dysfunction or takotsubo syndrome.

One of the few objective studies on this entity was performed by Reynolds et al. [27]. They prospectively evaluated all women who presented to the hospital with AMI per the universal definition of MI. Patients who had obstructive CAD or had recent vasospastic agent use (i.e. cocaine) were excluded. Eligible patients underwent intravascular ultrasound at the time of angiography and also cardiac MRI within 7 days of angiography. Fifty women were fully eligible and enrolled in the study. The suspected culprit vessel, based on electrocardiographic and wall motion evidence was studied with IVUS. Thirty-eight percent of patients were found to have plaque disruption by IVUS. Although there were no obstructive angiographic lesions, plaque rupture was found only in patients with some degree, albeit mild, of angiographic coronary artery disease and not in any patients with completely normal appearing angiograms. Of the patients that continued enrollment and underwent cardiac MRI, 39 % had at least one area of late gadolinium enhancement, correlating to the territory of infarction. Interestingly, out of the 14 patients with IVUS proven plaque rupture, only one of these patients had late gadolinium enhancement (LGE) but the majority had T2 signal hyperintensity, indicative of acute myocardial edema [27]. Among the 22 patients without any IVUS evidence of plaque rupture, 11 had LGE on cardiac MRI (Fig. 10.2). Thus, plaque rupture appears to be not uncommonly found in women who present with signs and symptoms suggesting a type 1 MI and yet with non-obstructive CAD. However, due to the limitations of angiography in evaluating atherosclerosis and positive remodeling, many of these

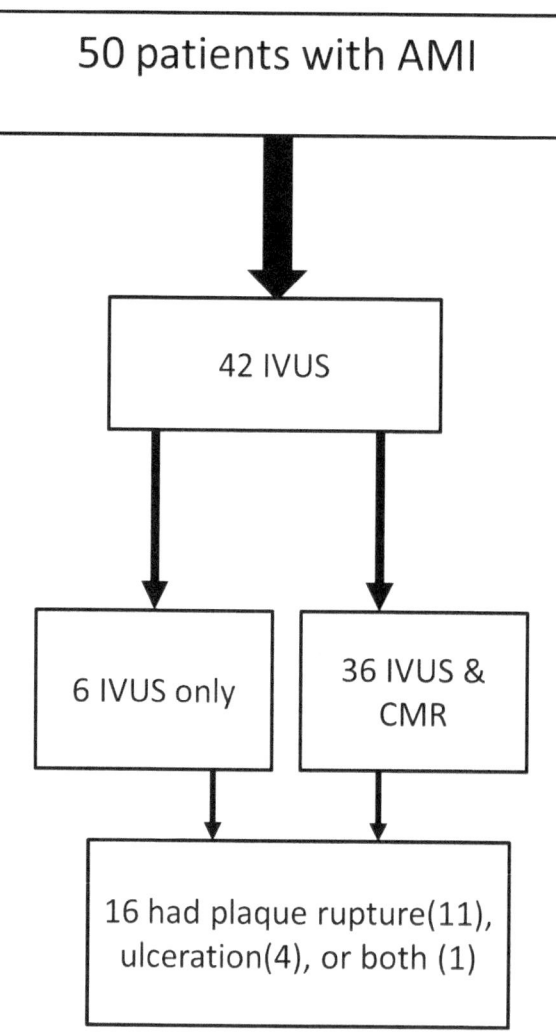

Fig. 10.2 Proportion of plaque disruption in women presenting with AMI [27]. *AMI* acute myocardial infarction, *IVUS* intravascular ultrasound, *CMR* cardiac magnetic resonance

lesions do not appear significant on luminal coronary angiography and require intravascular imaging to appreciate the lesion. But the fact that the majority of ischemic appearing LGE images on CMR corresponded to patients without any plaque disruption on IVUS point to possible other clinical syndromes such as microvascular coronary dysfunction, occult plaque disruption not visible with IVUS or possibly other etiologies yet to be identified.

Conclusions

Our evolving understanding of atherosclerotic coronary artery disease and the pathophysiology of myocyte necrosis has pioneered many advances in diagnosis and treatment of ischemic heart disease, but it has also exposed several areas of uncertainties. Based on the above discussion, we conclude the following:

1. The Universal Definition of AMI has helped clarify the diagnosis and etiology of AMI in the era of sensitive troponin assays.
2. Most troponin elevations do not meet criteria for AMI.
3. The diagnosis and treatment of type 2 MI is still unresolved. We believe that coronary angiography is necessary in most cases to rule out significant coronary artery disease in order to properly guide therapy, although more data in this area are needed.
4. When a myocardial infarction is diagnosed clinically but there is normal or non-obstructive coronary arteries, the diagnosis can still be elusive. These cases may require intravascular imaging and/or advanced non-invasive imaging such as cardiac MRI or CT angiography to elucidate a diagnosis as the appropriate treatment relies, in part, on establishing the causative etiology.

References

1. Thygesen K, Alpert JS, White HD, et al. Universal definition of myocardial infarction. Circulation. 2007;116:2634–53.
2. Pasotti M, et al. The pathology of myocardial infarction in the pre- and post-interventional era. Heart. 2006;92(11):1552–6.
3. Jaffe AS, Babuin L, Apple FS. Biomarkers in acute cardiac disease. J Am Coll Cardiol. 2006;48:1–11.
4. Apple FS, Collinson PO, IFCC Task Force on Clinical Applications of Cardiac Biomarkers. Analytical characteristics of high-sensitivity cardiac troponin assays. Clin Chem. 2012;58:54–61.
5. Thygesen K, Alpert JS, Jaffe AS, et al. Third universal definition of myocardial infarction. Circulation. 2012;126:2020–35.
6. Shave R, Baggish A, George K, et al. Exercise-induced cardiac troponin elevation: evidence, mechanisms, and implications. J Am Coll Cardiol. 2010;56:169–76.
7. Sabatine MS, Morrow DA, de Lemos JA, et al. Detection of acute changes in circulating troponin in the setting of transient stress test-induced myocardial ischaemia using an ultrasensitive assay: results from TIMI 35. Eur Heart J. 2009;30:162–9.

8. Katus HA, Remppis A, Scheffold T, Diederich KW, Kuebler W. Intracellular compartmentation of cardiac troponin T and its release kinetics in patients with reperfused and nonreperfused myocardial infarction. Am J Cardiol. 1991;67:1360–7.

9. Jaffe AS, Ravkilde J, Roberts R, Naslund U, Apple FS, Galvani M, Katus H. It's time for a change to a troponin standard. Circulation. 2000;102:1216–20.

10. Schwartz P, Piper HM, Spahr R, Spieckermann PG. Ultrastructure of cultured adult myocardial cells during anoxia and reoxygenation. Am J Pathol. 1984;115:349–61.

11. White HD. Pathobiology of troponin elevations: do elevations occur with myocardial ischemia as well as necrosis? J Am Coll Cardiol. 2011;57:2406–8.

12. Javed U, Aftab W, Ambrose JA, et al. Frequency of elevated troponin I and diagnosis of acute myocardial infarction. Am J Cardiol. 2009;104:9–13.

13. Ambrose JA, Loures-Vale A, Javed U, Buhari CF, Aftab W. Angiographic correlates in type 1 and 2 MI by the universal definition. JACC Cardiovasc Imaging. 2012;5:463–4.

14. Moussa ID, Klein LW, et al. Consideration of a new definition of clinically relevant myocardial infarction after coronary revascularization: an expert consensus document from the Society for Cardiovascular Angiography and Interventions (SCAI). Catheter Cardiovasc Interv. 2014;83(1):27–36.

15. Hochman JS, Tamis JE, Thompson TD, Weaver WD, White HD, VandeWerf F, Aylward P, Topol EJ, Califf RM. Sex, clinical presentation, and outcome in patients with acute coronary syndromes. N Engl J Med. 1999;341:226–32.

16. Gehrie ER, Reynolds HR, et al. Characterization and outcomes of women and men with non-ST-segment elevation myocardial infarction and nonobstructive coronary artery disease: results of the CRUSADE quality improvement initiative. Am Heart J. 2009;158:688–94.

17. Berger JS, Elliott L, et al. Sex differences in mortality following acute coronary syndromes. JAMA. 2009;302:874–82.

18. Chokshi NP, Iqbal SN, Berger RL, Hochman JS, Feit F, Slater JN, Pena-Sing I, Yatskar L, Keller NM, Babaev A, Attubato MJ, Reynolds HR. Sex and race are associated with the absence of epicardial coronary artery obstructive disease at angiography in patients with acute coronary syndromes. Clin Cardiol. 2010;33:495–501.

19. Hung MJ, Hu P, Hung M. Coronary artery spasm: review and update. Int J Med Sci. 2014;11:1161–71.

20. Sy F, Basraon J, Zheng H, Singh M, Richina J, Ambrose JA. Frequency of Takotsubo cardiomyopathy in postmenopausal women presenting with an acute coronary syndrome. Am J Cardiol. 2013;112:479–82.

21. Regan TJ, Wu CF, Weisse AB, et al. Acute myocardial infarction in toxic cardiomyopathy without coronary obstruction. Circulation. 1975;51:453–61.

22. Pasternak RC, Thibault GE, Savoia M, DeSanctis RW, Hutter AM. Chest pain with angiographically insignificant coronary arterial obstruction. Clinical presentation and long-term follow-up. Am J Med. 1980;68:813–7.

23. Reis SE, Holubkov R, Conrad Smith AJ, Kelsey SF, Sharaf BL, Reichek N, Rogers WJ, Merz CN, Sopko G, Pepine CJ; WISE Investigators. Coronary microvascular dysfunction is highly prevalent in women with chest pain in the absence of coronary artery disease: results from the NHLBI WISE study. Am Heart J. 2001;141(5):735–41.

24. Johnson BD, Shaw LJ, Buchthal SD, et al. Prognosis in women with myocardial ischemia in the absence of obstructive coronary disease, Results from the National Institutes of Health-National Heart, Lung, and Blood Institute-sponsored Women's Ischemia Syndrome Evaluation (WISE). Circulation. 2004;109:2993–9.

25. Samim A, Nugent L, Mehta PK, Shufelt C, Bairey Merz CN. Treatment of angina and microvascular coronary dysfunction. Curr Treat Options Cardiovasc Med. 2010;12(4):355–64.

26. Johnson BD, Shaw LJ, Pepine CJ, et al. Persistent chest pain predicts cardiovascular events in women without obstructive coronary artery disease: results from the NIH-NHLBI-sponsored Women's Ischaemia Syndrome Evaluation (WISE) study. Eur Heart J. 2006;27:1408–15.

27. Reynolds HR, Srichai MB, Iqbal SN, Slater JN, John GB. Mechanisms of myocardial infarction in women without angiographically obstructive coronary artery disease. Circulation. 2011;124:1414–25.

Chapter 11
New Therapeutic Options for Patients with Refractory Angina

Luís Henrique Wolff Gowdak and Eulógio E. Martinez

Abstract Despite the indisputable advances in medical treatment and revascularization procedures (percutaneous and surgical), many patients present debilitating symptoms related to myocardial ischemia which cannot be controlled by a combination of antianginal drugs due to progression of disease with arterial occlusion and diffuse involvement of previous grafts or post-angioplasty restenosis, preventing new attempts of myocardial revascularization. This condition is defined as refractory angina, which greatly impairs the quality of life of the affected. Recently, new therapeutic strategies are being either developed or already applied for the treatment of patients with refractory angina, including gene therapy, stem cell therapy, transmyocardial laser revascularization, enhanced external counterpulsation, spinal cord stimulation, and extracorporeal shockwave myocardial revascularization. However, many of the above techniques are still surrounded by a shadow of controversy, conflicting results between the basic science and clinical application, mixed feelings from the scientific community regarding their usefulness (beyond the placebo effect), and the appropriateness of the conducted clinical trials in which they have been tested. Common challenges in the field are, for example, the fact that there is no experimental model that exactly mimics the condition seen in patients with diffuse CAD; many promising new therapies, i.e. gene therapy, have succeeded in animal models of myocardial ischemia only to fail when rigorously tested in double-blind, placebo controlled trials. Finally, the scientific community should truly be committed regarding the rigor with which data are obtained and presented, so that science may steadily advance towards finding better, proven treatment options for patients with refractory angina.

L.H.W. Gowdak, MD, PhD, FESC
Laboratory of Genetics and Molecular Cardiology, Heart Institute, São Paulo, SP, Brazil
e-mail: luis.gowdak@incor.usp.br

E.E. Martinez, MD (✉)
Federal University of São Paulo Medical School, São Paulo, SP, Brazil

Department of Cardiac Catheterization and Interventional Cardiology, Hospital do Coração (HCor), São Paulo, SP, Brazil

Catheterization and Interventional Cardiology, Heart Institute (InCor), São Paulo, SP, Brazil

University of São Paulo, São Paulo, SP, Brazil

© Springer International Publishing Switzerland 2015
J.A. Ambrose, A.E. Rodríguez (eds.), *Controversies in Cardiology*,
DOI 10.1007/978-3-319-20415-4_11

147

Keywords Angina • Treatment • Gene therapy • Stem cell therapy • Laser • Shockwave • Counterpulsation • Neurostimulation

Introduction

Cardiovascular disease (CVD) is the leading cause of death worldwide. The World Health Organization [1] estimates that CVD alone was responsible for approximately 17.5 million deaths in 2012 (or 31.4 % of all deaths in that year). CVD deaths are mainly due to ischemic heart disease (7.3 million deaths) or stroke (6.7 million deaths).

One of the most common manifestations associated with ischemic heart disease (IHD) is stable coronary artery disease (CAD), which can be translated clinically by chest discomfort (or equivalent) evoked by different levels of physical activity depending on the extent of the disease. In the United States, approximately 7.8 million people live with the diagnosis of angina pectoris [2].

Despite the indisputable advances in medical treatment and revascularization procedures (percutaneous and surgical), many patients will present debilitating symptoms related to myocardial ischemia which cannot be controlled by a combination of antianginal drugs due to progression of disease with arterial occlusion and diffuse involvement of previous grafts or post-angioplasty restenosis, preventing new attempts of myocardial revascularization. This condition is defined as refractory angina [3]. The estimated annual incidence of patients with refractory angina is between 50,000 and 200,000 new cases in the United States [4] and between 30,000 and 100,000 in Europe [5]. Currently, between 600,000 and 1.8 million individuals are living with refractory angina in the United States [6].

The hallmark of this condition is the great impairment of quality of life [7, 8]. Their goal is to be able to perform any physical activity (no matter how trivial it seems like walking a few meters or even bathing) without anginal pain. Some patients are frequently awakened during the night by angina. Presently, all major Cardiology Societies (American Heart Association and American College of Cardiology [9], Canadian Cardiovascular Society [10] and the European Society of Cardiology [5]) acknowledge the need to seek new therapeutic strategies for this growing population of patients in whom maximally tolerated conventional treatment has failed. For these patients, the primary goal of treatment is to improve quality of life, to increase exercise tolerance, and to decrease the need for hospitalization and diagnostic or therapeutic procedures. In this chapter, we will briefly discuss the main non-pharmacological therapeutic strategies being either developed or already applied for the treatment of patients with refractory angina (Table 11.1) and consider any unrvesolved or controversial areas in therapy.

It is important to note, however, that many of the above techniques are still surrounded by a shadow of controversy, conflicting results between the basic science and clinical application, mixed feelings from the scientific community regarding their usefulness (beyond the placebo effect), and the appropriateness of the conducted clinical trials in which they have been tested. Table 11.2 shows a few examples of the controversial issues to be explored in the corresponding sessions in this Chapter.

Table 11.1 New therapeutic options for patients with refractory angina

Therapy	Current status for clinical use (class of recommendation/level of evidence)
Gene therapy	Investigational
Stem cell therapy	Investigational
Transmyocardial laser revascularization	Approved (IIb/B)[a]
Enhanced external counter-pulsation	Approved (IIb/B)[a] (IIa/B)[b]
Spinal cord stimulation	Approved (IIb/C)[a] (IIb/B)[b]
Extracorporeal shockwave myocardial revascularization	Approved in a few countries in Europe and Asia
	Investigational in the USA

[a]According to the American Heart Association/American College of Cardiology Guidelines
[b]According to the European Society of Cardiology Guidelines

Table 11.2 Controversial issues in therapeutic options for patients with refractory angina

Therapy	Controversy/unresolved issues
Gene therapy	Conflicting results between experimental models (success) and clinical application (disappointment)
	Moved to fast from bench to bedside (!)
	Placebo effect (?)
Stem cell therapy	Conflicting results between experimental models (success) and clinical application (failure or modest benefit)
	Moved to fast from bench to bedside (!)
	Placebo effect (?)
	Unanswered "burning" questions: best cell? Dosage? Route for delivery? Which patient? Long-term safety profile?
	The "miracle cure" for almost every disease known to man (false advertisement without robust scientific support)
Transmyocardial laser revascularization	Placebo effect (?)
	Class IIb/B in the USA versus a class III in Europe
Enhanced external counter-pulsation	Reduction in MACE (?)
Spinal cord stimulation	Reduction in MACE (?)
	Mechanism of action (?)
Extracorporeal shockwave myocardial revascularization	Placebo effect (?)
	Lack of randomized, double-blind, placebo-controlled, properly sized trial

Gene Therapy

Gene therapy can be defined as a medical intervention for transferring genetic material to somatic cells *in vivo*, allowing the *in situ* expression of the transferred gene [11] with therapeutic effect. Administration of therapeutic genes requires the use of a vehicle, called a vector, capable of carrying the gene of interest and guiding it to the target cell, thereby facilitating the transfer of genetic material into somatic cells [12] (Fig. 11.1).

The accumulation of knowledge about vascular growth and angiogenic cytokines and the parallel development of more efficient vectors allowed for testing the hypothesis that gene transfer of growth factors could mitigate the damage from myocardial ischemia by stimulating vascular growth, a strategy known as therapeutic angiogenesis [12].

From the late 1990s, many researchers including Losordo et al. [13], Symes et al. [14], Rosengart et al. [15] and others reported the results of the $VEGF_{165}$ gene transfer by direct intramyocardial injection in patients with refractory angina. During follow-up, they were able to document a significant reduction in the number of angina attacks, a significant decrease in the number of hypoperfused myocardial segments, and an increased Rentrop score (number of collateral vessels) in all patients. No procedure-related adverse effects were observed.

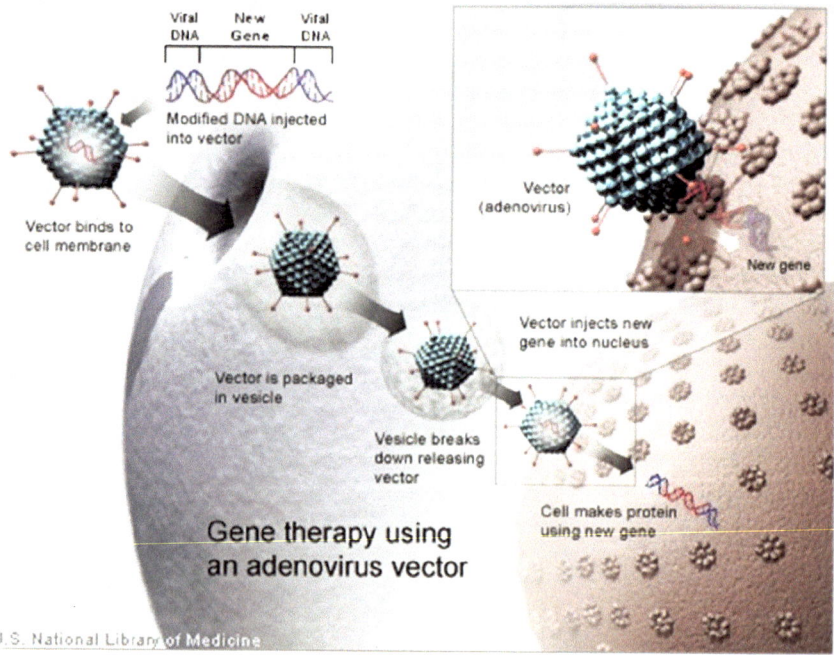

Fig. 11.1 Gene therapy using a modified virus as a vector for gene transfer into somatic cells (Source: United States National Library of Medicine)

Later on, the AGENT (*Angiogenic Gene Therapy*) trial [16], the first multicenter study to include 79 patients with symptomatic CAD to receive one of five escalating doses of viral vector encoding FGF_4 or placebo, was published. Although the analysis of the overall therapeutic effectiveness based on the exercise test did not show any differences between groups, analysis of the subgroup with greater initial functional impairment showed a significant increase in exercise tolerance. Subsequent studies like the AGENT-3 and -4 [17] trials involving more than 500 patients in several countries did not replicate the results originally obtained regarding better exercise tolerance after administration of FGF_4 in patients with stable angina and were, therefore, prematurely interrupted. Similar results were also obtained in the VIVA trial (*Vascular Endothelial Growth Factor in Ischemia for Vascular Angiogenesis*) [18]. In this trial, clinical evaluation performed at 120 days after treatment showed that the group receiving the highest dose of VEGF had a significant reduction in angina (functional class improvement) with only a favorable trend towards better exercise performance. Because of the lack of consistent, replicable data in terms of efficacy in controlled randomized clinical trials, much of the initial interest in gene therapy for the treatment of patients with refractory angina has faded away.

Cell Therapy

The therapeutic potential of transplantation of stem cells and/or progenitor cells has been explored experimentally for over a decade aiming to induce the growth of new blood vessels (angiogenesis) [19] and/or to regenerate cardiomyocytes after myocardial infarction [20].

Motivated by the initial success obtained in experimental models of myocardial ischemia, the first results of cell therapy applied to patients with CAD were reported in the last decade. Assmus et al. [22] transplanted bone marrow-derived or peripheral blood progenitor cells by means of intracoronary infusion in patients after acute MI. After 4 months, treated patients had improved the left ventricular ejection fraction and the regional wall motion in the infarct area was associated with a lower end-systolic volume and increased coronary flow reserve in the culprit, treated coronary artery was noted. No adverse events were observed.

The use of adult bone marrow-derived cells for treating severe CAD associated with heart failure was proposed by Perin et al. [23]. Fourteen patients underwent trans endocardial injection guided by electromechanical mapping in ischemic but viable areas (hibernating myocardium). The authors showed that, after 4 months, there was an improvement in functional class, significant reduction in perfusion defects assessed by SPECT, and an increase in ejection fraction from 20 to 29 % in treated patients.

Stamm et al. [24] proposed the use of intramyocardial injection of bone marrow-derived stem cells combined with CABG in 6 post-MI patients. Functional assessment revealed an increase in LV global motility (in 4 out of 6 patients) and increased perfusion in the infarct area (in 5 out of 6 patients). Gowdak et al. [25] tested a similar strategy for the treatment of patients with severe and diffuse CAD, refractory to medical therapy and not amenable to complete surgical revascularization strategy because of the extent of the disease. In 21 patients, autologous progenitor hematopoietic cells were injected during CABG in those areas previously identified as viable and ischemic. No adverse events related to the procedure were noted [26]. There was an increase in myocardial perfusion in the injected segments, which have not been grafted, along with improved regional contractility. A large randomized, double blind, controlled trial is underway to test the role of cell therapy as adjunctive therapy to incomplete myocardial revascularization in patients with stable angina [27].

The RENEW study, currently underway, will test the safety and efficacy of intramyocardial injection of autologous CD34+ cells in patients with refractory angina unresponsive to optimal medical therapy and who are not candidates for revascularization procedures [28]. Another study recently launched, the IMPACT-CABG [29], will test the safety and efficacy of intramyocardial injection of autologous CD133+ cells in patients undergoing CABG.

More recently, the angiogenic potential of adipose-derived mesenchymal cells began to be explored in patients with ischemic heart disease [30], acute myocardial infarction and heart failure [31]. These clinical trials will document the possibility, if successful, of using this abundant cell source for the treatment of patients with a large spectrum of CVD.

Finally, one of the last cell types to be tested in the treatment of patients with ischemic cardiomyopathy resulted from the identification of resident cardiac stem cells with the potential for myocardial regeneration [32]. Many preclinical studies have demonstrated the efficacy of these cells in the treatment of post-MI left ventricular dysfunction [33, 34]. In the SCIPIO [35] study, cardiac resident stem cells were obtained from the right atrial appendage during surgery for myocardial revascularization. Once isolated, the cells were expanded and infused via intracoronary about 4 months after surgery. Evaluation of cardiac function by magnetic resonance imaging showed a significant increase in LVEF in the treated group from 27.5 % (baseline) to 35.1 % and 41.2 %, 4 and 12 months after infusion of the cells, respectively, as well as a significant decrease in the area of infarction. However exciting these data might sound, caution must be exercised in the interpretation of these studies due to the small numbers of highly selected patients and intra- and inter-observer variability in infarct size measurements. Anatomical and histological examinations of large numbers of patients treated with these cells are necessary to confirm significant generation of myocytes and decreases in infarct size and fibrosis [36]. Moreover, as with any other form of novel therapy, the use of cardiac resident stem cells will have to face the challenge of a double-blind, randomized, placebo controlled clinical trial so that its contribution for myocardial repair can be determined. But even before that, a shadow of uncertainty was already casted on these preliminary data, as we learned that concerns about the integrity of certain data published have led to an internal investigational on the fairness of the study [37].

Transmyocardial Laser Revascularization (TMLR)

Mirhoseini and Cayton first proposed the use of laser beams for myocardial revascularization in 1981, after a successful experimental study in acute myocardial ischemia model by ligation of the left anterior descendent artery in dogs [38]. The same group published the first report of the clinical use of a CO_2 laser as an adjunct strategy to CABG [39]. Transmyocardial laser revascularization (TMLR) is a surgical procedure in which intramyocardial channels (1 mm in diameter) are created through the application of high-energy CO_2 laser beams on the heart, without cardiopulmonary bypass, through a left anterolateral thoracotomy. The procedure is based on the premise that myocardial perfusion will increase as blood flows from the myocardial ventricular cavity through the channels created to the ischemic areas (Fig. 11.2).

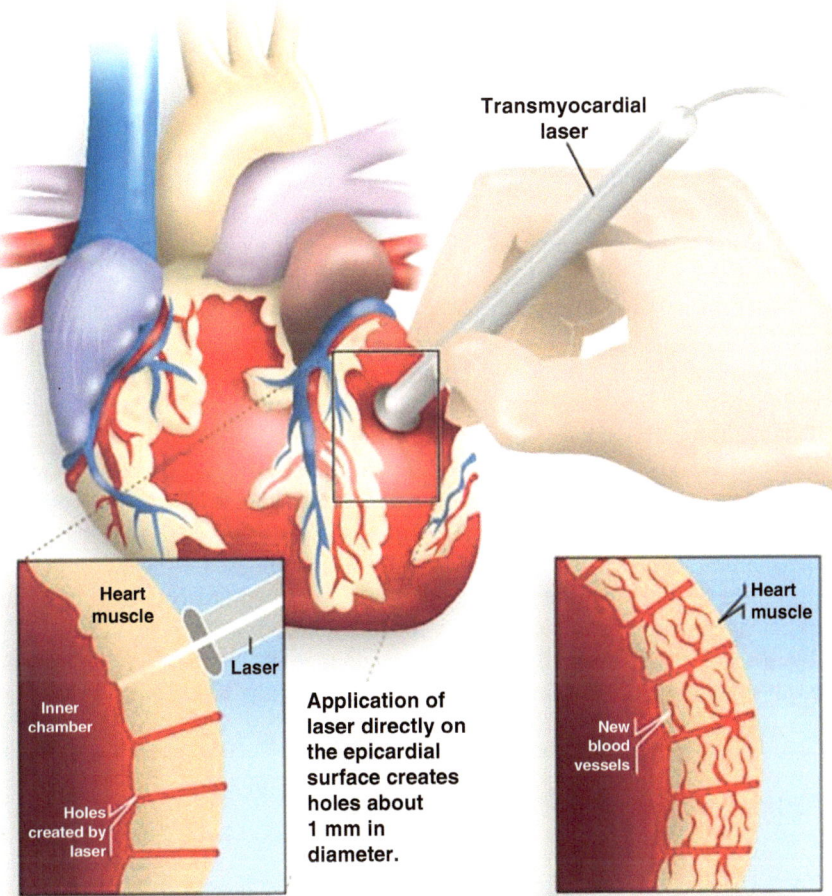

Fig. 11.2 Transmyocardial laser revascularization for the treatment of patients with inoperable CAD

In one of the early clinical experiences in a small series of patients, Frazier et al. [40] applied TMLR in 31 patients with refractory angina who were not candidates for conventional revascularization procedures. Their study showed a significant improvement in functional capacity, increased endocardial perfusion and LVEF after the procedure. The patency of the channels created by laser was documented for the first time in a post-mortem study on a patient who died 3 months after surgery [41]. On the other hand, Dallan and Oliveira [42] performing an autopsy in a patient who died 14 months after surgery demonstrated that the initially open intramyocardial channels were closed and replaced by interstitial fibrosis, perpendicular to the epicardium, extending towards the endocardium. Careful histological analysis revealed, however, in the same case, the presence of newly formed vessels, which could contribute to the beneficial effects observed, despite the late occlusion of the channels.

The evidence for benefit and safety of this technique was obtained from randomized clinical trials with adequate numbers of patients. The positive results initially seen in small series of patients were replicated in a larger study involving 200 patients with advanced, inoperable CAD and several centers in the United States [43]. A comparative study between TMLR and medical therapy in patients with refractory angina followed for 1 year showed that medical treatment-only was associated with a higher incidence of unstable angina and hospitalizations, worsening of functional class and worsening myocardial perfusion [44]. However, in a similar study by Schofield et al. with 188 refractory angina patients, TMLR was not able to significantly increase functional capacity (objectively assessed by exercise treadmill testing) or to offer any benefit on survival at 12 months of follow-up [45].

After many years in practice, the experience accumulated in numerous clinical studies was compiled in a recent meta-analysis involving more than 1000 patients showing that TMLR provides benefit in relieving symptoms and improving quality of life, with no appreciable impact on the incidence of cardiovascular events [46]. Thus, in the United States, TMLR received in the ACC/AHA guidelines, a Class IIb, level of evidence B [45, 47], and it therefore may be utilized for the relief of symptoms in patients with refractory angina, not candidates for conventional myocardial revascularization procedures. The association between TMLR and intramyocardial stem cell therapy has recently been proposed with the objective of exploring the potential synergistic angiogenic effect resulting from the combination of both techniques, to accelerate the recovery of the perfusion in ischemic areas [48, 49]. As with the stem cell therapy, large randomized controlled trials are needed to establish the role of the combined procedure for patients with refractory angina.

Enhanced External Counter-Pulsation

Enhanced external counterpulsation (EECP) is a noninvasive physical therapy designed to increase venous return, raise cardiac preload, increase cardiac output, and decrease systemic vascular resistance [50]. EECP therapy is usually offered at daily sessions with 1 h duration, five times a week for 7 weeks, totaling 35 sessions.

During each session, the patient's lower extremities are wrapped in three compressive pneumatic cuffs applied to the calves, lower thighs, and upper thighs/buttocks (Fig. 11.3). Leg compression occurs sequentially from distal to proximal in early diastole resulting in not only an increase in proximal diastolic aortic pressure but also in venous return. Next, the cuffs rapidly deflate just before the onset of systole, significantly reducing the heart's workload by lowering peripheral vascular resistance (Fig. 11.4) [51].

Fig. 11.3 A patient with refractory angina undergoing EECP (Reproduced from Braverman [51], with permission of Elsevier)

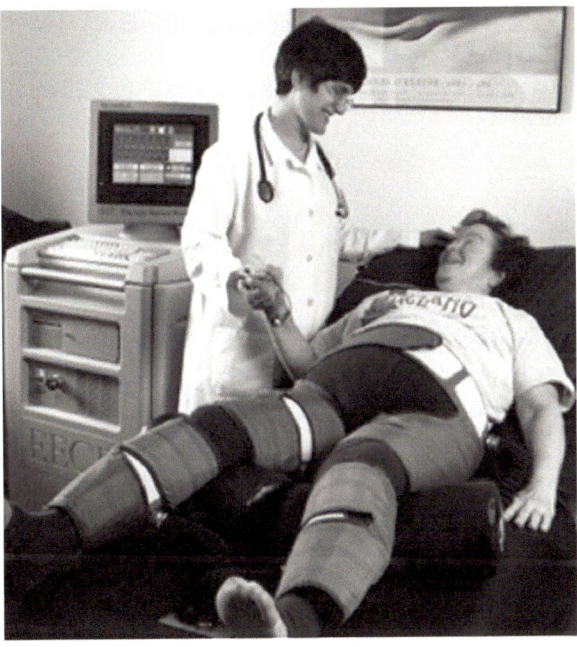

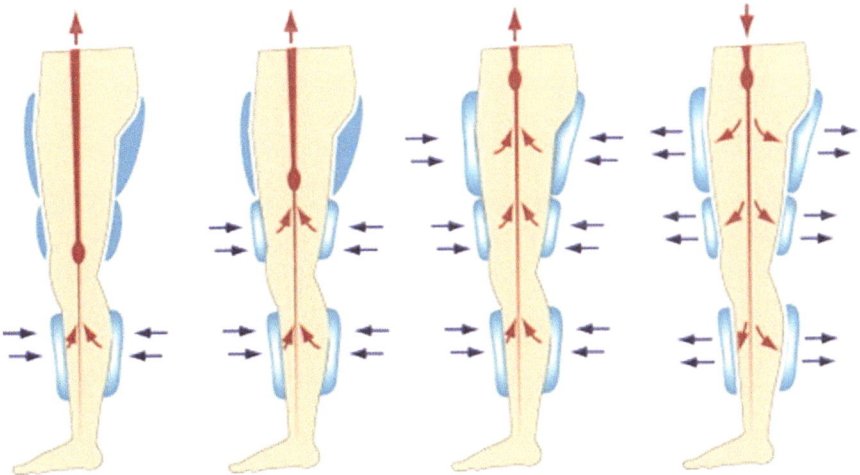

Fig. 11.4 Schematics of the EECP. Details in the text (Reproduced from Braverman [51], with permission of Elsevier)

Several mechanisms of action were postulated to explain the beneficial effects often observed with this therapy, both in the short and long term. Such mechanisms involve improved endothelial function, development of coronary collateral circulation, restauration of left ventricular function and improvement in peripheral circulation [52]. Clinical benefits were observed in over 80 % of those who underwent this therapeutic strategy including a decrease in the number of angina attacks and consumption of sublingual nitrate, increased exercise tolerance, improved quality of life, objectively demonstrable increase in time for the onset of ischemia and improvement in myocardial perfusion defects [53–55]. These benefits occur early after treatment initiation and can be sustained in many patients as long as up to 5 years [56]. In the United States, EECP therapy received a Class IIb, level of evidence B.

Spinal Cord Stimulation

Spinal cord stimulation (SCS) has been used from the 1960s for the treatment of neurogenic pain and, beginning in 1976, for the treatment of ischemic pain secondary to peripheral arterial disease. The clinical application of SCS for the treatment of refractory angina was proposed in the early 1990s [57] with many favorable results on the quality of life of those affected, improved exercise tolerance and decreased consumption of short action nitrates, although the mechanisms of action this technique are still under investigation.

In theory, SCS decreases myocardial ischemia by one or more of the following mechanisms: an increase of coronary blood flow, reduction of O_2 demand, and direct inhibition of nociception with consequent reduction in the consumption of O_2. One cannot rule out the contribution of neuromodulation to increase the pain threshold, possibly by redistributing coronary flow [58]. Briefly, this technique involves inserting a cable into the epidural space connected to an implanted stimulation pulse generator in the subcutaneous tissue. Electrical stimulation can be generated in a continuous, cyclical or intermittent mode.

The effectiveness of SCS was documented in several open clinical observational studies or randomized controlled trials. The Italian Prospective Registry [59] described improvement of >50 % in angina attacks in 73 % of treated individuals and at least one functional class of angina in 80 % of patients. Recently, randomized controlled studies have been published: one study demonstrated increased exercise capacity and improved ischemia recorded by 24-h Holter in 13 patients with refractory angina undergoing the procedure compared to a group kept on optimal medical therapy only. Another study confirmed similar clinical benefit (reduction in angina) between SCS and CABG, but with lower rates of cardiovascular morbidity and mortality in the SCS group [60]. Currently in the United States, SCS has received a Class IIb, level of evidence C, for symptomatic relief in patients with refractory angina.

Extracorporeal Shockwave Myocardial Revascularization

Extracorporeal shockwave myocardial revascularization (ESMR) is a noninvasive therapy that, through the application of low energy shock waves directed to the ischemic areas of the myocardium, the induction of growth of new blood vessels (neoangiogenesis) may occur, increasing tissue perfusion and leading to relief of symptoms (Fig. 11.5).

The mechanisms involved in the vascular growth involve the release of angiogenic cytokines such as VEGF, the enzyme endothelial NO synthase and the recruitment of progenitor endothelial cells [61–63]. A few experimental studies have shown that the application of shock waves increases the perfusion in ischemic myocardum [63] and improves left ventricular function after myocardial infarction [64]. Initial experience in small series of 9 patients [65] demonstrated the safety and efficacy of the procedure in relieving angina in patients with severe CAD. This study was followed by another study comprised of 18 patients with debilitating angina [66], in whom not only clinical improvement was observed (decreased number of angina attacks and lower consumption of short-acting nitrates), but also an improvement in left ventricular function. This technology is investigational in the United States, although it is being used in few countries in Europe and Asia.

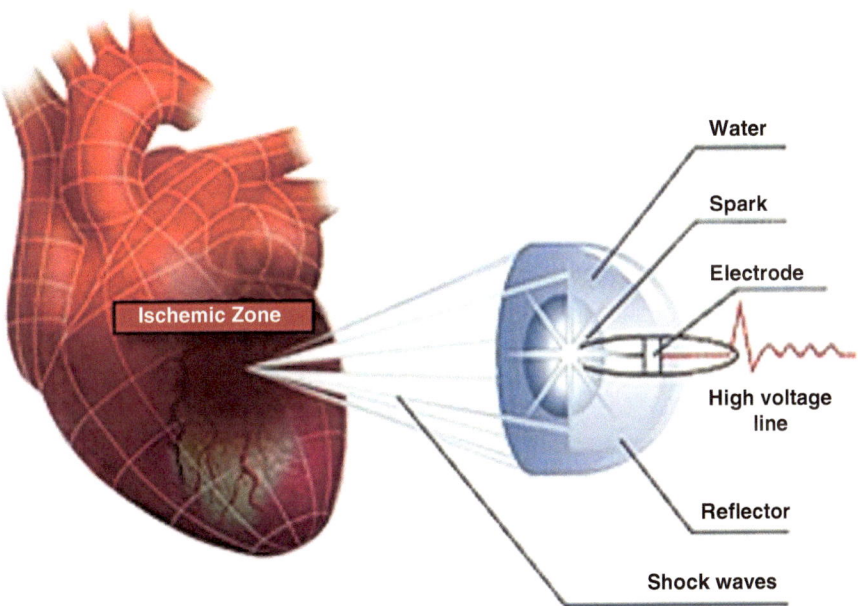

Fig. 11.5 Basic principle of extracorporeal shock-wave myocardial revascularization

Conclusion

As a result of the combination of a greater life expectancy, a decline in CVD mortality adjusted for age and an increased prevalence of risk factors (especially diabetes, obesity and hypertension), the number of patients living with chronic CVD is expected to grow in the coming years, particularly those with CAD. Moreover, these patients with CAD now have a longer life expectancy than three decades ago thanks to the many advances in medical therapy and interventional procedures. On the other hand, this allowed for the appearance of a population of patients in which the disease continues its relentless progression towards more advanced forms, with diffuse arterial involvement, also affecting grafts distally or previously implanted stents. Thus, we believe that new therapeutic strategies must be sought for those living with refractory angina. Accordingly, new therapeutic options are being tested in the treatment of this condition but they all have to deal with common challenges:

1. There is no experimental model that exactly mimics the condition seen in patients with diffuse CAD. We have to rely on approximate animal models to test new therapies.
2. Many promising new therapies, i.e. gene therapy, have greatly succeeded in animal models of myocardial ischemia and even in early, open label, uncontrolled clinical trials. When rigorously tested in double-blind, placebo controlled trials, they fell far short of expectations. On the other hand, there was criticism regarding many trial designs and chosen endpoints to prove the benefit of gene therapy, and that "*the baby was thrown away with the dirty water*".
3. The compelling need to relief symptoms and improve survival serve as the rational for quickly moving from an early experimental success in the bench to the bedside. If one considers stem cell therapy, we are still looking for the best cell, in the right concentration properly delivered for a great cell survival rate into the right patient. But clinical trials have been conducted beginning in the 2000s.
4. The lack of properly sized, double-blind, placebo controlled clinical trials may hamper the further application and development of conceptually interesting strategies such as external shockwave myocardial revascularization.
5. Perhaps the future will show that, indeed, a combined approach may work best for patients with refractory angina, i.e., TMR and stem cell therapy.
6. Finally, every single scientist involved in this field should keep the highest level of scientific commitment regarding the rigor with which data are obtained and presented, above any personal conflict of interest, so that science may steadily advance towards finding better treatment options for our patients. For they deserve to not only live longer but also and, equally important, live better.

References

1. World Health Organization. WHO methods and data sources for global causes of death 2000-2012 (2013). Available on: http://apps.who.int/gho/data/node.main.CODWORLD?lang=en.
2. Go AS, Mozaffarian D, Roger VL, Benjamin EJ, Berry JD, Borden WB, et al. Heart disease and stroke statistics – 2013 update: a report from the American Heart Association. Circulation. 2013;127(1):e6–245.
3. Jolicoeur EM, Cartier R, Henry TD, Barsness GW, Bourassa MG, McGillion M, et al. Patients with coronary artery disease unsuitable for revascularization: definition, general principles, and a classification. Can J Cardiol. 2012;28(2 Suppl):S50–9.
4. Mukherjee D, Bhatt DL, Roe MT, Patel V, Ellis SG. Direct myocardial revascularization and angiogenesis – how many patients might be eligible? Am J Cardiol. 1999;84(5):598–600.
5. Mannheimer C, Camici P, Chester MR, Collins A, DeJongste M, Eliasson T, et al. The problem of chronic refractory angina; report from the ESC Joint Study Group on the Treatment of Refractory Angina. Eur Heart J. 2002;23(5):355–70.
6. Bhatt AB, Stone PH. Current strategies for the prevention of angina in patients with stable coronary artery disease. Curr Opin Cardiol. 2006;21(5):492–502.
7. César LA, Gowdak LH, Mansur AP. The metabolic treatment of patients with coronary artery disease: effects on quality of life and effort angina. Curr Pharm Des. 2009;15(8):841–9.
8. Khan SN, Dutka DP. A systematic approach to refractory angina. Curr Opin Support Palliat Care. 2008;2(4):247–51.
9. Fraker TD Jr, Fihn SD, Writing on behalf of the 2002 Chronic Stable Angina Writing Committee. 2007 chronic angina focused update of the ACC/AHA 2002 guidelines for the management of patients with chronic stable angina: a report of the American College of Cardiology/American Heart Association task force on practice guidelines Writing Group to develop the focused update of the 2002 guidelines for the management of patients with chronic stable angina. J Am Coll Cardiol. 2007;50(23):2264–74.
10. McGillion M, L'Allier PL, Arthur H, Watt-Watson J, Svorkdal N, Cosman T, et al. Canadian Cardiovascular Society. Recommendations for advancing the care of Canadians living with refractory angina pectoris: a Canadian Cardiovascular Society position statement. Can J Cardiol. 2009;25(7):399–401.
11. Anderson WF. Human gene therapy. Nature. 1998;392(6679 Suppl):25–30.
12. Höckel M, Schlenger K, Doctrow S, Kissel T, Vaupel P. Therapeutic angiogenesis. Arch Surg. 1993;128(4):423–9.
13. Losordo DW, Vale PR, Symes JF, Dunnington CH, Esakof DD, Maysky M, et al. Gene therapy for myocardial angiogenesis: initial clinical results with direct myocardial injection of phVEGF165 as sole therapy for myocardial ischemia. Circulation. 1998;98(25):2800–4.
14. Symes JF, Losordo DW, Vale PR, Lathi KG, Esakof DD, Mayskiy M, et al. Gene therapy with vascular endothelial growth factor for inoperable coronary artery disease. Ann Thorac Surg. 1999;68(3):830–6.
15. Rosengart TK, Lee LY, Patel SR, Kligfield PD, Okin PM, Hackett NR, et al. Six-month assessment of a phase I trial of angiogenic gene therapy for the treatment of coronary artery disease using direct intramyocardial administration of an adenovirus vector expressing the VEGF121 cDNA. Ann Surg. 1999;230(4):466–70.
16. Grines CL, Watkins MW, Helmer G, Penny W, Brinker J, Marmur JD, et al. Angiogenic Gene Therapy (AGENT) trial in patients with stable angina pectoris. Circulation. 2002;105(11):1291–7.
17. Grines CL, Watkins MW, Mahmarian JJ, Iskandrian AE, Rade JJ, Marrott P, et al. A randomized, double-blind, placebo-controlled trial of Ad5FGF-4 gene therapy and its effect on myocardial perfusion in patients with stable angina. J Am Coll Cardiol. 2003;42(8):1339–47.
18. Henry TD, Annex BH, McKendall GR, Azrin MA, Lopez JJ, Giordano FJ, et al. The VIVA trial: vascular endothelial growth factor in ischemia for vascular angiogenesis. Circulation. 2003;107(10):1359–65.

19. Sunkomat JN, Gaballa MA. Stem cell therapy in ischemic heart disease. Cardiovasc Drug Rev. 2003;21:327–42.
20. Perin EC, Silva GV. Stem cell therapy for cardiac diseases. Curr Opin Hematol. 2004;11:399–403.
21. Kang HJ, Kim HS, Park YB. Stem cell therapy for myocardial infarction. Can Med Assoc J. 2004;171(5):442–3.
22. Assmus B, Schächinger V, Teupe C, Britten M, Lehmann R, Döbert N, et al. Transplantation of progenitor cells and regeneration enhancement in acute myocardial infarction (TOPCARE-AMI). Circulation. 2002;106:3009–17.
23. Perin EC, Dohmann HF, Borojevic R, Silva SA, Sousa AL, Mesquita CT, et al. Transendocardial, autologous bone marrow cell transplantation for severe, chronic ischemic heart failure. Circulation. 2003;107:2294–302.
24. Stamm C, Westphal B, Kleine HD, Petzsch M, Kittner C, Klinge H, et al. Autologous bone-marrow stem-cell transplantation for myocardial regeneration. Lancet. 2003;361:45–6.
25. Gowdak LH, Schettert IT, Rochitte CE, Lisboa LA, Dallan LA, César LA, et al. Early increase in myocardial perfusion after stem cell therapy in patients undergoing incomplete coronary artery bypass surgery. J Cardiovasc Transl Res. 2011;4:106–13.
26. Gowdak LH, Schettert IT, Baptista E, Lopes NL, Rochitte CE, Vieira ML, et al. Intramyocardial injection of autologous bone marrow cells as an adjunctive therapy to incomplete myocardial revascularization – safety issues. Clinics (Sao Paulo). 2008;63:207–14.
27. Tura BR, Martino HF, Gowdak LH, dos Santos RR, Dohmann HF, Krieger JE, et al. Multicenter randomized trial of cell therapy in cardiopathies – MiHeart Study. Trials. 2007;8:2.
28. Povsic TJ, Junge C, Nada A, Schatz RA, Harrington RA, Davidson CJ, et al. A phase 3, randomized, double-blinded, active-controlled, unblinded standard of care study assessing the efficacy and safety of intramyocardial autologous CD34+ cell administration in patients with refractory angina: design of the RENEW study. Am Heart J. 2013;165:854–61.
29. Forcillo J, Stevens LM, Mansour S, Prieto I, Salem R, Baron C, et al. Implantation of CD133+ stem cells in patients undergoing coronary bypass surgery: IMPACT-CABG pilot trial. Can J Cardiol. 2013;29:441–7.
30. Qayyum AA, Haack-Sørensen M, Mathiasen AB, Jørgensen E, Ekblond A, Kastrup J. Adipose-derived mesenchymal stromal cells for chronic myocardial ischemia (MyStromalCell Trial): study design. Regen Med. 2012;7:421–8.
31. Panfilov IA, De Jong R, Takashima S, Duckers HJ. Clinical study using adipose-derived mesenchymal-like stem cells in acute myocardial infarction and heart failure. Methods Mol Biol. 2013;1036:207–12.
32. Beltrami AP, Barlucchi L, Torella D, Baker M, Limana F, Chimenti S, et al. Adult cardiac stem cells are multipotent and support myocardial regeneration. Cell. 2003;114(6):763–6.
33. Dawn B, Stein AB, Urbanek K, Rota M, Whang B, Rastaldo R, et al. Cardiac stem cells delivered intravascularly traverse the vessel barrier, regenerate infarcted myocardium, and improve cardiac function. Proc Natl Acad Sci U S A. 2005;102(10):3766–71.
34. Tang XL, Rokosh G, Sanganalmath SK, Yuan F, Sato H, Mu J, et al. Intracoronary administration of cardiac progenitor cells alleviates left ventricular dysfunction in rats with a 30-day-old infarction. Circulation. 2010;121(2):293–305.
35. Bolli R, Chugh AR, D'Amario D, Loughran JH, Stoddard MF, Ikram S, et al. Stem cells in patients with ischaemic cardiomyopathy (SCIPIO): initial results of a randomised phase 1 trial. Lancet. 2011;378(9806):1847–57.
36. Henning RJ. Stem cells for cardiac repair: problems and possibilities. Future Cardiol. 2013;9(6):875–84.
37. The Lancet Editors. Expression of concern: the SCIPIO trial. Lancet. 2014;383(9925):1279.
38. Mirhoseini M, Cayton MM. Revascularization of the heart by laser. J Microsurg. 1981;2(4):253–60.
39. Mirhoseini M, Fisher JC, Cayton M. Myocardial revascularization by laser: a clinical report. Lasers Surg Med. 1983;3(3):241–5.

40. Frazier OH, Cooley DA, Kadipasaoglu KA, et al. Myocardial revascularization with laser. Preliminary findings. Circulation. 1995;92(9 Suppl):II58–65.
41. Cooley DA, Frazier OH, Kadipasaoglu KA, Pehlivanoglu S, Shannon RL, Angelini P. Transmyocardial laser revascularization. Anatomic evidence of long-term channel patency. Tex Heart Inst J. 1994;21(3):220–4.
42. Dallan LAO, Oliveira AS. Cirurgia de revascularização transmiocárdica a laser de CO_2. Rev Bras Cir Cardiovasc. 2000;15(2):89–104 [Article in Portuguese].
43. Horvath KA, Cohn LH, Cooley DA, Crew JR, Frazier OH, Griffith BP, et al. Transmyocardial laser revascularization: results of a multicenter trial with transmyocardial laser revascularization used as sole therapy for end-stage coronary artery disease. J Thorac Cardiovasc Surg. 1997;113(4):645–53.
44. March RJ. Transmyocardial laser revascularization with the CO_2 laser: one year results of a randomized, controlled trial. Semin Thorac Cardiovasc Surg. 1999;11(1):12–8.
45. Schofield PM, Sharples LD, Caine N, Burns S, Tait S, Wistow T, et al. Transmyocardial laser revascularisation in patients with refractory angina: a randomised controlled trial. Lancet. 1999;353(9152):519–24.
46. Liao L, Sarria-Santamera A, Matchar DB, Huntington A, Lin S, Whellan DJ, et al. Meta-analysis of survival and relief of angina pectoris after transmyocardial revascularization. Am J Cardiol. 2005;95(10):1243–5.
47. Fihn SD, Gardin JM, Abrams J, Berra K, Blankenship JC, Dallas AP, et al. 2012 ACCF/AHA/ACP/AATS/PCNA/SCAI/STS guideline for the diagnosis and management of patients with stable ischemic heart disease: a report of the American College of Cardiology Foundation/American Heart Association task force on practice guidelines, and the American College of Physicians, American Association for Thoracic Surgery, Preventive Cardiovascular Nurses Association, Society for Cardiovascular Angiography and Interventions, and Society of Thoracic Surgeons. J Am Coll Cardiol. 2012;60(24):e44–164.
48. Gowdak LH, Schettert IT, Rochitte CE, Lisboa LA, Dallan LA, César LA, et al. Cell therapy plus transmyocardial laser revascularization for refractory angina. Ann Thorac Surg. 2005;80(2):712–4.
49. Gowdak LH, Schettert IT, Rochitte CE, Rienzo M, Lisboa LA, Dallan LA, et al. Transmyocardial laser revascularization plus cell therapy for refractory angina. Int J Cardiol. 2008;127(2):295–7.
50. Michaels AD, Accad M, Ports TA, Grossman W. Left ventricular systolic unloading and augmentation of intracoronary pressure and Doppler flow during enhanced external counterpulsation. Circulation. 2002;106(10):1237–42.
51. Braverman DL. Enhanced external counterpulsation: a novel therapy for angina. Complement Ther Clin Pract. 2012;18(4):197–203.
52. Kitsou V, Xanthos T, Roberts R, Karlis GM, Padadimitriou L. Enhanced external counterpulsation: mechanisms of action and clinical applications. Acta Cardiol. 2010;65(2):239–47.
53. Masuda D, Nohara R, Hirai T, Kataoka K, Chen LG, Hosokawa R, et al. Enhanced external counterpulsation improved myocardial perfusion and coronary flow reserve in patients with chronic stable angina; evaluation by(13)N-ammonia positron emission tomography. Eur Heart J. 2001;22(16):1451–8.
54. Arora RR, Chou TM, Jain D, Fleishman B, Crawford L, McKiernan T, et al. The multicenter study of enhanced external counterpulsation (MUST-EECP): effect of EECP on exercise-induced myocardial ischemia and anginal episodes. J Am Coll Cardiol. 1999;33(7):1833–40.
55. Manchanda A, Soran O. Enhanced external counterpulsation and future directions: step beyond medical management for patients with angina and heart failure. J Am Coll Cardiol. 2007;50(16):1523–31.
56. Lawson WE, Hui JC, Cohn PF. Long-term prognosis of patients with angina treated with enhanced external counterpulsation: five-year follow-up study. Clin Cardiol. 2000;23(4):254–8.

57. de Jongste MJ, Staal MJ. Preliminary results of a randomized study on the clinical efficacy of spinal cord stimulation for refractory severe angina pectoris. Acta Neurochir Suppl (Wien). 1993;58:161–4.

58. Eckert S, Horstkotte D. Management of angina pectoris: the role of spinal cord stimulation. Am J Cardiovasc Drugs. 2009;9(1):17–28.

59. Di Pede F, Lanza GA, Zuin G, Alfieri O, Rapati M, Romanò M, et al. Immediate and long-term clinical outcome after spinal cord stimulation for refractory stable angina pectoris. Am J Cardiol. 2003;91(8):951–5.

60. Mannheimer C, Eliasson T, Augustinsson LE, Blomstrand C, Emanuelsson H, Larsson S, et al. Electrical stimulation versus coronary artery bypass surgery in severe angina pectoris: the ESBY study. Circulation. 1998;97(12):1157–63.

61. Wang CJ, Wang FS, Yang KD, Weng LH, Hsu CC, Huang CS, et al. Shock wave therapy induces neovascularization at the tendon-bone junction. A study in rabbits. J Orthop Res. 2003;21(6):984–9.

62. Aicher A, Heeschen C, Sasaki K, Urbich C, Zeiher AM, Dimmeler S. Low-energy shock wave for enhancing recruitment of endothelial progenitor cells: a new modality to increase efficacy of cell therapy in chronic hind limb ischemia. Circulation. 2006;114(25):2823–30.

63. Nishida T, Shimokawa H, Oi K, Tatewaki H, Uwatoku T, Abe K, et al. Extracorporeal cardiac shock wave therapy markedly ameliorates ischemia-induced myocardial dysfunction in pigs in vivo. Circulation. 2004;110(19):3055–61.

64. Uwatoku T, Ito K, Abe K, Oi K, Hizume T, Sunagawa K, et al. Extracorporeal cardiac shock wave therapy improves left ventricular remodeling after acute myocardial infarction in pigs. Coron Artery Dis. 2007;18(5):397–404.

65. Fukumoto Y, Ito A, Uwatoku T, Matoba T, Kishi T, Tanaka H, et al. Extracorporeal cardiac shock wave therapy ameliorates myocardial ischemia in patients with severe coronary artery disease. Coron Artery Dis. 2006;17(1):63–70.

66. Zuoziené G, Laucevicius A, Leibowitz D. Extracorporeal shockwave myocardial revascularization improves clinical symptoms and left ventricular function in patients with refractory angina. Coron Artery Dis. 2012;23(1):62–7.

Chapter 12
Medical and Invasive Management of Coronary Artery Disease in Patients on Anticoagulants

Ryan Berg and Nabil Shafi

Abstract The management of coronary artery disease in patients on anticoagulants represents a difficult clinical scenario. As more intense therapy is given, patients are expected to have less ischemic/thrombotic events, but they will have increased bleeding risks. In this chapter we examine the evidence base of the risks and benefits of combining antiplatelet therapy and anticoagulant therapy in both the primary and secondary prevention settings. While most of these data concern warfarin as the primary anticoagulant, we will review any data on the novel oral anticoagulants (NOACs) as well.

Keywords Aspirin • Clopidogrel • Warfarin • Coronary artery disease • Triple therapy • Novel oral anticoagulants

Introduction

The management of coronary artery disease (CAD) in patients on anticoagulants represents a difficult clinical scenario. This has been previously described as a "Yin-Yang" paradigm of balancing anti-ischemic efficacy and bleeding risk when combining more potent antithrombotic/anticoagulant therapy [1]. As more intense therapy is given, patients are expected to have less ischemic/thrombotic events, however, in return they are at risk for increased bleeding. There is further potential risk when a recent coronary stent is placed in a patient on an anticoagulant due to the concern for stent thrombosis with early discontinuation of antiplatelet therapy if a bleeding episode occurs. To further complicate the matter, there are now multiple antiplatelet agents available (ticagrelor, clopidogrel, prasugrel, ticlopidine, aspirin) as well as multiple oral anticoagulants (warfarin, dabigatran, rivaroxaban, and

R. Berg, MD (✉) • N. Shafi, MD
UCSF Fresno Department of Cardiology, Community Regional Medical Center,
Fresno, CA, USA
e-mail: medrberg@hotmail.com

© Springer International Publishing Switzerland 2015
J.A. Ambrose, A.E. Rodríguez (eds.), *Controversies in Cardiology*,
DOI 10.1007/978-3-319-20415-4_12

apixaban). This chapter examines the evidence base in both primary and secondary prevention and considers the controversies and unresolved issues surrounding the use of triple therapy. While most of these data utilized warfarin as the primary anti-coagulant, we will review any data on the novel oral anticoagulants (NOACs) as well.

Aspirin for Primary Prevention of Cardiovascular Disease in addition to anticoagulation

Aspirin (ASA) has been the mainstay of pharmacotherapy for the secondary prevention of cardiovascular events by reducing mortality and decreasing subsequent cardiac events [2]. Aspirin's antithrombotic effect is through the irreversible inhibition of COX-1 and 2, which prevents the generation of prostaglandins including thromboxane A2 that induce platelet aggregation. Consequently, the principle effect of ASA is the inhibition of platelet-mediated thrombus formation in the arterial circulation [2–4]. The prophylactic use of ASA for the primary prevention of coronary artery disease (CAD) events has been extensively investigated over the last 25 years and the data are less certain than the secondary prevention data. Questions remain regarding the efficacy, safety and the degree of cardiovascular risk associated with the most favorable benefit: risk ratio for its use in primary prevention of CAD.

A meta-analysis carried out by the Anti-Thrombotic Trialists (ATT) Collaboration in 2009 [5] included the first six primary prevention trials [6–11] (n=95,000) and demonstrated ASA significantly reduced the incidence of serious vascular events, defined as a combined end point of MI, death from a vascular cause or stroke (0.51 versus 0.57 %/year). This significant reduction was attributable principally to a significant reduction in the first non-fatal MI (0.18 versus 0.23 %/year). ASA therapy was associated with six fewer myocardial infarctions (MI) per 1000 low-risk persons treated over a 10 year period (5 % CAD risk at 10 years according to the Framingham risk categories). For persons at moderate (15 %) and high (25 %) CVD risk, ASA led to a reduction of 19 and 31 MIs per 1000 patients treated, respectively [12]. However, this benefit came at the expense of a bleeding event rate that was higher as a function of cardiovascular risk. Compared with placebo, the high risk population would experience 22 more bleeds per 1000 persons treated with ASA versus 4 more bleeds per 1000 persons treated with ASA in the low-risk population [12]. The meta-analysis by the ATT Collaboration found that allocation to ASA increased major GI and other extracranial bleeds (defined as a bleed requiring transfusion or resulting in death) by about 50 % (0.10 %/year vs. 0.07 %/year; risk ratio: 1.54 [95 % CI: 1.30–1.82], p<0.0001). Furthermore, ASA also increased the risk of hemorrhagic stroke. A meta-analysis of 16 placebo-controlled RCTs, comprising a total of 55,462 patients, showed that treatment with aspirin was associated with a relative risk of hemorrhagic stroke of 1.84 (p<0.001) [13].

With respect to mortality, the ATT Collaboration showed aspirin compared with placebo did not reduce all-cause mortality, cardiovascular mortality, non-vascular mortality or deaths of unknown cause [4]. Four more recent meta-analyses have been performed by other groups, and published in 2011–2012 [14–17]. In all of them, three additional trials were included: the JPAD (Japanese Primary Prevention of Atherosclerosis With Aspirin for Diabetes), POPADAD (Prevention of Progression of Arterial Disease and Diabetes), and AAA (Aspirin for Asymptomatic Atherosclerosis) trials [18–20]. These meta-analyses had the same unified message that ASA use did not reduce cardiovascular related death or overall mortality. However, ASA use was associated with a 12 % proportional reduction in major vascular events, translating to a number needed to treat (NNT) of about 2000 in low risk individuals to prevent one non-fatal myocardial infarction [21]. In the 2012 meta-analysis, the net cardiovascular benefit exceeded the bleeding risk at higher baseline CAD events rates [17]. In summary, ASA use in the primary prevention of CAD events has been shown to reduce the risk of a first MI (particularly in high risk patients), but coming at a significant expense of an increased risk of both gastrointestinal bleeding and hemorrhagic stroke [7]. As a result, current guidelines differ substantially in their recommendations for ASA's use in primary prevention of CAD, reflecting the uncertainty of a clear risk/benefit ratio in this population [12, 22–24] (see Table 12.1).

As there is already a concern of increased bleeding with aspirin alone for primary prevention, it is no surprise that combining with an anticoagulant in primary prevention leads to even further increases in bleeding. There are limited data that assess combination therapy in the primary prevention cohort. One meta-analysis of ten randomized controlled trials performed by Dentali et al. assessed the treatment of combination warfarin-ASA compared to warfarin alone primarily in patients where the indication for aspirin was the primary prevention of cardiovascular disease (both CAD and stroke) [25]). Six of the trials used low dose aspirin (<100 mg), and four of the trials had higher doses of aspirin. The risk for cardiovascular events

Table 12.1 Summary of major society recommendations for aspirin use in primary prevention of CVD

American Heart Association (AHA)/American College of Cardiology (ACC)/American Diabetes Association (ADA) [22]
1. Aspirin is reasonable in diabetic patient whose 10 year risk of events is >10 % and who are not at increased risk of bleeding
2. Aspirin may be considered for diabetic patients with intermediate risk of cardiovascular events (younger patients with at least risk factor, older patients with no risk factors, or patients with a 10-year risk of 5–10 %)
American College of Chest Physicians (ACCP) [12]
Aspirin (75–100 mg daily) for persons age 50 years or older without symptomatic CVD (Grade 2B)
US Preventative Services Task Force [23]
Low dose Aspirin for men 45–79 years and women 55–79 years when the potential benefit due to reduction of MI outweighs the potential harm due to increase in gastrointestinal hemorrhage (Grade A). Risk factor calculator for available at http://cvdrisk.nhlbi.nih.gov/calculator.asp
European Society of Cardiology [24]
Aspirin is not recommended in individuals without cardiovascular or cerebrovascular disease due to increased risk of major bleeding (Class III, Level of Evidence: B)

was significantly reduced by combination warfarin-ASA therapy (OR=0.66; 95 % CI: 0.52–0.84). However, this therapeutic benefit was driven by five studies involving patients with mechanical heart valves (OR=0.27; 95 % CI: 0.15–0.49). There was no statistically significant cardiovascular event reduction in the other studies where the warfarin was given for other indications. The aforementioned meta-analysis also assessed the risk for major bleeding associated with combination warfarin-ASA compared with warfarin alone. There was an increased risk for major bleeding with warfarin-ASA over warfarin alone, with an annual risk of 2.3 % vs. 1.3 %, a difference that was clinically relevant, although it was of borderline statistical significance (OR=1.43; 95 % CI: 1.00–2.02).

In the ORBIT AF registry, it was found that despite this known evidence, it is common in up to 35 % of patients in atrial fibrillation in modern practice to be on combination therapy with an antiplatelet on top of an anticoagulant [26]. A significant proportion of this population (39 %) was on the antiplatelet agent for primary prevention only. As this was a more modern study, most (89 %) patients were on an 81 mg dose of aspirin. This study also confirmed what was postulated in the prior meta-analysis: combination therapy was associated with more major bleeding (adjusted hazard ratio, 1.53; 95 % confidence interval, 1.20–1.96 p=0.0006) with no benefit in preventing ischemic outcomes leading toward a trend in increased mortality in the dual therapy group (adjusted hazard ratio 1.26 (0.98–1.63) p=.08).

Overall, there does not appear to be compelling evidence that warfarin-ASA combination therapy is more effective than warfarin alone for the prevention of cardiovascular events in patients with atrial fibrillation. There is, however, consistent evidence that warfarin-ASA therapy increases serious bleeding, irrespective of the patient population studied. As stated above, the group of patients with mechanical heart valves should be considered separately as combination therapy has shown net clinical benefit. Patients with mechanical valve prostheses require long-term anticoagulation and aspirin administration due to the inherent risk of thromboembolism. This is primarily due to abnormal flow conditions (stagnation and shear stress flow) imposed by the prosthetic heart valves, increasing both the risk of thrombosis and thromboembolism [27]. In a Cochrane report, 13 studies involving 4122 patients were reviewed [28]. Compared with anticoagulation alone, the addition of an antiplatelet agent (either dipyridamole or ASA) reduced the risk of thromboembolic events (odds ratio (OR) 0.43, 95 % confidence interval (CI) 0.32–0.59; P<0.00001). This came at the expense of an increase in major bleeding (OR 1.58, 95 % CI 1.14–2.18; P=0.006), despite the fact that low dose aspirin (<100 mg) was used in a majority of the trials that included aspirin as the antiplatelet agent. However, the net clinical benefit favored the combination of an anticoagulant plus an antiplatelet, as there was shown to be decreased mortality (OR 0.57, 95 % CI 0.42–0.78; P=0.0004). In summary, patients with mechanical heart valves derive a net therapeutic benefit with warfarin-ASA as the reduction in thromboembolic events outweighs the increase in the risk for serious bleeding and this combination is endorsed by the latest American College of Cardiology (ACC) 2014 guidelines on Valvular heart disease [29].

Secondary Prevention

While it is fairly clear from primary prevention that the risk of bleeding outweighs the benefit of a combination of antiplatelet therapy and anticoagulation, there is much more controversy in the realm of secondary prevention. There are many different secondary prevention scenarios (stable CAD, acute coronary syndromes, patients after recent coronary artery bypass surgery (CABG), and patients after recent stenting) each of which have different ischemic risk profiles in which to balance the bleeding risk. As we make our decision as to what regimen to give, we are always balancing a risk/benefit ratio of ischemic efficacy vs bleeding risk. The ischemic benefit of the antiplatelet therapy on top of the anticoagulants is quite different in each of those secondary prevention scenarios. Unfortunately, there are not enough data available to cover every different drug in every different clinical scenario. However, we must examine these clinical scenarios separately and review the data that are available and the subsequent guideline recommendations from the major medical societies.

Secondary Prevention of Stable CAD

The ACC guidelines on secondary prevention in stable ischemic heart disease state that aspirin monotherapy (or other antiplatelet if allergic) is a Class I indication to continue lifelong [30]. For a patient on anticoagulation for thrombotic disease, the anticoagulants are more efficacious as compared to antiplatelet agents in preventing a thrombotic event in the common clinical scenarios of deep vein thrombosis (DVT), pulmonary embolism (PE), and atrial fibrillation [31]. It is common in up to 11 % of the population with stable coronary artery to have an indication for anticoagulation [32]. In this situation, it is common for practitioners to combine an antiplatelet agent with an anticoagulant with the thought that they are treating two separate diseases with two separate targeted therapies. However, recent real world registries have shown that the combination can lead to serious bleeding which is an independent predictor of mortality [32, 33]. In the CORONOR trial, over 4000 patients with stable CAD (at least 1 year out from any acute coronary syndrome or revascularization procedure) were prospectively studied over a 2 year period [32]. Patients on an anticoagulant in addition to an antiplatelet had a 7.3 times increased risk of bleeding in comparison to antiplatelet monotherapy. This trial only assessed significant (Bleeding Academic Research Consortium (BARC) 3 or higher) bleeding, and indeed the bleeding events were an independent predictor of mortality in this stable CAD population. There was no downside (no increased ischemic stroke, myocardial infarction or cardiovascular death) to being on a single anticoagulant alone as compared to being on an anticoagulant plus an antiplatelet agent. Therefore, this study clearly shows the benefit of only taking anticoagulation alone (without the addition of any antiplatelet agent) in a stable coronary artery disease patient that is at least 1 year out from an acute coronary syndrome or any type of revascularization that has a definite indication for anticoagulation. One limitation of this study was that the dosing of aspirin was not reported. A larger observational cohort study of 8700 Danish patients with both atrial fibrillation and stable coronary artery disease backs up this hypothesis as well [33]. They showed that relative to warfarin mono-therapy, there was no decrease in the risk of MI or coronary death associated with the use of warfarin plus an antiplatelet agent. In fact, if triple combination therapy was used, there was actually an increase in this ischemic risk. There was also comparative benefit in all of these groups in terms of preventing thromboembolism. On the flip side, bleeding risk hazard ratios were significantly (50–80 %) higher on dual therapy and up to 100 % higher with triple therapy as compared with monotherapy with warfarin alone. Bleeding was also shown to be an independent predictor of mortality in this study as well. What about trying antiplatelet therapy alone in this population? This population had over 95 % of the patients with a $CHADS_2VASC_2$ score of ≥ 2. Antiplatelet therapy alone did have decreased bleeding risks, but in exchange there was increased MI, cardiovascular death, thromboembolism and mortality. Therefore, this is not an acceptable alternative. One limitation of this large data set was that the exact aspirin dosing was not reported and broken down to the individual endpoints, although it was stated that all doses were <150 mg i.e. a relatively low dose. A second limitation was that there were no patients on NOACS or new antiplatelet agents in this trial. However, the combination of dual or single antiplatelet therapy in addition to NOACs has been shown to have a similarly increased bleeding risk without additional stroke prevention benefit [34, 35]. Current guidelines do not provide guidance on combination therapy in this stable ischemic heart disease population.

Secondary Prevention after Acute Coronary Syndrome (ACS) or Percutaneous Coronary Intervention (PCI)

Most ACS patients will undergo an early invasive strategy which frequently leads them to revascularization by CABG or stenting. It is clear from the early stent trials that antiplatelet therapy is more efficacious in preventing stent thrombosis than warfarin alone or with warfarin with a single antiplatelet agent [36–39]. However, these trials involved early generation bare metal stents that were not necessarily deployed appropriately and would be expected to be at a higher risk of thrombosis than current stent deployment techniques with thin strut bare metal stent systems or second /third generation drug eluting stent (DES) systems. On the other hand, it is also clear that dual antiplatelet therapy alone is not a substitute for anticoagulation in those patients at risk of stroke [40]. Therefore, it is important to assess newer trials in the DES area to see where the net clinical benefit of multiple pharmacologic regimens lie.

Initial registry data (n = 239) showed the combination of warfarin plus clopidogrel as having no stent thrombosis compared to a 15 % rate with warfarin plus aspirin, as well as a higher MI rate of 18.2 % vs 11 % [41]. This was followed by the large Danish registry assessing over 12,000 patients with atrial fibrillation that had a recent MI or PCI on various anticoagulant regimens [42]. This registry showed no increased risk of an ischemic coronary event in double therapy (anticoagulant plus single antiplatelet) vs triple therapy (dual antiplatelet plus anticoagulant). On the other hand, the bleeding risk was lower with dual therapy as compared to triple therapy. When clopidogrel was the antiplatelet agent, this lower bleeding risk was not statistically significant, compared to aspirin which did have statistically significant lower bleeding. One limitation of this trial was that aspirin dosing was not reported. All-cause mortality was statistically significantly lower with the combination of an oral anticoagulant plus clopidogrel in comparison to an oral anticoagulant plus aspirin. As a whole, these registry data are hypothesis-generating suggesting that a combination of clopidogrel plus an oral anticoagulant alone might be the best combination when a stent is placed and both an anticoagulant and an antiplatelet is needed.

The warfarin and clopidogrel combination was more definitively tested in the multicenter, randomized WOEST trial [43]. The WOEST trial studied 573 patients who were on long term anticoagulation for multiple clinical indications (majority of patient had atrial fibrillation) and who were undergoing PCI (25–30 % with acute coronary syndromes). Patients were randomized to receive triple therapy (aspirin at a dose of 80–100 mg, clopidogrel 75 mg, and warfarin) versus dual therapy with warfarin plus clopidogrel. The primary endpoint was any bleeding which occurred more in the triple therapy group (44.4 %) as compared to the double therapy group (19.4 % p < .0001). Severe bleeding (BARC 3) was twice as high with triple therapy as compared to double therapy and this was statistically significant. There was no difference in ischemic/thrombotic outcomes in either of the groups. However, there was lower mortality with double therapy (2.5 %) vs triple therapy (6.3 % p = .027). While these data are impressive, the study was not powered to consider the ischemic and mortality endpoints and must only be considered hypothesis-generating.

One limitation of these studies was that warfarin was used as the anticoagulant and not the NOACS. However, based on other evidence, it is reasonable to expect similar increased bleeding risk with NOACS as part of a triple therapy combination. For example, in post ACS patients, triple therapy with apixaban was associated with worsening bleeding but no better thromboembolic protection leading to premature discontinuation of the APPRAISE-2 clinical trial [44]. When all studies of NOACs in ACS were included in multiple meta-analyses, a similar trend was seen with at least a doubling of bleeding rate with triple therapy as compared to dual antiplatelet therapy with only a very mild decrease in ischemic events [45, 46].

The newest 2014 ACC guidelines on atrial fibrillation give a IIb recommendation for choosing bare metal stents to minimize the duration of dual antiplatelet therapy in atrial fibrillation patients as compared to DES [47]. There is also a IIb recommendation to use clopidogrel alone plus an oral anticoagulant for those with a $CHADS_2VASC_2$ scores ≥2. This is in contrast to the European guidelines on revascularization [48] and their consensus document on atrial fibrillation in the setting of PCI or ACS [49]. These provide more detail depending on the patient's

Recommendations	Class[a]	Level[b]
In patients with a firm indication for oral anticoagulation (e.g. atrial fibrillation with CHA_2DS_2-VASc score ≥2, venous thromboembolism, LV thrombus, or mechanical valve prosthesis), oral anticoagulation is recommended in addition to antiplatelet therpay.	I	C
New-generation DES are preferred over BMS among patients requiring oral anticoagulation if bleeding risk is low (HAS-BLED ≤2).	IIa	C
In patients with SCAD and atrial fibrillation with CHA_2DS_2-VASc score ≥2 at low bleeding risk (HAS-BLED ≤2), inital triple therapy of (N)OAC and ASA (75–100 mg/day) and clopidogrel 75 mg/day should be considered for a duration of at least one month after BMS or new-generation DES followed by dual therapy with (N)OAC and aspirin 75–100 mg/day or clopidogrel (75 mg/day) continued up to 12 months.	IIa	C
DAPT should be considered as alternative to initial triple therapy for patients with SCAD and atrial fibrillation with a CHA_2DS_2-VASc score ≤1.	IIa	C
In patients with ACS and atrial fibrillation with low bleeding risk (HAS-BLED ≤2), inital triple therapy of (N)OAC and ASA (75–100 mg/day) and clopidogrel 75 mg/day should be considered for a duration of 6 months irrespective of stent type followed by (N)OAC and aspirin 75–100 mg/day or clopidogrel (75 mg/day) continued up to 12 months.	IIa	C
In patients requiring oral anticoagulation at high bleeding risk (HAS BLED ≥3), triple therapy of (N)OAC and ASA (75–100 mg/day) and clopidogrel 75 mg/day should be considered for a duration of one month followed by (N)OAC and aspirin 75–100 mg/day or clopidogrel (75 mg/day) irrespective of clinical setting (SCAD or ACS) and stent type (BMS or new-generation DES).	IIa	C
Dual therapy of (N)OAC and clopidogrel 75 mg/day may be considered as a alternative to initial triple therapy in selected patients.	IIb	B
The use of ticagrelor and prasugrel as part of initial triple therapy is not recommended	III	C

Fig. 12.1 2014 European Guideline recommendations for antithrombotic treatment in patients undergoing PCI who require oral anticoagulation. *a* class of recommendation, *b* level of evidence, *DAPT* dual antiplatelet therapy, *SCAD* stable coronary artery disease (Modified from Windecker et al. [48], with permission of Oxford University Press)

$CHADS_2VASC_2$ score and HAS BLED score (see Fig. 12.1). Triple therapy was the preferred strategy for at least 1 month. These recommendations were based mostly on expert opinion. Like the ACC guidelines, they endorsed the WOEST strategy of dual therapy right away as only a IIb indication. They do clarify that prasugrel or ticagrelor should not be used as a part of triple therapy because of the greater risk of major bleeding [50].

Conclusion

Based on the current guidelines and the data presented above, in a patient with an indication for anticoagulation, we recommend the following:

1. No additional antiplatelet regimen should be used for primary prevention of coronary artery disease or for secondary prevention in stable coronary artery disease patients (at least 1 year out from revascularization or ACS). Anticoagulation alone should be given.
2. In a patient with a recent acute coronary syndrome or a recently placed stent, we endorse the individualized approach of the ESC guidelines in which the exact regimen should be based on weighing their thrombotic risk ($CHADS_2VASC_2$ score) vs the bleeding risk (HAS BLED) score (Fig. 12.1).
3. In patients with mechanical heart valves, combination therapy of both aspirin and warfarin should be given, regardless of cardiovascular disease status.
4. It is important to realize the limitations of most of the data that have been presented. First, it is important to realize that most of the data comes from patients

with the indication for anticoagulation being atrial fibrillation. When considering atrial fibrillation, the risk of stroke using the $CHADS_2VASC_2$ risk algorithm might be low (score = 0 or 1) and these patients could benefit from antiplatelet therapy alone. This was shown convincingly in the MUSICA prospective registry. Low risk atrial fibrillation patients (CHADS of 0 or 1) had no adverse cardiovascular events, including stroke, on dual antiplatelet therapy alone whereas any combination with an anticoagulant showed more bleeding and worsening cardiovascular events in this low risk subset [51]. Another limitation is that the exact dosing of aspirin wasn't known in many of the large registries and meta-analyses that make up a bulk of the data. Also, when considering bleeding risk, there are multiple definitions of bleeding that vary from minor nuisance bleeding to a major intracranial bleed that could be life threatening. Therefore, all bleeding "endpoints" don't carry the same clinical weight within and between trials. It is important for the physician to make sure they are comparing "major" ischemic events that they are trying to prevent (like stroke and myocardial infarction) to "major" bleeding events. It is sometimes necessary to go back to the individual clinical trial to sort this out. Therefore, even with the current evidence and guideline recommendations, it is always necessary for a physician to individualize care to their particular patient, and it is often necessary to go outside of the guidelines when the evidence base that made up the guidelines didn't include that particular demographic in their trials.

5. Clearly, there is currently an incomplete evidence base and we look forward to the publication of further trials Redual PCI (looking at dabigatran in various combination regimens), Pioneer AF-PCI (examining rivaroxaban in various combination regimens, Isar Triple (looking at 6 weeks of triple therapy vs 6 months of triple therapy after DES implantation)) and the creation of new larger randomized trials to help further guide best practices in this controversial area.

References

1. Lardizabal J, Joshi B, Ambrose J. The balance between anti-ischemic efficacy and bleeding risk of antithrombotic therapy in percutaneous coronary intervention: a Yin-Yang paradigm. J Invasive Cardiol. 2010;22:284–92.
2. Collaborative meta-analysis of randomised trials of antiplatelet therapy for prevention of death, myocardial infarction, and stroke in high risk patients. BMJ. 2002;324:71–86.
3. Hamberg M, Svensson J, Samuelsson B. Thromboxanes: a new group of biologically active compounds derived from prostaglandin endoperoxides. Proc Natl Acad Sci. 1975;72:2294–8.
4. Fitzgerald GA. Mechanisms of platelet activation: thromboxane A2 as an amplifying signal for other agonists. Am J Cardiol. 1991;68:11B–5.
5. Baigent C, Blackwell L, Collins R, et al. Aspirin in the primary and secondary prevention of vascular disease: collaborative meta-analysis of individual participant data from randomised trials. Lancet. 2009;373:1849–60.
6. Peto R, Gray R, Collins R, et al. Randomised trial of prophylactic daily aspirin in British male doctors. Br Med J. 1988;296:313–6.
7. Ridker PM, Cook NR, Lee IM, et al. A randomized trial of low-dose aspirin in the primary prevention of cardiovascular disease in women. N Engl J Med. 2005;352:1293–304.

8. Collaborative Group of the Primary Prevention Project. Low-dose aspirin and vitamin E in people at cardiovascular risk: a randomised trial in general practice. Collaborative Group of the Primary Prevention Project. Lancet. 2001;357:89–95.

9. Steering Committee of the Physicians' Health Study Research Group. Final report on the aspirin component of the ongoing Physicians' Health Study. N Engl J Med. 1989;321:129–35.

10. The Medical Research Council's General Practice Research Framework. Thrombosis prevention trial: randomised trial of low-intensity oral anticoagulation with warfarin and low-dose aspirin in the primary prevention of ischaemic heart disease in men at increased risk. Lancet. 1998;351:233–41.

11. Hansson L, Zanchetti A, Carruthers SG, et al. Effects of intensive blood-pressure lowering and low-dose aspirin in patients with hypertension: principal results of the Hypertension Optimal Treatment (HOT) randomised trial. Lancet. 1998;351:1755–62.

12. Vandvik PO, Lincoff AM, Gore JM, et al. Primary and secondary prevention of cardiovascular disease: antithrombotic Therapy and Prevention of Thrombosis, 9th edition: American College of Chest Physicians Evidence-Based Clinical Practice Guidelines. Chest. 2012;141: e637S–68.

13. He J, Whelton PK, Vu B, et al. Aspirin and risk of hemorrhagic stroke: a meta-analysis of randomized controlled trials. JAMA. 1998;280:1930–5.

14. Bartolucci AA, Tendera M, Howard G. Meta-analysis of multiple primary prevention trials of cardiovascular events using aspirin. Am J Cardiol. 2011;107:1796–801.

15. Raju N, Sobieraj-Teague M, Hirsh J, et al. Effect of aspirin on mortality in the primary prevention of cardiovascular disease. Am J Med. 2011;124:621–9.

16. Berger JS, Lala A, Krantz MJ, et al. Aspirin for the prevention of cardiovascular events in patients without clinical cardiovascular disease: a meta-analysis of randomized trials. Am Heart J. 2011;162:115–24.

17. Seshasai SR, Wijesuriya S, Sivakumaran R, et al. Effect of aspirin on vascular and nonvascular outcomes: meta-analysis of randomized controlled trials. Arch Intern Med. 2012;172:209–16.

18. Ogawa H, Nakayama M, Morimoto T, et al. Low-dose aspirin for primary prevention of atherosclerotic events in patients with type 2 diabetes: a randomized controlled trial. JAMA. 2008;300:2134–41.

19. Fowkes FG, Price JF, Stewart MC, et al. Aspirin for prevention of cardiovascular events in a general population screened for a low ankle brachial index: a randomized controlled trial. JAMA. 2010;303:841–8.

20. Belch J, MacCuish A, Campbell I, et al. The prevention of progression of arterial disease and diabetes (POPADAD) trial. BMJ. 2008;337:a1840.

21. Patrono C. Low-dose aspirin in primary prevention: cardioprotection, chemoprevention, both, or neither? Eur Heart J. 2013;34:3403–11.

22. Pignone M, Alberts MJ, Colwell JA, et al. Aspirin for primary prevention of cardiovascular events in people with diabetes: a position statement of the American Diabetes Association, a scientific statement of the American Heart Association, and an expert consensus document of the American College of Cardiology Foundation. Circulation. 2010;121:2694–701.

23. Wolff T, Miller T, Ko S. Aspirin for the primary prevention of cardiovascular events: an update of the evidence for the US Preventative Services Task Force. Ann Intern Med. 2009;150:405–10.

24. Perk J, De Backer G, Gohlke H, et al. European Guidelines on cardiovascular disease prevention in clinical practice (version 2012). The Fifth Joint Task Force of the European Society of Cardiology and Other Societies on Cardiovascular Disease Prevention in Clinical Practice (constituted by representatives of nine societies and by invited experts). Eur Heart J. 2012;33:1635–701.

25. Dentali F, Douketis JD, Lim W, Crowther M. Combined aspirin-oral anticoagulant therapy compared with oral anticoagulant therapy alone among patients at risk for cardiovascular disease. Arch Intern Med. 2007;167:117–1241.

26. Steinberg B, Kim S, Piccini J, et al. Use and associated risks of concomitant aspirin therapy with oral anticoagulation in patients with atrial fibrillation: insights from the Outcomes Registry for Better Informed Treatment of Atrial Fibrillation (ORBIT-AF) Registry. Circulation. 2013;128:721–8.
27. Butchart EG. Prosthetic heart valves. Cardiovascular thrombosis. 2nd ed. 1998. p. 395–414.
28. Massel D, Little S. Antiplatelet and anticoagulation for patients with prosthetic heart valves. Cochrane Database Syst Rev. 2013 (7):CD003464.
29. Nishimura RA, Otto CM, Bonow RO, et al. 2014 AHA/ACC guideline for the management of patients with valvular heart disease: a report of the American College of Cardiology/American Heart Association Task Force on Practice Guidelines. J Am Coll Cardiol. 2014;63(22): e57–185.
30. Fihn S, Gardin J, Abrams J, et al. 2012 ACCF/AHA/ACP/AATS/PCNA/SCAI/STS guideline for the diagnosis and management of patients with stable ischemic heart disease. J Am Coll Cardiol. 2012;60:e44–164.
31. Hart R, Pearce L, Aguilar M. Meta-analysis: antithrombotic therapy to prevent stroke in patients who have nonvalvular atrial fibrillation. Ann Intern Med. 2007;146:857–67.
32. Hamon M, Lemesle G, Tricot O, et al. Incidence, source, determinants, and prognostic impact of major bleeding in outpatients with stable coronary artery disease. J Am Coll Cardiol. 2014;64:1430–6.
33. Lamberts M, Gislason G, Lip G, et al. Antiplatelet therapy for stable coronary artery disease in atrial fibrillation patients taking an oral anticoagulant. Circulation. 2014;129:1577–85.
34. Dans A, Connolly S, Wallentin L, et al. Concomitant use of antiplatelet therapy with dabigatran or warfarin in the Randomized Evaluation of Long-Term Anticoagulation Therapy (RE-LY) trial. Circulation. 2013;127:634–40.
35. Alexander J, Lopes R, Thomas L, et al. Apixaban vs. warfarin with concomitant aspirin in patients with atrial fibrillation: insights from the ARISTOTLE trial. Eur Heart J. 2014;35:224–32.
36. Schömig A, Neumann FJ, Kastrati A, et al. A randomized comparison of antiplatelet and anticoagulant therapy after the placement of coronary-artery stents. N Engl J Med. 1996;334:1084–9.
37. Leon MB, Baim DS, Popma JJ, et al. A clinical trial comparing three antithrombotic-drug regimens after coronary-artery stenting. N Engl J Med. 1998;339:1665–71.
38. Bertrand ME, Legrand V, Boland J, et al. Randomized multicenter comparison of conventional anticoagulation versus antiplatelet therapy in unplanned and elective coronary stenting. The Full Anticoagulation Versus Aspirin and Ticlopidine (FANTASTIC) Study. Circulation. 1996;98:1597–603.
39. Urban P, Macaya C, Rupprecht H, et al. Randomized evaluation of anticoagulation versus antiplatelet therapy after coronary stent implantation in high-risk patients. The Multicenter Aspirin and Ticlopidine Trial after Intracoronary Stenting (MATTIS). Circulation. 1998;98:2126–32.
40. Connolly S, Pogue J, Hart R, et al. Clopidogrel plus aspirin versus oral anticoagulation for atrial fibrillation in the Atrial fibrillation Clopidogrel Trial with Irbesartan for prevention of Vascular Events (ACTIVE W): a randomised controlled trial. Lancet. 2006;367:1903–12.
41. Karjalainen PP, Porela P, Ylitalo A, et al. Safety and efficacy of combined antiplatelet-warfarin therapy after coronary stenting. Eur Heart J. 2007;28:726–32.
42. Lamberts M, Gislason G, Olesen J, et al. Oral anticoagulation and antiplatelets in atrial fibrillation patients after myocardial infarction and coronary intervention. J Am Coll Cardiol. 2013;62:981–9.
43. Dewilde W, Oirbans T, Verheugt F, et al. Use of clopidogrel with or without aspirin in patients taking oral anticoagulant therapy and undergoing percutaneous coronary intervention: an open-label, randomized, controlled trial. Lancet. 2013;381:1107–15.
44. Alexander JH, Lopes RD, James S, et al. Apixaban with antiplatelet therapy after acute coronary syndrome. N Engl J Med. 2011;365:699–708.

45. Oldgren J, Wallentin L, Alexander J, et al. New oral anticoagulants in addition to single or dual antiplatelet therapy after an acute coronary syndrome: a systematic review and meta-analysis. Eur Heart J. 2013;34:1670–80.
46. Komocsi A, Vorobcsuk A, Kehl D, et al. Use of new-generation oral anticoagulant agents in patients receiving antiplatelet therapy after an acute coronary syndrome: systematic review and meta-analysis of randomized controlled trials. Arch Intern Med. 2012;172:1537–45.
47. January C, Wann L, Alpert J, et al. AHA/ACC/HRS guideline for the management of patients with atrial fibrillation. J Am Coll Cardiol. 2014;64(21):e1–76.
48. Windecker S, Kolh P, Alfonso F, et al. 2014 ESC/EACTS guideline on myocardial revascularization. Eur Heart J. 2014;35(37):2541–619. doi:10.1093/eurheartj/ehu278. Epub 2014 Aug 29.
49. Lip G, Windecker S, Hubert K, et al. Management of antithrombotic therapy in atrial fibrillation patients presenting with acute coronary syndrome and/or undergoing percutaneous coronary or valve interventions: a joint consensus document of the European Society of Cardiology Working Group on Thrombosis, European Heart Rhythm Association (EHRA), European Association of Percutaneous Cardiovascular Interventions (EAPCI) and European Association of Acute Cardiac Care (ACCA) endorsed by the Heart Rhythm Society (HRS) and Asia-Pacific Heart Rhythm Society (APHRS). Eur Heart J. 2014;35(45):3155–79.
50. Sarafoff N, Martischnig A, Wealer J, et al. Triple therapy with aspirin, prasugrel, and vitamin K antagonists in patients with drug-eluting stent implantation and an indication for oral anticoagulation. J Am Coll Cardiol. 2013;61:2060–6.
51. Sambola A, Ferreira-Gonzalez I, Angel J, et al. Therapeutic strategies after coronary stenting in chronically anticoagulated patients: the MUSICA study. Heart. 2009;95:1483–8.

Chapter 13
Managing Intracoronary Thrombus During PCI

David Antoniucci

Abstract Occlusive or nonocclusive thrombosis triggered by a disrupted or eroded atherosclerotic plaque is the anatomic substrate of most acute coronary syndromes including ST-segment elevation myocardial infarctions (AMI). For this pathological substrate, macro- and microembolization during percutaneous coronary intervention (PCI) in the setting of AMI is frequent and may result in obstruction of the microvessel network, and decreased efficacy of reperfusion and myocardial salvage. Thrombus may complicate other complex anatomic conditions associated with an altered flow such as ectatic or aneurysmatic coronary arteries, degenerated venous grafts, or coronary stents. Removal of thrombus before any other intervention may dramatically decrease the risk of no-flow, and has the potential for improvement in survival. Many types of thrombectomy removal or protection devices are currently available, from low technology catheters based on manual thrombus aspiration, including proximal or distal antiembolic protection devices, to high technology devices using mechanical energy allowing fragmentation and removal of thrombus. Studies on thrombectomy before stenting have produced conflicting results and there is no consensus as to their routine use in lesions containing thrombus. Other procedural approaches include specific covered and self-expandable stents for thrombus jailing, or deferred stenting after prolonged infusion of antithrombotic drugs.

Keywords Thrombectomy • Myocardial infarction • Primary percutaneous coronary intervention

Introduction

Occlusive or nonocclusive thrombosis triggered by a disrupted or eroded atherosclerotic plaque is the anatomic substrate of most acute coronary syndromes including ST-segment elevation myocardial infarctions (AMI). For this pathological

D. Antoniucci, MD
Division of Cardiology, Department of Cardiology, Careggi Hospital,
Largo Brambilla 3, Florence 50121, Italy
e-mail: david.antoniucci@virgilio.it

© Springer International Publishing Switzerland 2015   175
J.A. Ambrose, A.E. Rodríguez (eds.), *Controversies in Cardiology*,
DOI 10.1007/978-3-319-20415-4_13

substrate, macro- and microembolization during percutaneous coronary intervention (PCI) in the setting of AMI is frequent and may result in obstruction of the
microvessel network, and decreased efficacy of reperfusion and myocardial salvage
[1]. Thrombus may complicate other complex anatomic conditions associated with
an altered flow such as ectatic or aneurysmatic coronary arteries, degenerated
venous grafts, or coronary stents. In this conditions frequently the thrombotic burden is large and the risk of extensive macro- and micro-vessel network disruption
and myocardial infarction due to embolization during PCI is very high. Removal of
thrombus before any other intervention may dramatically decrease the risk of no-
flow, and has the potential for improvement in survival. A specific procedural
approach to thrombus removal should be considered in the large majority of patients
with AMI and in patients with angiographic evidence of thrombus and a large area
at risk, or pre-existing severe left ventricular dysfunction, since in these patients
no-reflow due to embolization is associated with a very high mortality rate [2].

Many types of thrombectomy removal or protection devices are currently available, from low technology catheters based on manual thrombus aspiration, including proximal or distal antiembolic protection devices, to high technology devices
using mechanical energy allowing fragmentation and removal of thrombus. Studies
on thrombectomy before stenting have produced conflicting results and there is no
consensus as to their routine use in lesions containing thrombus. Other procedural
approaches include specific covered and self-expandable stents for thrombus jailing, or deferred stenting after prolonged infusion of antithrombotic drugs.

Antiembolic Protection Devices (Table 13.1)

Antiembolic protection devices include distal and proximal occlusive devices and
filters. All studies on these devices in the setting of AMI have failed to show any
reduction in infarct size and improvement in clinical outcome [3–7]. Conversely,
their use in the treatment of degenerated venous grafts is supported by the positive
results of several trials [8–10].

Manual Aspiration Catheters

The majority of published studies on thrombectomy in patients with AMI used aspiration catheters [11–17]. A major advantage of manual aspiration catheters is the
ease of use. Two major limitations of these devices are the unpredictability of the
efficacy, since in 30 % of cases of successful lesion crossing by the catheter, the
aspiration is completely negative, and the high profile of the catheters that may
promote embolization when the occlusion is crossed or prevent their utilization in
tortuous, calcified, or small vessels. The routine use of manual aspiration catheters
in the setting of AMI was supported by the positive results of some single center

Table 13.1 Summary of studies on antiembolic protection devices

	Setting	Device	End point	Result
Stone et al. [3]	AMI (n=496)	GuardWire[a]	Infarct size, ST-segment resolution	Negative
Muramatsu et al. [4]	AMI (n=341)	Guardwire[a]	Blush score 3	Negative
Gick et al. [5]	AMI (n=200)	FilterWire[b]	Adenosine-induced Doppler flow velocity	Negative
Guetta et al. [6]	AMI (n=100)	FilterWire[b]	TIMI flow, myocardial blush, ST-segment resolution	Negative
Cura et al. [7]	AMI (n=140)	FilterWire[b]	ST-segment resolution	Negative
Baim et al. [8]	SVG (n=801)	GuardWire[a]	30-day MACE	Positive
Stone et al. [9]	SVG (n=651)	FilterWire[b] vs GuardWire[a]	30-day MACE	Positive
Grube et al. [10]	SVG (n=103)	GuardWire[a]	TIMI flow grade 3	Positive[c]

AMI acute myocardial infarction, *MACE* major adverse cardiac events, *SVG* saphenous venous graft
[a]Distal occlusive device
[b]Nonocclusive device
[c]Nonrandomized trial

studies. In the Thrombus Aspiration during Percutaneous coronary intervention in Acute myocardial infarction (TAPAS) trial 1,071 patients were randomized to manual aspiration or conventional PCI, and 10 % of patients randomized to thrombus aspiration crossed to conventional PCI since the operator considered the target vessel too small or tortuous to allow the use of the aspiration catheter [15]. Thus, in this study any traumatic attempt to cross the lesion with the aspiration catheter in patients with a difficult anatomy was avoided. Despite the exclusion from aspiration of patients with difficult anatomy, particles could be retrieved in only 72.9 % of cases randomized to aspiration, and manual aspiration was associated with a better myocardial reperfusion as assessed by the surrogate angiographic primary end point of myocardial blush [15]. At 1 year follow-up, patients randomized to manual aspiration had a better survival than patients randomized to conventional PCI: the mortality rates were 3.6 and 6.7 %, respectively [16]. However, it should be outlined that the study was not powered for survival and the differences in survival could have been due to chance.

The results of the TAPAS trial were not confirmed by the TASTE trial, that was the largest trial comparing manual aspiration with conventional angioplasty in patients with AMI and sufficiently powered for clinical outcome [18, 19]. This multicenter study randomized 7,244 patients to manual aspiration or conventional PCI. Randomization to manual aspiration was not associated with improved survival at 1 month and at 12 months. The 30-day mortality rates were 3.0 % in the standard PCI arm and 2.8 % in the manual aspiration arm (HR 0.94 95 % CI 0.72–1.20, p =0.63). At 1 year, there were no difference in the composite of death, myocardial infarction and stent thrombosis between the 2 arms (17.7 % in the standard PCI arm, and 16.3 % in the manual aspiration arms). Another ongoing trial comparing manual aspiration with standard PCI is enrolling 10,700 patients and will provide a definite answer to the usefulness or futility of routine use of manual aspiration catheter in AMI (TOTAL; ClinicalTrials.gov number, NCT01149044).

Mechanical Thrombectomy Devices

The rheolytic thrombectomy (RT) system (AngioJet, Boston Scientific, Minneapolis, MN) consists of a dual lumen catheter with an external pump providing pressurized saline solution via the effluent lumen to the catheter tip. Multiple saline jets from the distal part of the catheter travel backwards at 390 mph, and create a localized negative pressure zone that draws thrombus where the jets fragment it and propels the small particles to the evacuation lumen of the catheter. The first 5 F generation catheter for coronary use was associated with a substantial device failure rate due to the inability to cross the lesion by the large and poorly trackable catheter, embolization, and vessel perforation. In a post-hoc analysis in a series of 70 patients with AMI enrolled in the VEGAS 1 and 2 trials, the device failure rate was 22 % [20, 21]. The second generation AngioJet catheter (XMI) and the more recent third generation catheter (Spiroflex) that are available are 4 F in size and have an improved design of the profile and of the opening of the jets allowing easy and nontraumatic navigation also in complex anatomy (tortuous or calcified vessels), and the ability to remove quickly large amount of fresh thrombus. The last generation catheter can cross the lesion without the need for pre-dilation in more than 95 % of the cases.

Four randomized trials tested the efficacy and safety of RT in different settings (Table 13.2). The efficacy of RT in decreasing procedural embolization and subsequent clinical adverse events was demonstrated by the VeGAS-2 trial that enrolled patients with a very high risk of embolization, such as patients with diseased venous grafts or native vessels with angiographic evidence of large thrombus [21]. Patients with AMI were excluded. The study, based on a sample of 352 patients compared RT with intravessel infusion of urokinase and showed a > 50 % reduction in 1-month major adverse events in patients randomized to thrombectomy (16 %and 33 % respectively, P < 0.001). The Florence-AngioJet randomized trial was a mechanistic small study based on a sample of 100 patients with a first AMI and the end points of the study were early ST-segment resolution, the corrected TIMI frame count, and the infarct size as assessed by technetium-99 m sestamibi scintigraphy at 1 month [22]. All end points were met. Patients randomized to thrombectomy before direct stenting had a higher incidence of early ST-segment elevation resolution (90 % vs 72 %, P=0.022), lower corrected TIMI frame counts (18.2±7.7 vs 22.5±11.0, P=0.032), and smaller infarcts (13.0±11.6 % vs 21.2±18.0 %, P=0.010) as compared to patients randomized to direct stenting alone. By multivariate analysis, the only variables related to the early ST-segment resolution were randomization to

Table 13.2 Randomized studies on rheolytic thrombectomy

	Setting	Patients	End point	Result
Kuntz et al. [21]	SVG and native vessel with thrombus	352[a]	30-day MACE	Positive
Antoniucci et al. [22]	AMI	100	cTIMI frame count, ST segment resolution, infarct size	Positive
Ali et al. [23]	AMI	480	Infarct size	Negative
Migliorini et al. [24]	AMI	501	ST-segment resolution and infarct size	Negative for infarct size, positive for ST-segment resolution and clinical outcome

AMI acute myocardial infarction, *MACE* major adverse cardiac events, *SVG* saphenous vein graft
[a]Comparison of rheolytic thrombectomy with local infusion of urokinase

thrombectomy (OR 3.56, 95 % CI 1.11–11.42, P=0.032), and diabetes mellitus (OR 0.24, 95 % CI 0.07–0.86, P=0.029). At 1 month, no patient died, or had reinfarction, and the 6-month clinical outcomes were identical in the 2 arms: the mortality rate was 2 % in both groups, and no patient had reinfarction.

The AIMI trial is a multicenter randomized trial that compared RT before stenting of the infarct artery with conventional PCI and was based on a sample of 480 patients [23]. The primary end point of the study was infarct size as assessed by sestamibi scintigraphy at 14–28 days after the procedure. The study showed larger infarcts in the thrombectomy arm as compared to the control arm (12.5±12.13 % and 9.8±10.92 % respectively, P=0.03), and more importantly, an unexpected higher mortality in the thrombectomy arm at 1 month (4.6 % vs 0.8 %, P=0.02) and at 6 months (6.7 % vs 1.7 %, P=0.01). Final TIMI grade 3 flow was seen more frequently in the control arm as compared to the thrombectomy arm (97 % and 91.8 % respectively, P<0.02). Several concerns in study design and in RT technique may explain the negative and harmful results of the study. The enrollment criteria did not include angiographically visible thrombus, and moderate to large thrombus (grade 3 and 4 according to TIMI thrombus score) was present in an unrealistic minority of patients at baseline angiography (21.3 % in the thrombectomy arm and 19.6 % in the control arm). This figure suggests a selection bias against the enrollment of patients with a large amount of thrombus and who could derive the strongest benefit from thrombectomy before coronary stenting. Unfortunately, the authors did not provide a screen fail registry, but other characteristics of the study patient cohort strengthen this suspicion. More than 1/3 of patients (35 %) had an already open infarct artery at baseline angiography, and more importantly the infarct size was very small in both arms, with similar normal left ventricular ejection fraction at the time of scintigraphic assessment (51.3±11.53 % in the thrombectomy arm, and 52.3±10.89 % in the control arm). Another concern of the study design was the exclusion from enrollment of patients with severe left ventricular dysfunction and cardiogenic shock. The exclusion of these high-risk patients is not easily explained considering that just in this type of patients a no-reflow due to PCI embolization may be immediately fatal.

Finally, the nonuniformity of treatment may have introduced confounding effects favoring the control arm. Eight percent of patients randomized to thrombectomy did not have the treatment, procedural variables that may have a significant impact on the risk of no-reflow, such as predilation, or postdilation, or stent type were left to the discretion of the operator, as well as the thrombectomy technique, with a distal-to proximal approach used in 48 % of cases. The thrombectomy retrograde technique should be considered as inappropriate since with this technique, the activation of the thrombectomy catheter is made only after the positioning of the device across the occlusion favoring embolization before thrombectomy.

The JETSTENT trial was a multicenter trials that enrolled 501 patients with AMI and angiographic evidence of thrombus TIMI grade 3–5, and compared RT before direct infarct artery stenting with direct stenting alone [24]. The co-primary end points of the study were early ST-segment elevation resolution and infarct size as assessed by ^{99m}Tc-sestamibi scintigraphy. The ST-segment resolution was more frequent in the RT arm as compared with the DS alone arm: 85.8 % and 78.8 %, respectively (p=0.043), while no significant differences between groups were revealed in infarct size and the other surrogate angiographic end points. The 6-month major adverse cardiovascular events rate was 11.2 % in the thrombectomy arm and 19.4 % in the direct stenting alone arm (p=0.011). The 1-year event-free survival rates were 85.2 ± 2.3 % for the RT arm, and 75.0 ± 3.1 % for the direct stenting alone arm (p=0.009). At multivariable analysis, RT was independently related to early ST-segment elevation resolution (OR 1.70, 95 % CI 1.03–2.82, p=0.0039) and to major adverse cardiovascular events at 1 year (HR 0.55, 95 % CI 0.35–0,86, p=0.008). Although the primary efficacy end points were not met, the results of this study support the use of RT before infarct artery stenting in patients with acute myocardial infarction and evidence of coronary thrombus.

A small randomized study including 80 patients with AMI, the SMART trial, compared the efficacy of RT with manual aspiration catheter [25]. The primary end point of the study was residual thrombus burden after thrombectomy and before direct infarct artery stenting as assessed by optical coherence tomography. The study showed large residual thrombus burden more frequently in the manual aspiration arm as compared to RT (patients with number of quadrants containing thrombus above the median value were 60 % in the manual aspiration arm and 37 % in the rheolytic thrombectomy arm, p=0.039). All surrogate markers of reperfusion were better in the RT arm and at 6 months, the percentage of malapposed stent struts in the manual aspiration arm was higher than the RT arm (2.7 ± 4.5 %, and 0.8 ± 1.6 %, respectively, p 0.019). More importantly, the study showed that both techniques do not allow for the complete removal of thrombus (only 1 out of 80 patients did not have residual thrombus after thrombectomy). It is unknown if the residual more organized thrombus after thrombectomy has a decreased potential for embolization after infarct artery stenting.

Alternative energies such as laser and ultrasound have shown, despite the rationale for the use of these energies to destroy the thrombus, negative and harmful results in the clinical setting, due to the poor trackability of the catheters, the low efficacy of thrombus ablation, and the high rate of major procedural complications (dissection, perforation, embolization).

Self-Expanding Stents

The rationale for the use of a self-expanding stent in the setting of AMI is that thrombus and vasoconstricion can result in undersizing the stent with subsequent stent malapposition when the jailed thrombus is resolved, and an increased risk of thrombosis and restenosis. On the other hand, an aggressive post dilatation after stent deployment may result in an increased risk of embolization and no-reflow. A small randomized study including 80 patients compared stent malapposition after self-expanding stent (Stentys, Stentys S.A., Paris, France) with a balloon expandable stent utilizing optical coherence tomography. At 3 days after implantation, there was a better apposition of the self-expanding stent and no difference in the clinical outcome at 6 months [26]. A large multicenter registry including 1000 patients with AMI treated with the self-expanding stent Stentys showed a low rate of major adverse cardiac events and cardiac mortality at 12 months (9.3 % and 3.2 %, respectively) and a definite or probable stent thrombosis rate of 3.4 % [27]. In this registry, stent post-dilation was at the discretion of the operator, and the rate of definite or probable stent thrombosis was high (5 %) in patients who did not receive post-dilation.

Covered Stents

A specific covered stent for the treatment of patients with AMI and lesion containing thrombus is the M-Guard stent (InspireMD, Tel Aviv, Israel). This stent comprises a balloon-expandable, thin-strut stainless steel (316 L) or chromium cobalt alloy bare metal stent platform with mesh sleeve fibers of polyethylene erephtalate (fiber width of 20 μm) attached to its outer surface. These fibers act like a net preventing distal embolization of the plaque debris/thrombus placed between the vessel wall and the stent. A randomized trial including 422 patients with AMI, the MASTER trial, compared this device with a standard balloon expandable stent [28]. The primary end point of the study was complete (>70 %) ST-segment elevation resolution. The primary end point rate was reached in 57.8 % in the M-Guard arm and 44.7 % in the control arm (p=0.008). No difference between arms was found in the 30-day clinical outcome or surrogate angiographic end points.

Deferred Stenting

An alternative strategy for the treatment of lesion containing thrombus in patients with AMI is to defer infarct artery stenting after the recanalization of the infarct artery in order to decrease the thrombus burden with a prolonged infusion of antithrombotic drugs. This strategy was tested in the DEFER- STEMI trial that compared immediate infarct artery stenting with deferred stenting in 101 patients with AMI and a high risk of no-reflow [29]. The study hypothesis was that after the initial achievement of a normal TIMI flow by wiring or nonaggressive balloon angioplasty or aspiration, a brief deferral of stenting (4–16 h) and simultaneous infusion of glycoprotein IIb/IIIa and low weight heparin could result in a decreased thrombotic burden and risk of no-reflow. The deferred stenting strategy resulted in a dramatic decrease in the no/slow- reflow rate (5.9 % vs 28.6 %, OR 0.16 [0.03–0.63], p = 0.005), and more importantly, the prevention of the no/slow-reflow according to the mechanistic design of the study, was associated with improved myocardial reperfusion and myocardial salvage as shown by all angiographic, electrocardiographic and magnetic resonance imaging parameters. Recurrence of AMI due to infarct artery reocclusion in the deferred stenting group was very low: only two patients had reocclusion of the infarct artery and both were treated successfully with bailout stenting. Indirectly, the study confirms the inability of manual thrombus aspiration to decrease the risk of embolization and no/slow-reflow since the large majority of patients in both arms (>85 %) received this treatment. Using the short temporal window of 4–16 h from the restoration of a normal flow, the logistic constraints in the application of this strategy are not impossible. However, the increased costs of a second procedure should be balanced by the demonstration of improved clinical outcome by a large clinical randomized trial.

Conclusions

According to the available evidence, I believe the following points are valid:

1. The routine use of manual aspiration catheters in the setting of AMI is not recommended due to the complete ineffectiveness of this technique in approximately 40 % of cases, and the high rate of a large residual thrombus burden in most cases.
2. Rheolytic thrombectomy is more effective than manual aspiration in thrombus removal and can be used also in difficult and complex coronary anatomies but data from randomized studies are insufficient to recommend its routine use in the setting of AMI.
3. Other specific approaches in the setting of AMI such as self-expandable stents and covered mesh stents can be considered in individual patients, but data from studies are insufficient to recommend their routine use.
4. In case of a large thrombus burden complicating a coronary aneurysm or degenerated vein grafts, antiembolic protection devices or rheolytic thrombectomy should be considered as a first option treatment, and in these cases a multi device approach can be considered as the most appropriate (Fig. 13.1).
5. Deferred stenting in patients with a restored normal flow and a predicted high risk of no-reflow after stenting is an attractive option.

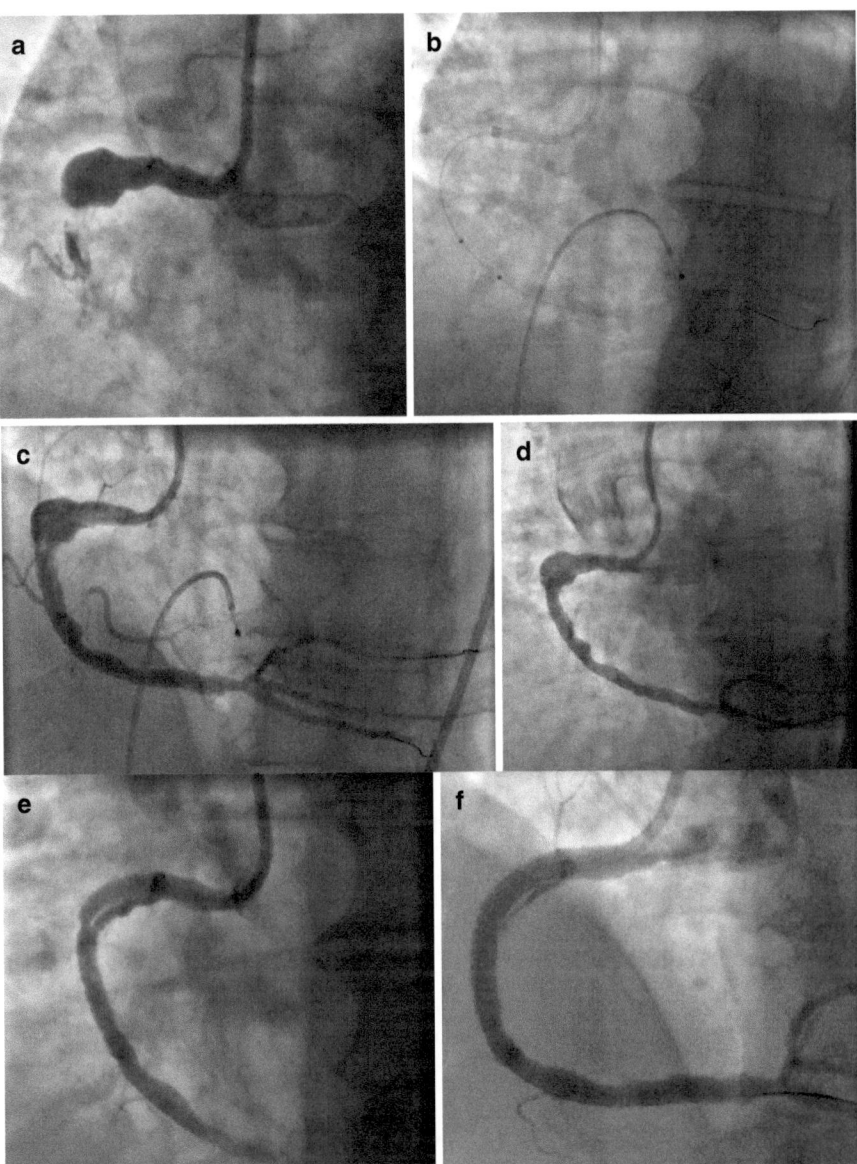

Fig. 13.1 (**a**) Acute myocardial infarction due to the thrombotic occlusion complicating a big aneurysm of the proximal right coronary artery. (**b**) The 4 French Angiojet catheter (2 radiopaque markers) navigating in the vessel. (**c**) Restoration of a normal flow. (**d**) Implantation of 2 covered stent (3,5 mm/ 14 mm in length, covering of bovine pericardium) and partial exclusion of the aneurysm. (**e**) shifting of the stents due to malapposition and evidence of 2 channels. (**f**) jailing and fixing of the 2 covered stent by a self-expandable stent with complete exclusion of the aneurysm

References

1. Topol EJ, Yadav JS. Recognition of the importance of embolization in atherosclerotic vascular disease. Circulation. 2000;101:570–80.
2. Antoniucci D, Valenti R, Migliorini A. Thrombectomy during percutaneous coronary intervention for acute myocardial infarction: are the randomized trial data relevant to patients who really need this technique? Catheter Cardiovasc Interv. 2008;71:863–9.
3. Stone GW, Webb J, Cox DA, et al. Distal microcirculatory protection during percutaneous coronary intervention in acute ST-segment elevation myocardial infarction: a randomized controlled trial. JAMA. 2005;293:1063–72.
4. Muramatsu T, Kozuma K, Tsukahara R, et al. Comparison of myocardial perfusion by distal protection before and after primary stenting for acute myocardial infarction: angiographic and clinical results of a randomized controlled trial. Catheter Cardiovasc Interv. 2007;70:677–82.
5. Gick M, Jander N, Bestehorn HP, et al. Randomized evaluation of the effects of filter-based distal protection on myocardial perfusion and infarct size after primary percutaneous catheter intervention in myocardial infarction with and without ST-segment elevation. Circulation. 2005;112:1462–9.
6. Guetta V, Mosseri M, Shechter M, et al. Safety and efficacy of the FilterWire EZ in acute ST-segment elevation myocardial infarction. Am J Cardiol. 2007;99:911–5.
7. Cura FA, Escudero AG, Berrocal D, et al. Protection of distal embolization in high-risk patients with acute ST-segment elevation myocardial infarction (PREMIAR). Am J Cardiol. 2007;99:357–63.
8. Baim DS, Wahr D, George B, et al. Randomized trial of a distal embolic protection device during percutaneous intervention of saphenous vein aorto-coronary bypass grafts. Circulation. 2002;105:1285–90.
9. Stone GW, Rogers C, Hermiller J, et al. Randomized comparison of distal protection with a filter-based catheter and a balloon occlusion and aspiration system during percutaneous intervention of diseased saphenous vein aorto-coronary bypass grafts. Circulation. 2003;108:548–53.
10. Grube E, Schofer J, Webb J, For the Saphenous Vein Graft Angioplasty Free of Emboli (SAFE), et al. Evaluation of a balloon occlusion and aspiration system for protection from distal embolization during stenting in saphenous vein grafts. Am J Cardiol. 2002;89:941–5.
11. Burzotta F, Trani C, Romagnoli E, et al. Manual thrombus-aspiration improves myocardial reperfusion: the randomized evaluation of the effect of mechanical reduction of distal embolization by thrombus-aspiration in primary and rescue angioplasty (REMEDIA) trial. J Am Coll Cardiol. 2005;46:371–6.
12. Silva-Orrego P, Colombo P, Bigi R, et al. Thrombus aspiration before primary angioplasty improves myocardial reperfusion in acute myocardial infarction: the DEAR-MI (Dethrombosis to Enhance Acute Reperfusion in Myocardial Infarction) study. J Am Coll Cardiol. 2006;48:1552–9.
13. De Luca L, Sardella G, Davidson CJ, et al. Impact of intracoronary aspiration thrombectomy during primary angioplasty on left ventricular remodelling in patients with anterior ST elevation myocardial infarction. Heart. 2006;92:951–7.
14. Kaltoft A, Bøttcher M, Nielsen SS, et al. Routine thrombectomy in percutaneous coronary intervention for acute ST-segment-elevation myocardial infarction: a randomized, controlled trial. Circulation. 2006;114:40–7.
15. Svilaas T, Vlaar PJ, van der Horst IC, et al. Thrombus aspiration during primary percutaneous intervention. N Engl J Med. 2008;358:557–67.
16. Vlaar PJ, Svilaas T, van der Horst IC, et al. Cardiac death and reinfarction after 1 year in the Thrombus Aspiration during Percutaneous coronary intervention in Acute myocardial infarction Study (TAPAS): a 1-year follow-up study. Lancet. 2008;371:1915–20.
17. Sardella G, Mancone M, Bucciarelli-Ducci C, et al. Thrombus aspiration during primary percutaneous coronary intervention improves myocardial reperfusion and reduces infarct size: the

EXPIRA (thrombectomy with Export catheter in Infarct-Related Artery during primary percutaneous coronary intervention) prospective randomized trial. J Am Coll Cardiol. 2009;53: 309–15.

18. Fröbert O, Lagerqvist B, Olivecrona GK, et al. Thrombus aspiration during ST-segment elevation myocardial infarction. N Engl J Med. 2013;369:1587–97.

19. Lagerqvist B, Fröbert O, Olivecrona GK, et al. Outcomes 1 year after thrombus aspiration for myocardial infarction. N Engl J Med. 2014;371:1111–20.

20. Rinfret S, Katsiyiammis PT, Ho KK, et al. Effectiveness of rheolytic coronary thrombectomy with the AngioJet catheter. Am J Cardiol. 2002;90:470–6.

21. Kuntz RE, Baim DS, Cohen DJ, et al. A trial comparing rheolytic thrombectomy wiyth intracoronary urokinase for coronary and vein graft thrombus (the Vein Graft Angiojet Study [VeGAS 2]). Am J Cardiol. 2002;89:326–30.

22. Antoniucci D, Valenti R, Migliorini A, et al. Comparison of rheolytic thrombectomy before direct infarct artery stenting versus direct stenting alone in patients undergoing percutaneous coronary intervention for acute myocardial infarction. Am J Cardiol. 2004;93:1033–5.

23. Ali A, Cox D, Dib N, et al. Rheolytic thrombectomy with percutaneous coronary intervention for infarct size reduction in acute myocardial infarction: 30-day results from a multicenter randomized study. J Am Coll Cardiol. 2006;48:244–52.

24. Migliorini A, Stabile A, Rodriguez AE, et al. Comparison of AngioJet rheolytic thrombectomy before direct infarct artery stenting with direct stenting alone in patients with acute myocardial infarction. The JETSTENT Trial. J Am Coll Cardiol. 2010;56:1298–306.

25. Parodi G, Valenti R, Migliorini A, et al. Comparison of manual thrombus aspiration with rheolytic thrombectomy in acute myocardial infarction. Circ Cardiovasc Interv. 2013;6:224–30.

26. van Geuns RJ, Tamburino C, Fajadet J, et al. Self-expanding versus balloon-expandable stents in acute myocardial infarction: results from the APPOSITION II study: self-expanding stents in ST- segment elevation myocardial infarction. JACC Cardiovasc Interv. 2012;5:1209–19.

27. Koch Kt Stellbrink C, Le Heuzey JY, et al. One year clinical autcomes of the STENTYS Self - Apposing coronary stent in patients presenting with ST elevation myocardial infartions: results from the APPOSITION III registry Eurointervention. 2015;11(3):264–71.

28. Stone GW, Abizaid A, Silber S, et al. Prospective, randomized, multicenter evaluation of a polyethylene terephthalate micronet mesh–covered stent (MGuard) in ST-Segment Elevation Myocardial Infarction The MASTER Trial. J Am Coll Cardiol. 2012;60:1975–84.

29. Carrick D, Oldroyd KG, McEntegart M, et al. A randomized trial of deferred stenting versus immediate stenting to prevent no- or slow-reflow in acute ST-segment elevation myocardial infarction (DEFER-STEMI). J Am Coll Cardiol. 2014;63:2088–98.

Chapter 14
Coronary Stenting Remains the First Revascularization Option in Most Patients with a Clinical Indication for Myocardial Revascularization

Juan Mieres, Nicolás Herscovich, and Alfredo E. Rodríguez

Abstract In the past, randomized clinical trials (RCT) either with the use of plain old balloon angioplasty or bare metal stents (BMS) did not show a survival advantage with coronary artery graft surgery (CABG) in spite of a greater number of repeat revascularization procedures (TVR) with angioplasty. Moreover, meta-analysis from RCT in the BMS era showed similar survival and the incidence of myocardial infarction (MI) between PCI and CABG including diabetic patients.

With the introduction of drug eluting stents (DES) in the past decade, the incidence of TVR and restenosis was significantly reduced, although the high incidence of stent thrombosis in the very late period after DES implantation introduced a cause of concern.

Recently, long term follow up of new RCTs between PCI with 1st generation DES versus CABG showed poor survival and a high incidence of MI when they were treated with 1st generation DES in comparison with CABG. However, patients treated with surgery had a threefold increase in stroke.

J. Mieres, MD
Department of Interventional Cardiology, Otamendi Hospital and Sanatorio Las Lomas, Buenos Aires, Argentina
e-mail: juanmieres@centroceci.com.ar

N. Herscovich, MD
Department of Cardiology, Otamendi Hospital, Buenos Aires, Argentina
e-mail: nicoherscov@hotmail.com

A.E. Rodríguez, MD, PhD, FACC, FSCAI (✉)
Cardiac Unit, Department of Interventional Cardiology, Revista Argentina de Cardioagiologia Intervencionista (RACI), Otamendi Hospital, Buenos Aires, Argentina

Interventional Cardiology Unit, Department of Interventional Cardiology, Otamendi Hospital, Buenos Aires, Argentina

Otamendi Hospital, Post Graduate Buenos Aires School of Medicine, Buenos Aires, Argentina

Director, Cardiovascular Research Center (CECI), Buenos Aires, Argentina
e-mail: arodriguez@centroceci.com.ar

© Springer International Publishing Switzerland 2015
J.A. Ambrose, A.E. Rodríguez (eds.), *Controversies in Cardiology*,
DOI 10.1007/978-3-319-20415-4_14

Simultaneously with these studies, a large improvement in the design of DES platforms was observed which significantly enhanced the safety profile of these devices. Several well conducted RCT and also large registries demonstrated the safety profile of these new DES platforms, including biocompatible or biodegradable polymers or complete bioabsorbable stents. All showed a remarkably low rate of adverse events with these new DES designs, either in comparison to 1st generation DES or BMS. Furthermore, the incidence of very late stent thrombosis was almost zero.

In summary, the current safety gap between PCI and CABG in complex lesion subsets, three vessel CAD and diabetics, should not be closed until new RCT with the last generation of DES have been conducted.

Keywords Coronary artery bypass surgery • Stents • Drug eluting stents • Randomized trials • Myocardial revascularization • Coronary artery disease

Introduction

In the past, several randomized comparisons between percutaneous coronary interventions (PCI), either with balloon angioplasty (POBA) or bare metal stents (BMS), versus coronary artery bypass graft (CABG) in patients with a clinical indication for myocardial revascularization showed a similar comparative long term incidence of death and myocardial infarction (MI), in spite of a greater number of repeat revascularization procedures (TVR) with PCI. In those trials, the extent of coronary artery disease (CAD) was not associated with a better survival with CABG, and only diabetic patients had an inferior survival after percutaneous procedures [1–8].

With the introduction of drug eluting stents (DES) during coronary angioplasty, the incidence of TVR was significantly reduced compared to BMS although, the high incidence of stent thrombosis (SET) present with 1st generation DES including very late SET years after stent implantation introduced a new cause for concern [9–11]. In the past decade, new randomized comparisons between PCI with DES versus CABG in complex patient subsets such as 3 vessel CAD, unprotected left main and diabetics were designed and launched [12–19]. End points of these trials were, in general, a composite of hard clinical end points such as death, MI and cerebrovascular accident (CVA) with 1, 3 and 5 years of follow up. One of these included diabetic and non- diabetic patients [12–14] whereas the last three included only patients with diabetes [15–19]. The 5 year follow up from the two largest (FREEDOM and SYNTAX) showed a lower incidence of death, cardiac death and MI with CABG in spite of higher CVA rates with surgery. Surprisingly, long term follow up of these DES vs CABG studies did not show any improvement in comparison to the old results with BMS vs CABG [20, 21]. This chapter explores these studies and the reasons for these intriguing differences are considered. Do we really know that all diabetics do better with CABG and that CABG is always preferred with complex multi vessel disease?

Randomized Comparisons Among PCI and CABG: From Balloon Angioplasty to BMS and DES

We can summarize the data from early RCT between PCI either POBA or BMS, analyzing the results from 2 meta-analysis from individual patient pooled data [22]. One included 10 randomized studies [23], either with the archaic techniques of POBA and or BMS, whereas the other analysis included only studies using BMS as a default strategy in the PCI arm [23]. Hlatky et al. reported long term results, 6 years or beyond, of these two revascularization techniques, where only diabetics had a survival advantage with CABG. As the authors pointed out in their conclusion, the extent of coronary artery disease was not a predictor of better survival with surgery [24]. In addition, they [23] observed that over a median follow-up of 5.9 years, the effect of CABG vs. PCI on mortality varied according to age with an adjusted CABG: PCI hazard ratios (HR) of 1.23 (0.95–1.59) in the youngest tertile, 0.89 (0.73–1.10) in the middle tertile, and 0.79 (0.67–0.94) in the oldest tertile. In their analysis, younger diabetic patients had a similar survival independent of revascularization treatment, 19 % with CABG and PCI: HR 0.93 (0.55–1.55) p = 0.77.

In the same way, Daemen et al. also reported 5 years results from the combined data of the studies that used only BMS (Table 14.1). In this meta-analysis [22] there were no differences in freedom of death and MI between both revascularization strategies; 1533 were randomized to CABG and 1520 to BMS. The cumulative

Table 14.1 Meta-analysis of the 4 randomized clinical trials between BMS and CABG in multiple vessel disease

| Variables | Crude event rates % | | | Kaplan-Meier estimates % | | | |
	PCI (n = 1518)	CABG (n = 1533)	p	PCI (n = 1518)	CABG (n = 1533)	HR (95 % CI)	p
Death	8.5(129/1518)	8.2 (125/1533)	0.74	8.5	8.2	0.95 (0.73–1.23)	0.69
Stroke	2.5 (38/1518)	2.9 (45/1533)	0.51	3.1	3.6	1.16 (0.73–1.83)	0.54
MI	6.6 (100/1518)	6.1 (94/1533)	0.66	7.3	7.6	0.91 (0.68–1.23	0.54
TVR	25.0 (379/1518)	6.3 (96/1533)	0.001	29.0	7.9	0.23 (0.18–0.29)	<0.001
Death, stroke, or MI	14.2 (215/1518)	14.6 (224/1533)	0.76	16.7	16.9	1.04 (0.86–1.27)	0.69
Death, stroke, MI, or TVR	34.2 (519/1518)	19.6 (301/1533)	<0.001	39.2	23.0	0.53 (0.45–0.61)	<0.001

Adapted from Daemen J, et al. [26] with permission of Wolters Kluwer Health
BMS bare metal stent, *PCI* percutaneous coronary intervention, *CABG* coronary artery bypass graft, *MI* myocardial infarction, *TVR* target vessel revascularization

incidence of death, MI and CVA was similar in the randomized group of patients treated with PCI versus the corresponding group treated with CABG (16:7 % versus 16:9 %, respectively; p = 0.69) with a low statistical heterogeneity. As expected, a significantly higher frequency of repeat revascularization for the group treated with PCI was observed (29:0 % vs 7:9 % of the CABG group; p < 0:001); furthermore, there was no interaction in this analysis in the diabetic patient cohort, p = 0.70. An unexpected finding was that diabetics had a similar incidence in the composite of death, MI or CVA, 20.9 % in PCI and 21.4 % in CABG arms, in spite of a higher recurrence of revascularization with PCI [22].

In the last decade, with the introduction of 1st generation DES, we were able to significantly reduce angiographic and clinical in stent restenosis and improve outcomes compared to BMS technology. Therefore, one expected that any new randomized comparison between PCI versus CABG would be now more favorable to PCI [25].

During 2004/2008, 4 randomized clinical trials (RCT) have been conducted to compare 1st generation DES versus CABG in patients with multi vessel disease including left main stenosis and diabetics. We will briefly illustrate the study design and results from these latest trials [14, 15, 17, 19] (Table 14.2).

Table 14.2 Trial design and baseline characteristics of recent randomized clinical trials between 1st generation DES versus CABG. [14,15,17,19]

	CARDIa	SYNTAX	FREEDOM	VA CARDS
Enrolment period	2002–2007	2005–2007	2005–2010	2006–2010
Patients (n)	254	903	699	101
Mean age (y)	64	65	63	62
Men (%)	74	71	71	99
Diabetes (%)	100	26	100	100
Hypertension (%)	79	70	NA	96
Smokers (%)	24	16	16	24
Hyper cholesterol (%)	90	82	NA	NA
Previous MI (%)	NA	32	26	41
PVD (%)	4	15	NA	14
Congestive heart failure (%)	NA	7	NA	8[a]
Severe LV dysfunction (%)	1	3[c]	3[b]	7[d]
Three vessel disease (%)	62	83	83	NA
Left main disease (%)	Excluded	29	Excluded	Excluded
Stents (%)	100	100	100	100
DES (%)	69	100	100	100
Glycoprotein IIb/IIIa inhibitor (%)	Routine	34	Recommended	100

BMS bare metal stent, *DES* drug eluting stent, *LV* left ventricule, *MI* myocardial infarction, *NA* not available, *PCI* percutaneous coronary intervention, *PVD* peripheral vascular disease
[a]Class III congestive heart failure
[b]LVEF <40 %
[c]LVEF <30 %
[d]LVEF <35 %

SYNTAX

The study design included patients with three vessels (71 %) and left main stenosis (29 %) in diabetic and non- diabetic populations [12–14]. SYNTAX was a non-inferiority trial and the primary end point of major adverse cardiac and cerebrovascular events at 1 year was not met due to the higher rate of TVR in the PCI arm. Secondary end points included the same end points at 5 years, rates of each individual component and rates of SET or graft occlusion. Taxus Express stents (Boston Scientific, Natick, MA, USA) were used in all PCI patients; 4.6 stents per patient were used and per protocol, all vessels with a reference diameter>2.0 mm should be treated.

At 5 years, adverse events were higher in the PCI arm compared to CABG (37.3 and 26.9 %, respectively, p<0.001). This difference between arms was driven by the higher rate of TVR, MI and cardiac death, although this benefit was more pronounced in patients with 3 vessel CAD (death: 14.6 and 8.2 % with DES and CABG respectively p<0.001; MI: 10.6 and 6.1 % with DES and CABG respectively p=0.003). On the contrary, in most patients with left main stenosis, long term outcomes were similar between both revascularization strategies. The authors made a post hoc subgroup analysis using a risk /benefit angiographic score called "Syntax Score", and they found that patients with low scores (<22) had similar composite end points with both revascularization strategies . In contrast, in patients with an intermediate or high "Syntax score", the benefit was in favor of bypass surgery. One might argue that, since the primary end point of the study was not met, these subgroup analyses should not be allowed.

Analyzing the subgroup of 452 patients with treated diabetes, CABG had a better survival and lower incidence of MI only in the subgroup with insulin dependent diabetes (IDDM), whereas in non- insulin dependent diabetes (NDDM), the differences between PCI and CABG were only driven by a greater number of revascularization procedures with PCI.

This study had potential limitations:

1. unpublished data showed an extreme variability in the performance of the centers involved in the study: among the 85 sites, the incidence of the primary end point ranged from 0 to more than 40 % in patients randomized to CABG (11 centers without adverse events; 1 top enroller center with>40 % of adverse events) or PCI (3 centers without adverse events; 1 center with>50 % of them).
2. There was a disparity in the follow-up rate between groups at long term. Originally, 897 patients were randomized to CABG and 903 to PCI; after 1 year 849 patients randomized to CABG remained in the study (40 patients withdrew or were lost), while 891 randomized to PCI remained in the study (7 withdrew and 5 were lost). At 5 years, only 805 CABG patients remained in the study compared to 871 in the PCI group. Consequently, 92 (10.2 %) patients out of 897 randomized to CABG withdrew consent or were lost, while only 32 (3.5 %) from the PCI arm with the same situation. Sensitivity analysis showed that if all non-evaluable patients (withdrawn or lost) were thought dead, the 5-year mortality rate was lower in the PCI arm than the CABG arm [26].

3. The Taxus Express, a 1st generation DES which is now considered largely out-of-date, as reflected in the results of randomized trials and registries with new generations DES [27, 28] was used.
4. The sample size in diabetics was too small to achieve any conclusion.

FREEDOM trial

The FREEDOM trial was a multicenter, open-label prospective randomized superiority trial of PCI/DES versus CABG in 1900 diabetic patients in whom revascularization was indicated with stenoses of more than 70 % in 2 or more major epicardial vessels involving ≥2 separate coronary-artery territories and without left main stenosis. In the PCI arm, DES was used in 100 % of the cases and Taxus and Cypher (Johnson & Jonhson, Cordis, Miami Lakes, FL, USA) were the predominant stents [15, 16].

Recently, the FREEDOM trial results at 5 years have shown that for diabetics and multiple vessel disease, CABG was superior to PCI with DES in that CABG significantly reduced death rates and MI, albeit with a higher rate of non- fatal CVA. Similar to SYNTAX, the primary end point of death, MI and CVA became significant in the CABG arm only after the second year of follow up. The composite end point was 13 % vs 10.9 %, p=ns, at the 2nd year of follow up. It rose to 26.6 % vs 18.7 %, in PCI and CABG respectively at 5 years, making the differences highly significant in favor of CABG, p=0.005. At 5 years, the advantage of CABG over PCI was seen in both IDDM and NIDM; an increase of 33 and 57 % in the combined end point of mortality and MI respectively with PCI, in spite of the 54 % increase in non- fatal CVA with surgery [15, 16]. The stroke risk was higher with CABG in both groups of diabetic patients-NIDM (1,7 % vs 4.3 % with PCI and CABG respectively) and IDDM (3.7 % vs 7.5 % with PCI and CABG respectively) although the differences were not significant - 5 years stroke HR, PCI vs CABG was 0.51 (0.25–1.06) in NIDM and 0.60 (0.28–1.30) in IDDM. Repeat revascularization procedures were low with CABG [16]. In FREEDOM, the advantages with surgery were independent of the SYNTAX score, underscoring the potential limitations of this score to predict outcome in all groups.

In FREEDOM, there were geographic differences in the results. The primary end point was reached in favor to CABG only in USA and Canada sites; death/MI/CVA was 16 and 28 % with DES and CABG respectively, from a population of 770 patients. Conversely, non-USA and Canada sites, from a population of 1130 patients, the primary end point was 25 % with DES and 21 % with CABG which was not statistically significant, with a p=0.05 for interaction between North American and outside North American sites. These observed geographic disparities between PCI and CABG in FREEDOM should not be a surprise as regional differences in results between PCI and CABG were also seen in RCTs in the BMS era. Moreover, 2 South American studies -ERACI II and MASS II- showed similar mortality with both revascularization strategies in non- diabetic and diabetic patients treated either with BMS or CABG [RR 1 (0.27–3.72) and 0.95 (0.41–2.22) in ERACI II and MASS II, respectively] [5, 6]. In contrast, another European BMS/CABG trial showed significant survival advantages with CABG at 6 years [8] and the advantages were driven by extremely low in-hospital mortality with surgery.

Therefore, both old (ERACI, MASS and SOS) [5, 6, 8] and new RCTs (FREEDOM and SYNTAX) [12, 15] have shown large geographic inconsistencies in the results between PCI and CABG. These differences may profoundly affect the interpretation of these trials.

CARDia

In this trial, 510 diabetic patients were randomized to either PCI or CABG. The first year of follow up was published and the 5 years was reported [17, 18]. This was a non-inferiority trial that compared, as the primary end point, a composite of death, MI and CVA. In the PCI arm, DES was used in 69 % and BMS in 31 %.

At 5 years, PCI was non inferior to CABG. Death, MI and CVA were 20.5 % with CABG and 26.6 % with PCI (p = 0.11). However, significant differences in MI, 6.3 % with CABG and 14 % with PCI, p = 0.007, and a repeat revascularization rate of 8.3 % with CABG vs 21.9 % with PCI p < 0.001 was seen. Overall death and non-fatal CVA were similar. A major limitation was the small sample size with lack of power to detect end point differences between groups [18].

VA CARDS

This study randomized 198 patients, 97 to surgery and 101 to PCI, and it was terminated due to low recruitment rate, and at that point no significant differences between groups were found [19].

Major limitation: the VA CARDS was severely underpowered for its primary endpoint and therefore no firm conclusions about the comparable effectiveness of CABG and PCI were possible. However, at 2 years, a 76 % reduction of death was noted in CABG group. On the other hand, the incidence of MI, was significantly higher in CABG group. Similarly to the FREEDOM trial [12], SYNTAX score did not predict differences in outcome (Table 14.2).

Randomized Clinical Trials of Stents Versus CABG: ARTS, ERACI II, MASS II, SoS, CARDia, FREEDOM, SYNTAX and VA CARDS; Lack of Benefit with 1st Generation DES

We have now the opportunity to analyze results from the 8 RCT comparing stents versus CABG; a first meta-analysis showed a significant safety advantage of bypass surgery over PCI only in patients with diabetes with the penalty of a threefold increase stroke risk with CABG (RR 1.84: 1.18–2.53). As we can see in Table 14.3, death in the overall group was significantly lower with CABG (0.79 [0.69–0.90] p < 0.001), although this benefit was only driven by significant differences in the diabetic subgroup of patients. On the contrary, survival was almost identical with PCI or CABG in the non-diabetic group (8.9 and 9.1 % with CABG and PCI respectively, p = 0.80). The same findings were seen with the composite of death/MI/CVA-a significant benefit with CABG only driven by the outcome in diabetics (p < 0.001), Table 14.3.

If we compare the results of CABG from the 8 trials with only those achieved with BMS (4 trials), there is no significant difference between both revascularization strategies, neither in diabetics (9.5 and 12.4 %, with CABG and BMS, respectively, p = 0.14) nor in non- diabetics (8.9 and 7.7 % with CABG and BMS, respectively, p = 0.34). Similar finding were observed with the composite of death/MI/CVA between CABG and BMS, all differences were not significant. Diabetics had non-significant lower mortality but 46 % higher risk of CVA with surgery, 4.6 % (58/1248) with CABG vs. 2.5 % with BMS (38/1518), p < 0.001 [21, 22] (Table 14.3).

On the contrary, comparing CABG results from the 4 of the 8 trials utilizing only DES, survival was better with CABG, including diabetics (9.5 % with CABG and 14.3 with DES, p < 0.001) and non-diabetics (8.9 % with CABG and 11.8 % with DES, p = 0.028) (Fig. 14.1); similar results were observed when we analyzed the composite of death/MI/CVA. All data were significantly in favor of CABG, independent of diabetes status (p < 0.001 in both subgroups). These results were obtained in spite of a significant increase in CVA [12, 15, 17] with surgery.

What might explain these differences that seemingly favor BMS in these comparisons? The completeness of revascularization [29] does not seem to explain these differences, taking in account that in all randomized studies, CABG always achieved a higher completeness of revascularization than PCI with either DES or BMS. We may argue that BMS data included different patient populations. However [12], if

Table 14.3 Indirect comparison among randomized clinical trials of BMS vs CABG (ARTS, ERACI II, MASS II and SoS) and 1st generation DES versus CABG (CARDia, FREEDOM, SYNTAX and VA CARDS) in diabetics and non diabetics population [7, 5, 6, 8, 14, 15, 17, 19]

	CABG (%)	BMS (%)	DES (%)	CABG: BMS	CABG:DES	BMS:DES
Death non diabetics	8.9	7.7	11.8	1.15 (0.90–1.46) p = 0.23	0.75 (0.58–0.97) p = 0.031	0.65 (0.49–0.87) p = 0.003
Death diabetics	9.5	12.4	14.3	0.77 (0.54–1.09) p = 0.14	0.66 (0.55–0.80) p < 0.001	0.86 (0.61–1.21) p = 0.39
Death, MI or stroke non diabetics	13.9	12.6	19.5	1.10 (0.91–1.32) p = 0.29	0.71 (0.58–0.85) p = 0.001	0.64 (0.52–0.79) p < 0.001
Death, MI or stroke in diabetics	17.6	21.5	23.4	0.81 (0.63–1.04) p = 0.12	0.75 (0.65–0.86) p < 0.001	0.91 (0.71–1.17) p = 0.48

DES drug eluting stent, *CABG* coronary artery bypass graft, *MI* myocardial infarction

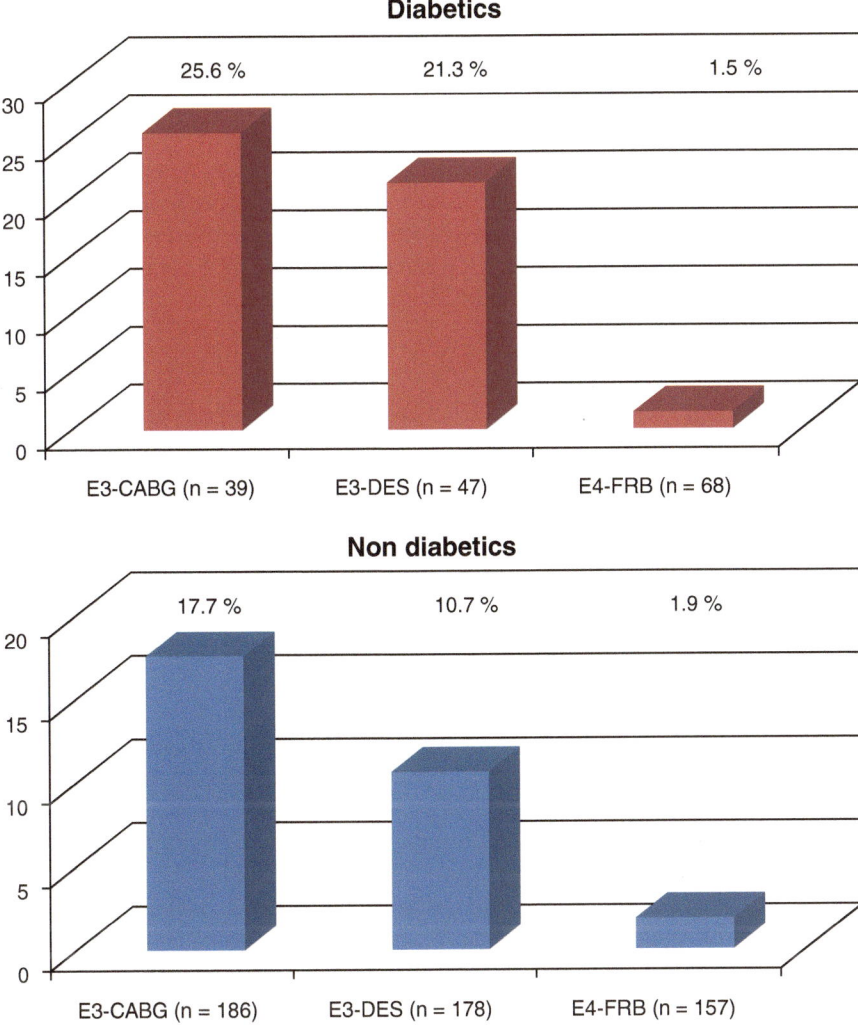

Fig. 14.1 Outcome of patients included in the registry. MACCE rate with 2nd generation DES Firebird 2 are similar between diabetics and no-diabetics. As we can see in the figure the MACE was similar between the two populations. This has not been observed in previous studies. *MACCE* major adverse cardiovascular events, *MI* myocardial infarction, *CVA* cerebrovascular accident, *TVR* target vessel revascularization, *E3-CABG* coronary artery bypass graft arm from ERACI 3 Study, *E3-DES* drug eluting stent arm from ERACI 3 study, *E4-FRB2* ERACI 4 Registry

we analyzed only those patients having 3 vessel CAD, any cause of death with BMS was 10.2 % in 548 patients, lower than the 14.6 % in the 456 patients treated with 1st generation DES from Syntax, p < 0.03. Moreover, this lack of benefit with 1st generation DES was seen in diabetic and non-diabetic populations. In fact, the observed incidence in the composite of death, MI and CVA in FREEDOM at 5 years was 20 % higher than previously seen in diabetic patients randomized in BMS/CABG trials [3, 7, 12].

It is clear that this indirect comparison has limitations: 1- we are including a non-simultaneous series of patients with one decade of difference between BMS and DES data; 2- baseline and angiographic characteristics between groups may be different; 3-adjunctive medical therapy changed and we have now better medical therapies for prevention/progression.

However, the reason for this comparison is to demonstrate a potential major flaw *of SYNTAX* [12] *and FREEDOM* [15] *which was likely the stent design used in most patients. C*onsequently, any definitive conclusion of the advantages of CABG therapy over PCI is questionable when the results with these DES appear to be worse than those obtained years ago with BMS.

Randomized Comparison with the Latest Generation DES

In the past few years, several RCT either comparing 2nd or 3rd generation DES versus the 1st generation were conducted. All consistently showed a significant reduction in the incidence of cardiac late events including cardiac death and/or MI, death/MI and very late stent thrombosis with the newer DES [30–34]. Randomized studies with everolimus-eluting stents (EES) with a durable polymer, versus paclitaxel-eluting stents (PES/ Taxus, Boston Scientific Corp) showed a significant reduction in death/MI ($p < 0.02$), SET and target lesion revascularization (TLR) ($p < 0.001$ for both) in the non- diabetic population (Table 14.4).

In the randomized SPIRIT V diabetic study, late lumen loss and 1-year cardiac death or MI was also significantly reduced with EES. Recently, the randomized ESSENCE-DIABETES study found an extremely low ID-TLR rate with EES [35] which is in agreement with the Bern-Rotterdam registry [36] in diabetic patients. In addition, with the introduction of absorbable polymer or complete bioabsorbable stents (BVS), we are observing promising results in the diabetic patient cohort. Pooled results from individual patient-level data from RCT -ISAR-TEST 3, ISAR-TEST 4 and LEADERS- comparing biodegradable polymer DES with durable polymer SES, reported at 4 years a significant reduction of SET, definite or probable, in diabetic patients treated with biodegradable polymer DES and the difference was driven by significantly lower SET with biodegradable polymer DES between 1 and 4 years (0.4% vs. 2.8% $p = 0.02$) [33]. Furthermore, a pooled analysis from the 1 year-follow up of diabetics from several trials using a 2nd generation permanent polymer and EES: SPIRIT FIRST, SPIRIT II, SPIRIT III, SPIRIT IV versus a 3rd generation bioabsorbable DES (BVS): ABSORB Cohort B and ABSORB EXTEND trial, showed that in diabetes treated with BVS, the incidence of target lesion failure (TLF), cardiac death, MI, and ID-TLR was -for the first time in the stent era lower when compared to non-diabetics. The cumulative incidence of adverse events at 1 year did not differ between diabetic and non-diabetic patients treated with BVS (3.7% vs. 5.1%, $p = 0.64$), whereas SET between diabetics and non-diabetics was also equal (0.7%) [37]. The role of restoring vasomotor function and the potential for "stabilizing" vulnerable plaques with BVS might be of great interest in diabetics where endothelial dysfunction and plaque rupture are common [38].

Table 14.4 Randomized clinical trials among different DES designs [30–34]

DES	Spirit III 2 years			Spirit IV 3 years			ISAR test 4 3 years						Pool data			SCAAR registry 2 years		
	EES (n=642)	PES (n=309)	P	EES (n=2458)	PES (n=1.229)	P	EES (n=652)	SES (n=652)	P	BP (n=1299)	DP (n=1304)	P	BP (n=2358)	DP (n=1704)	P	BMS (n=42773)	oDES (n=12153)	nDES (n=6425)
Death	2.0 %	2.6 %	0.64	3.2 %	5.1 %	0.02	9.3 %	10.3 %	0.57	9.3 %	9.8 %	0.71	9.3 %	10.0 %	0.32	6.8 %	3.4 %	1.9 %
MI	3.0 %	5.9 %	0.08	3.0 %	4.6 %	0.02	4.1 %	4.7 %	0.60	4.6 %	4.4 %	0.77	6.0 %	6.8 %	0.74	NA	NA	NA
TVR	10.1 %	13.9 %	0.10	10.1 %	10.6 %	0.64	NA	NA	NA	NA	NA	NA	NA	NA	NA	NA	NA	NA
TLR	NA	NA	NA	NA	NA	NA	12.8 %	15.5 %	0.15	13.9 %	14.2 %	0.79 %	12 %	13.7 %	0.02	5.5 %	4.9 %	3.1 %
ST	1.0 %	1.7 %	0.35	0.59 %	1.6 %	0.003	1.4 %	1.9 %	0.51	1.2 %	1.7 %	0.32	1.3 %	2.8 %	0.01	1.4 %	1.3 %	0.6 %
MACCE	7.7 %	13.8 %	0.005	NA	NA	NA	NA	NA	NA	NA	NA	NA	19 %	21.6 %	0.02	NA	NA	NA

DES drug eluting stent, *EES* everolimus eluting stent, *PES* paclitaxel eluting stent, *SES* sirolimus eluting stent, *BP* biodegradable polymer, *DP* durable polymer, *BMS* bare metal stent, *oDES* old generation drug eluting stent, *nDES* new generation drug eluting stent, *MI* myocardial infarction, *TVR* target vessel revascularization, *TLR* target lesion revascularization, *ST* stent thrombosis, *MACCE* major adverse cardiovascular events

Table 14.5 ERACI IV 9 months follow up of the three arms, ERACI III-DES (Taxus and Cypher); ERACI III-CABG; ERACI IV-Firebird 2 stents

Overall outcome	ERACI III DES (225)	ERACI III CABG (225)	ERACI IV firebird (225)	ERACI III DES vs ERACI IV FB (p value)	ERACI III CABG vs ERACI IV FB (p value)
Any death	17 (7.6 %)	7 (3.1 %)	1 (0.4 %)	<0.001	0.03
MI	14 (6.2 %)	6 (2.7 %)	1 (0.4 %)	<0.001	0.057
Non fatal stroke	2 (0.9 %)	5 (2.2 %)	0 (0 %)	0.47	0.07
Death/MI/stroke	33 (14.7 %)	15 (6.7 %)	2 (0.8 %)	<0.001	0.001
TVR	11 (4.9 %)	20 (8.9 %)	3 (1.3 %)	0.03	<0.001
MACCE (Death/MI/ stroke/TVR)	44 (19.1 %)	27 (12 %)	4 (1.8 %)	<0.001	<0.001

DES drug eluting stent, *CABG* coronary artery bypass graft, *MI* myocardial infarction, *TVR* target vessel revascularization, *MACCE* major adverse cardiovascular events

Also, in all of these new DES designs, stent strut coverage and the incidence of late stent mal-apposition were significantly improved [39]. New data suggest that long term dual antiplatelet therapy with these newer generation stents may be preferable for 30 months after implantation [40].

Recent data from a multicenter prospective and controlled registry, ERACI IV, with a "real world" patient population of 2 or 3 vessel disease and /or unprotected left main, 60 % with acute coronary syndromes including 67 % in Braunwald class III B/C, over 30 % of diabetics, bifurcations in 17 %, overlapping stents in 29 % etc. showed interesting results. All were treated with a second generation DES, Firebird −2 (Microport Inc, Shangai, China), a rapamycin-eluting coronary stent with a cobalt chromium platform and a polyolefin polymer. This prospective registry showed, at 9 months of follow-up, a remarkably low incidence of death/MI/CVA, 1.8 %. An indirect comparison with results obtained in the previous ERACI III study demonstrated either in comparison with CABG or 1st generation DES, a significant reduction of MACE (p < 0.001 and p = 0.004 respectively), and these advantages were also seen in diabetics, p = 0.04 vs. CABG and p = 0.02 vs 1st generation DES [41]. (Table 14.5) Noteworthy, for the first time in our large experience with PCI in complex multi-vessel disease, MACE rate in diabetics and non- diabetics patients were similar 1.5 % and 1.9 % respectively with a cumulative incidence of definite/ probable SET of 0.4 % (Fig. 14.1).

Conclusions and Highlights

1. *In non-diabetic patients, coronary angioplasty with stent implantation compared to CABG had both similar death rates and the composite of death, MI and CVA at 5 years of follow up. These results remain when the comparison included patients with 2, 3 vessel or left main disease CAD.*

2. *In diabetes, coronary angioplasty with DES had a higher risk of death and the composite of death, MI and CVA compared to CABG. Thus, CABG has become the preferred revascularization strategy in diabetic patients with multi vessel CAD. However, the threefold increased risk of stroke with CABG, could balance the final decision, particularly in young patients or patients with comorbidities.*
3. *CABG is associated with a significant reduction of repeat revascularization procedures at 5 years compared to PCI, either if they used DES or BMS.*
4. *Randomized and observational studies with new generation DES demonstrate a significant improvement in safety profile compared to the 1st generation in terms of MACE, cardiac death, myocardial infarction, SET, stent strut coverage, late stent mal-apposition and restoration of endothelial dysfunction. Therefore, the safety gap between PCI with CABG observed in FREEDOM [15] and SYNTAX [12], cannot be closed until new trials with the latest generation DES have been conducted.*
5. *All the RCT mentioned in this manuscript met clinical, angiographic or functional appropriateness revascularization criteria [42]. Thus, if medical treatment alone was an option, those patients were mostly excluded from these trials.*

In conclusion in most non- diabetic patients with clinical indication of myocardial revascularization, PCI with stent deployment remains the first therapeutic option if an equivalent completeness of revascularization can be achieved. We believe, as mentioned above, that the diabetic strategy remains to be determined.

References

1. Bari Investigators. The final 10-years follow up results from the BARI randomized trial. J Am Coll Cardiol. 2007;49(15):1600–6.
2. Hamm CW, et al. A randomized study of coronary angioplasty compared with bypass surgery in patients with symptomatic multivessel coronary disease. German Angioplasty Bypass Surgery Investigation (GABI). N Engl J Med. 1994;331(16):1037–43.
3. CABRI Trial Participants. First-year results of CABRI (Coronary Angioplasty versus Bypass Revascularisation Investigation). Lancet. 1995;346(8984):1179–84.
4. King SB, et al. Eight-year mortality in the Emory Angioplasty Versus Surgery Trial (EAST). J Am Coll Cardiol. 2000;35(5):1116–21.
5. Rodriguez AE, et al. Five-year follow-up of the Argentine randomized trial of coronary angioplasty with stenting versus coronary bypass surgery in patients with multiple vessel disease (ERACI II). J Am Coll Cardiol. 2005;46(4):582–8.
6. Hueb W, et al. Five-year follow-up of the Medicine, Angioplasty, or Surgery Study (MASS II): a randomized controlled clinical trial of 3 therapeutic strategies for multivessel coronary artery disease. Circulation. 2007;115(9):1082–9.
7. Serruys PW, et al. Five-year outcomes after coronary stenting versus bypass surgery for the treatment of multivessel disease: the final analysis of the Arterial Revascularization Therapies Study (ARTS) randomized trial. J Am Coll Cardiol. 2005;46(4):575–81.
8. Booth J, et al. Randomized, controlled trial of coronary artery bypass surgery versus percutaneous coronary intervention in patients with multivessel coronary artery disease: six-year follow-up from the Stent or Surgery Trial (SoS). Circulation. 2008;118:381–91.

9. Kirtane AJ, et al. Safety and efficacy of drug-eluting and bare metal stents: comprehensive meta-analysis of randomized trials and observational studies. Circulation. 2009;119(25): 3198–206.

10. Stettler C, et al. Outcomes associated with drug-eluting and bare-metal stents: a collaborative network meta-analysis. Lancet. 2007;370:937–48.

11. Stone GW, et al. Selection criteria for drug-eluting versus bare-metal stents and the impact of routine angiographic follow-up: 2-year insights from the HORIZONS-AMI (Harmonizing Outcomes With Revascularization and Stents in Acute Myocardial Infarction) trial. J Am Coll Cardiol. 2010;56(19):1597–604.

12. Serruys PW, et al. Percutaneous coronary intervention versus coronary-artery bypass grafting for severe coronary artery disease. N Engl J Med. 2009;360(10):961–72.

13. Kappetein AP, et al. Comparison of coronary bypass surgery with drug-eluting stenting for the treatment of left main and/or three-vessel disease: 3-year follow-up of the SYNTAX trial. Eur Heart J. 2011;32(17):2125–34.

14. Mohr FW, et al. Coronary artery bypass graft surgery versus percutaneous coronary intervention in patients with three-vessel disease and left main coronary disease: 5-year follow-up of the randomised, clinical SYNTAX trial. Lancet. 2013;381(9867):629–38.

15. Farkouh ME, et al. FREEDOM trial investigators. Strategies for multivessel revascularization in patients with diabetes. N Engl J Med. 2012;367(25):2375–84.

16. Dangas GD, et al. FREEDOM Investigators. Long-Term Outcome of PCI versus CABG in insulin and non-insulin-treated diabetic patients: results from the FREEDOM trial. J Am Coll Cardiol. 2014;64(12):1189–97.

17. Kapur A, et al. Randomized comparison of percutaneous coronary intervention with coronary artery bypass grafting in diabetic patients. 1-year results of the CARDia (Coronary Artery Revascularization in Diabetes) trial. J Am Coll Cardiol. 2010;55(5):432–40.

18. Hall R. CARDia: coronary artery revascularisation in diabetes trial. ESC Congress. 2012; Session number 710009–710010.

19. Kamalesh M, et al. Percutaneous coronary intervention versus coronary bypass surgery in United States veterans with diabetes. J Am Coll Cardiol. 2013;61:808–16.

20. Rodriguez AE. Are drug-eluting stents superior to bare metal stents when compared to coronary artery bypass surgery? Show me the data. Cardiovasc Revasc Med. 2013;14(2):90–2.

21. Rodriguez AE. Coronary artery bypass grafting vs percutaneous coronary intervention in multivessel disease. JAMA Intern Med. 2014;174(6):1007.

22. Daemen J, et al. Long-term safety and efficacy of percutaneous coronary intervention with stenting and coronary artery bypass surgery for multivessel coronary artery disease: a meta-analysis with 5-year patient-level data from the ARTS, ERACI-II, MASS-II, and SoS trials. Circulation. 2008;118(11):1146–54.

23. Flather M, et al. The effect of age on outcomes of coronary artery bypass surgery compared with balloon angioplasty or bare-metal stent implantation among patients with multivessel coronary disease. A collaborative analysis of individual patient data from 10 randomized trials. J Am Coll Cardiol. 2012;60(21):2150–7.

24. Hlatky MA, et al. Coronary artery bypass surgery compared with percutaneous coronary interventions for multivessel disease: a collaborative analysis of individual patient data from ten randomised trials. Lancet. 2009;373(9670):1190–7.

25. Caixeta A, et al. 5-Year clinical outcomes after sirolimus-eluting stent implantation insights from a patient-level pooled analysis of 4 randomized trials comparing sirolimus-eluting stents with bare-metal stents. J Am Coll Cardiol. 2009;54(10):894–902.

26. Antoniucci D. SYNTAX mistakes. Revista Argentina de Cardioangiología Intervencionista. 2013;4(03):0151–4.

27. Valenti R, et al. Clinical and angiographic outcomes of patients treated with everolimus-elutingstents or first-generation paclitaxeleluting stents for unprotected left main disease. J Am Coll Cardiol. 2012;60(14):1217–22.

28. Farooq V, et al. Short and long term clinical impact of stent thrombosis and graft occlusion in the synergy between percutaneous coronary intervention with Taxus and cardiac surgery trial: the SYNTAX Trial at 5 years. J Am Coll Cardiol. 2013;62(25):2360–9.

29. Garcia S, et al. Outcomes after complete versus incomplete revascularization of patients with multivessel coronary artery disease: a meta-analysis of 89,883 patients enrolled in randomized clinical trials and observational studies. J Am Coll Cardiol. 2013;62(16):1421–31.

30. Stone GW, et al. Randomized comparison of everolimus-eluting and paclitaxel-eluting stents: two-year clinical follow-up from the Clinical Evaluation of the Xience V Everolimus Eluting Coronary Stent System in the Treatment of Patients With De Novo Native Coronary Artery Lesions (SPIRIT) III trial. Circulation. 2009;119:680–6.

31. Brener SJ, et al. Everolimus-eluting stents in patients undergoing percutaneous coronary intervention: final 3-year results of the clinical evaluation of the XIENCE V everolimus eluting coronary stent system in the treatment of subjects with de novo native coronary artery lesions trial. Am Heart J. 2013;166(6):1035–42.

32. Byrne RA, et al. Intracoronary stenting and angiographic results: test efficacy of 3 limus-eluting stents (ISAR-TEST-4) investigators. Randomized, noninferiority trial of three limus agent-eluting stents with different polymer coatings: the intracoronary stenting and angiographic results: test efficacy of 3 limus-eluting stents (ISAR-TEST-4) trial. Eur Heart J. 2009;30(20):2441–9.

33. Stefanini GG, et al. Biodegradable polymer drug-eluting stents reduce the risk of stent thrombosis at 4 years in patients undergoing percutaneous coronary intervention: a pooled analysis of individual patient data from the ISAR-TEST 3, ISAR-TEST 4, and LEADERS randomized trials. Eur Heart J. 2012;33(10):1214–22.

34. Sarno G, et al. Lower risk of stent thrombosis and restenosis with unrestricted use of 'new-generation' drug-eluting stents: a report from the nationwide Swedish coronary angiography and angioplasty registry (SCAAR). Eur Heart J. 2012;33(5):606–13.

35. Park GM, et al. Comparison of zotarolimus-eluting stent versus sirolimus-eluting stent for de novo coronary artery disease in patients with diabetes mellitus from the ESSENCE-DIABETES II trial. Am J Cardiol. 2013;112(10):1565–70.

36. Simsek C, et al. Long-term outcome of the unrestricted use of everolimuseluting stents compared to sirolimus-eluting stents and paclitaxel-eluting stents in diabetic patients: the Bern–Rotterdam diabetes cohort study. Int J Cardiol. 2013;170:36–42.

37. Muramatsu T, et al. 1-year clinical outcomes of diabetic patients treated with everolimus-eluting bioresorbable vascular scaffolds: a pooled analysis of the ABSORB and the SPIRIT trials. J Am Coll Cardiol Intv. 2014;7:482–93.

38. Brugaletta S, et al. Endothelial-dependent vasomotion in a coronary segment treated by ABSORB everolimus-eluting bioresorbable vascular scaffold system is related to plaque composition at the time of bioresorption of the polymer: indirect finding of vascular reparative therapy? Eur Heart J. 2012;33:1325–33.

39. Choi HH, et al. Favorable neointimal coverage in everolimus-eluting stent at 9 months after stent implantation: comparison with sirolimus-eluting stent using optical coherence tomography. Int J Cardiovasc Imaging. 2012;28(3):491–7.

40. Mauri L, et al. Twelve or 30 months of dual antiplatelet Therapy after drug eluting stents. N Engl J Med. 2014;371(23):2155–66.

41. Haiek C, et al. Revascularization strategies for patients with multiple vessel disease and unprotected left main with a cobalt-chromium rapamycin eluting stent (ERACI IV Registry). European Congress of Cardiology, Abstract Presentation 303, Barcelona, Spain, August 31 2014.

42. Patel MR, et al. ACCF/SCAI/STS/AATS/AHA/ASNC/HFSA/SCCT 2012 Appropriate use criteria for coronary revascularization focused update: a report of the American College of Cardiology Foundation Appropriate Use Criteria Task Force, Society for Cardiovascular Angiography and Interventions, Society of Thoracic Surgeons, American Association for Thoracic Surgery, American Heart Association, American Society of Nuclear Cardiology, and the Society of Cardiovascular Computed Tomography. J Am Coll Cardiol. 2012; 59(9):857–81.

Chapter 15
Optimal Management of Multivessel CAD: PCI Versus CABG Surgery Versus Medical Therapy Alone

William E. Boden

Abstract Over the past decade, landmark randomized clinical trials comparing initial management strategies in stable ischemic heart disease (SIHD) have demonstrated no significant reduction in "hard" endpoints (all-cause mortality, cardiac death, or myocardial infarction [MI]). The main advantage derived from early revascularization is improved short-term angina relief and improved quality of life, and often a reduction in myocardial ischemia. Nonetheless, questions remain regarding how best to approach the initial management of SIHD patients, such as when (or if) cardiac catheterization should be performed, whether one or more high-risk subgroups (defined either by coronary anatomy or functional ischemic burden) could be identified that benefit from early revascularization, and if not, when should revascularization be performed to improve symptoms alone and/or quality of life. The NIH-funded ISCHEMIA trial is designed to address many of these scientific questions by randomizing SIHD patients with at least moderate ischemia to an initial conservative strategy of optimal medical therapy (OMT) or an initial invasive strategy of OMT plus cardiac catheterization and revascularization.

Keywords Stable ischemic heart disease • Optimal medical therapy • Coronary bypass surgery • Percutaneous coronary intervention

Introduction

Since the first percutaneous coronary intervention (PCI) was performed almost 40 years ago, there have been profound and sustained evolutions in catheter-based revascularization that has shifted the treatment of patients with coronary artery disease (CAD) largely away from an initial pharmacologic approach to one that has

W.E. Boden, MD, FACC, FAHA
Department of Medicine, Albany Medical College, Samuel S. Stratton VA Medical Center
and Albany Medical Center, 113 Holland Avenue, Albany, NY 12208, USA
e-mail: william.boden@va.gov

© Springer International Publishing Switzerland 2015
J.A. Ambrose, A.E. Rodríguez (eds.), *Controversies in Cardiology*,
DOI 10.1007/978-3-319-20415-4_15

increasingly embraced a more anatomically-driven management strategy. Because there are abundant clinical trial data that support the benefit of urgent/emergent PCI in patients with ST-segment elevation myocardial infarction or non-ST-segment elevation acute coronary syndromes (ACS) in reducing death or myocardial infarction (MI) [1–6], there has been an understandable and appropriately-expanding use of PCI and coronary stenting that has revolutionized patient management and improved significantly clinical outcomes in these high-risk patients.

By contrast, patients with stable CAD—or perhaps using the more encompassing descriptive term, stable ischemic heart disease (SIHD)—do not appear to derive the same clinical benefit of cardiovascular event (CV) reduction with PCI. On the other hand, in randomized trials that have compared clinical outcomes in patients with multivessel CAD, particularly among those subjects with more extensive epicardial coronary disease and among diabetics, who have undergone coronary artery bypass graft (CABG) surgery—either when compared to PCI or medical therapy—these patients appear to derive significant CV event reduction with CABG surgery.

It is against this therapeutic backdrop that clinicians frequently are faced with discordant evidence from clinical trials that complicate decision-making for patients with symptomatic CAD. Clinical intuition would suggest that adverse clinical outcomes (i.e., all-cause mortality, cardiac death and MI) associated with ischemic myocardium or high-grade coronary stenoses could be avoided with prompt revascularization in SIHD patients, as this is clearly what is observed in patients with ACS. However, landmark clinical trials over the past decade – implementing aggressive lifestyle interventions and comprehensive aggressive contemporary optimal medical therapy – have challenged this paradigm [7–9][1,2,3]. COURAGE, BARI-2D, and FAME-2 have provided the clinical community robust evidence that the benefit from early revascularization in most SIHD patients is only symptomatic, with no survival benefit.

Differing Pathobiology Between ACS and SIHD

One important factor that may explain the apparent differences in clinical outcomes with revascularization between patients with ACS and SIHD is the likely difference in pathobiology that underlies these two clinical expressions of CAD. Clearly, there have been major advances in our understanding of the pathophysiology of ACS and the recognition of the significance that predisposing non-flow-limiting coronary stenoses are more prone to rupture, as well as increasing insight into plaque and patient vulnerability. Clearly, in the context of an acute plaque rupture associated with total or subtotal coronary occlusion, mechanical dilatation of the infarct-related coronary

---

[1] Boden et al., 2007—The original COURAGE trial article that conceptualized and demonstrated that OMT + PCI did not lead to improved outcomes in SIHD patients.

[2] BARI-2D Study Group 2009—One of the original landmark trials comparing OMT against revascularization with CABG or PCI.

[3] De Bruyne et al., 2012—The original FAME-2 trial results comparing FFR-guided PCI versus OMT demonstrating no benefit with PCI in regards to hard cardiovascular outcomes.

artery results in a significant improvement in both long-term death and the composite of late death or MI. This improved understanding of the pathobiology of ACS has led directly to the more aggressive use of appropriately targeted pharmacologic agents and an evolution in what constitutes contemporary optimal medical therapy (OMT). Moreover, these same observations of the benefits associated with PCI in ACS patients, based on the pathobiology of plaque rupture causing obstructive lesions that cause increased death or MI, provide important insight into why PCI may not reduce clinical events (death or MI) in SIHD patients. In the chronic angina or SIHD patient, progressive, fibrotic and calcified coronary stenoses cause angina, exercise-induced myocardial ischemia, and increased calcium scores on CT imaging studies, but these stenotic/fibrotic lesions with small lipid cores and thick fibrous caps are much less likely to result in acute plaque ruptures of thin-capped fibroatheromas. Conversely (and perhaps paradoxically), the late events that occur in SIHD patients are generally associated with plaque ruptures in native, non-instrumented coronary arteries where stenosis diameter is less than 50–60 %. Thus, it is plausible to understand why PCI for stable CAD does not necessarily confer clinical benefit, since such non-flow-limiting coronary stenoses are not amenable to PCI in the first place, and successful PCI of flow-limiting coronary stenoses may reduce the propensity for ischemic complications or clinical events, but only in those stented coronary segments.

Evolution of Contemporary Optimal Medical Therapy (OMT)

Perhaps less well-recognized and appreciated over the past two decades has been concomitant evolution and refinement in medical therapy, which has become increasingly robust by contemporary standards and now includes the routine use of evidence-based "disease-modifying" secondary prevention therapies (e.g., aspirin, thienopyridines, statins, inhibitors of the renin-angiotensin system, and beta-blockers for post-MI patients)—all of which have been shown in placebo-controlled, randomized controlled trials (RCTs) to reduce death and MI in CAD patients. Additionally, important treatments directed primarily toward anginal symptoms and relief of ischemia (e.g., beta-blockers for angina, calcium channel blockers, long-acting nitrates, and ranolazine) are widely-utilized clinically. When these proven therapies are combined with lifestyle interventions (heart-healthy diet and weight loss/maintenance, smoking cessation, and regular physical exercise), the aggregation of these complementary and additive management approaches is frequently referred to as OMT.

Clinical Conundrum Facing Clinicians

Many clinicians are left with an uncomfortable paradox: diseased epicardial coronary anatomy underlies future adverse cardiovascular events, but prophylactic revascularization of such lesions may not necessarily produce better clinical outcomes [10]. Thus, these landmark clinical trials comparing optimal medical therapy

(OMT) alone versus OMT plus revascularization have met substantial resistance in changing practice patterns [11]. The difficulty in translating these clinical trials into practice may arise from misinterpreting trial results: COURAGE, BARI-2D and FAME-2 should be viewed as evaluating *initial* management strategies for SIHD patients, with OMT considered a safe and effective *initial* treatment option while revascularization can be reserved for those with refractory symptoms or an Acute Coronary Syndrome (ACS) [12]. The results of these trials do not cast doubt on whether revascularization is appropriate when necessary, but question *when* revascularization should be employed, if at all, in the individual patient who has had a trial of intensive optimal medical therapy and is showing signs of symptom improvement and/or ischemia reduction.

In this chapter, a careful review of the evidence comparing an initial conservative strategy versus an invasive approach in SIHD management will be undertaken. Additionally, the strengths and limitations of each trial and scientific questions that remain to be answered – i.e., is there an ischemic threshold above which prompt revascularization provides a death or MI benefit over an initial course of medical therapy will be addressed. Finally, a concluding discussion of the ongoing ISCHEMIA (International Study of Comparative Health Effectiveness with Medical and Invasive Approaches) trial, designed to provide clarity to SIHD management by addressing the gaps in knowledge following previous SIHD strategy trials will be provided.

What Do the Current SIHD Guidelines Recommend?

The 2012 ACCF/AHA/ACP/AATS/PCNA/SCAI/STS Guidelines for the Diagnosis and Management of Patients with SIHD recommend revascularization for a survival benefit in patients with three-vessel CAD with >70 % stenosis or two-vessel CAD including the proximal LAD, regardless of extent of ischemic burden or symptom status [13][4]. For those patients with two-vessel disease, the guideline recommendation is to utilize various noninvasive stress testing modalities to detect inducible ischemia, allowing clinicians to risk stratify those patients who would benefit from revascularization. Despite endorsing the use of ischemic burden to guide the revascularization decision, the 2012 guidelines loosely identify an ischemic threshold at which point revascularization would be indicated, instead describing situations of "large ischemic burden"(i.e., ≥10 % of the left ventricle), regardless of stress test results, as grounds to proceed with invasive coronary angiography and potential revascularization [13]. Several early observational cohort studies proposed that the severity of ischemic burden, measured by imaging modalities such as stress single-photon emission computed tomography (SPECT), can identify subsets of patients who may benefit from early revascularization, leading to overall better prognosis.

---

[4]Fihn et al., 2012—Current professional society based guidelines for the management of SIHD patients.

However, many observational studies justifying this premise predated the common use of contemporary disease-modifying OMT [14–16], and more recent studies further challenge this well-established paradigm [17–19][5].

The aforementioned 2012 SIHD management guidelines [13] and the 2013 European Society of Cardiology (ESC) guidelines [20] recommend coronary angiography to risk stratify those SIHD patients with signs and symptoms of heart failure, high risk features or inconclusive findings on noninvasive testing, or refractory symptoms despite OMT. The 2014 focused update by the ACC/AHA further delineates the role of coronary angiography – but with substantial room for interpretation [21]. The evidence base to determine when to perform cardiac catheterization in SIHD patients is inconclusive, and is currently being addressed by the ISCHEMIA trial.

Clinical Trials Comparing Initial Revascularization Versus Conservative Strategies

Before the modern era of OMT, randomized clinical trials (RCTs) from the 1980s suggested coronary artery bypass grafting (CABG) had a survival benefit as compared with medical therapy for certain patient subsets with high risk anatomy [22]. Medical therapy in those trials was relatively minimal and consisted principally of aspirin, beta-blockers and nitrates [23–25]. Clearly, those early trials are outdated historically, as effective secondary prevention with lifestyle and pharmacologic interventions are now firmly established with a combination of robust secondary prevention therapies and lifestyle interventions.

As cited previously, recent clinical trials have rigorously compared revascularization plus medical therapy with medical therapy alone and shown that neither strategy is superior. The findings from COURAGE, BARI-2D, and FAME-2 assure us that in SIHD patients – particularly those without significant left main coronary disease, refractory angina, and with preserved left ventricular function – a trial of OMT is a justifiable and appropriate initial strategy [7–9]. The results and limitations of these RCTs are discussed in further detail below.

The COURAGE Trial

The COURAGE trial investigators randomized 2,287 patients with SIHD to either an initial strategy of PCI+OMT or a conservative strategy of OMT alone [7]. A pre-randomization diagnostic angiogram was required, and only patients with objective evidence of inducible ischemia and a ≥70 % coronary artery stenosis plus evidence of inducible ischemia were included in the trial. In the approximately

---

[5] Mancini et al. 2014—COURAGE trial post hoc analysis demonstrating anatomic burden of disease better prognosticates future cardiovascular events compared to ischemic burden.

10 % of patients who presented with Canadian Cardiovascular Society Class 3 symptoms at baseline, and for whom stress testing was considered not indicated clinically, an ≥80 % coronary artery stenosis was required for inclusion. After a median 4.6 year follow-up, there was no significant difference in the rate of the primary endpoint of all-cause mortality and non-fatal MI in the PCI+OMT group versus the OMT alone group (19 % vs. 18.5 % of patients; HR, 1.05, 95 % CI, 0.87–1.27; P=0.62). Additionally, there were no significant differences in the composite of death, MI, stroke, and hospitalization for unstable angina between the two study groups. In a 2008 analysis investigating quality of life of COURAGE participants, 53 % of patients in the PCI group and 42 % in the medical therapy group were angina-free (P<0.001) at 3 months, with those patients with more severe angina at baseline deriving the greatest benefit [26]. The difference in symptom control was greatest at 3 months, but at 3 years there was no difference between the quality of life in the PCI and OMT groups.

The COURAGE trial forms the foundation of a growing evidence base demonstrating that PCI can be safely deferred until a later time without risk of increased death and overall rate of MI, compared with earlier intervention [27]. Nonetheless, COURAGE does have some limitations. With randomization occurring *after* angiography, some patients with severe lesions may have been revascularized during catheterization and excluded from the study, unintentionally skewing results by eliminating high-risk groups who may have most benefitted from revascularization [12]. DES was not widely available during enrollment, as they were not FDA-approved until mid-2003, which was approximately 6 months before enrollment ended in January 2004. Eligibility criteria excluded patients with significant left main coronary disease, an ejection fraction (EF) <30 %, refractory heart failure, and those with persistent Canadian Cardiovascular Society (CCS) Class IV angina. In regards to inducible ischemia, a minimal threshold (1.0- to 1.5-mm ST segment depression) was required for enrollment, and of the 1,381 randomized patients who underwent stress SPECT imaging, 34 % had moderate to severe ischemia at baseline [28] while approximately two-thirds had "mild ischemia". As such, the results of COURAGE cannot be generalized to all SIHD patients.

The BARI-2D Trial

The BARI-2D investigators randomized 2,368 patients with type 2 diabetes mellitus and SIHD to revascularization (either with PCI, n=798, or CABG, n=378) with OMT or OMT alone (n=1192) [8]. The primary endpoint, survival at 5 years, was similar in the revascularization arm of the study and the conservative management group (88.3 % vs. 87.8 %; an absolute difference of 0.5 %, 95 % CI, −2.0 to 3.1; P=0.97). The composite of mortality, MI, or stroke (i.e., major cardiovascular events) also showed no statistically significant difference between the revascularization and medical therapy arms (22.8 % vs. 24.1 %; P=0.70). The trial design allowed comparison of PCI+OMT versus OMT alone, and again, no significant difference was reported in terms of all-cause mortality (10.8 % vs. 10.2 %; P=0.48) and major cardiovascular events (23 % vs. 21.1 %; P=0.15). In the CABG treatment arm of BARI-2D, all-cause mortality was similar to the OMT group (13.6 % vs. 16.4 %; P=0.33). However, the secondary endpoint (i.e., death, MI and stroke) was lower in the CABG group (22.4 % vs. 30.5 %; P=0.01), with a reduction in the number of non-fatal MIs driving the difference in the composite secondary endpoint.

After 3 years of follow-up, 66 % of revascularization patients and 58 % of all patients randomized to OMT were free of angina (P=0.003; at baseline 21 % of all patients were angina-free) [29]. In the angioplasty stratum, PCI halted the development of worsening angina and increased the percentage of angina-free patients after the first year of follow-up. Thereafter and at the 5-year follow-up, there was no difference in reported angina symptoms between the PCI and OMT groups in the angioplasty stratum. In the CABG stratum, a reduced rate of worsening angina and increased percentage of angina-free patients was also seen at 1 year and was sustained through the 5-year follow-up.

As with COURAGE, all patients underwent catheterization before randomization, which has led to the criticism that once coronary anatomy is defined those patients most suitable for revascularization fail to be enrolled. Additionally, patients were not randomized to a revascularization strategy; rather, enrollees were chosen for CABG or PCI based on the treating physician's interpretation of the pre-randomization angiogram. BARI-2D is also limited by the fact that the trial was conducted during a period when DES were all first-generation and less frequently used by treating cardiologists [8].

The FAME-2 Trial

In the FAME-2 trial, 888 SIHD patients were randomized to an initial strategy of FFR-guided PCI plus OMT versus an initial strategy of OMT alone [9][6]. Those patients with angiographic evidence of flow-limiting stenoses with an FFR ≤ 0.80 were included, while patients with an FFR > 0.80 were treated medically and followed in a registry. The Data and Safety Monitoring Board (DSMB) halted recruitment for the trial after 7 months of follow-up due to a significant difference in the rate of the primary endpoint (i.e., a composite of all-cause mortality, non-fatal MI, or unplanned hospitalization leading to emergent revascularization) between the FFR-guided PCI and the OMT arms (4.3 % vs. 12.7 %; P<0.001). The driving force behind the difference was attributed to the lower rates of urgent revascularization in the FFR-guided PCI group (1.6 % vs. 11.1 % at 7 months, P<0.001; 4.0 % vs 16.3 % at 2 years, P<0.001). But hard cardiovascular endpoints were similar in the revascularization and medical therapy arms: death (0.2 % vs. 0.7 % at 7 months, P=0.31) or non-fatal MI (3.4 % vs. 3.2 % at 7 months, P=0.89). Results at 2 years of follow-up again demonstrated a statistically significant difference in the primary

---

[6] De Bruyne et al., 2012—The updated FAME-2 trial results form 2014 demonstrating a potential benefit with FFR-guided PCI in regards to rates of MI.

endpoint driven solely by urgent revascularization, favoring PCI over OMT (8.1 % vs. 19.5 %; P<0.001) [30].

In the original publication, FAME-2 investigators stated angina symptoms initially were less in the FFR-guided PCI group but became equivalent to the OMT arm by 12 months of follow-up. In the provocative 2-year follow-up of FAME-2, investigators reported that, contrary to prior analyses, at all follow-up evaluations (including 12 months), patients who underwent FFR-guided PCI+OMT actually had significantly less angina symptoms. In the landmark analysis, the authors also demonstrated that the rate of death or MI from 8 days to 2 years was lower in the PCI group than in the medical-therapy group (4.6 % vs. 8.0 %; HR, 0.56, 95 % CI, 0.32-0.97; P=0.04) [30]. However, within 7 days of randomization, there were more primary endpoint events in the PCI group than the medical therapy arm, with 6 out of 10 events being peri-procedural MI (2.2 % vs 0.9 %; HR, 2.49, 95 % CI, 0.78 – 8.00; P=0.11).

FAME-2 has many limitations that warrant comment [9, 31][7]. The absolute number of cardiac deaths was exceptionally low (3 in each group) with no statistically significant difference in the overall number of MIs (26 vs. 30, P=0.56) at 2 years [30], suggesting that the study population was skewed towards low-risk patients. Only 24 % of patients in the FAME-2 population had multi-vessel disease, compared to 69 % of patients in the COURAGE trial. Additionally, FAME-2 trial investigators intended to enroll well over 1,600 patients, but the trial was terminated after little over 50 % of planned enrollment due to the large discrepancy in urgent revascularization between the groups, resulting in a significantly underpowered sample size. Given the unblinded nature of the trial, selection bias may have been a factor in the results the authors reported, as 52 % of the unscheduled revascularizations were done solely on the basis of reported clinical symptoms without any supporting biochemical or electrocardiographic evidence of ischemia [9]. Among OMT patients undergoing urgent revascularization, no data were provided to show whether culprit lesions were in the same vascular territories deemed to be flow limiting by FFR versus involving diseased territories elsewhere not previously deemed significant. Without objective findings of inducible ischemia through non-invasive testing at follow-up, worsening angina symptoms cannot be ascribed to a specific vascular bed.

The MASS II Trial

The earlier Medicine, Angioplasty, or Surgery Study II (MASS II) trial, a small, single-site, 3-armed study of 611 patients with stable multi-vessel CAD and preserved left ventricular ejection fraction, (LVEF) randomized subjects to medical therapy (n=203), PCI (n=205), or CABG (n=203) [32]. The primary endpoint (a composite of all-cause mortality, Q-wave MI, and refractory angina requiring

---

[7]Boden 2012—An editorial outlining the salient differences between FAME-2 and COURAGE, especially considering trial design.

non-randomized revascularization) occurred at a rate of 33.0 % in the CABG arm, 42.4 % in the PCI arm, and 59.1 % in the OMT group, while mortality rates were not significantly different between the different strategies at 10 years [32, 33]. However, the trial was notably underpowered to detect any meaningful differences between the management strategies, and was a single-center study conducted during an era (i.e., enrollment was between 1995 and 2000) when OMT and modern DES had not fully come of age [34].

A recent MASS II post-hoc analysis evaluated serial LVEF measurements in the 350 enrollees surviving at 10 years to assess the widespread belief that revascularization is more effective than OMT in preserving LVEF [35]. After the 10-year follow-up period, LV systolic function was preserved (LVEF of 0.56 ± 0.11, 0.55 ± 0.11, 0.55 ± 0.12; P=0.675, respectively in the PCI, CABG, and OMT arms) and only declined minimally from baseline regardless of the initial treatment strategy applied, except among SIHD patients who had suffered an MI either prior to or after revascularization [34]. This post-hoc analysis is limited by its sample size and potential selection bias. Patients who died prior to the 10-year follow-up evaluation were excluded from the analysis, thus eliminating a subset of patients with potentially lower EFs from analysis. Nevertheless, results support an initial trial of OMT with deferred revascularization in SIHD patients, as there is no significant difference between treatment strategies in clinical outcomes or objective markers of heart function, such as LVEF. The ISCHEMIA trial requires baseline evaluation of LV systolic function and long-term follow-up of trial participants, which will allow further investigation of which initial management strategy best preserves systolic function [34].

SYNTAX Trial

In the Synergy between Percutaneous Coronary Intervention with Taxus and Cardiac Surgery (SYNTAX) trial, 1,800 patients with three-vessel or left main coronary artery disease, determined to be equally amenable to coronary-artery bypass grafting (CABG) or PCI with a drug-eluting stent, were randomly assigned to either treatment and followed for 12 months for a non-inferiority comparison [36]. The primary end point was a composite of major adverse cardiac or cerebrovascular events, so-called MACCE that consisted of death from any cause, stroke, MI, or repeat revascularization. At 12 months of follow-up, the rate of MACCE was significantly more frequent with PCI vs. CABG (17.8 %, vs. 12.4 %; P=0.002), largely due to the need for repeat revascularization (13.5 % vs. 5.9 %, P<0.001). Rates of death and MI were similar between the two groups, but stroke was significantly more likely to occur with CABG (0.6 % vs. 2.2 %; P=0.003). Thus, even with contemporary PCI techniques, CABG was shown to be preferable for most cases of complex or extensive, multivessel CAD, while the benefits of PCI were largely restricted to those of symptom-relief in patients with less extensive anatomic CAD, generally those with single-vessel or two-vessel angiographic CAD and in those with low or intermediate SYNTAX scores.

At 5-years of follow-up, 26.9 % of CABG and 37.3 % of PCI patients reached the composite endpoint (P<0.001) of death (11.4 % vs. 13.9 %; P=0.10), MI (3.8 % vs. 9.7 %; P<0.001), stroke (3.7 % vs. 2.4 %; P=0.09), or repeat revascularization (13.7 % vs. 25.9 %; P<0.001) [37]. Because PCI failed to reach the pre-specified criteria for non-inferiority, all other findings can only be regarded as observational and hypothesis generating. Nevertheless, in 1,095 patients with three-vessel CAD, CABG reduced the risk of death (9.2 % vs. 14.6 %; P=0.006), MI (3.3 % vs. 10.6 %; P<0.001) and need for repeat revascularization (12.6 % vs. 25.4 %; P<0.001) without an increase in the risk of stroke (3.4 % vs. 3 %; P=0.66). When analyzed by severity of CAD, as judged by SYNTAX scores, patients with intermediate (between 23–32) and higher (>32) scores had an absolute survival advantage with CABG (by 6.7 % and 9 %, respectively) as well as highly significant reductions in the incidence of MI and need for repeat revascularization. Only in those with scores <22 was there a similar mortality between CABG and PCI, although CABG still resulted in significantly fewer MIs and repeat revascularizations. This is an important distinction as 79 % of all patients with three-vessel CAD in SYNTAX (1,095 in the RCT and 570 in the registry) had SYNTAX scores >22. However, when the SYNTAX results were analyzed according to patients with three-vessel CAD and no left main disease, as compared with the 705 patients with left main disease, a different pattern of response emerges. In contrast to the situation for three-vessel CAD, the respective 5-year rates of death (14.6 % vs. 12.8 %; P=0.53) and MI (4.8 % vs. 8.2 %; P=0.10) were similar, whereas those who underwent CABG had a lower risk of repeat revascularization (15.5 % vs. 26.7 %; P<0.001) but a higher rate of stroke (4.3 % vs. 1.5 %; P=0.03). In patients with SYNTAX scores >32, CABG resulted in lower mortality (14.1 % vs. 20.9 %; P=0.01) and the need for repeat revascularization (11.6 % vs. 34.1 %; P<0.001), but at the expense of a higher risk of stroke (4.9 % vs. 1.6 %; P=0.13). In contrast, in the lower two SYNTAX score tertiles, PCI appeared to have superior outcomes to CABG in terms of reduced mortality.

FREEDOM Trial

This trial randomized 1,900 patients with diabetes and multivessel CAD already receiving aggressive medical therapy to either CABG or DES. The 5-year primary composite outcome occurred in 26.6 % of the PCI group and 18.7 % of the CABG group (P=0.005). Crucially, the benefit of CABG was driven by highly significant absolute reductions in both death (5.4 %; P=0.049) and myocardial infarction (7.9 %; P<0.001), but with a higher risk of stroke in the CABG group (5.2 % vs. 2.4 %; P=0.03). Some reassurance that these findings are likely to be real is that they are entirely.

consistent with the previous collaborative analysis reporting a hazard ratio for death of 0.7 in patients with diabetes undergoing CABG rather than PCI [38]. The findings from the FREEDOM Trial likewise buttress the results of the BARI-2D Trial, which showed that among diabetics with SIHD, CABG surgery was associated with a significant reduction of the secondary composite endpoint of death, MI, or stroke as compared with OMT—with these favorable findings being driven largely by a significant reduction in the incidence of MI.

Is there an Ischemic Threshold?

Observational data from prior to the contemporary era of OMT suggests there is a survival benefit with early revascularization over medical therapy in patients with moderate to severe ischemic burden (i.e., >10 %) on stress myocardial perfusion imaging (MPI) [14–16]. Incremental increases in ischemic burden potentially may be linked with survival, but whether revascularization to mitigate ischemia improves prognosis remains unknown. RCTs to date have evaluated the advantage with an early revascularization strategy compared with medical therapy after angiography, but less evidence exists evaluating the benefit of revascularization following baseline stress testing [12].

A 2008 COURAGE Trial substudy of 314 patients who receiving SPECT imaging before randomization and a second scan 1 year later demonstrated that mean total perfusion defect (i.e., a measure of ischemic reduction) was greater with PCI (2.7 %) than with medical therapy (0.5 %), and the percentage of OMT patients achieving ≥5 % ischemia reduction was 19 % as compared with 33 % in the PCI group [39]. For the 105 patients (conservative and invasive groups combined) whose pretreatment perfusion scan revealed moderate-to-severe ischemia, lower rates of death and MI were seen with significant ischemia reduction compared to patients without a reduction (16 % vs. 34 %; adjusted multivariate P=0.08). Though a graded relationship between ischemic burden and mortality/MI is suggested by this nuclear substudy, it is simply too underpowered to make any definitive statements about the relationship between ischemia severity and the potential clinical benefit of early revascularization. A second COURAGE trial nuclear substudy of 1,381 patients, all of whom had a pre-randomization SPECT scan with or without a subsequent second follow-up scan, showed no difference in mortality or overall rate of MI between the PCI+OMT and OMT arms in both the no-to-mild ischemia (19 and 18 %, P=0.92) and moderate-to-severe ischemia (22 and 19 %, P=0.53) subsets, respectively [28]. Thus, two nuclear subsets analyses from the same trial showed discordant results as to whether moderate-severe ischemia was a driver of increased CV events and was associated with a lower event rate following revascularization. Further research is needed to answer if there is an ischemic threshold that must be met for revascularization to demonstrate a benefit over medical therapy in SIHD patients [40]. Investigators leading the International Study of Comparative Health Effectiveness with Medical and Invasive Approaches (ISCHEMIA) trial hope to answer this question (ClinicalTrials.gov Identifier: NCT01471522).

Finally, a recent 2014 COURAGE trial post-hoc analysis of 621 SIHD patients revealed that when both anatomic burden and ischemic burden were measured at baseline, ischemia did not independently predict death, nonfatal MI, or non-ST segment elevation acute coronary syndromes (NSTE-ACS) [17]. However, anatomic burden defined by coronary anatomy and LVEF appeared to better and more reliably predict long-term clinical outcomes. Though the analysis is relatively underpowered and the cohort studied was not a pre-specified subgroup, it has important implications for the ISCHEMIA trial, which will include higher-risk patients. The hypothesis that "anatomy trumps physiology" challenges the dogma that inducible ischemia should be used to guide revascularization decisions. The blinded baseline coronary computed tomographic angiogram (CCTA) in the ISCHEMIA trial will allow investigators to conduct a post-hoc analysis to more reliably determine whether anatomic burden or ischemic burden has greater prognostic importance [41].

Future Perpsective: The Ischemia Trial [42]

The primary objective of the ISCHEMIA Trial is to determine whether an initial management strategy of revascularization (PCI or CABG) plus OMT versus a conservative strategy of OMT alone with revascularization reserved for a failure of OMT in SIHD patients with *at least* moderate ischemia on baseline testing favorably reduces the primary end point, a composite of cardiovascular death or nonfatal MI. ISCHEMIA is the first trial to require an ischemic threshold for entry. Directly addressing prior criticisms of referral bias, patients in the ISCHEMIA trial will be randomized prior to cardiac catheterization. To ensure patient safety and reassure treating physicians, patients with normal renal function will have a blinded CCTA prior to randomization to exclude patients with significant left main coronary artery disease. The main secondary end point is angina-related quality of life, as measured by the Seattle Angina Questionnaire (SAQ). Other secondary end points include all-cause death, cardiovascular death, nonfatal MI, resuscitated cardiac arrest, hospitalization for unstable angina or heart failure, and stroke. Health resource utilization, associated costs, and cost-effectiveness will be compared between the two arms. ISCHEMIA seeks to randomize 8,000 participants, making it the largest SIHD strategy trial ever conducted.

Only patients with at least moderate ischemia are included, defined on stress testing by nuclear myocardial perfusion (≥ 10 % ischemic myocardium), echocardiography or cardiac magnetic resonance (CMR) wall motion abnormalities ($\geq 3/16$ segments with stress-induced severe hypokinesis or akinesis), CMR perfusion (≥ 12 % ischemic myocardium), or ischemia at a low workload on a non-imaging exercise tolerance test. Subjects randomized to the invasive strategy will undergo complete ischemic revascularization using optimal revascularization modalities (i.e., DES, FFR, and CABG). These features distinguish ISCHEMIA from all prior SIHD strategy trials.

General Principles to Guide Patient Selection for Revascularization

Each of the following considerations may be used to guide decisions regarding the indications for (as well as the approach to) revascularization: (1) the presence and severity of symptoms; (2) physiological significance of coronary lesions and other anatomic considerations; (3) extent of myocardial Ischemia and the presence of LV dysfunction; (4) other medical conditions which influence the risks of percutaneous or surgical revascularization; and (5) the potential risks of the procedure.

Some general principles regarding the choice of treatment in patients with SIHD should also be considered:

1. For the majority of patients with chronic angina, revascularization should not constitute the initial management strategy before evidence-based medical therapy (pharmacologic anti-anginal therapy, disease-modifying treatments, and therapeutic lifestyle intervention) is initiated and optimized.
2. When improvement in survival is not a relevant consideration, the severity of angina or impairment in health status should play a significant role in determining whether revascularization is appropriate (i.e., limiting angina on optimal medical therapy is a more compelling indication than episodic, exertional angina on minimal medical therapy).
3. The patient's treatment preferences and socio-demographic/clinical circumstances should always be a consideration in choosing which treatment strategy should be employed.
4. In certain clinical circumstances, it may be difficult to reliably ascertain whether anginal symptoms or anginal equivalents such as exertional dyspnea or fatigue are a direct manifestation of underlying CAD, especially in patients with significant obesity, those who are sedentary, or who may have co-existing chronic obstructive pulmonary disease. Such symptoms that are either atypical or non-diagnostic for obstructive CAD may not necessarily improve with revascularization, even when such symptoms co-exist with physiologically significant CAD.
5. The decision to proceed with myocardial revascularization in the SIHD patient should entail a thoughtful, transparent discussion of all potential treatment options, with full disclosure of the anticipated benefits and potential risks associated with PCI or CAG surgery, relative to guideline-directed medical therapy. In an elective setting where urgent/emergent PCI is not being contemplated to reduce death or MI, the employment of a "heart team", as cited above, is both prudent and clinically appropriate. While it is often very common to undertake adhoc PCI once the patient's coronary anatomy is defined in the catheterization laboratory, frequently it is difficult to have the type of discussion that would involve a "heart team" in this setting. It has been suggested that a "time out", or hitting the "therapeutic pause button", might facilitate a more thorough understanding of what is best for a particular patient, particularly the patient with

extensive multivessel CAD. In summary, treatment decisions must be individualized according to the specific clinical features and personal preferences of a given patient (often in collaboration with family members and the patient's referring physician) with informed discussion about the potential risks and benefits of all three therapeutic options.

Conclusions

1. Unless there are compelling reasons not to do so, optimal medical therapy and lifestyle intervention should be the initial approach to management the majority of patients with SIHD, particularly those who have not been treated previously medically and in those who do not have objective evidence of moderate-to-severe ischemia. Such treatment decisions need to be individualized, as highlighted in the previous section.
2. However, it is also important to clarify that there are clear indications for coronary revascularization in selected patient subsets: (1) those subjects with significant left main CAD; (2) patients with significant multivessel CAD, particularly when involving the LAD coronary artery; (3) diabetic patients with multivessel CAD; (4) CAD patients refractory to OMT.
3. Among the first 3 subsets of CAD patients, the data from BARI-2D and SYNTAX would generally support the benefit of CBG surgery vs. multivessel PCI, particularly if CV event reduction is the goal of therapy (i.e., to prolong survival or to reduce MI). For patients who refuse surgery or in whom the risk would likely outweigh the benefit of symptom-relief, PCI remains a viable and, at times, a desirable alternative.
4. Outside of these subsets, clinicians will need to await the results of the ISCHEMIA trial to answer which approach, invasive or conservative medical therapy, is the most effective initial strategy in managing SIHD patients with at least moderate inducible ischemia at baseline. Until then, the use of revascularization for SIHD should be made judiciously and individualized based upon clinical need and the response to medical therapy.

References

1. Cannon CP, Weintraub WS, Demopoulos LA, Vicari R, Frey ML, Lakkis N, Neumann F-J, Robertson DH, DeLucca PT, DiBatistte P, Gibson CM, Braunwald E. Comparison of early invasive and conservative strategies in patients with unstable coronary syndromes treated with the glycoprotein IIb/IIIa inhibitor tirofiban. N Engl J Med. 2001;344:1879–87.
2. Fox KA, Poole-Wilson PA, Henderson RA, Clayton TC, Chamberlain DA, Shaw TR, Wheatley DJ, Pocock SJ, et al. Interventional versus conservative treatment for patients with unstable angina or non-ST-elevation myocardial infarction: the British heart foundation RITA 3 randomised trial. Randomized intervention trial of unstable angina. Lancet. 2002;360:743–51.

3. Keeley EC, Boura JA, Grines CL. Primary angioplasty versus intravenous thrombolytic therapy for acute myocardial infarction: a quantitative review of 23 randomised trials. Lancet. 2003;361:13–20.
4. Kushner FG, Hand M, Smith SC, King SB, Anderson JL, Antman EM, Bailey SR, Bates ER, Blankenship JC, Casey DE, Green LA, Hochman JA, Jacobs AK, Krumholz HM, Morrison DA, Ornato JP, Pearle DL, Peterson ED, Sloan MA, Whitlow PL, Williams DO. 2009 focused updates; ACC/AHA guidelines for the management of patients with ST-elevation myocardial infarction (updating the 2004 guidelines and 2007 focused update) and ACC/AHA/SCAI guidelines on percutaneous coronary intervention (Updating the 2005 guidelines and 2007 focused update). J Am Coll Cardiol. 2009;54:2205–41.
5. Mehta SR, Cannon CP, Fox KAA, Wallentin L, Boden WE, Spacek R, Widimsky P, McCullough PA, Hunt D, Braunwald E, Yusuf S. Routine versus selective invasive strategies in patients with acute coronary syndromes: a collaborative meta-analysis of randomized trials. JAMA. 2005;293:2908–17.
6. Wallentin L, et al. Invasive compared with non-invasive treatment in unstable coronary-artery disease: FRISC II prospective randomised multicentre study. FRagmin and Fast Revascularisation during Instability in Coronary artery disease Investigators. Lancet. 1999;354:708–15.
7. Boden WE, O'Rourke RA, Teo KK, et al. Optimal medical therapy with or without PCI for stable coronary disease. N Engl J Med. 2007;356(15):1503–16. doi:10.1056/NEJMoa070829.
8. BARI 2D Study Group, Frye RL, August P, Brooks MM, Hardison RM, Kelsey SF, et al. A randomized trial of therapies for type 2 diabetes and coronary artery disease. N Engl J Med. 2009;360(24):2503–15.
9. De Bruyne B, Pijls NH, Kalesan B, et al. Fractional flow reserve-guided PCI versus medical therapy in stable coronary disease. N Engl J Med. 2012;367(11):991–1001.
10. Desai KP, Sidhu MS, Boden WE. Evaluation of the stable coronary artery disease patient: anatomy trumps physiology. Trends Cardiovasc Med. 2014;24(8):332–40. doi:10.1016/j.tcm.2014.08.003.
11. Borden WB, Redberg RF, Mushlin AI, Dai D, Kaltenbach LA, Spertus JA. Patterns and intensity of medical therapy in patients undergoing percutaneous coronary intervention. JAMA. 2011;305(18):1882–9.
12. Mecklai A, Bangalore S, Hochman J. How and when to decide on revascularization in stable ischemic heart disease. Curr Treat Options Cardiovasc Med. 2013;15(1):79–92. doi:10.1007/s11936-012-0214-5. PubMed.
13. Fihn SD, Gardin JM, Abrams J, Berra K, Blankenship JC, Dallas AP, et al. 2012 ACCF/AHA/ACP/AATS/PCNA/SCAI/STS guideline for the diagnosis and management of patients with stable ischemic heart disease: executive summary: a report of the American College of Cardiology Foundation/American Heart Association task force on practice guidelines, and the American College of Physicians, American Association for Thoracic Surgery, Preventive Cardiovascular Nurses Association, Society for Cardiovascular Angiography and Interventions, and Society of Thoracic Surgeons. Circulation. 2012;126(25):3097–137.
14. Hachamovitch R, Berman DS, Shaw LJ, Kiat H, Cohen I, Cabico JA, et al. Incremental prognostic value of myocardial perfusion single photon emission computed tomography for the prediction of cardiac death: differential stratification for risk of cardiac death and myocardial infarction. Circulation. 1998;97(6):535–43.
15. Hachamovitch R, Hayes SW, Friedman JD, Cohen I, Berman DS. Comparison of the short-term survival benefit associated with revascularization compared with medical therapy in patients with no prior coronary artery disease undergoing stress myocardial perfusion single photon emission computed tomography. Circulation. 2003;107(23):2900–7.
16. Hachamovitch R. Risk assessment of patients with known or suspected CAD using stress myocardial perfusion SPECT: Part I: the ongoing evolution of clinical evidence. Rev Cardiovasc Med. 2000;1(2):91–102.
17. Mancini GB, Hartigan PM, Shaw LJ, et al. Predicting outcome in the COURAGE trial (Clinical Outcomes Utilizing Revascularization and Aggressive Drug Evaluation): coronary anatomy

versus ischemia. JACC Cardiovasc Interv. 2014;7(2):195–201. doi:10.1016/j.jcin.2013.10.017. Epub 2014 Jan 15.

18. Panza JA, Holly TA, Asch FM, She L, Pellikka PA, Velazquez EJ, et al. Inducible myocardial ischemia and outcomes in patients with coronary artery disease and left ventricular dysfunction. J Am Coll Cardiol. 2013;61(18):1860–70.

19. Aldweib N, Negishi K, Hachamovitch R, Jaber WA, Seicean S, Marwick TH. Impact of repeat myocardial revascularization on outcome in patients with silent ischemia after previous revascularization. J Am Coll Cardiol. 2013;61:1616–23.

20. Montalescot G, Achenbach S, Andreotti F, et al. 2013 ESC guidelines on the management of stable coronary artery disease: the task force on the management of stable coronary artery disease of the European Society of Cardiology. Eur Heart J. 2013. doi:10.1093/eurheartj/eht296.

21. Fihn SD, Blankenship JC, Alexander KP, Bittl JA, Byrne JG, Fletcher BJ, et al. 2014 ACC/AHA/AATS/PCNA/SCAI/STS focused update of the guideline for the diagnosis and management of patients with stable ischemic heart disease: a report of the American College of Cardiology/American Heart Association Task Force on Practice Guidelines, and the American Association for Thoracic Surgery, Preventive Cardiovascular Nurses Association, Society for Cardiovascular Angiography and Interventions, and Society of Thoracic Surgeons. J Am Coll Cardiol. 2014;64(18):1929–49.

22. Yusuf S, Zucker D, Peduzzi P, Fisher LD, Takaro T, Kennedy JW, Davis K, Killip T, Passamani E, Norris R, et al. Effect of coronary artery bypass graft surgery on survival: overview of 10-year results from randomised trials by the Coronary Artery Bypass Graft Surgery Trialists Collaboration. Lancet. 1994;344(8922):563–70. Erratum in: Lancet 1994 Nov 19;344(8934):1446. PubMed.

23. Passamani E, Davis KB, Gillespie MJ, Killip T. A randomized trial of coronary artery bypass surgery. Survival of patients with a low ejection fraction. N Engl J Med. 1985;312(26):1665–71.

24. Varnauskas E. Twelve-year follow-up of survival in the randomized European Coronary Surgery Study. N Engl J Med. 1988;319(6):332–7.

25. Veterans Affairs Cooperative Study. Eleven-year survival in the Veterans Administration randomized trial of coronary bypass surgery for stable angina. The Veterans Administration Coronary artery Bypass Surgery Cooperative Study Group. N Engl J Med. 1984;311(21):1333–9. doi:10.1056/NEJM198411223112102.

26. Weintraub WS, Spertus JA, Kolm P, Maron DJ, Zhang Z, Jurkovitz C, Zhang W, Hartigan PM, Lewis C, Veledar E, Bowen J, Dunbar SB, Deaton C, Kaufman S, O'Rourke RA, Goeree R, Barnett PG, Teo KK, Boden WE, COURAGE Trial Research Group, Mancini GB. Effect of PCI on quality of life in patients with stable coronary disease. N Engl J Med. 2008;359(7):677–87. doi:10.1056/NEJMoa072771.

27. Diamond GA, Kaul S. COURAGE under fire: on the management of stable coronary disease. J Am Coll Cardiol. 2007;50(16):1604–9.

28. Shaw LJ, Weintraub WS, Maron DJ, et al. Baseline stress myocardial perfusion imaging results and outcomes in patients with stable ischemic heart disease randomized to optimal medical therapy with or without percutaneous coronary intervention. Am Heart J. 2012;164:243–50.

29. Dagenais GR, Lu J, Faxon DP, et al. Effects of optimal medical treatment with or without coronary revascularization on angina and subsequent revascularizations in patients with type 2 diabetes mellitus and stable ischemic heart disease. Circulation. 2011;123(14):1492–500. doi:10.1161/CIRCULATIONAHA.110.978247. Epub 2011 Mar 28.

30. De Bruyne B, Fearon WF, Pijls NH, et al. Fractional flow reserve-guided PCI for stable coronary artery disease. N Engl J Med. 2014;371(13):17. doi:10.1056/NEJMoa1408758. Epub 2014 Sep 1.

31. Boden WE. Which is more enduring–FAME or COURAGE? N Engl J Med. 2012;367(11):1059–61. doi:10.1056/NEJMe1208620.

32. Hueb W, Lopes NH, Gersh BJ, et al. Five-year follow-up of the medicine, angioplasty, or surgery study (MASS II): a randomized controlled clinical trial of 3 therapeutic strategies for multivessel coronary artery disease. Circulation. 2007;115(9):1082–9. doi:10.1161/CIRCULATIONAHA.106.625475.

33. Hueb W, Lopes N, Gersh BJ, et al. Ten-year follow-up survival of the medicine, angioplasty, or surgery study (MASS II): a randomized controlled clinical trial of 3 therapeutic strategies for multivessel coronary artery disease. Circulation. 2010;122(10):949–57. doi:10.1161/CIRCULATIONAHA.109.911669.

34. Sidhu MS, Boden WE. Optimal medical therapy vs. revascularization on long-term LV function. Eur Heart J. 2013;34(43):3339–41. doi:10.1093/eurheartj/eht297.

35. Garzillo CL, Hueb W, Gersh BJ, Lima EG, Rezende PC, Hueb AC, et al. Long-term analysis of left ventricular ejection fraction in patients with stable multivessel coronary disease undergoing medicine, angioplasty or surgery: 10-year follow-up of the MASS II trial. Eur Heart J. 2013;34(43):3370–7. doi:10.1093/eurheartj/eht201. Epub 2013 Jul 4.

36. Serruys PW, Morice M-C, Kappetein AP, Colombo A, Holmes DR, Mack MJ, et al. Percutaneous coronary intervention versus coronary artery bypass grafting for severe coronary arte disease. N Engl J Med. 2009;360:961–72.

37. Mohr FW, Morice M-C, Kappetein AP, Feldman TE, Stahle E, Colombo A, et al. Coronary artery bypass graft surgery versus percutaneous coronary intervention in patients with three-vessel disease and left main coronary disease: 5-year follow-up of the randomised, clinical SYNTAX trial. Lancet. 2013;381:629–38.

38. Hlatky MA, Boothroyd DB, Bravata DM, et al. Coronary artery bypass surgery compared with percutaneous coronary interventions for multivessel disease: a collaborative analysis of individual patient data from ten randomised trials. Lancet. 2009;373:1190–7.

39. Shaw LJ, Berman DS, Maron DJ, Mancini GB, Hayes SW, Hartigan PM, et al. Optimal medical therapy with or without percutaneous coronary intervention to reduce ischemic burden: results from the clinical outcomes utilizing revascularization and aggressive drug evaluation (COURAGE) trial nuclear substudy. Circulation. 2008;117(10):1283–91.

40. Bangalore S, Messerli FH. Is there an ischemic threshold beyond which percutaneous coronary intervention is beneficial in the clinical outcomes utilizing revascularization and aggressive drug evaluation (COURAGE) Trial? Am J Cardiol. 2007;100:1495.

41. King SB. 3rd. Is it form or function?: the "COURAGE" to ask. JACC Cardiovasc Interv. 2014;7(2):202–3. doi:10.1016/j.jcin.2013.10.018. Epub 2014 Jan 15.

42. International Study of Comparative Health Effectiveness with Medical and Invasive Approaches (ISCHEMIA) home page. Available at: http://www.clinicaltrials.gov/ct2/show/NCT01471522, NIH Grant: 1U01HL105907. Accessed Dec 2014.

Chapter 16
Percutaneous Coronary Intervention in Unprotected Left Main Stenosis: Medical Evidence from Randomized and Observational Studies

Carlos Fernández-Pereira and Alfredo E. Rodríguez

Abstract Left main disease (LMD) is a stenosis of ≥50 %, and occurs in 3–5 % of patients, associated with multi-vessel coronary artery disease (CAD) in more than 75 %. With bare metal stents (BMS), left main stenting became more popular and the technique was used mainly in high risk patients such as acute myocardial infarction (AMI) or with contraindications for coronary artery bypass grafts (CABG). There was an initial low incidence of adverse events with this approach, but with concerns regarding restenosis-related events, drug eluting stents (DES) became the preferred option. Comparative studies with CABG and DES showed that both had similar mortality and incidence of MI but with higher recurrence of repeat revascularization procedures with DES. CABG had a higher stroke risk. Percutaneous Coronary intervention (PCI) should be a good option in most patients with LMD without bifurcation disease, in those with a small diameter circumflex artery and /or low or intermediate anatomic risk score. The latest European guidelines recommended PCI with DES implantation as a class I indication in certain subgroups of patients with LMD. On the other hand, CABG is still the "gold standard" and has remained a better option when the SYNTAX score is ≥33, with severe multi-vessel coronary disease, total occlusions of ≥2 major coronary epicardial vessels, severe calcifications or tortuosity, and in those with a contraindication to antiplatelet therapy.

C. Fernández-Pereira, MD, PhD
Department of Interventional Cardiology, Otamendi Hospital, Buenos Aires, Argentina
e-mail: cfernandezpereira@centroceci.com.ar

A.E. Rodríguez, MD, PhD, FACC, FSCAI (✉)
Cardiac Unit, Department of Interventional Cardiology, Revista Argentina de Cardioagiologia Intervencionista (RACI), Otamendi Hospital, Buenos Aires, Argentina

Interventional Cardiology Unit, Department of Interventional Cardiology, Otamendi Hospital, Buenos Aires, Argentina

Otamendi Hospital, Post Graduate Buenos Aires School of Medicine, Buenos Aires, Argentina

Director, Cardiovascular Research Center (CECI), Buenos Aires, Argentina

© Springer International Publishing Switzerland 2015
J.A. Ambrose, A.E. Rodríguez (eds.), *Controversies in Cardiology*,
DOI 10.1007/978-3-319-20415-4_16

Keywords Coronary disease • Left main • Bare metal stents • Drug eluting stents • Bifurcation lesions • Coronary by pass graft • Registry • Randomized trial • Meta analysis

Introduction

Significant left main disease (LMD) is defined as a stenosis of ≥50 %, and is associated with multi-vessel coronary artery disease (CAD) in more than 75 % of patients. LMD occurs in 3–5 % of patients undergoing coronary angioplasty [1]. Coronary artery bypass graft surgery (CABG) has remained as the standard of care therapy for patients with LMD mostly because the long-term outcomes, including mortality, were superior to those of medical treatment [2, 3].

Percutaneous coronary intervention (PCI) in LMD was first performed during the balloon angioplasty era although because of the risk of acute closure, this became a contra indication to PCI. With the introduction of bare metal stents (BMS) during PCI, left main stenting became more popular and the technique was reported in observational studies and registries mainly in high risk patients such as those with acute myocardial infarction (AMI) or with contraindications for myocardial revascularization with CABG [4, 5]. Observational studies reported an initial low incidence of adverse events with this approach [4] since BMS lowered the incidence of abrupt vessel closure, but concerns arose regarding high rates of restenosis-related events particularly for those lesions located distally and involving the bifurcation. Drug eluting stents (DES) have significantly decreased the risk of restenosis and target lesion revascularization (TLR) compared to BMS. Therefore, their introduction routinely during PCI has enhanced the mid and long -term outcomes of PCI for LMD [5, 6]. In this chapter, we will discuss the most relevant aspects about PCI in LMD analyzing mid and long term results from observational studies as well as randomized trials and meta-analyses, focusing studies mainly on DES designs.

PCI with Stenting

DES Versus BMS in Observational Studies and Registries

There are several observational studies comparing BMS and DES in LMD. In most, event free survival was improved with DES. In the LE MANS [7] (Left MaiN coronary artery Stenting) registry, performed in Poland, 252 patients were enrolled during 11 years between 1997 and 2008 with 58 % having a non ST segment elevation acute coronary syndrome, diabetics in 26.4 % and a distal location of the stenosis in 56 % [8]. Between 1997 and 2001 only BMS were used. After that, DES was recommended for the LM with a reference diameter ≤3.8 mm. First generation DES [paclitaxel (PES) and sirolimus (SES)] were implanted in 36.2 % of patients. The Euro score surgery risk was 6±2.

Major adverse cardiovascular and cerebral events (MACCE) defined as death, myocardial infarction (MI), TLR, stent thrombosis (ST) or cerebrovascular accident (CVA) stroke occurred in 12 (4.8 %) patients during the 30-day follow-up period. During long-term follow-up (mean 3.8 years, range 1–11 years) MACCE rates were 25.4 % and 13.9 % of patients died. The 5- and 10-year survival rates were 78.1 % and 68.9 % respectively. Despite more favorable baseline characteristics in patients treated with BMS, unmatched analysis showed a significantly lower MACCE rate in DES patients (25.9 % vs. 14.9 %, respectively p=0.039). This difference was strengthened even further after propensity score matching. DES lowered both mortality and MACCE for distal LMD lesions when compared to BMS. Ejection fraction <50 % was the only independent risk factor influencing long-term survival.

The Italian Society of Invasive Cardiology ran a multicenter retrospective registry [9] in 19 high volumes centers enrolling 1453 consecutive patients who underwent PCI on LMD between January 2002 and December 2006. Four hundred and seventy-nine received either first generation DES (334 patients) or BMS (145 patients) but only for lesions located at the ostium or shaft, without any distal involvement. After propensity score matching was performed, baseline covariates between the two yielded 119 well-matched pairs. At 3-year follow-up, risk-adjusted survival rates were higher in patients treated with DES than in those treated with BMS, although the adjusted 3-year rates of TLR were not significantly lower with DES compared to BMS (P=0.60).

Our group began to perform left main stenting in the early 1990s soon after PCI with BMS became a default strategy [4]. In 1996, the ERACI II study [10, 11] became the first randomized revascularization trial that included unprotected LMD patients. This included about 5 % of the overall population, 4 % in CABG and 5.8 % in the PCI arms. Moreover, in Argentina in 2013, a multicenter registry was published in patients with unprotected LMD [12]. Two hundred and eighty-one consecutive patients treated between 2002 and 2012 were included. Baseline characteristics included mean age of 67.1 years, diabetes in 18.5 %, a Euro SCORE of 5.5, acute coronary syndromes in 72.9, 25.4 % of them with ST elevation MI (STEMI) and distal LMD stenosis in 49.8 %. 391 stents were implanted, BMS and DES in 49 % and 51 % respectively. During a mean follow-up 3.2±2.7 years, death occurred in 9.6 and 6.0 % had an MI; 14.5 % had death/MI/CVA and 30 % MACCE (Fig. 16.1). Compared to proximal

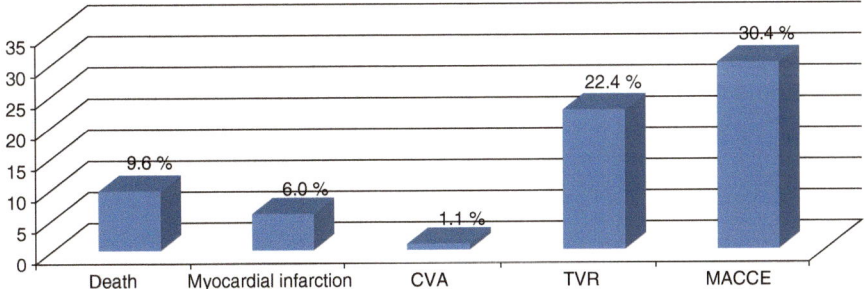

Fig. 16.1 Left main Argentine CECI registry, overall results at 3.2 years of follow-up (mean). *CECI* Cardiovascular Research Center, *CVA* cerebrovascular accident, *TVR* target vessel revascularization, *MACCE* major adverse cardiovascular events: death, MI, CVA and TVR

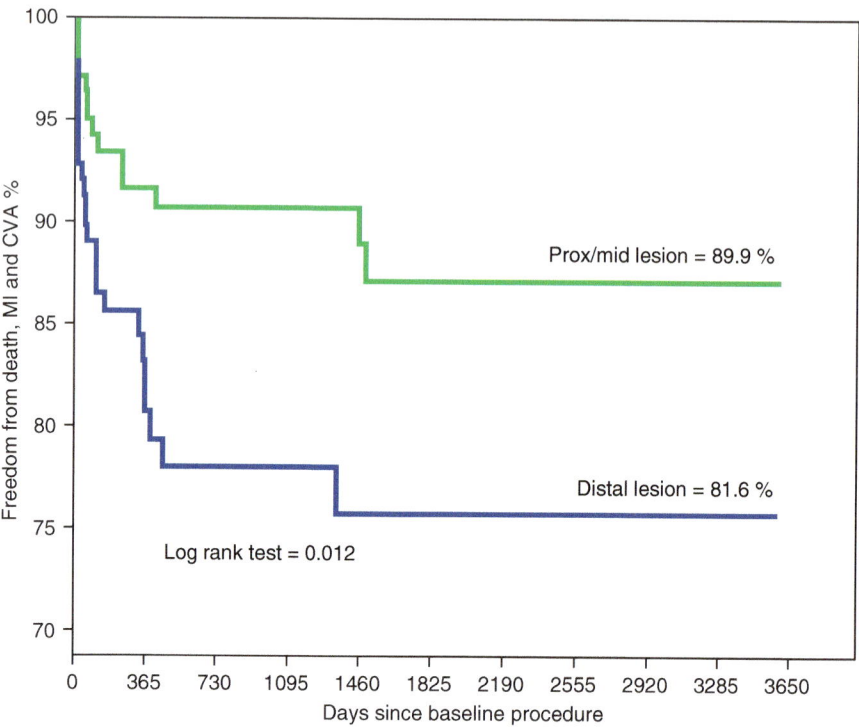

Fig. 16.2 Kaplan-Meier Death, myocardial infarction and cerebrovascular accident curve at 3.2±2.7 years follow- up comparing distal vs. proximal lesions (n=281). *Prox/mid* proximal and/ or mid left main coronary lesions. *MI* myocardial infarction

lesions, distal lesions had a significantly worse freedom from death/MI/CVA (81.9 % vs. 89 %, respectively=0.012) (Fig. 16.2) and MACCE (66.7 % vs. 77.7 %, respectively p=0.02). Patients receiving a DES had less MACCE than with BMS (p=0.025). Those treated with BMS also had poorer outcomes with distal lesions (Fig. 16.3). Better event free survival with DES was also observed in patients treated for an acute MI with ostial LAD or LCX involvement. Thus, DES implantation had become the default strategy in left main PCI [13]. Further pooled data from several trials suggested better outcomes with DES compared to BMS. A meta-analysis [14] with 10,342 patients from 44 studies assessed the incidence of death/MI, TVR/TLR and MACCE at 3 years. Mortality (8.8 and 12.7 %, p=0.01), TVR/TLR (8.0 and 16.4 % with DES and BMS: p=0.01), and MACCE (21.4 and 31.6 %, p=0.12) were all lower with DES.

DES Stent Selection

There are few studies that compared different DES designs in LMD. A randomized trial [14] and two observational studies [15, 16] suggested that outcomes were comparable between both first generations DES. However, now we are using second

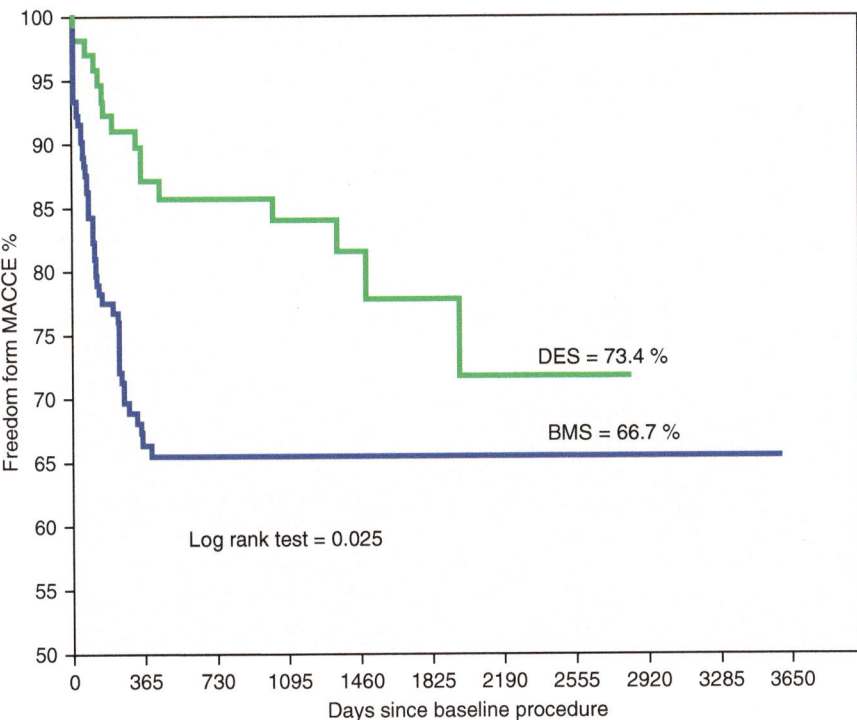

Fig. 16.3 Kaplan-Meier MACCE survival curve at 3.2±2.7 follow-up comparing DES vs. BMS. *MACCE* major adverse cardiovascular events (death, myocardial infarction, cerebrovascular accident and target vessel revascularization); *DES* drug eluting stent, *BMS* bare metal stent

and third generation drug- (limus family mostly, sirolimus, everolimus, zotarolimus and biolimus) eluting stents with new polymers, including biocompatible or biodegradable polymers. In the Florence registry, 390 patients underwent PCI with DES implantation, 224 received a paclitaxel eluting stent (PES) and 166 an everolimus-eluting stent (EES) [17]. At 9 months, coronary restenosis by angiography was 5.2 % in EES and 15.6 % in PES (p=0.002). Among 166 propensity matched pairs, the rate of MACCE at 2 years was significantly higher with PES (20.4 versus 10.2 %, respectively, p=0.010).

In the Left main Taxus and left main Xience (LEMAX) non-randomized registry, 173 patients treated with an EES were compared with a historical cohort of 291 patients treated with PES. At 12-month clinical follow-up, the EES was associated with a lower rate of target lesion failure, MACCE and ST compared with PES [18]. The ISAR-LEFT-MAIN 2 study compared the safety and efficacy of the zotarolimus-eluting stent (ZES) versus EES [19]. Patients were randomly assigned to receive either a ZES (n=324) or an EES (n=326). The primary endpoint was the combined incidence of death, MI and TLR at 1 year. Secondary endpoints were definite or probable ST at 1 year and angiographic restenosis based on analysis of the left main coronary artery area at follow-up angiography. At 1 year, the cumulative incidence of the primary endpoint was 17.5 % in the ZES group and 14.3 % in the EES group (p=0.25). Three patients in the ZES group (0.9 %) and 2 patients in the EES group (0.6 %) experienced definite or probable ST (p<0.99). All-cause mortality at 1 year was equal in the 2 groups (5.6 %). Angiographic restenosis occurred in 21.5 % in the ZES group and 16.8 % in the EES group (p=0.24). The results suggested that the use of second-generation EES and ZES had comparable outcomes to those noted with the use of first-generation DES, and both stent types appeared to afford similar results at 1-year follow-up.

PCI Versus CABG

Observational Studies

There are several non-randomized studies and registries (Table 16.1) comparing DES to CABG for patients with LMD [21–23]. The DELTA multicenter registry [20] included consecutive "all comers" with LMD treated either with PCI and a 1st generation DES or CABG between April 2002 and April 2006. Patients treated in 14 centers were retrospectively analyzed in this worldwide registry. A propensity score analysis was performed to adjust for baseline differences in the overall cohort. In total 2775 patients were included: 1874 were treated with PCI and 901 with CABG. At 1295 days (range: 928–1713), there were no differences, in the adjusted analysis, in the primary composite endpoint of death, cerebrovascular accidents, AMI, or the composite endpoint of death and AMI . An advantage of CABG over PCI was observed in the composite secondary endpoint of MACCE (p=0.0001), driven exclusively by the higher incidence of TVR with PCI.

The MAIN COMPARE registry in patients with LMD evaluated 2240 patients who received coronary stents (n=1102; 318 with BMS and 784 with DES) or underwent CABG (n=1138) at 12 major cardiac centers in Korea between January 2000 and June 2006 and for whom complete follow-up data were available for at least 3–9 years (median 5.2 years) [24]. From January 2000 through May 2003, coronary stenting was performed exclusively with BMS, whereas from May 2003 through June 2006, DES was used exclusively. The 5-year adverse outcomes (death, a composite outcome of death, Q-wave MI, or stroke and TVR) were compared with the use of the inverse probability of treatment weighted method and propensity-score matching.

After adjustment for differences in baseline risk factors, the 5-year risk of death (hazard ratio [HR]: 1.13; 95 % confidence interval [CI]: 0.88–1.44, p=0.35) and the combined risk of death, Q-wave MI, or stroke (HR: 1.07; 95 % CI: 0.84–1.37, p=0.59) were not significantly different for patients undergoing stenting versus CABG. The risk of TVR was significantly higher in the stenting group versus the CABG group (HR: 5.11; 95 % CI: 3.52–7.42, p<0.001). Similar results were obtained in compari-

Table 16.1 Randomized clinical trials and registries comparing CABG vs. PCI for the treatment of unprotected left main disease

Trial	Design	CABG	PCI (DES%)	Primary endpoint	Follow-up (primary endpoint)	Remarks	Authors main conclusion
LEMANS Registry [7]	Observational	1849	252 (37 %)	All-cause of death	3.8 years (range 1–11 years)	DES decreased the risk of long-term MACCE, particularly in distal lesions.	PCI is feasible and offers good long-term outcome.
DELTA [20]	Observational	901	1874 (100 %)	All-cause death, CVA, MI and repeat revascularization.	1295 days (range 928–1713)	It was an all-comers registry	No differences were observed in death, CVA and MI between groups.
Lee et al. [21]	Observational	123	50 (100 %)	MACCE	6 months	More than 50 % of high risk patients (Parsonnet >15)	PCI was not associated with an increase in immediate or medium-term complications.
Chieffo et al. [22]	Observational	142	107 (100 %)	Death; death/MI; death/MI/CVA; repeat revascularization; MACCE	12 months	In-hospital results were significantly in favor of PCI	There were no differences between groups.
Seung et al. [23]	Observational	1138	1102 (71 %)	Death; death/QMI or CVA; repeat revascularization.	1017 (688–1451) days	Even with DES, PCI was associated with higher TVR	No differences in death, MI or CVA.
MAIN-COMPARE [24]	Observational	1138	1102 (71 %)	Death; death, MI and CVA; and repeat revascularization	5.2 years (range 3–9 years)	Similar results comparing DES vs CABG and BMS vs CABG	PCI had similar death, MI and CVA with greater rates of TVR

(continued)

Table 16.1 (continued)

Trial	Design	CABG	PCI (DES%)	Primary endpoint	Follow-up (primary endpoint)	Remarks	Authors main conclusion
LEMANS Randomized [25]	RCT	53	52 (67 %)	LVEF	12 months	Late FU (>2 years) MACCE-free survival was similar in both groups.	LVEF had improved significantly only in PCI arm.
Precombat [26]	RCT	300	300 (100 %)	All-cause death, CVA, MI, and	Precombat [26]	RCT	300
SYNTAX Left Main [27]	RCT	348	357 (100 %)	All-cause death, CVA, MI, and repeat revascularization	5 years	This was a pre-specified subanalysis	No differences in primary endpoint between groups.
Boudriot et al. [28]	RCT	101	100 (100 %)	Cardiac death, MI and repeat revascularization	12 months	Hard endpoints (death/MI) where favorable to PCI	PCI did not show non-inferiority to CABG.

CABG coronary artery by-pass grafting, *PCI* percutaneous coronary intervention, *DES* drug eluting stent, *MACCE* major adverse cardiovascular events, *CVA* cerebrovascular accident, *MI* myocardial infarction, *TVR* target vessel revascularization, *BMS* bare metal stent, *RCT* randomized clinical trials, *LVEF* left ventricular ejection fraction sons of BMS or DES with concurrent CABG. Comparing DES with CABG in patients with a low-risk SYNTAX score, the rates of death (6.1 versus 16.2; HR 0.52. 95 % CI 0.21–1.28) and the composite of death, Q-wave MI, or stroke (6.4 for versus 16.2 %; HR 0.54, 95 % CI 0.22–1.34) favored DES but were not statistically significant. Comparing DES with CABG in patients with high-risk SYNTAX scores, the rates of death (26.9 versus 17.8; HR 1.46, 95 % CI 0.92–2.3) and the composite of death, Q-wave MI, stroke (27.6 versus 19.5 %; HR 1.26, 95 % CI 0.87–2.12) favored CABG but were not statistically significant. In patients with intermediate SYNTAX scores, the safety outcomes were similar in the two groups. TVR was significantly more frequent in patients who received DES, irrespective of the SYNTAX score.

Randomized Clinical Trials

DES Versus CABG

The LE MANS study [25] from Poland randomly assigned 105 patients with LMD to PCI in 52 patients and CABG in 53 patients. DES was used in 35 % of cases when the LMD was less than 3.8 mm, similar criteria used in the registry. PCI had favorable early outcomes in comparison with the CABG group. At 1 year, Left Ventricular Ejection Fraction (LVEF) had improved significantly only in the PCI group. After more than 2 years, MACCE-free survival was similar in both groups with a trend toward improved survival after PCI.

The PRECOMBAT trial, another LMD trial performed in Korea randomly assigned patients to undergo CABG (300 patients) or PCI with SES (300 patients). Using a wide margin for non -inferiority, they compared the groups with respect to the primary composite end point of MACCE (death from any cause, myocardial infarction, stroke, or ischemia-driven TVR) at 1 year. Event rates at 2 years were also compared between the two groups [26].

The primary end point was not statistically significant between both groups at 1 and 2 years although there was a trend in favor to CABG driven by a significantly lower incidence of TVR (9 % and 4.2 % in PCI and CABG respectively p = 0.02). The composite rate of death, MI, or CVA at 2 years occurred in 13 and 14 patients in the two groups, respectively (cumulative event rate, 4.4 % and 4.7 %, respectively P = 0.83). Limitations of this study were the lower than expected event rates, making less confident the finding of non-inferiority and the routine angiographic follow up in the PCI group, that may have led to a greater number of "ischemia-driven TVR" than would have been detected clinically.

The SYNTAX trial was a prospective, multinational, randomized (Synergy between Percutaneous Coronary Intervention with TAXUS stent and Cardiac Surgery) trial that was designed to evaluate the optimal revascularization strategy between PCI and CABG, for patients with LMD and/or 3-vessel coronary disease [29]. Our focus will be on the results of the pre-specified subgroup of 705 randomized patients who had LMD, among the 1800 patients included. MACCE rates at

1 year in LMD patients were similar for CABG and PCI (13.7 % versus 15.8 %; 2.1 % [95 % confidence interval 3.2–7.4 %]; p = 0.44). At 1 year, CVA was significantly higher in the CABG arm (2.7 % versus 0.3 %) p = 0.009, whereas repeat revascularization was significantly higher in the PCI arm (6.5 % versus 11.8 %); p = 0.02; there was no difference between groups for other end points. When patients were scored for anatomic complexity, those with higher baseline SYNTAX scores had significantly worse outcomes with PCI than did patients with low or intermediate SYNTAX scores; outcomes for patients with CABG did not correlate with baseline SYNTAX score, but interestingly, baseline Euro SCORE significantly predicted outcomes for both treatments. In summary at 1 year, patients with LM disease in this study with revascularization with PCI had safety and efficacy outcomes comparable to CABG.

At 5-years follow up, MACCE was 36.9 % in PCI patients and 31.0 % in CABG patients, p = 0.12 [27] Mortality was 12.8 and 14.6 % in PCI and CABG patients, respectively (p = 0.53). Stroke was significantly increased in the CABG group (PCI 1.5 % vs. CABG 4.3 %), p = 0.03 and repeat revascularization in the PCI arm (26.7 % vs. 15.5 %, p ≤ 0.01). MACCE was similar between arms in patients with low/intermediate SYNTAX Scores but significantly increased in PCI patients with high scores (≥33:46.5 versus 29.7 %). However, independently of the SYNTAX score, in patients with isolated LMD or LMD plus one vessel disease, the MACCE rate at 5 years was low with PCI.

This well conducted randomized study, however, had several potential limitations [30]: (1) the study was not powered to analyzed subgroups of patients according to risk scores, (2) there was a disparity in follow-up rate between the randomized arms: 92 patients out of 897 randomized to CABG withdrew consent or were lost, while only 55 patients randomized to PCI withdrew consent or were lost, (3) operator disparities between sites in MACCE rates, (4) a possible inappropriate PCI strategy- all side branches >1.5 mm should be treated and (5) complete obsolescence of the TAXUS stent utilized compared with the latest generation DES.

Meta-analysis DES Versus CABG

In recent years, a well conducted meta-analysis from RCT and observational registries evaluated the efficacy of CABG to PCI with 1st-generation DES among patients with LMD disease [31]. In general, CABG reduced revascularization risk (RR: 0.60, 95 % CI: 0.46–0.78) at the price of an increased stroke risk (RR: 2.89, 95 % CI: 1.15–7.27) without differences in death and AMI. Another large meta-analysis from Cleveland Clinic analyzed 24 studies comprising 14,203 patients [32].. Again, there was no significant difference for all-cause mortality between PCI or CABG- at 1 year (odds ratio [OR]: 0.792, 95 % confidence interval [CI]: 0.53–1.19), 2 years (OR: 0.920, 95 % CI: 0.67–1.26), 3 years (OR: 0.94, 95 % CI:

0.60–1.48), 4 years (OR: 0.84, 95 % CI: 0.53–1.33), and 5 years (OR: 0.79, 95 % CI: 0.57–1.08). The need for TVR was significantly higher in patients undergoing PCI at all time points. The occurrence of stroke, however, was significantly less frequent in patients treated with PCI. The occurrence of nonfatal MI showed a statistically significant trend towards a lower incidence in CABG patients at 1 year (OR: 1.62, 95 % CI: 1.05–2.50), 2 years (OR: 1.60, 95 % CI: 1.09–2.35), and 3 years (OR: 2.06, 95 % CI: 1.36–3.1). There was no significant difference in the combined MACCE between the 2 groups. Finally a 3rd meta-analysis by Capodanno et al. [33] from the 4 RCTs, Syntax Left Main, LEMANS, Boudriot et al. [28] and PRECOMBAT reported that in the 1597 patients, PCI had a non significantly lower risk of death (2, 9 % vs. 4 % OR 0.74 CI 0.42–1.28) with a significantly higher number of repeat revascularization procedures (OR 2.24 CI 1.52–3.28 p<0.000) . On the contrary, CABG increased the risk of stroke (1.7 % with CABG and 0.1 % with PCI, p=0.013) Table 16.2

Current Revascularization Guidelines in LMD

The 2011 ACC/AHA/SCAI guidelines made a strong recommendation about treatment in LMD patients [34]. In those with significant disease (>50 % diameter stenosis), PCI received a Class IIa recommendation in patients at increased risk for surgical revascularization with ostial or mid shaft left main disease, or in those with low SYNTAX scores (<23) (Table 16.3). A Class IIa recommendation was also made for PCI in NSTEMI acute syndromes if a patient was not a candidate for CABG or in the setting of ST-elevation AMI, if coronary flow was compromised and PCI could be performed more quickly and safely than CABG. There was a Class IIb recommendation for PCI in patients with bifurcation disease, low-intermediate SYNTAX scores (<33), and increased surgical risk. However, CABG is still considered the gold standard and a Class I indication in all other cases.

The European Society of Cardiology (ESC) and European Association for Cardio-Thoracic Surgery (EACTS) recently released their latest guideline statement for myocardial revascularization in 2014 (Table 16.4) [35] These guidelines gave a Class I recommendation, level B for PCI in the setting of LMD and Syntax scores ≤22. If the Syntax score was 23–32, it was a IIa recommendation. A class III recommendation was given for PCI and a Syntax score >33. CABG received a Class I recommendation in all of these scenarios. Both the American and European guidelines recommend strongly that the patient should seek opinions from a Heart Team involving interventional cardiologists and surgeons to determine the best revascularization strategy. Thus, patient preference should be included in decision making.

Current studies such as the EXCEL trial will help to clarify the contemporary role of PCI in the treatment of LMD with latest generation DES [36].

Table 16.2 Clinical outcome from the meta-analysis comparing Randomized Clinical data from 4 trials comparing PCI vs CABG for the treatment of ULMD [33]

	PCI, n (%)	CABG, n (%)	Odds ratio	Confidence Interval 95 %		P value
				Lower limit	Upper limit	
Death	24/807 (3.0)	32/790 (4.0)	0.74	0.42	1.28	0.28
MI	23/807 (2.8)	21/790 (2.6)	0.98	0.54	1.78	0.95
CVA	1/707 (0.14)	12/689 (1.7)	0.15	0.03	0.67	0.012
Repeat revascularization	92/807 (11.4)	43/790 (5.4)	2.24	1.53	3.28	<0.001
Death, MI or CVA	35/655 (5.3)	43/636 (6.7)	0.76	0.48	1.22	0.26
MACCE	117/807 (14.5)	93/790 (11.7)	1.27	0.95	1.75	0.10

PCI percutaneous coronary intervention, *CABG* coronary artery bypass grafting, *ULMD* unprotected left main disease, *MI* myocardial infarction, *CVA* cerebrovascular accident, *MACCE* major adverse cardiovascular events

Table 16.3 ACCF/AHA/SCAI recommendations for the use of percutaneous coronary intervention for unprotected left main disease

Recommendations according to extent of CAD		2011	
		Class[a]	Level[b]
Stable Ischemic Heart Disease	Ostial or trunk left main CAD	IIa	B
	Bifurcation left main CAD	IIb	B
	Low SYNTAX score <23	IIa	B
	Low-intermediate SYNTAX score <33	IIb	B
	High SYNTAX score ≥33	NC	
Acute Coronary Syndromes	For UA/NSTEMI if not a CABG candidate	IIa	B
	For STEMI when distal coronary flow is TIMI flow grade <3 and PCI can be performed more rapidly and safety than CABG	IIa	C

ACCF American College of Cardiology Foundation, *AHA* American Heart Association, *SCAI* Society for Cardiovascular Angiography and Interventions, *CAD* coronary artery disease, *NC* No comments on the guidelines, *SYNTAX* Synergy between percutaneous coronary intervention with TAXUS and Cardiac Surgery, *UA/NSTEMI* unstable angina/non-ST elevation myocardial infarction, *STEMI* ST-elevation myocardial infarction, *CABG* Coronary artery bypass grafting
[a]Class of recommendation
[b]Level of evidence

Table 16.4 Recommendation for the type of revascularization (CABG or PCI) in patients with SCAD with suitable coronary anatomy for both procedures and low predicted surgical mortality

Recommendations according to extent of CAD	CABG		PCI	
	Class[a]	Level[b]	Class[a]	Level[b]
One or two-vessel disease without proximal LAD stenosis	IIb	C	I	C
One-vessel disease with proximal LAD stenosis.	I	A	I	A
Two-vessel disease with proximal LAD stenosis.	I	B	I	C
Left main disease with a SYNTAX score 22.	I	B	I	B
Left main disease with a SYNTAX score 23–32.	I	B	IIa	B
Left main disease with a SYNTAX score >32.	I	B	III	B
Three-vessel disease with a SYNTAX score 22.	I	A	I	B
Three-vessel disease with a SYNTAX score 23–32.	I	A	III	B
Three-vessel disease with a SYNTAX score >32.	I	A	III	B

CABG coronary artery bypass grafting, *LAD* left anterior descending coronary artery, *PCI* percutaneous coronary intervention, *SCAD* stable coronary artery disease
[a]Class of recommendation
[b]Level of evidence

Conclusions

1. *PCI with stent implantation has become a viable revascularization strategy in certain groups of patients with LMD. The use of DES as compared to BMS significantly reduced adverse events.*
2. *Compared to CABG, PCI with DES stents in LMD has had similar mortality and incidence of MI but with a higher recurrence of repeat revascularization procedures.*
3. *Compared to PCI, CABG has had a higher risk of stroke in LMD.*
4. *PCI appears to be a rational revascularization option in most patients with LMD either without a significant bifurcation stenosis, or with a small diameter circumflex artery and /or low or intermediate anatomic risk scores.*
5. *CABG has remained a better option in complex coronary anatomy (SYNTAX score ≥33 due to LMD lesion associated with severe multi-vessel coronary disease, total occlusions of ≥2 major coronary epicardial vessels, severe calcifications or tortuosity), and also in those with absolute or relative contraindications to antiplatelet therapy.*
6. *The latest guidelines from ESC included PCI with DES implantation as a class I in certain low risk subgroups of patients with LMD. In the ACC/AHA guidelines, PCI has a Class IIa recommendation particularly when the surgical risk is high.*

References

1. Cherro A, Fernández Pereira C, Torresani E, et al. Primary Outcomes and Morbi-mortality Associated Factors in the Coronary Angioplasty Argentine Registry – RadAC. Rev Argent Cardiol. 2012;80:461–70.
2. El-Menyar AA, Al Suwaidi J, Holmes Jr DR, et al. Left main coronary artery stenosis: state-of-the-art. Curr Probl Cardiol. 2007;32:103–93.
3. Conley MJ, Ely RL, Kiss J, et al. The prognostic spectrum of left main stenosis. Circulation. 1978;57:947.
4. Bernardi V, Fernández Pereira C, Saavedra S, et al. Unprotected left main angioplasty. In-Hospital and long term follow up in the stent era. Rev Argen Cardiol. 1998;66:627–34.
5. Park SJ, Kim YH, Lee BK, et al. Sirolimus-eluting stent implantation for unprotected left main coronary artery stenosis: comparison with bare metal stent implantation. J Am Coll Cardiol. 2005;45:351–6.
6. Chieffo A, Stankovic G, Bonizzoni E, et al. Early and mid-term results of drug-eluting stent implantation in unprotected left main. Circulation. 2005;111:791.
7. Buszman PE, Buszman PP, Kiesz RS, et al. Early and long-term results of unprotected left main coronary artery stenting: the LE MANS (Left Main Coronary Artery Stenting) registry. J Am Coll Cardiol. 2009;54(16):13.
8. Mehilli J, Kastrati A, Byrne RA, et al. Paclitaxel- versus sirolimus-eluting stents for unprotected left main coronary artery disease. J Am Coll Cardiol. 2009;53:1760.
9. Tamburino C, Di Salvo ME, Capodanno D, et al. Are drug-eluting stents superior to bare-metal stents in patients with unprotected non bifurcation left main disease? Insights from a multicentre registry. Eur Heart J. 2009;30:1171–9.
10. Rodriguez A, Bernardi V, Navia J, et al. Argentine randomized study: coronary angioplasty with stenting versus coronary bypass surgery in patients with Multiple-Vessel Disease (ERACI II): 30-day and one-year follow-up results. ERACI II Investigators. J Am Coll Cardiol. 2001;37(1):51–8.
11. Rodríguez AE, Baldi J, Fernández Pereira C, et al. Five-year follow-up of the argentine randomized trial of coronary angioplasty with stenting versus coronary bypass surgery in patients with multiple vessel disease (ERACI II). J Am Coll Cardiol. 2005;46(4):582–8.
12. Fernández-Pereira C, Mieres J, Rodríguez-Granillo AM, et al. In-hospital results and long term follow up in unprotected left main angioplasty performed at Interventional Cardiology Research Center (CECI). Rev Argent Cardioangiología Intervencionista. 2013;4(3):155–63.
13. Fernández-Pereira C, Rifourcat I, Mieres J, et al. TCT-577 revascularization strategies for patients with multiple vessel coronary disease and unprotected left main. Mid term results from a Prospective, Multicenter and Controlled Argentina Registry with a Cobalt- Chromium Rapamycin Eluting Stent, FIREBIRD 2® (ERACI 4). J Am Coll Cardiol. 2014;64(11_S).
14. Pandya SB, Kim YH, Meyers SN, et al. Drug-eluting stents versus bare metal stents in unprotected left main coronary artery stenosis: a meta-analysis. JACC Cardiovasc Interv. 2010;3(6):602–11.
15. Lee JY, Park DW, Yun SC, et al. Long-term clinical outcomes of sirolimus- versus paclitaxel-eluting stents for patients with unprotected left main coronary artery disease: analysis of the MAIN-COMPARE (revascularization for unprotected left main coronary artery stenosis: comparison of percutaneous coronary angioplasty versus surgical revascularization) registry. J Am Coll Cardiol. 2009;54:853.
16. Valgimigli M, Malagutti P, Aoki J, et al. Sirolimus-eluting versus paclitaxel-eluting stent implantation for the percutaneous treatment of left main coronary artery disease: a combined RESEARCH and T-SEARCH long-term analysis. J Am Coll Cardiol. 2006;47:507.
17. Valenti R, Migliorini A, Parodi G, et al. Clinical and Angiographic outcomes of patients treated with everolimus-eluting stents or first generation Paclitaxel-eluting stents for unprotected left main diseased. J Am Coll Cardiol. 2012;60:1217–22.

18. Moynagh A, Salvatella N, Harb T, et al. Two-year outcomes of everolimus vs. paclitaxel-eluting stent for the treatment of unprotected left main lesions: a propensity score matching comparison of patients included in the French Left Main Taxus (FLM Taxus) and the LEft MAin Xience (LEMAX) registries. EuroIntervention. 2013;9:452–62.
19. Mehilli J, Richardt G, Valgimigli M, et al. Zotarolimus- versus everolimus-eluting stents for unprotected left main coronary artery disease. J Am Coll Cardiol. 2013;62:2075.
20. Chieffo A, Meliga E, Latib A, et al. Drug-eluting stent for left main coronary artery disease. The DELTA registry: a multicenter registry evaluating percutaneous coronary intervention versus coronary artery bypass grafting for left main treatment. J Am Coll Cardiol Intv. 2012;5:718–27.
21. Lee MS, Kapoor N, Jamal F, et al. Comparison of coronary artery bypass surgery with percutaneous coronary intervention with drug-eluting stents for unprotected left main coronary artery disease. J Am Coll Cardiol. 2006;47:864.
22. Chieffo A, Morici N, Maisano F, et al. Percutaneous treatment with drug-eluting stent implantation versus bypass surgery for unprotected left main stenosis: a single-center experience. Circulation. 2006;113:2542.
23. Seung KB, Park DW, Kim YH, et al. Stents versus coronary-artery bypass grafting for left main coronary artery disease. N Engl J Med. 2008;358:1781.
24. Park DW, Seung KB, Kim YH, et al. Long-term safety and efficacy of stenting versus coronary artery bypass grafting for unprotected left main coronary artery disease. 5-year results from the MAIN-COMPARE (revascularization for unprotected left main coronary artery stenosis: comparison of percutaneous coronary angioplasty versus surgical revascularization). J Am Coll Cardiol. 2010;56(2):117–24.
25. Buszman PE, Kiesz SR, Bochenek A, et al. Acute and late outcomes of unprotected left main stenting in comparison with surgical revascularization. J Am Coll Cardiol. 2008;51:538–45.
26. Park SJ, Kim YH, Park DW, et al. Randomized trial of stents versus bypass surgery for left main coronary artery disease. N Engl J Med. 2011;364:1718–27.
27. Morice MC, Serruys PW, Kappetein AP, et al. Year outcomes in patients with left main disease treated with either percutaneous coronary intervention or coronary artery bypass grafting in the SYNTAX trial. Circulation. 2014;129:2388–94.
28. Boudriot E, Thiele H, Walther T, et al. Randomized comparison of percutaneous coronary intervention with sirolimus-eluting stents versus coronary artery bypass grafting in unprotected left main stem stenosis. J Am Coll Cardiol. 2011;57:538–45.
29. Morice MC, Serruys PW, Kappetein AP, et al. Outcomes in patients with De novo left main disease treated with either percutaneous coronary intervention using paclitaxel-eluting stents or coronary artery bypass graft treatment in the Synergy Between Percutaneous Coronary Intervention with Taxus and Cardiac Surgery (SYNTAX) trial. Circulation. 2010;121:2645–53.
30. Antoniucci D. Syntax mistakes. Rev Argent Cardioangiología Intervencionista. 2013; 4(3):151–4.
31. Jang JS, Choi KN, Jin HY, et al. Meta-analysis of three randomized trials and nine observational studies comparing drug-eluting stents versus coronary artery bypass grafting for unprotected left main coronary artery disease. Am J Cardiol. 2012;110(10):1411–8.
32. Athappan G, Patvardhan E, Tuzcu ME, et al. Left main coronary artery stenosis: a meta-analysis of drug-eluting stents versus coronary artery bypass grafting. JACC Cardiovasc Interv. 2013;6(12):1219–30.
33. Capodanno D, Stone GW, Morice MC, et al. Percutaneous coronary intervention versus coronary artery bypass graft surgery in left main coronary artery disease: a meta-analysis of randomized clinical data. J Am Coll Cardiol. 2011;58(14):1426–32.
34. Levine GN, Bates ER, Blankenship JC, et al. 2011 ACCF/AHA/SCAI guideline for percutaneous coronary intervention: a report of the American College of Cardiology Foundation/American Heart Association Task Force on Practice Guidelines and the Society for Cardiovascular Angiography and Interventions. Circulation. 2011;124, e574.

35. Windecker S, Kolh P, Alfonso F, et al. 2014 ESC/EACTS Guidelines on myocardial revascu-
    larization: The Task Force on Myocardial Revascularization of the European Society of
    Cardiology (ESC) and the European Association for Cardio-Thoracic Surgery (EACTS)
    Developed with the special contribution of the European Association of Percutaneous
    Cardiovascular Interventions (EAPCI). Eur Heart J. 2014;35(37):2541–619.
36. Serruys PW. Excel trial: rationale, design, endpoints and timelines. Presented at: EuroPCR, 26
    May 2010, Paris.

Chapter 17
Technical Aspects of Left Main Stem Percutaneous Coronary Intervention

Neil Ruparelia, Alaide Chieffo, and Antonio Colombo

Abstract Significant (>50 %) unprotected left main stem disease (ULMS) is found in 5–7 % of all patients undergoing coronary angiography and is of prognostic importance by virtue of the large volume of myocardium that it supplies. With advances in technology, coupled with increased operator experience, percutaneous coronary intervention (PCI) of ULMS is not only feasible, but has been shown to be safe and effective in this patient group. Diagnosis with the use of angiography, intravascular imaging and coronary physiology indices to characterize LMS plaque and determine its functional significance is critical to planning the optimal percutaneous strategy. Based on anatomical considerations of the location of disease and branch anatomy, the appropriate stent strategy and equipment required can be selected. Lesion preparation is fundamental to optimal outcomes irrespective of which stenting strategy is decided upon. In general a single (provisional) strategy is preferred but in selected circumstances a 2-stent strategy should be used. Finally, post-stent implantation optimisation with intravascular imaging is mandatory to ensure the best possible outcome in addition to the correct adjunctive pharmacotherapy.

Keywords Left main stem • Angioplasty • Percutaneous coronary intervention • Stent • Fractional flow reserve • Optical coherence tomography • Intravascular ultrasound • Bifurcation

N. Ruparelia, BSc, MBBS, DPhil, MRCP
Department of Invasive Cardiology, San Raffaele Scientific Institute, Milan, Lombardy, Italy

Imperial College, London, UK

A. Chieffo, MD
Department of Invasive Cardiology, San Raffaele Scientific Institute, Milan, Lombardy, Italy

A. Colombo, MD (✉)
Department of Invasive Cardiology, San Raffaele Scientific Institute, Milan, Lombardy, Italy

EMO-GV Centro Cuore Columbus, Via Buonarroti 48, Milan 20145, Italy
e-mail: info@emocolumbus.it; antonio.colombo@hsr.it

© Springer International Publishing Switzerland 2015
J.A. Ambrose, A.E. Rodríguez (eds.), *Controversies in Cardiology*,
DOI 10.1007/978-3-319-20415-4_17

237

Introduction

Significant (>50 %) unprotected left main stem disease (ULMS) is found in 5–7 % of all patients undergoing coronary angiography [1] and is of prognostic importance by virtue of the large volume of myocardium that it supplies. Treated medically, patients have a 3-year mortality rate of 50 % [2, 3]. Revascularisation by coronary artery bypass grafting (CABG) has been shown to confer significant benefits in comparison to medical therapy alone [4, 5] and until very recently has been regarded as the 'gold standard' treatment for this patient group. With advances in technology, coupled with increased operator experience, percutaneous coronary intervention (PCI) of ULMS is not only feasible, but has been shown to be safe and effective in this patient group [6–9]. This is also reflected in the recently updated European Society of Cardiology (ESC) [10] and American Heart Association (AHA)/American College of Cardiology (ACC) [11] guidelines where LMS PCI is **currently** regarded as an alternative to CABG in patients without complex anatomy. There are many considerations **and several unresolved issues** that need to be taken into account when contemplating ULMS PCI and during the course of this chapter we shall discuss the technical aspects of this procedure.

Diagnosis and Assessment of LMS Stenosis

The diagnosis of the LMS stenosis and subsequent characterisation of disease is surprisingly challenging. Invasive coronary angiography has been the gold standard for many years to define the severity of disease. The first indications of LMS disease are a drop in both systolic and diastolic pressures on intubation of the ostium with the coronary catheter (catheter pressure damping) or the absence of contrast dye backflow into the aorta on first injection. However, there are limitations of angiography in assessing the LMS and this approach is associated with the greatest amount of inter-observer variability [12, 13]. Common anatomical variables including a short LMS, overlapping vessels, foreshortening, presence of calcification and diffuse disease (no reference point) all contribute to difficulty in accurate assessment. The utilisation of additional tools including intravascular imaging techniques and assessment of fractional flow reserve (FFR) are thus essential in the accurate diagnosis of LMS, its functional significance and subsequent optimal procedural planning.

Intravascular Ultrasound

Approximately 90 % of patients that have normal angiographic appearances of LMS have atherosclerotic disease following intravascular ultrasound (IVUS) evaluation [14]. Even the presence of angiographic stenosis does not accurately reflect minimal luminal area (MLA). The exact 'cut-off' for significance with regards to MLA is currently debated. A MLA of <6 mm^2 has generally been considered as significant on the basis of comparisons of IVUS findings with fractional flow reserve (FFR) [15] and clinical outcome, although more recently, a 'cut-off' of <4.8 mm² has been proposed and found to strongly **correlate** with a FFR of <0.8 although this study was limited by a small number of patients, exclusion of patients with significant downstream stenosis and no clinical outcome data with this 'cut-off' [16]. In an IVUS study of intermediate LMS lesions as assessed by angiography, 33 % of LMS lesions with <30 % stenosis had a MLA by IVUS of <6 mm² and 43 % of LMS lesions with >50 % stenosis had a MLA of >6 mm² [17]. In addition to confirmation of diagnosis, IVUS is helpful **in** lesion characterization with information obtained regarding plaque morphology and composition and appropriate vessel sizing which can aid the procedural planning with regards to lesion preparation and stent selection [18] (Fig. 17.1). Following stent implantation, it is also essential in confirming appropriate stent expansion [19, 20] (Fig. 17.1). However it is important to consider some technical considerations using IVUS in LMS. It is important to try and keep the IVUS catheter as coaxial as possible both when assessing distal bifurcation disease when **the** most coaxial branch should be selected and also in the assessment of ostial disease where additionally the guiding catheter should be disengaged to enable appropriate interrogation.

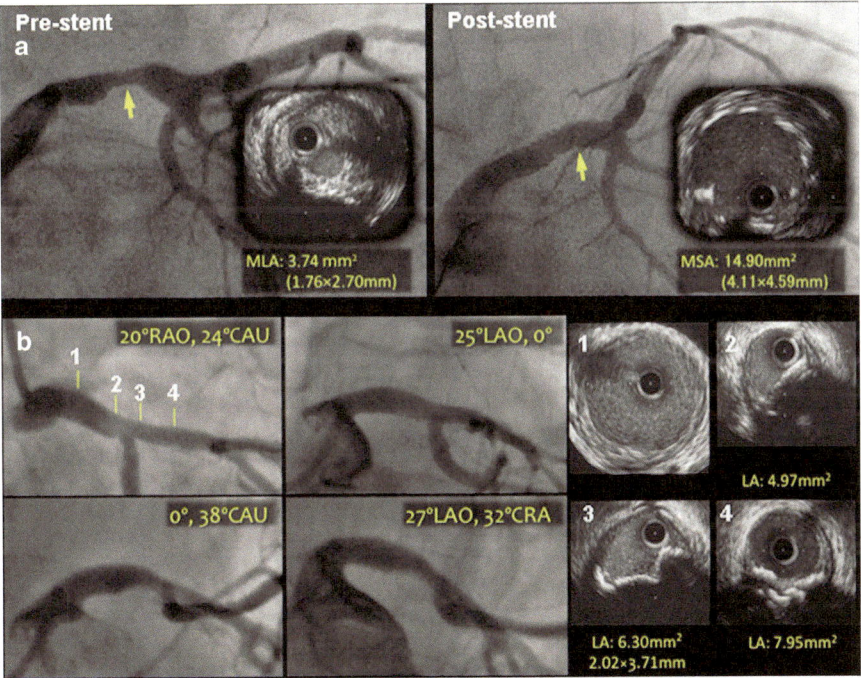

Fig. 17.1 Intravascular imaging (IVUS) in left main stem coronary intervention. Mid-shaft LMS stenosis with IVUS imaging (*arrows*) to assess composition of plaque and to aid in vessel sizing (**a**, *left panel*). Following PCI, IVUS demonstrates excellent stent dilation with good strut apposition to vessel wall (**a**, *right panel*). When there is diagnostic uncertainty with regards to **the** presence of disease after multiple angiographic angles, (**b**, *left panels*), IVUS can be used to confirm final diagnosis (**b** *right panels*)

Optical Coherence Tomography

Optical coherence tomography has many advantages with regards to characterisation of intravascular disease by virtue of its high resolution [21]. However, it has poor depth penetration and requires adequate clearance of blood by contrast in the vessel of interest to obtain optimal imaging [21]. In the LMS assessment, **while** the use of OCT has been shown to be comparable to IVUS findings [22], the vessel diameters are often too large to be adequately imaged by OCT and often does not allow for adequate interrogation of ostial disease. For these reasons, OCT has limited value in the pre-intervention assessment of LMS stem prior to intervention.

Fractional Flow Reserve

The utilisation of fractional flow reserve (FFR) in determining the functional significance of a lesion in the LMS and has been shown to be useful in managing revascularisation strategies [23]. **While** LMS disease was an exclusion criteria within the DEFER (deferral versus performance of PCI of non-ischaemia-stenoses [24] and FAME (FFR versus angiography for multivessel evaluation)) [25] trials, FFR has been used successfully to determine the physiological significance of intermediate lesions. Only a minority of patients demonstrate isolated LMS disease (9 %) [26] and it is therefore important to appreciate the effect that this will have on the FFR [27] when interrogating a LMS stenosis. In the presence of concomitant disease in the left anterior descending artery or circumflex artery, it is important to appreciate that this may artificially raise the FFR reading obtained at the LMS. However, if the pressure wire is placed in a non-stenosed downstream vessel and the other vessel does not have a critical proximal stenosis [28] then the results can be interpretable (Fig. 17.2). There are however currently no large randomised studies investigating the role of FFR in the management of LMS disease and the long-term safety and effect of outcomes of FFR-guided revascularisation of the LMS.

Equipment Selection

Guiding Catheter

The correct choice of guiding catheter is important both to maximise support but also with regards to stenting strategies in particular when 2-stent bifurcation techniques are being considered for distal LMS disease. For ostial lesions, a 6 French (Fr) catheter is usually sufficient for the majority of cases. When planning intervention of distal bifurcation lesions, it is helpful to determine strategy if possible following lesion assessment. If two stents are being considered, it is possible to perform two stent strategies using a 6 Fr. guiding catheter with the majority of current techniques such as culotte, T and two-step crush stenting. However, at least a 7 Fr.

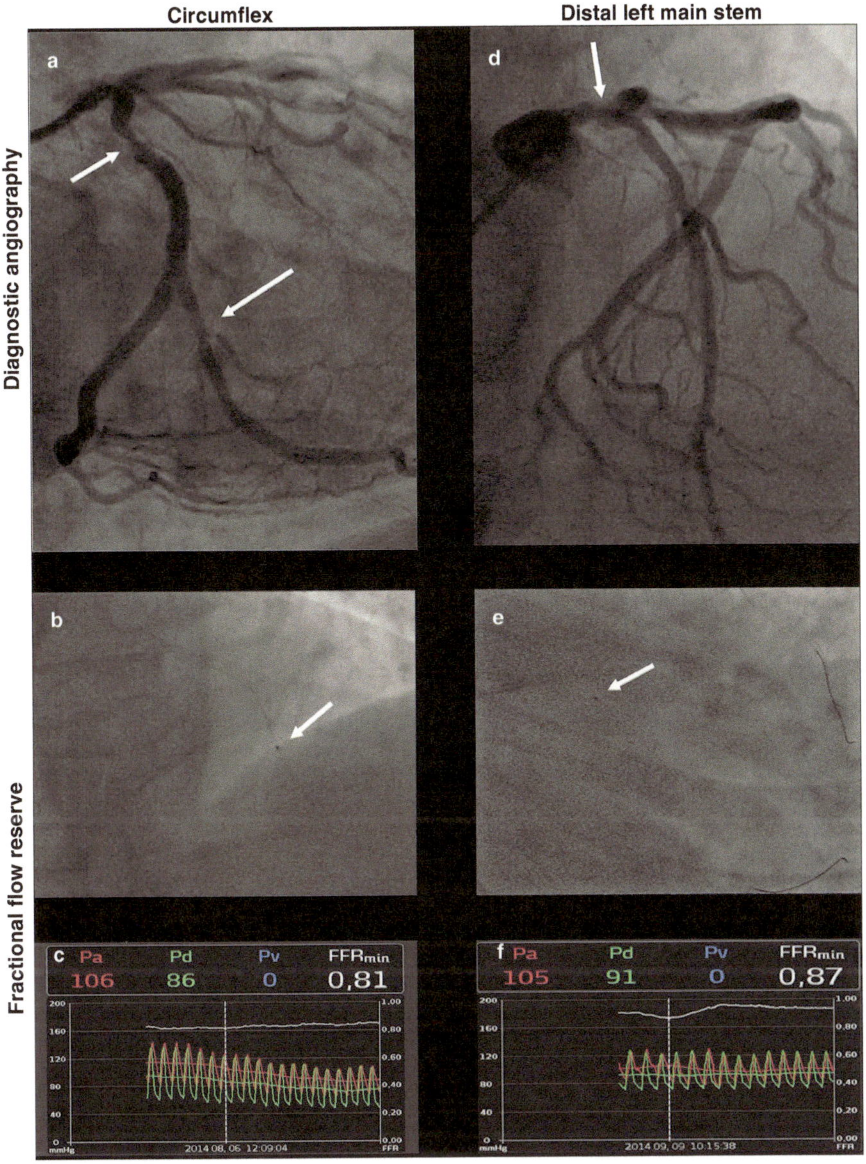

Fig. 17.2 Fractional flow reserve (FFR) in left main stem coronary lesion evaluation. Diagnostic angiography demonstrated stenosis of circumflex artery (*arrows*, **a**) and distal left main stem (*arrows*, **d**). Fractional flow measurements carried out with ACIST-Navvus catheter (Bracco, MN, USA) in both circumflex (*arrow*, **b**) and left main stem (*arrow*, **e**). Both FFR of circumflex (**c**) and left main stem (**f**) were negative and so this patient was **managed** with aggressive medical therapy without the need for revascularisation

catheter is required if V stenting and standard crush-mini crush strategies are required. Additionally, the use of a larger guide catheter also provides better support, visualisation and accommodation of all sizes of burr if rotablation is required.

Hemodynamic Support

Hemodynamic support is not mandatory, but should be considered in patients deemed at high risk for developing instability peri-procedurally with an estimated 8 % risk of this occurrence [29]. High-risk features include impaired left ventricular (LV) function, complex bifurcation strategy or patients with persistent angina or ischaemia on maximal medical therapy and elective intra-aortic balloon pump (IABP) placement in this setting may be beneficial [29]. Other options for **hemodynamic** support include Impella (Abiomed, Danvers, MA, USA) or Tandem Heart (CardiacAssist Inc. Pittsburgh, PA, USA).

Lesion Preparation

As with all percutaneous coronary interventions, appropriate lesion preparation is essential to ensuring a good outcome and is even more important in the setting of ULMS intervention where the sequelae of any complication (e.g. acute stent thrombosis) are likely to be fatal. Information obtained from IVUS with regards to characterisation of disease can be invaluable. In the setting of extensive calcific disease, rotational atherectomy can be performed, whereas extensive fibrosis **or** diffuse calcification may demand more aggressive pre-dilatation with non-compliant balloons. On the other hand, identification of uncomplicated, soft plaque may permit direct stenting.

Stent Choice

DES are generally preferred in ULMS PCI, and in comparison to bare metal stents (BMS), are associated with lower rates of mortality, myocardial infarction and revascularisation [30, 31]. There are currently no data to support the use of bioresorbable vascular scaffolds (BVS) in ULMS PCI. The main limitation of the current devices is their maximal diameter that presently cannot exceed 4 mm.

There does not appear to be a difference between various designs or type of drug/polymer DES. The ISAR-LEFT MAIN (Intracoronary Stenting and Angiographic Results: Drug-Eluting Stents for Unprotected Coronary Left Main Lesions) study that randomised patients to either a paclitaxel-eluting stent (PES) or a sirolimus-eluting stent (SES) did not demonstrate a difference with regards to death, myocardial infarction or target lesion revascularisation at 1 year [31]. Similarly the more recent ISAR-LEFT MAIN 2 that examined the use of second-generation DES and randomised patients to zotarolimus-eluting stent (ZES) or everolimus-eluting stent (EES) again did not demonstrate any differences at 1 year, which has also been supported by findings from other registries [32–36]. A practical consideration is when a 2-stent strategy is opted for in the presence of large branches (>3.5 mm), stents with an open cell design may be preferable to facilitate re-crossing and maintain patency of branches.

Anatomical Considerations

The location of LMS disease determines the interventional strategy and **while** the overall rate of restenosis is low after stenting for LMS, the distal LMS is the usual site of restenosis and the ostium of the circumflex is particularly vulnerable to recurrence [37]. The distal LMS is involved in the majority of cases, and the results of PCI for these patients are worse than for those patients with lesions located at the ostium or mid-shaft likely representing the more complex nature of this disease [38, 39]. This is reflected in the current guidelines which by using the SYNTAX score to determine anatomical complexity, recommend PCI as an equivalent alternative to CABG for patients with a low score (SYNTAX score ≤22) and as an option in patients with an intermediate score (SYNTAX 22-32). In patients with complex anatomy (SYNTAX >32) CABG is the recommended revascularisation option.

Ostial LMS Disease

Disease isolated to the LMS ostium occurs in a minority of patients [40]. It is important to accurately assess the size of the reference vessel (often exceeds 4 mm). The extent of disease should be checked in a number of different projections (left anterior oblique caudal projection is useful for the assessment of distal extent of disease from the bifurcation) and to aid in the choice of stent length (Fig. 17.1). The stent should be allowed to protrude 1–2 mm into the aorta (the right anterior oblique cranial view is helpful in determining protrusion of the proximal stent into the aorta) while distally it should not involve the distal bifurcation. If the stent is too short there is a risk of dislodgement especially during post-dilatation and on-going catheter manipulation. When selecting a stent to be implanted in this location, devices with minimal longitudinal deformation should be selected.

Mid-Shaft LMS Disease

Treating mid-shaft disease is very similar to that of ostial lesions, with particular attention made to not **involve** the distal bifurcation. If this is not possible due to distal extension of disease close **to** the bifurcation with risk of plaque shift following stent deployment, a reasonable strategy, that should be used liberally, is to extent the stent into the LAD with protection of the SB with a second wire (see section "Provisional stenting strategy" below).

Distal Bifurcation LMS Disease

Distal bifurcation disease can be treated either by a 1-stent (provisional strategy) or a 2-stent technique. From observational non-randomized studies the provisional strategy, when possible, appears to be superior to a 2-stent technique with regards to the rate of target lesion revascularisation in 2-stent procedures [38, 39, 41] although, the use of 2 stents may simply reflect more complex disease and therefore be associated with worse outcomes. However, a provisional strategy is not always appropriate - for example in the setting of severe and diffuse disease in the ostium of the side branch. In these cases, a 2-stent strategy should be employed. There are a number of different techniques and these are outlined below.

Provisional Stenting Strategy

The provisional strategy is a single-stent strategy and allows for the placement of a second stent if required. This strategy is most appropriate if plaque is limited to the LMS and main vessel (MV) alone. The MV (almost always the left anterior descending artery (LAD)) is wired and a second wire is placed in the side branch (SB). A stent is then placed from the LMS into the LAD and post-dilated as required with the wire 'jailed' in the SB. Depending on the appearances, the SB **may be** left untouched, or treated with a 'kissing' balloon inflation. In the case of a suboptimal result such as SB dissection or significant residual stenosis (>50 %), a second stent may be deployed into the side branch with a 'kissing' inflation to complete the procedure. If a second stent needs to be implanted on the SB, the preferred technique is the T and protrusion (TAP).

Two-Stent Strategies

In instances where disease extends into both the MV and diffusely and significantly in the ostium of the SB then elective double stenting should be considered. The most important determining factor with regards to which strategy to use is the internal angle between the MV and the SB. Y-shaped bifurcations demonstrate an angle of <70° whilst T-shaped bifurcations have an angle of >70°. The majority of distal bifurcation lesions are T-shaped. This is important because a large angle may not allow for easy wire access to the SB or the passing of an additional wire, balloon or stent after MV stenting and is a predictor for SB occlusion. Finally, in the presence of a wide angle between the LMS-left circumflex artery (LCx) or a narrow angle between the LAD-LCx, the SB ostium area is by definition greater and this might be best treated with stents with large cells. The double-stent strategies are outlined below and illustrated in Fig. 17.3. Which technique is superior in LM bifurcations

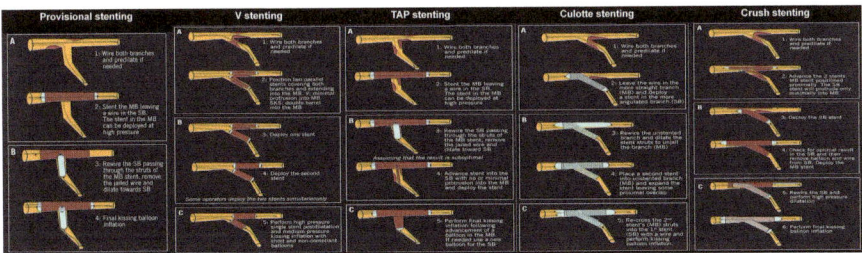

Fig. 17.3 Schematic of bifurcation techniques. Schematic diagrams of bifurcation techniques that can be considered when attempting PCI to distal LMS bifurcation (Adapted and reprinted from Ielasi and Chieffo [42] Copyright 2011, with permission from Europa Edition)

is currently unclear with outcome success most likely determined by anatomical considerations and operator experience [43].

V-Stenting

The V stent technique (or 'kissing' stent technique) involves the simultaneous deployment of stents in both the MV and the SB. This technique is particularly applicable for Medina 0.1.1 lesions that can be treated with a minimal and very short neo-carina and in case of **hemodynamic** instability of the patient.

T-Stenting

This technique is most useful when the angle between the MV and the SB is close to 90°. Both the MV and SB are wired and the SB is stented first with the careful deployment of the stent to ensure that the ostium of the SB is covered with only minimal protrusion into the MV. The LMS-LAD is then stented followed by final 'kissing balloon' inflation.

The T and Protrusion (TAP) Technique

This technique is applicable to the majority of LMS bifurcation lesions and it is the preferred technique to switch from a 1 to a 2-stent strategy. After both the MV and SB are wired, the LMS-LAD is stented first. A stent is then placed into the SB with a balloon left inside the MV (LAD). After careful positioning of the second stent ensuring that the proximal edge of the stent protrudes 1–2 mm into the MV the side branch stent is deployed at high pressure while keeping the deflated balloon in the MV. Final 'kissing' balloon inflation is then performed to complete the procedure to reshape the carina.

Culotte-Stenting

This technique is useful if the angle between the MV and SB is shallow (<60°) and the two vessels are of similar diameter. After wiring both vessels, the SB is stented. The MB is then re-wired and a second stent is placed through the stent struts, leaving an overlap of both stents in the LMS. Following deployment of the second stent, the SB is then re-wired and final 'kissing' balloon inflation is performed to reshape the carina [44] (Fig. 17.4a). The operator can also choose to perform a reverse Culotte **with** stenting first the MB.

Crush Stenting Techniques

This strategy can be used when there is a size mismatch between the MV (usually larger) and the SB (usually smaller) and the angle between the branches is <60° (to facilitate re-wiring of the SB). In the crush stenting technique, after wiring of both branches and pre-dilatation if required, two stents are advanced into both the MV and the SB. The SB is first stented and then after removal of the wire and balloon the MV is then stented. The SB is then re-wired through the crushed stent and final 'kissing' balloon inflation is performed [45] (Fig. 17.4b). An evolution of this technique is the mini-crush technique where the overlap of the 2 stents in the MB is minimal and 2-step final kissing balloon inflation is performed: first the post-dilatation with a non compliant balloon of the SB and then a final kissing balloon inflation on MB and SB [46]. A variation of this technique is the DK-crush (double-kiss crush) where two 'kissing' balloon inflations are carried out both after stenting of the SB before MV stenting and at the end of the procedure [47].

Final Optimisation

IVUS imaging is central to the assessment of the LMS following stent implantation. Specifically, stent expansion and apposition, side-branch ostium assessment, final vessel size and the presence of proximal or distal dissection are important. A subgroup from the MAIN-COMPARE (Revascularisation for Unprotected Left Main Coronary Stenosis: Comparison of Percutaneous Coronary Angioplasty Versus Surgical Revascularisation) registry reported that IVUS guidance was associated with improved 3-year mortality compared with conventional angiography-guided procedures after adjustment with propensity matching [48]. OCT has also been used in the evaluation of LMS following PCI [49] although due to the limitations as previously described in particular with regards to the diameter of the vessel and difficulty in obtaining high quality imaging, IVUS is currently recommended as the preferable intravascular imaging modality.

A: Culotte stenting

B: Crush stenting

C: Mini-crush stenting

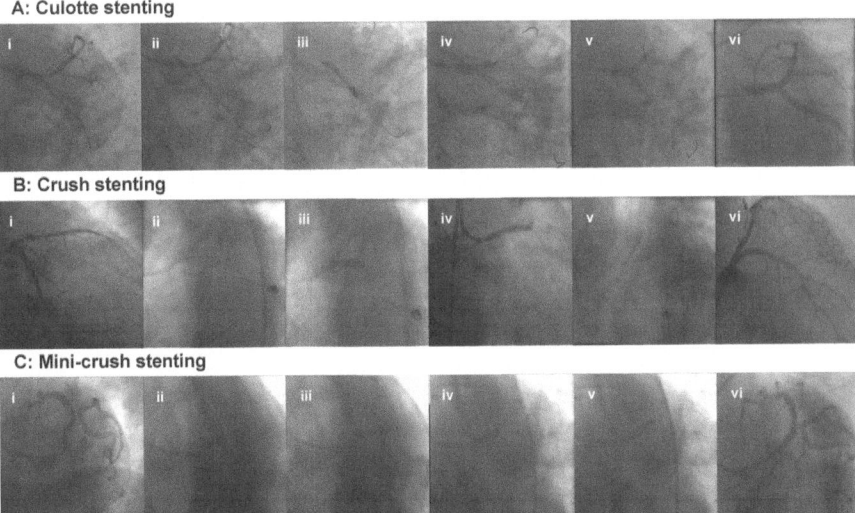

Fig. 17.4 Examples of bifurcation 2-stent strategies. (**a**) Culotte stenting. Suitable when both branches of a bifurcation are of similar diameter with a shallow angle (*i*). Both branches are wired (*ii*). The side branch is stented first (*iii*). The main branch is re-wired and then stented (*iv*), followed by a kissing balloon post-dilation (*v*) resulting in excellent final angiographic result (*vi*). (**b**) Crush stenting. Suitable when there is a size mismatch between the main branch and the side branch (*i*). After wiring of both branches, both stents are advanced (*ii*); the side branch is stented first (*iii*). The wire and balloon are removed and the main branch is stented (*iv*). There is a final kissing balloon post-dilation after the SB is re-wired through the crushed stent (*v*) resulting in an excellent angiographic result (*vi*). (**c**) Mini-crush stenting. Suitable when there is a size mismatch between the two branches (*i*). Both branches are wired and both stents are advanced (*ii*). The side branch stent is deployed with minimal protrusion of the proximal stent struts into the main branch (*iii*). After post-dilation of the side branch stent, the main vessel is stented crushing the first stent (*iv*). The side branch is re-wired and final kissing balloon inflation is performed (*v*) resulting in an excellent angiographic result (*vi*)

Complications

A number of complications can occur during ULMS PCI. There are a number of technical aspects that can be utilised to reduce the likelihood of occurrence and also strategies that can be employed to manage them when they do occur. These are outlined in Table 17.1.

Post-procedure

Following ULMS PCI, patients should be prescribed dual anti-platelet therapy (DAPT). The optimal duration of DAPT in this patient cohort is still to be determined and the continued use beyond 6 or 12 months **is** unclear in this patient group

Table 17.1 Complications and management strategies in left main stem percutaneous coronary intervention

Complication	Management strategy
LMS dissection	Catheter manipulation
	Prompt intervention with PCI ideally
LMS perforation	Treatment with covered stent
	CABG if unsuccessful
	Be aware of possibility of tamponade and treat with pericardiocentesis if required
Catheter induced LMS spasm	Change catheter position
	Nitrate or calcium channel blocker
Stent loss	Retrieval of lost stent
Thrombotic occlusion	Anti-platelet, anti-thrombotic agents
	Aspiration
	Flushing catheter away from ostium

LMS left main stem, *PCI* percutaneous coronary intervention

[50, 51]. The current guidelines [10] suggest a minimum of 12 months DAPT after implantation of a DES, although there maybe additional benefit of continued DAPT beyond 1 year but at the risk of increased bleeding [52].

Finally, patients may also represent with LMS in-stent restenosis. The appropriate treatment is debated but options include, treatment with repeat DES implantation, treatment with a drug-eluting balloon, plain old balloon angioplasty (POBA) or coronary artery bypass grafting (CABG). Repeat PCI in this setting appears to be safe and effective with favourable 2-year outcomes [53].

Conclusions

1. In patients presenting with significant LMS stenosis, PCI is a potential management strategy that is technically feasible and associated with favourable short and medium term outcomes.
2. The diagnosis of LMS disease with the use of adjunctive tools to accurately delineate plaque composition and its functional significance is critical to procedural planning. Anatomical considerations including involvement of the bifurcation determine the stenting strategy employed.
3. Following stent implantation, intravascular imaging is essential in confirming an acceptable response and maximising longer term outcomes.

References

1. DeMots H, Rosch J, McAnulty JH, Rahimtoola SH. Left main coronary artery disease. Cardiovasc Clin. 1977;8(2):201–11.

2. Taylor HA, Deumite NJ, Chaitman BR, Davis KB, Killip T, Rogers WJ. Asymptomatic left main coronary artery disease in the Coronary Artery Surgery Study (CASS) registry. Circulation. 1989;79(6):1171–9.

3. Cohen MV, Gorlin R. Main left coronary artery disease. Clinical experience from 1964-1974. Circulation. 1975;52(2):275–85.

4. Yusuf S, Zucker D, Peduzzi P, Fisher LD, Takaro T, Kennedy JW, Davis K, Killip T, Passamani E, Norris R, et al. Effect of coronary artery bypass graft surgery on survival: overview of 10-year results from randomised trials by the Coronary Artery Bypass Graft Surgery Trialists Collaboration. Lancet. 1994;344(8922):563–70.

5. Caracciolo EA, Davis KB, Sopko G, Kaiser GC, Corley SD, Schaff H, Taylor HA, Chaitman BR. Comparison of surgical and medical group survival in patients with left main equivalent coronary artery disease. Long-term CASS experience. Circulation. 1995;91(9):2335–44.

6. Seung KB, Park DW, Kim YH, Lee SW, Lee CW, Hong MK, Park SW, Yun SC, Gwon HC, Jeong MH, Jang Y, Kim HS, Kim PJ, Seong IW, Park HS, Ahn T, Chae IH, Tahk SJ, Chung WS, Park SJ. Stents versus coronary-artery bypass grafting for left main coronary artery disease. N Engl J Med. 2008;358(17):1781–92. doi:10.1056/NEJMoa0801441.

7. Park DW, Seung KB, Kim YH, Lee JY, Kim WJ, Kang SJ, Lee SW, Lee CW, Park SW, Yun SC, Gwon HC, Jeong MH, Jang YS, Kim HS, Kim PJ, Seong IW, Park HS, Ahn T, Chae IH, Tahk SJ, Chung WS, Park SJ. Long-term safety and efficacy of stenting versus coronary artery bypass grafting for unprotected left main coronary artery disease: 5-year results from the MAIN-COMPARE (Revascularization for Unprotected Left Main Coronary Artery Stenosis: Comparison of Percutaneous Coronary Angioplasty Versus Surgical Revascularization) registry. J Am Coll Cardiol. 2010;56(2):117–24. doi:10.1016/j.jacc.2010.04.004.

8. Serruys PW, Morice MC, Kappetein AP, Colombo A, Holmes DR, Mack MJ, Stahle E, Feldman TE, van den Brand M, Bass EJ, Van Dyck N, Leadley K, Dawkins KD, Mohr FW, Investigators S. Percutaneous coronary intervention versus coronary-artery bypass grafting for severe coronary artery disease. N Engl J Med. 2009;360(10):961–72. doi:10.1056/NEJMoa0804626.

9. Athappan G, Patvardhan E, Tuzcu ME, Ellis S, Whitlow P, Kapadia SR. Left main coronary artery stenosis: a meta-analysis of drug-eluting stents versus coronary artery bypass grafting. JACC Cardiovasc Interv. 2013;6(12):1219–30. doi:10.1016/j.jcin.2013.07.008.

10. Windecker S, Kolh P, Alfonso F, Collet JP, Cremer J, Falk V, Filippatos G, Hamm C, Head SJ, Juni P, Kappetein AP, Kastrati A, Knuuti J, Landmesser U, Laufer G, Neumann FJ, Richter DJ, Schauerte P, Sousa Uva M, Stefanini GG, Taggart DP, Torracca L, Valgimigli M, Wijns W, Witkowski A, Authors/Task Force m. 2014 ESC/EACTS guidelines on myocardial revascularization: the Task Force on Myocardial Revascularization of the European Society of Cardiology (ESC) and the European Association for Cardio-Thoracic Surgery (EACTS)Developed with the special contribution of the European Association of Percutaneous Cardiovascular Interventions (EAPCI). Eur Heart J. 2014;35(37):2541–619. doi:10.1093/eurheartj/ehu278.

11. Fihn SD, Blankenship JC, Alexander KP, Bittl JA, Byrne JG, Fletcher BJ, Fonarow GC, Lange RA, Levine GN, Maddox TM, Naidu SS, Ohman EM, Smith PK. 2014 ACC/AHA/AATS/PCNA/SCAI/STS focused update of the guideline for the diagnosis and management of patients with stable ischemic heart disease: a report of the American College of Cardiology/American Heart Association Task Force on Practice Guidelines, and the American Association for Thoracic Surgery, Preventive Cardiovascular Nurses Association, Society for Cardiovascular Angiography and Interventions, and Society of Thoracic Surgeons. Circulation. 2014;130(19):1749–67. doi:10.1161/CIR.0000000000000095.

12. Isner JM, Kishel J, Kent KM, Ronan Jr JA, Ross AM, Roberts WC. Accuracy of angiographic determination of left main coronary arterial narrowing. Angiographic–histologic correlative analysis in 28 patients. Circulation. 1981;63(5):1056–64.

13. Lindstaedt M, Spiecker M, Perings C, Lawo T, Yazar A, Holland-Letz T, Muegge A, Bojara W, Germing A. How good are experienced interventional cardiologists at predicting the functional significance of intermediate or equivocal left main coronary artery stenoses? Int J Cardiol. 2007;120(2):254–61. doi:10.1016/j.ijcard.2006.11.220.

14. Nissen SE, Yock P. Intravascular ultrasound: novel pathophysiological insights and current clinical applications. Circulation. 2001;103(4):604–16.

15. Jasti V, Ivan E, Yalamanchili V, Wongpraparut N, Leesar MA. Correlations between fractional flow reserve and intravascular ultrasound in patients with an ambiguous left main coronary artery stenosis. Circulation. 2004;110(18):2831–6. doi:10.1161/01.CIR.0000146338.62813.E7.

16. Kang SJ, Lee JY, Ahn JM, Song HG, Kim WJ, Park DW, Yun SC, Lee SW, Kim YH, Mintz GS, Lee CW, Park SW, Park SJ. Intravascular ultrasound-derived predictors for fractional flow reserve in intermediate left main disease. JACC Cardiovasc Interv. 2011;4(11):1168–74. doi:10.1016/j.jcin.2011.08.009.

17. de la Torre Hernandez JM, Hernandez Hernandez F, Alfonso F, Rumoroso JR, Lopez-Palop R, Sadaba M, Carrillo P, Rondan J, Lozano I, Ruiz Nodar JM, Baz JA, Fernandez Nofrerias E, Pajin F, Garcia Camarero T, Gutierrez H, LITRO Study Group. Prospective application of pre-defined intravascular ultrasound criteria for assessment of intermediate left main coronary artery lesions results from the multicenter LITRO study. J Am Coll Cardiol. 2011;58(4): 351–8. doi:10.1016/j.jacc.2011.02.064.

18. Huo Y, Finet G, Lefevre T, Louvard Y, Moussa I, Kassab GS. Optimal diameter of diseased bifurcation segment: a practical rule for percutaneous coronary intervention. EuroIntervention J EuroPCR Collaboration Working Group Interv Cardiol Eur Soc Cardiol. 2012;7(11):1310–6. doi:10.4244/EIJV7I11A206.

19. Jang JS, Song YJ, Kang W, Jin HY, Seo JS, Yang TH, Kim DK, Cho KI, Kim BH, Park YH, Je HG, Kim DS. Intravascular ultrasound-guided implantation of drug-eluting stents to improve outcome: a meta-analysis. JACC Cardiovasc Interv. 2014;7(3):233–43. doi:10.1016/j. jcin.2013.09.013.

20. McDaniel MC, Eshtehardi P, Sawaya FJ, Douglas Jr JS, Samady H. Contemporary clinical applications of coronary intravascular ultrasound. JACC Cardiovasc Interv. 2011;4(11):1155–67. doi:10.1016/j.jcin.2011.07.013.

21. Prati F, Regar E, Mintz GS, Arbustini E, Di Mario C, Jang IK, Akasaka T, Costa M, Guagliumi G, Grube E, Ozaki Y, Pinto F, Serruys PW, Expert's OCT Review Document. Expert review document on methodology, terminology, and clinical applications of optical coherence tomography: physical principles, methodology of image acquisition, and clinical application for assessment of coronary arteries and atherosclerosis. Eur Heart J. 2010;31(4):401–15. doi:10.1093/eurheartj/ehp433.

22. Fujino Y, Bezerra HG, Attizzani GF, Wang W, Yamamoto H, Chamie D, Kanaya T, Mehanna E, Tahara S, Nakamura S, Costa MA. Frequency-domain optical coherence tomography assessment of unprotected left main coronary artery disease-a comparison with intravascular ultrasound. Catheter Cardiovasc Interv Off J Soc Card Angiogr Interv. 2013;82(3):E173–83. doi:10.1002/ccd.24843.

23. Hamilos M, Muller O, Cuisset T, Ntalianis A, Chlouverakis G, Sarno G, Nelis O, Bartunek J, Vanderheyden M, Wyffels E, Barbato E, Heyndrickx GR, Wijns W, De Bruyne B. Long-term clinical outcome after fractional flow reserve-guided treatment in patients with angiographically equivocal left main coronary artery stenosis. Circulation. 2009;120(15):1505–12. doi:10.1161/CIRCULATIONAHA.109.850073.

24. Bech GJ, De Bruyne B, Pijls NH, de Muinck ED, Hoorntje JC, Escaned J, Stella PR, Boersma E, Bartunek J, Koolen JJ, Wijns W. Fractional flow reserve to determine the appropriateness of angioplasty in moderate coronary stenosis: a randomized trial. Circulation. 2001;103(24):2928–34.

25. Tonino PA, De Bruyne B, Pijls NH, Siebert U, Ikeno F, van' t Veer M, Klauss V, Manoharan G, Engstrom T, Oldroyd KG, Ver Lee PN, MacCarthy PA, Fearon WF, FAME Study Investigators. Fractional flow reserve versus angiography for guiding percutaneous coronary intervention. N Engl J Med. 2009;360(3):213–24. doi:10.1056/NEJMoa0807611.

26. Ragosta M, Dee S, Sarembock IJ, Lipson LC, Gimple LW, Powers ER. Prevalence of unfavorable angiographic characteristics for percutaneous intervention in patients with unprotected left main coronary artery disease. Catheter Cardiovasc Interv Off J Soc Card Angiogr Interv. 2006;68(3):357–62. doi:10.1002/ccd.20709.

27. Puri R, Kapadia SR, Nicholls SJ, Harvey JE, Kataoka Y, Tuzcu EM. Optimizing outcomes during left main percutaneous coronary intervention with intravascular ultrasound and fractional flow reserve: the current state of evidence. JACC Cardiovasc Interv. 2012;5(7):697–707. doi:10.1016/j.jcin.2012.02.018.

28. Yong AS, Daniels D, De Bruyne B, Kim HS, Ikeno F, Lyons J, Pijls NH, Fearon WF. Fractional flow reserve assessment of left main stenosis in the presence of downstream coronary stenoses. Circ Cardiovasc Interv. 2013;6(2):161–5. doi:10.1161/CIRCINTERVENTIONS.112.000104.

29. Briguori C, Airoldi F, Chieffo A, Montorfano M, Carlino M, Sangiorgi GM, Morici N, Michev I, Iakovou I, Biondi-Zoccai G, Colombo A. Elective versus provisional intraaortic balloon pumping in unprotected left main stenting. Am Heart J. 2006;152(3):565–72. doi:10.1016/j.ahj.2006.02.024.

30. Pandya SB, Kim YH, Meyers SN, Davidson CJ, Flaherty JD, Park DW, Mediratta A, Pieper K, Reyes E, Bonow RO, Park SJ, Beohar N. Drug-eluting versus bare-metal stents in unprotected left main coronary artery stenosis a meta-analysis. JACC Cardiovasc Interv. 2010;3(6): 602–11. doi:10.1016/j.jcin.2010.03.019.

31. Mehilli J, Kastrati A, Byrne RA, Bruskina O, Iijima R, Schulz S, Pache J, Seyfarth M, Massberg S, Laugwitz KL, Dirschinger J, Schomig A, LEFT-MAIN Intracoronary Stenting and Angiographic Results: Drug-Eluting Stents for Unprotected Coronary Left Main Lesions Study Investigators. Paclitaxel- versus sirolimus-eluting stents for unprotected left main coronary artery disease. J Am Coll Cardiol. 2009;53(19):1760–8. doi:10.1016/j.jacc.2009.01.035.

32. Mehilli J, Richardt G, Valgimigli M, Schulz S, Singh A, Abdel-Wahab M, Tiroch K, Pache J, Hausleiter J, Byrne RA, Ott I, Ibrahim T, Fusaro M, Seyfarth M, Laugwitz KL, Massberg S, Kastrati A, ISAR-LEFT-MAIN 2 Study Investigators. Zotarolimus- versus everolimus-eluting stents for unprotected left main coronary artery disease. J Am Coll Cardiol. 2013;62(22):2075–82. doi:10.1016/j.jacc.2013.07.044.

33. Takagi K, Ielasi A, Shannon J, Latib A, Godino C, Davidavicius G, Mussardo M, Ferrarello S, Figini F, Carlino M, Montorfano M, Chieffo A, Nakamura S, Colombo A. Clinical and procedural predictors of suboptimal outcome after the treatment of drug-eluting stent restenosis in the unprotected distal left main stem: the Milan and New-Tokyo (MITO) registry. Circ Cardiovasc Interv. 2012;5(4):491–8. doi:10.1161/CIRCINTERVENTIONS.111.964874.

34. Almudarra SS, Gale CP, Baxter PD, Fleming SJ, Brogan RA, Ludman PF, de Belder MA, Curzen NP, National Institute for Cardiovascular Outcomes Research. Comparative outcomes after unprotected left main stem percutaneous coronary intervention: a national linked cohort study of 5,065 acute and elective cases from the BCIS Registry (British Cardiovascular Intervention Society). JACC Cardiovasc Interv. 2014;7(7):717–30. doi:10.1016/j.jcin.2014.03.005.

35. Salvatella N, Morice MC, Darremont O, Tafflet M, Garot P, Leymarie JL, Chevalier B, Lefevre T, Louvard Y, Boudou N, Dumonteil N, Carrie D. Unprotected left main stenting with a second-generation drug-eluting stent: one-year outcomes of the LEMAX Pilot study. EuroIntervention J EuroPCR Collaboration Working Group Interv Cardiol Eur Soc Cardiol. 2011;7(6):689–96. doi:10.4244/EIJV7I6A111.

36. Bernelli C, Chieffo A, Buchanan GL, Montorfano M, Carlino M, Latib A, Figini F, Takagi K, Naganuma T, Maccagni D, Colombo A. New-generation drug-eluting stent experience in the percutaneous treatment of unprotected left main coronary artery disease: the NEST registry. J Invasive Cardiol. 2013;25(6):269–75.

37. Baim DS, Mauri L, Cutlip DC. Drug-eluting stenting for unprotected left main coronary artery disease: are we ready to replace bypass surgery? J Am Coll Cardiol. 2006;47(4):878–81. doi:10.1016/j.jacc.2005.12.016.

38. Toyofuku M, Kimura T, Morimoto T, Hayashi Y, Ueda H, Kawai K, Nozaki Y, Hiramatsu S, Miura A, Yokoi Y, Toyoshima S, Nakashima H, Haze K, Tanaka M, Take S, Saito S, Isshiki T, Mitsudo K, j-Cypher Registry Investigators. Three-year outcomes after sirolimus-eluting stent implantation for unprotected left main coronary artery disease: insights from the j-Cypher registry. Circulation. 2009;120(19):1866–74. doi:10.1161/CIRCULATIONAHA.109.873349.

39. Palmerini T, Sangiorgi D, Marzocchi A, Tamburino C, Sheiban I, Margheri M, Vecchi G, Sangiorgi G, Ruffini M, Bartorelli AL, Briguori C, Vignali L, Di Pede F, Ramondo A, Inglese L, De Carlo M, Bolognese L, Benassi A, Palmieri C, Filippone V, Barlocco F, Lauria G, De Servi S. Ostial and midshaft lesions vs. bifurcation lesions in 1111 patients with unprotected left main coronary artery stenosis treated with drug-eluting stents: results of the survey from the Italian Society of Invasive Cardiology. Eur Heart J. 2009;30(17):2087–94. doi:10.1093/eurheartj/ehp223.

40. Chieffo A, Park SJ, Valgimigli M, Kim YH, Daemen J, Sheiban I, Truffa A, Montorfano M, Airoldi F, Sangiorgi G, Carlino M, Michev I, Lee CW, Hong MK, Park SW, Moretti C, Bonizzoni E, Rogacka R, Serruys PW, Colombo A. Favorable long-term outcome after drug-eluting stent implantation in nonbifurcation lesions that involve unprotected left main coronary artery: a multicenter registry. Circulation. 2007;116(2):158–62. doi:10.1161/CIRCULATIONAHA.107.692178.

41. Koh YS, Kim PJ, Chang K, Park HJ, Jeong MH, Kim HS, Jang Y, Gwon HC, Park SJ, Seung KB. Long-term clinical outcomes of the one-stent technique versus the two-stent technique for non-left main true coronary bifurcation disease in the era of drug-eluting stents. J Interv Cardiol. 2013;26(3):245–53. doi:10.1111/joic.12025.

42. Ielasi A, Chieffo A. Tools & techniques: left main coronary artery percutaneous coronary intervention. EuroIntervention J EuroPCR Collaboration Working Group Interv Cardiol Eur Soc Cardiol. 2011;6(8):1020–1. doi:10.4244/EIJV6I8A176.

43. Latib A, Colombo A, Sangiorgi GM. Bifurcation stenting: current strategies and new devices. Heart. 2009;95(6):495–504. doi:10.1136/hrt.2008.150391.

44. Chevalier B, Glatt B, Royer T, Guyon P. Placement of coronary stents in bifurcation lesions by the "culotte" technique. Am J Cardiol. 1998;82(8):943–9.

45. Colombo A, Stankovic G, Orlic D, Corvaja N, Liistro F, Airoldi F, Chieffo A, Spanos V, Montorfano M, Di Mario C. Modified T-stenting technique with crushing for bifurcation lesions: immediate results and 30-day outcome. Catheter Cardiovasc Interv Off J Soc Card Angiogr Interv. 2003;60(2):145–51. doi:10.1002/ccd.10622.

46. Galassi AR, Colombo A, Buchbinder M, Grasso C, Tomasello SD, Ussia GP, Tamburino C. Long-term outcomes of bifurcation lesions after implantation of drug-eluting stents with the "mini-crush technique". Catheter Cardiovasc Interv Off J Soc Card Angiogr Interv. 2007;69(7):976–83. doi:10.1002/ccd.21047.

47. Chen SL, Ye F, Zhang JJ, Zhu ZS, Lin S, Shan SJ, Liu ZZ, Liu Y, Duan BX, Ge JB. DK crush technique: modified treatment of bifurcation lesions in coronary artery. Chin Med J (Engl). 2005;118(20):1746–50.

48. Park SJ, Kim YH, Park DW, Lee SW, Kim WJ, Suh J, Yun SC, Lee CW, Hong MK, Lee JH, Park SW, Investigators M-C. Impact of intravascular ultrasound guidance on long-term mortality in stenting for unprotected left main coronary artery stenosis. Circ Cardiovasc Interv. 2009;2(3):167–77. doi:10.1161/CIRCINTERVENTIONS.108.799494.

49. Parodi G, Maehara A, Giuliani G, Kubo T, Mintz GS, Migliorini A, Valenti R, Carrabba N, Antoniucci D. Optical coherence tomography in unprotected left main coronary artery stenting. EuroIntervention J EuroPCR Collaboration Working Group Interv Cardiol Eur Soc Cardiol. 2010;6(1):94–9.

50. Colombo A, Chieffo A, Frasheri A, Garbo R, Masotti M, Salvatella N, Oteo Dominguez JF, Steffanon L, Tarantini G, Presbitero P, Menozzi A, Pucci E, Mauri J, Cesana BM, Giustino G, Sardella G. Second generation drug-eluting stents implantation followed by six versus twelve-month – dual antiplatelet therapy- the SECURITY randomized clinical trial. J Am Coll Cardiol. 2014. doi:10.1016/j.jacc.2014.09.008.

51. Valgimigli M, Campo G, Monti M, Vranckx P, Percoco G, Tumscitz C, Castriota F, Colombo F, Tebaldi M, Fuca G, Kubbajeh M, Cangiano E, Minarelli M, Scalone A, Cavazza C, Frangione A, Borghesi M, Marchesini J, Parrinello G, Ferrari R, Prolonging Dual Antiplatelet Treatment After Grading Stent-Induced Intimal Hyperplasia Study Investigators. Short- versus long-term duration of dual-antiplatelet therapy after coronary stenting: a randomized multicenter trial. Circulation. 2012;125(16):2015–26. doi:10.1161/CIRCULATIONAHA.111.071589.

52. Mauri L, Kereiakes DJ, Yeh RW, Driscoll-Shempp P, Cutlip DE, Steg PG, Normand SL, Braunwald E, Wiviott SD, Cohen DJ, Holmes Jr DR, Krucoff MW, Hermiller J, Dauerman HL, Simon DI, Kandzari DE, Garratt KN, Lee DP, Pow TK, Lee PV, Rinaldi MJ, Massaro JM, the DAPT Study Investigators. Twelve or 30 months of dual antiplatelet therapy after drug-eluting stents. N Engl J Med. 2014. doi:10.1056/NEJMoa1409312.
53. Sheiban I, Sillano D, Biondi-Zoccai G, Chieffo A, Colombo A, Vecchio S, Margheri M, Gunn JP, Raina T, Liistro F, Bolognese L, Lee MS, Tobis J, Moretti C. Incidence and management of restenosis after treatment of unprotected left main disease with drug-eluting stents 70 restenotic cases from a cohort of 718 patients: FAILS (Failure in Left Main Study). J Am Coll Cardiol. 2009;54(13):1131–6. doi:10.1016/j.jacc.2009.06.018.

Chapter 18
DAPT After Stenting in Stable and Acute Coronary Syndromes- Does the Drug Combination Really Matter?

Dimitrios Alexopoulos

Abstract Dual antiplatelet treatment (DAPT) represents the standard of care in stable coronary artery disease and in acute coronary syndrome (ACS) patients undergoing stenting. Aspirin is the cornerstone of adjunctive medical therapy and a P2Y12 inhibitor is the second component of DAPT, with clopidogrel being the most widely used agent. In stable patients clopidogrel can be used in the overwhelming majority of them. The well recognized variability to clopidogrel response raises concerns about the usefulness of high-dose clopidogrel, prasugrel or ticagrelor in patients with high on-clopidogrel platelet reactivity or high risk angiographic features. However, randomized trials involving mainly stable patients with intensification of antiplatelet action have failed to improve outcome. In ACS patients, prasugrel and ticagrelor are more efficient than clopidogrel regarding ischemic events and may be preferred. Special attention should be given to the higher bleeding potential of prasugrel (mainly) and ticagrelor compared with clopidogrel. Subgroups have been identified in which the hazard ratio of ischemic events is particularly favorable, like ST-segment elevation myocardial infarction and diabetic patients treated with prasugrel and patients with renal dysfunction treated with ticagrelor. Clinical head-to-head comparisons between prasugrel and ticagrelor do not exist, though indirect comparisons, pharmacodynamic and registry data may assist the choice of the one agent over the other. In case of an increased bleeding risk, selection of the less potent clopidogrel seems prudent. Overall the appropriate DAPT should be defined for the individual patient following a balance between thrombotic and bleeding risk.

Keywords Antiplatelet drug • Clopidogrel • Prasugrel • Ticagrelor • Stable angina • Acute coronary syndrome • Percutaneous coronary intervention • Adjunctive pharmacotherapy

Dr. Alexopoulos has received payment for lectures from AstraZeneca.

D. Alexopoulos, MD, FACC, FESC
Department of Cardiology, Patras University Hospital, Rion, Patras 26500, Greece
e-mail: dalex@med.upatras.gr

J.A. Ambrose, A.E. Rodríguez (eds.), *Controversies in Cardiology*,
DOI 10.1007/978-3-319-20415-4_18

Dual antiplatelet treatment (DAPT) represents the standard of care in stable coronary artery disease and in acute coronary syndrome (ACS) patients undergoing percutaneous coronary intervention (PCI) with stent implantation [1–4]. Aspirin is the cornerstone of adjunctive medical therapy with its role very rarely challenged, like in cases of hypersensitivity to aspirin. A P2Y12 inhibitor is the second component of DAPT, with clopidogrel being the most widely used agent. However, the well recognized variability to clopidogrel response [5] raises concerns for identifying patients with high on-clopidogrel platelet reactivity (HPR), particularly in subpopulations with an increased risk for stent thrombosis. Clinical scenarios (e.g. diabetes, chronic kidney disease) and PCI anatomic features of high risk might challenge clopidogrel choice as the second antiplatelet agent. Genotypes associated with HPR or HPR itself can be identified and 'treated' either by increasing clopidogrel dose or, more effectively by novel oral P2Y12 inhibitors prasugrel and ticagrelor [6, 7]. But does this really matter in stable CAD patients? Prasugrel and ticagrelor have been introduced in clinical practice because of their antiischemic superiority vs clopidogrel as proven in TRITON-TIMI 38 (Trial to Assess Improvement in Therapeutic Outcomes by Optimizing Platelet Inhibition with Prasugrel-Thrombolysis In Myocardial Infarction 38), and in PLATO (PLATelet inhibition and patient Outcomes) trial, respectively [8, 9]. Both trials involved ACS patients and therefore the clinical role of the potent agents seems to be restricted only in such patients. Both trials identified subgroups where the hazard ratio (HR) of ischemic events was particularly favorable like ST-segment elevation myocardial infarction (STEMI) and diabetic patients in TRITON or in patients with renal dysfunction in PLATO. Selection of a new agent is particularly attractive in these cohorts, even for the conservative cardiologist who does not adopt a 'one size fits all' approach for using new agents in the absence of contraindications or concerns about bleeding risk and increased cost over clopidogrel.

In ACS patients undergoing PCI and treated with a novel agent, data for preferential use of prasugrel vs ticagrelor and vice versa are scarce. There have been no randomized clinical head-to-head comparison between prasugrel and ticagrelor. However, indirect comparisons, pharmacodynamic and registry data may assist the choice of the one agent over the other. The issue of pre-hospital administration of prasugrel and ticagrelor has been recently investigated in nonSTEMI and STEMI patients respectively [10, 11]. In STEMI patients undergoing primary PCI a delay in the onset of antiplatelet activity has been observed for both prasugrel and ticagrelor, delineating a gap for which an intravenous P2Y12 inhibitor like cangrelor seems particularly attractive [12, 13].

Regarding bleeding potential, although special warning for precaution of prasugrel and ticagrelor are quite similar to those for clopidogrel for conditions carrying an increased bleeding risk, a choice of the less potent clopidogrel appears prudent in such scenarios. Finally, the number and type of antiplatelet agents needed post PCI in patients requiring oral anticoagulation remains unresolved.

Aspirin Hypersensitivity

Background therapy with aspirin continues to be the unwavering, cornerstone of antiplatelet therapy. Hypersensitivity to aspirin can be a challenge, while isolated catastrophic events with stent thrombosis have been described [14]. Hypersensitivity to aspirin occurs very rarely (0.3–0.9 %) in the general population and rapid oral desensitization and subsequent aspirin administration have been proposed to overcome it [15, 16]. In primary PCI patients with aspirin hypersensitivity or in cases of failed initial aspirin desensitization the use of low thrombogenicity stents like endothelial progenitor cell capture stents has been described [17, 18]. Alternatively, antiplatelet treatment with clopidogrel and indobufen has also been suggested in ACS patients with hypersensitivity to aspirin undergoing coronary stenting [19].

Stable CAD Patients

The first oral antiplatelet agent used in addition to aspirin in PCI patients was ticlopidine [20]. This was quickly replaced by clopidogrel due to better tolerability and at least equivalent efficacy [21]. In the CREDO (Clopidogrel for the Reduction of Events During Observation) trial the benefit of clopidogrel pre-treatment as well as long-term DAPT were demonstrated [22, 23]. Clopidogrel is administered irrespective of the type of implanted stent (bare metal or drug eluting), the latter affecting the suggested duration of treatment but not the P2Y12 inhibitor choice. A loading dose of 600 mg is proposed followed by 75 mg maintenance dose [1].

Clopidogrel, however, has several limitations, including a delay in onset of antiplatelet action, variability in response, and modest potency [5]. HPR while on clopidogrel has been associated with major adverse cardiovascular events post PCI, including stent thrombosis, although results of studies exclusively in stable CAD patients have been contradictory. In 1069 patients taking clopidogrel and undergoing elective PCI with stenting, on-treatment platelet reactivity was measured by different platelet function assays. The primary end point (defined as a composite of all-cause death, nonfatal acute myocardial infarction, stent thrombosis, and ischemic stroke) occurred more frequently in patients with HPR by four assays. However, the predictive accuracy of these four tests was only modest [24]. In 1095 ACS patients and 1329 stable CAD patients treated with PCI on-clopidogrel HPR was measured by the VerifyNow P2Y12 assay (Accumetrics, San Diego, CA). During a 22 months follow up, HPR was associated with higher risks of the primary end point (a composite of death, myocardial infarction, stent thrombosis, or stroke) in patients with ACS with a HR, 95 % confidence interval (CI 2.03, 1.30–3.18, p=0.002) but not in those with stable CAD, HR, 95 % (CI 1.00, 0.71–1.39, p=0.98) [25]. In a collaborative meta-analysis of 6 studies with 3059 patients (2/3 of them with stable CAD) the level of on-treatment platelet reactivity was associated with long-term cardiovascular events after PCI, including death, myocardial infarction, and stent thrombosis [26]. In the prospective, multicentre, large-scale ADAPT-DES registry involving 8583 patients with 48.3 % of them with stable CAD patients, HPR identified with the VerifyNow assay was an independent predictor of both early (HR, 95 % CI 3.00, 1.39–6.49, p=0.005) and 1-year stent thrombosis (HR, 95 % CI 2.49, 1.43–4.31, p=0.001) [27]. The risk associated with HPR was greater in patients with ACS than in patients undergoing PCI for stable angina. For the latter, this risk was non-significant. Low event rates have been implicated for these findings [28].

Platelet function testing can easily be performed even with a point-of care assay. Genotyping also for the CYP2C19*2 dysfunctional allele can identify patients with high probability for HPR. The latter can be 'treated' either by increasing clopidogrel dose or, more effectively, by novel oral P2Y12 inhibitors prasugrel and ticagrelor [29, 30]. But does this really matter in stable CAD patients? Three randomised trials [GRAVITAS (Gauging Responsiveness With A VerifyNow Assay-Impact On Thrombosis And Safety), TRIGGER-PCI (Testing Platelet Reactivity In Patients Undergoing Elective Stent Placement on Clopidogrel to Guide Alternative Therapy With Prasugrel) and ARCTIC (Assessment by a Double Randomization of a Conventional Antiplatelet Strategy versus a Monitoring-guided Strategy for Drug-Eluting Stent Implantation and of Treatment Interruption versus Continuation One Year after Stenting)] have examined the utility of more potent P2Y12 inhibition in patients with HPR while on clopidogrel, but were unable to show a reduction in stent thrombosis or myocardial infarction with this approach [31–33]. Of note, these trials included mostly or exclusively stable CAD patients constituting therefore a low risk population with low events rate. Different results have been obtained in a recent observational study in 923 stable or non-ST elevation ACS patients undergoing PCI and exhibiting on-clopidogrel HPR by multiple electrode aggregometry [34]. During a median follow-up of 571 days, intensifying antiplatelet therapy by doubling clopidogrel maintenance dose or switching to prasugrel or ticagrelor reduced the risk of the composite of cardiovascular death, myocardial infarction, stroke, or stent thrombosis to a level equivalent to that of patients exhibiting normal platelet reactivity (HR, 95 % CI, 1.08, 0.59–1.99).

Overall, in stable patients after uncomplicated PCI, standard-dose clopidogrel should be preferred and routine platelet function testing or genotyping is not recommended. We feel however, that the use of novel agents might be considered, preferably based on platelet function results, in cases with high risk PCI anatomy e.g. left main, bifurcation/proximal left anterior descending artery, last remaining patent vessel. This may be particularly relevant in clinical scenarios with expected high prevalence of on-clopidogrel HPR like in diabetic or chronic kidney disease patients [35, 36].

Finally, in the rare event of stable patients undergoing PCI and presenting with allergy to clopidogrel the novel P2Y12 inhibitors have been successfully used as an alternative solution [37, 38].

Patients with ACS

In the randomized, double-blind PCI CURE (Clopidogrel in Unstable angina to prevent Recurrent Events) trial in 2658 patients with non-ST-elevation ACS undergoing PCI a strategy of clopidogrel pre-treatment followed by long-term therapy was proven beneficial in reducing major cardiovascular events, compared with placebo [39]. The primary endpoint -a composite of cardiovascular death, myocardial infarction, or urgent target-vessel revascularization- within 30 days of PCI occurred in 4.5 and 6.4 % of patients in the clopidogrel group and placebo group, respectively [relative risk (95 % CI) 0.70 (0.50–0.97), p=0.03]. Clopidogrel was subsequently introduced as a mainstay treatment in addition to aspirin in such patients.

In the TRITON-TIMI 38 trial, prasugrel (60 mg loading dose, 10 mg maintenance dose) has been compared with clopidogrel (300 mg loading dose, 75 mg maintenance dose) for 6–15 months in 13,608 clopidogrel-naïve, moderate-to-high-risk ACS patients undergoing PCI [8]. The primary composite efficacy end point of cardiovascular death, non-fatal myocardial infarction or non-fatal stroke occurred less frequently among patients assigned to prasugrel as compared with those treated with clopidogrel [9.9 % vs 12.1 %, HR (95 % CI) 0.81 (0.73–0.90), p<0.001]. Lower rates of myocardial infarction [7.4 % vs 9.7 %, HR (95 % CI) 0.76 (0.67–0.85), p<0.001] and stent thrombosis [1.1 % vs 2.4 %, HR (95 % CI) 0.48 (0.36–0.64), p<0.001] were observed in patients receiving prasugrel. No difference in mortality rates was found between patients treated with prasugrel or clopidogrel [3.0 % vs 3.2 %, HR (95 % CI) 0.95 (0.78–1.16), p=0.64]. The benefit of prasugrel came at the expense of an increased rate of major bleedings [2.4 % vs 1.8 %, HR (95 % CI) 1.32 (1.03–1.68), p=0.03)] as well as life-threatening and fatal bleeding. In post hoc subgroup analyses, patients with a history of stroke/ transient ischemic attack (TIA) had net harm and elderly patients ≥75 years, and patients with a body weight <60 kg experienced no net clinical benefit with prasugrel as compared with clopidogrel. Although the design of the TRITON–TIMI 38 trial had some limitations, including comparison with 300 mg of clopidogrel and lack of pre-treatment, prasugrel was introduced as an alternative for clopidogrel in clopidogrel-naive patients, without a history of stroke/TIA and without excess risk for bleeding. Prasugrel should be given no later than 1 h after PCI, once coronary anatomy is defined and a decision is made to proceed with PCI. There is a special warning for precaution in elderly patients ≥75 years, and patients with a body weight <60 kg. Particular consideration for prasugrel may be given in patients with STEMI and in those with diabetes, where the balance of benefit and risk should be maximized [40, 41].

In the PLATO trial ticagrelor (180 mg loading dose, 90 mg twice daily maintenance dose) has been compared with clopidogrel (300–600 mg loading dose, 75 mg maintenance dose) in 18,624 patients with ACS managed either invasively or medically [9]. DAPT was initiated prior to PCI in the majority of patients. At 12 months of follow-up, the rate of a composite of cardiovascular death, myocardial infarction and stroke was lower among patients in ticagrelor arm as compared with clopidogrel arm [9.8 % vs 11.7 %, HR (95 % CI) 0.84 (0.77–0.92), p<0.001]. A remarkable reduction in death from vascular causes was observed with ticagrelor vs clopidogrel (4.0 % vs. 5.1 %, p=0.001). While there were no differences in the overall rates of major bleeding (11.6 % vs 11.2 %, p=0.43), patients treated with ticagrelor had a higher risk of major bleeding not related to coronary artery bypass grafting [4.5 % vs 3.8 %, HR (95 % CI) 1.19 (1.02–1.38), p=0.03]. Among 13,408 (72. 0 %) of PLATO patients in whom an invasive strategy was planned, the primary composite endpoint occurred in fewer patients in the ticagrelor group than in the clopidogrel group [HR (95 % CI) 0.84 (0.75–0.94), p=0.0025] [42]. Cardiovascular death rate was reduced by ticagrelor vs clopidogrel [HR (95 % CI) 0.82 (0.68–0.98), p=0.025]. There was no difference between clopidogrel and ticagrelor groups in the rates of total major bleeding. Of note, 10,298 (76.8 %) of patients with planned invasive strategy underwent PCI before discharge. Patients with renal dysfunction and elderly patients were particularly benefited by ticagrelor over clopidogrel [43, 44]. Ticagrelor was introduced into clinical practice as an alternative to clopidogrel for ACS patients with moderate-to high risk for ischemic events (e.g. troponin eleva-tion), including those pre-treated with clopidogrel. In a recently published pre-specified PLATO substudy the benefit of ticagrelor over clopidogrel was present irrespective of the increase in high-sensitivity troponin T in the invasively but not in the non-invasively managed patients [45].

Regarding the benefit of platelet function testing to adjust therapy in ACS patients undergoing stenting, there is no evidence for a routine role. Out of the 3 relevant randomized trials mentioned above the GRAVITAS and the ARCTIC stud-ies included ACS patients as well, with the previously discussed results. In a pro-spective registry of 741 ACS patients undergoing PCI and pretreated with clopidogrel, patients with HPR by the Multiplate device were switched to prasugrel or treated with high-dose clopidogrel [46]. Switching to treatment with prasugrel reduced thrombotic and bleeding events to a level similar to that of those without HPR, while patients treated with high-dose clopidogrel presented a higher risk of both thrombotic and bleeding complications. Of interest, in a recent study in non-STEMI patients, HPR was associated with increased rates of ischemic events only in patients with a high SYNTAX score, suggesting a possible role of platelet func-tion testing according to angiographic disease severity [47].

Despite the demonstrated antiischemic superiority of the novel antiplatelet agents over clopidogrel, concerns about their bleeding potential and increased cost, particularly when compared to generic clopidogrel, have hampered their penetra-tion in general practice worldwide. In ESC Guidelines for the management of ACS in patients presenting without persistent ST-segment elevation (2011) clopidogrel was suggested in patients who cannot receive prasugrel or ticagrelor (class I, level of evidence A, recommendation), and in the respective ones for patients with ST-segment elevation (2012) clopidogrel was suggested preferably when prasugrel or ticagrelor was either not available or contraindicated (class I, level of evidence C, recommendation) [48, 49]. On the other hand, it was only in the very recently released AHA/ACC Guidelines for the management of patients with Non-ST-Elevation ACS when a choice of prasugrel or ticagrelor over clopidogrel was considered reasonable, with IIa, level of evidence B, recommendation [2].

There are several recent reports in the literature of switching initial P2Y12 inhibitor choice, mostly in the mode of clopidogrel to prasugrel or ticagrelor [50, 51]. Of note, special warnings for precautions concerning bleeding potential of the 3 oral P2Y12 inhibitors appear rather similar in their prescribing information. However, in real practice a choice of the less potent clopidogrel is selected in case of such a clinical condition [52]. Of importance, recent preliminary results from an observational study of prasugrel vs. clopidogrel at 233 U.S. hospitals involving 12,227 myocardial infarction patients treated with PCI revealed at 12 months lower major adverse events (composite of all-cause death, myocardial infarction, stroke, or unplanned coronary revascularization) in patients receiving prasugrel vs. clopidogrel in unadjusted comparison. This difference was no longer significant following adjustment. Prasugrel was associated with significantly lower adjusted risk of stent thrombosis. Bleeding adjusted risk was higher with prasugrel compared with clopidogrel, though differences were not significant among patients more likely to be treated with prasugrel in community practice [53].

In case of stent thrombosis in a patient treated with clopidogrel, switching treatment to a potent agent either prasugrel or ticagrelor is a widely applied practice. This ideally- though not necessary- should be guided by platelet function testing which documents laboratory and clinical 'resistance' to clopidogrel.

A personal view of oral P2Y12 inhibitor choice for stable or ACS patients undergoing PCI and stenting is shown in Table 18.1. Associated bleeding risk should significantly impact on antiplatelet choice, while a bleeding risk score like that proposed by Mehran et al. may be applied for event prediction [54, 55].

Prasugrel or Ticagrelor?

No direct randomized comparison between prasugrel and ticagrelor has been performed to date with clinical outcome. Data from network meta-analyses suggested similar safety and efficacy of the two drugs, but indicated better protection from stent thrombosis with prasugrel at the expense of a higher rate of bleeding [56, 57].

Table 18.1 Oral P2Y12 inhibitor selection post PCI

| | Stable CAD | | ACS | | | |
| | | | Usual TR | | High TR | |
	Usual TR	High TR/low BR	Usual BR	High BR	Usual BR	High BR
Clopidogrel	+++	+++	+	++	−	++[a]
Prasugrel	−	+/−	+++	−	+++	−
Ticagrelor	−	+/−	+++	++	+++	+++

High TR may include patients with diabetes, renal failure, HPR on clopidogrel, carriers of CYP2C19*2 or with anatomic features for high risk PCI. STEMI patients also carry a high TR
BR bleeding risk, *TR* thrombotic risk
[a]With the exemption of stent thrombosis, when ticagrelor should be preferred

However, differences between TRITON-TIMI 38 and PLATO designs and the context of the two trials limit comparability of these findings. The ongoing ISAR-REACT (iNtracoronary Stenting and Antithrombotic Regimen: Rapid Early Action for Coronary Treatment)-5 clinical outcome trial will elucidate this issue [58]. So far, in a direct, randomized, pharmacodynamic comparison of prasugrel vs ticagrelor in ACS patients post stenting with HPR while on-clopidogrel, ticagrelor reduced platelet reactivity by VerifyNow more than prasugrel (32.9 PRU, 95 % CI 18.7–47.2 vs 101.3 PRU, 95 % CI 86.8–115.7, respectively, p<0.001), Fig. 18.1 [59]. Similar results have been obtained in diabetic patients [60]. The clinical relevance of this pharmacodynamic difference is unclear. In an observational study of bleeding events following 1-month maintenance treatment with either ticagrelor or prasugrel and following propensity matching, BARC type 1 bleeding rate was marginally higher in ticagrelor vs prasugrel treated patients (35.7 % vs 27.1 %, p=0.05), though BARC type ≥ 2 events did not differ between groups [61]. As ticagrelor appears to have fewer contraindications/ special warnings for precaution than prasugrel, it has been suggested that a STEMI protocol using ticagrelor allows a higher proportion of patients to receive a novel P2Y12 inhibitor compared to a protocol based on prasugrel and a higher adhesion to the protocol by emergency practitioners [52, 62].

In STEMI patients undergoing primary PCI, direct, randomized, pharmacodynamic comparisons between ticagrelor and prasugrel did not reveal any significant difference between them regarding platelet reactivity during the first 24 h [12, 63]. However, a delay in the onset of antiplatelet action from what expected from stable or ACS patients data was observed for the first 2 h for both agents, likely due to a delayed absorption.

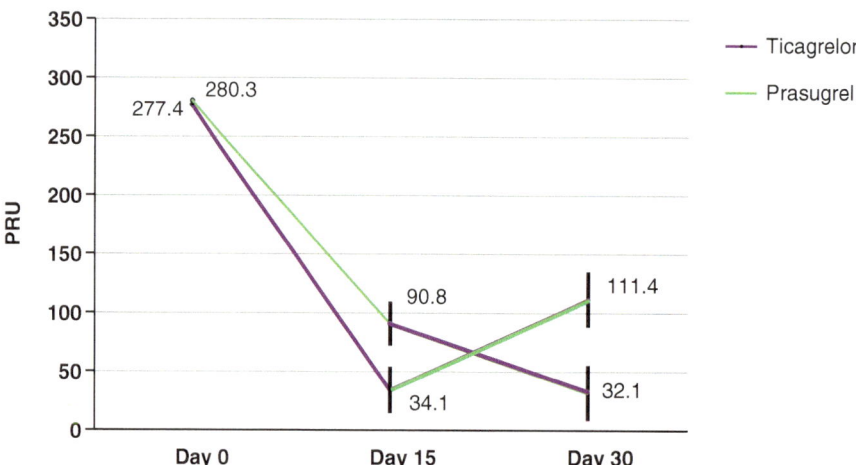

Fig. 18.1 PR (in PRU) by treatment sequence. PR is significantly lower in patients receiving ticagrelor compared with prasugrel. Least squares estimates and 95 % confidence intervals are presented. *PR* indicates platelet reactivity, *PRU* indicates platelet reactivity unit(s) (Reprinted, following permission, from Ref. [59])

The issue of pre-treatment with prasugrel or ticagrelor has been addressed by two recent trials. In the ACCOAST (Comparison of Prasugrel at the Time of Percutaneous Coronary Intervention (PCI) or as Pretreatment at the Time of Diagnosis in Patients with Non-ST Elevation Myocardial Infarction) trial 4033 patients with NSTE ACS and a positive troponin level were randomized to pre-treatment with prasugrel 30 mg (and additional 30 mg at the time of PCI) vs placebo and 60 mg of prasugrel at the time of PCI. The rate of the primary efficacy end point did not differ between arms, while the rate of the key safety end point of all Thrombolysis in Myocardial Infarction (TIMI) major bleeding episodes through day 7 was increased with pre-treatment [hazard ratio (95 % CI) 1.90 (1.19–3.02), p=0.006] [10]. Following these results, prasugrel received a class III recommendation in the recent ESC guidelines for revascularization [4]. In the ATLANTIC (Administration of Ticagrelor in the Cath Lab or in the Ambulance for New ST Elevation Myocardial Infarction to Open the Coronary Artery) study in 1862 patients with on-going STEMI, pre-hospital administration of ticagrelor loading dose (180 mg) was not associated with any difference in ST resolution before PCI or TIMI flow at initial angiography compared to in-hospital administration [11]. A lower stent thrombosis rate was observed with the pre-hospital administration, a finding that however should be considered as exploratory. Major bleeding events did not differ between groups. Pre-hospital administration of ticagrelor appears therefore safe and supports its administration at first medical contact in patients with STEMI.

Finally, the unusual event of HPR while on prasugrel leading to stent thrombosis can be successfully managed by ticagrelor [64].

Role of an Intravenous Antiplatelet Agent

Cangrelor is an intravenous, reversible P2Y12 inhibitor with rapid (within minutes) onset and offset of action which is currently undergoing regulatory review for approval in the US and Europe. In the Cangrelor Versus Standard Therapy to Achieve Optimal Management of Platelet Inhibition (CHAMPION PHOENIX) trial, 10,942 P2Y12 inhibitor naïve patients with stable CAD or ACS undergoing PCI were randomized to receive clopidogrel 300 or 600 mg LD or cangrelor 30 mcg/kg bolus + 4 mcg/kg/min for 2–4 h, initiated just before the PCI. Cangrelor reduced the 48-h primary endpoint (a composite of death, myocardial infarction, ischemia-driven revascularization, or stent thrombosis) from 5.4 to 4.1 % [odds ratio (95 % CI) 0.75 (0.63–0.90), p=0.002]. Diagnosis at presentation (stable angina, nonSTE-ACS, STEMI) did not affect this outcome (p for interaction=0.98). There was no increase in the incidence of severe bleeding with cangrelor, although moderate bleeding was increased [13]. Cangrelor may therefore appear as an attractive alternative to clopidogrel particularly suitable for patients not pre-treated, heavily sedated, vomiting or intubated patients, or those treated with therapeutic hypothermia after cardiac arrest. Cangrelor's role in the early hours of STEMI in comparison with potent agents deserves further elucidation.

Concomitant Need for Oral Anticoagulants

One of the 'hottest' areas of interest is DAPT in the context of triple antithrombotic treatment. Long-term oral anticoagulation is required in approximately 7 % of PCI patients and triple antithrombotic treatment carries undoubtedly a several-fold increased bleeding risk. Apart from the duration, the ideal type of DAPT is unclear. The safety and efficacy of clopidogrel alone compared with clopidogrel plus aspirin was investigated in the WOEST randomised trial involving 573 patients on oral anticoagulants and undergoing PCI. The primary outcome of any bleeding episode within 1 year of PCI occurred less frequently in the double compared to triple therapy group [HR (95 % CI) 0.36 (0.26–0.50) p < 0.0001] without concomitant increase in the rate of thrombotic events [64]. The ISAR-TRIPLE trial randomized 614 patients to receive aspirin and a vitamin-K antagonist plus 6 weeks or 6 months of clopidogrel [65]. Following 9-months, no difference in the primary endpoint (death, myocardial infarction, stent thrombosis, stroke or TIMI major bleeding) was observed between groups. WOEST and ISAR-TRIPLE therefore, suggested a strategy of omitting aspirin or clopidogrel beyond the 6th week, respectively. Prasugrel- instead of clopidogrel- has been studied as a part of triple therapy in an observational registry, with an unacceptably high rate of bleeding events, and should not be given in this setting [66].

Conclusion

There are several controversial and unresolved issues remaining when prescribing DAPT following stenting.

1. In stable CAD patients undergoing PCI, clopidogrel can be used in the overwhelming majority.
2. In patients with documented or in high risk for HPR while on-clopidogrel and in those with anatomic features for high risk PCI one may think of using a novel agent, although data from available randomized studies were not positive for such a strategy.
3. In ACS patients, prasugrel and ticagrelor should be preferred over clopidogrel, particularly if a high thrombotic and a usual bleeding risk are present. Prasugrel should not be used if the bleeding risk is high, in which case clopidogrel or ticagrelor may be preferred. The latter is, likely, a better choice in cases carrying a high thrombotic risk.
4. The role of cangrelor and the antiplatelet constituents of triple antithrombotic therapy if needed, requires further elucidation.
5. The appropriate DAPT should be defined for the individual patient following a balance between thrombotic and bleeding risk. Overall, a treatment strategy tailored to post PCI patients should have outcome improvement as the ultimate objective.

References

1. Levine GN, Bates ER, Blankenship JC, et al. 2011 ACCF/AHA/SCAI guideline for percutaneous coronary intervention. A report of the American College of Cardiology Foundation/American Heart Association Task Force on Practice Guidelines and the Society for Cardiovascular Angiography and Interventions. J Am Coll Cardiol. 2011;58:e44–122.
2. Amsterdam EA, Wenger NK, Brindis RG, et al. 2014 AHA/ACC guideline for the management of patients with non-ST-elevation acute coronary syndromes: a report of the American College of Cardiology/American Heart Association Task Force on Practice Guidelines. J Am Coll Cardiol. 2014;64(24):e139–228. pii: S0735-1097(14)06279-2. doi:10.1016/j.jacc.2014.09.017.
3. O'Gara PT, Kushner FG, Ascheim DD, et al. 2013 ACCF/AHA guideline for the management of ST-elevation myocardial infarction: a report of the American College of Cardiology Foundation/American Heart Association Task Force on Practice Guidelines. J Am Coll Cardiol. 2013;61:e78–140.
4. Windecker S, Kolh P, Alfonso F, et al. 2014 ESC/EACTS guidelines on myocardial revascularization: The Task Force on Myocardial Revascularization of the European Society of Cardiology (ESC) and the European Association for Cardio-Thoracic Surgery (EACTS) Developed with the special contribution of the European Association of Percutaneous Cardiovascular Interventions (EAPCI). Eur Heart J. 2014;35:2541–619.
5. Gurbel PA, Bliden KP, Hiatt BL, O'Connor CM. Clopidogrel for coronary stenting: response variability, drug resistance, and the effect of pretreatment platelet reactivity. Circulation. 2003;107:2908–13.
6. Holmes Jr DR, Dehmer GJ, Kaul S, Leifer D, O'Gara PT, Stein CM. ACCF/AHA clopidogrel clinical alert: approaches to the FDA "boxed warning": a report of the American College of Cardiology Foundation Task Force on clinical expert consensus documents and the American Heart Association endorsed by the Society for Cardiovascular Angiography and Interventions and the Society of Thoracic Surgeons. J Am Coll Cardiol. 2010;56:321–41.
7. Angiolillo DJ, Ferreiro JL, Price MJ, et al. Platelet function and genetic testing. J Am Coll Cardiol. 2013;62:S21–31.
8. Wiviott SD, Braunwald E, McCabe CH, et al.; for the TRITON-TIMI 38 Investigators. Prasugrel versus clopidogrel in patients with acute coronary syndromes. N Engl J Med 2007;357:2001–15.
9. Wallentin L, Becker RC, Budaj A, et al.; for the PLATO Investigators, Freij A, Thorsén M. Ticagrelor versus clopidogrel in patients with acute coronary syndromes. N Engl J Med 2009;361:1045–57.
10. Montalescot G, Bolognese L, Dudek D, et al.; ACCOAST Investigators. Pretreatment with prasugrel in non-ST-segment elevation acute coronary syndromes. N Engl J Med. 2013;369:999–1010.
11. Montalescot G, van 't Hof AW, Lapostolle F, et al. ATLANTIC Investigators. Prehospital ticagrelor in ST-segment elevation myocardial infarction. N Engl J Med. 2014;371:1016–27.
12. Alexopoulos D, Xanthopoulou I, Gkizas V, et al. Randomized assessment of ticagrelor versus prasugrel antiplatelet effects in patients with ST-segment-elevation myocardial infarction. Circ Cardiovasc Interv. 2012;5:797–804.
13. Bhatt DL, Stone GW, Mahaffey KW, et al.; CHAMPION PHOENIX Investigators. Effect of platelet inhibition with cangrelor during PCI on ischemic events. N Engl J Med. 2013;368:1303–13.
14. Patanè S, Marte F, Di Bella G. Catastrophic early drug eluting stents thrombosis and aspirin hypersensitivity. Int J Cardiol. 2008;131:e25–7.
15. Jenneck C, Juergens U, Buechler M, et al. Pathogenesis, diagnosis, and treatment of aspirin intolerance. Ann Allergy Asthma Immunol. 2007;99:13–21.
16. Rossini R, Angiolillo DJ, Musumeci G, et al. Aspirin desensitization in patients undergoing percutaneous coronary interventions with stent implantation. Am J Cardiol. 2008;101:786–9.

17. Wieczorek P, Parma R, Tendera M, Wojakowski W. Primary PCI with endothelial progenitor cell-capture stent in patient with skull base fracture and aspirin allergy. Kardiol Pol. 2013;71:210.

18. Jim MH, Yung AS, Tang GK, Fan KY, Chow WH. Successful use of endothelial progenitor cell capture stents in a coronary artery disease patient with aspirin hypersensitivity who failed initial aspirin desensitization. Int J Cardiol. 2011;148:350–1.

19. Barillà F, Pulcinelli FM, Mangieri E, et al. Clopidogrel plus indobufen in acute coronary syndrome patients with hypersensitivity to aspirin undergoing percutaneous coronary intervention. Platelets. 2013;24:183–8.

20. Schomig A, Neumann FJ, Kastrati A, et al. A randomized comparison of antiplatelet and anticoagulant therapy after the placement of coronary-artery stents. N Engl J Med. 1996;334:1084–9.

21. Bhatt DL, Bertrand ME, Berger PB, et al. Meta-analysis of randomized and registry comparisons of ticlopidine with clopidogrel after stenting. J Am Coll Cardiol. 2002;39:9–14.

22. Steinhubl SR, Berger PB, Mann III JT, et al. Early and sustained dual oral antiplatelet therapy following percutaneous coronary intervention: a randomized controlled trial. JAMA. 2002;288:2411–20.

23. Steinhubl SR, Berger PB, Brennan DM, et al. Optimal timing for the initiation of pre-treatment with 300 mg clopidogrel before percutaneous coronary intervention. J Am Coll Cardiol. 2006;47:939–43.

24. Breet NJ, van Werkum JW, Bouman HJ, et al. Comparison of platelet function tests in predicting clinical outcome in patients undergoing coronary stent implantation. JAMA. 2010;303:754–62.

25. Park DW, Ahn JM, Song HG, et al. Differential prognostic impact of high on-treatment platelet reactivity among patients with acute coronary syndromes versus stable coronary artery disease undergoing percutaneous coronary intervention. Am Heart J. 2013;165:34–42.

26. Brar SS, ten Berg J, Marcucci R, et al. Impact of platelet reactivity on clinical outcomes after percutaneous coronary intervention: a collaborative meta-analysis of individual participant data. J Am Coll Cardiol. 2011;58:1945–54.

27. Stone GW, Witzenbichler B, Weisz G, et al. Platelet reactivity and clinical outcomes after coronary artery implantation of drug-eluting stents (ADAPT-DES): a prospective multicentre registry study. Lancet. 2013;382:614–23.

28. Kirtane AJ, Rinaldi M, Parise H, et al. Impact of point-of-care platelet function testing among patients with and without acute coronary syndromes undergoing PCI with drug-eluting stents: an ADAPT-DES substudy. J Am Coll Cardiol. 2012;59, E291.

29. Alexopoulos D, Xanthopoulou I, Davlouros P, et al. Prasugrel overcomes high on-clopidogrel platelet reactivity in chronic coronary artery disease patients more effectively than high dose (150 mg) clopidogrel. Am Heart J. 2011;162:733–9.

30. Gurbel PA, Bliden KP, Butler K, et al. Response to ticagrelor in clopidogrel nonresponders and responders and effect of switching therapies: the RESPOND study. Circulation. 2010;121:1188–99.

31. Price MJ, Berger PB, Teirstein PS, et al.; for the GRAVITAS Investigators. Standard- vs high-dose clopidogrel based on platelet function testing after percutaneous coronary intervention: the GRAVITAS randomized trial. JAMA. 2011;305:1097–105.

32. Trenk D, Stone GW, Gawaz M, et al. A randomized trial of prasugrel versus clopidogrel in patients with high platelet reactivity on clopidogrel after elective percutaneous coronary intervention with implantation of drug-eluting stents: results of the TRIGGER-PCI (Testing Platelet Reactivity In Patients Undergoing Elective Stent Placement on Clopidogrel to Guide Alternative Therapy with Prasugrel) study. J Am Coll Cardiol. 2012;59:2159–64.

33. Collet JP, Cuisset T, Range G, et al.; for the ARCTIC Investigators. Bedside monitoring to adjust antiplatelet therapy for coronary stenting. N Engl J Med. 2012;367:2100–9.

34. Paarup Dridi N, Johansson PI, Lønborg JT, et al. Tailored antiplatelet therapy to improve prognosis in patients exhibiting clopidogrel low-response prior to percutaneous coronary intervention for stable angina or non-ST elevation acute coronary syndrome. Platelets. 2015;26(6):521–9. doi: 10.3109/09537104.2014.948837. Epub 2014 Aug 28.

35. Angiolillo DJ, Jakubowski JA, Ferreiro JL, et al. Impaired responsiveness to the platelet P2Y12 receptor antagonist clopidogrel in patients with type 2 diabetes and coronary artery disease. J Am Coll Cardiol. 2014;64:1005–14.
36. Htun P, Fateh-Moghadam S, Bischofs C, et al. Low responsiveness to clopidogrel increases risk among CKD patients undergoing coronary intervention. J Am Soc Nephrol. 2011;22:627–33.
37. Felix-Getzik E, Sylvia LM. Prasugrel use in a patient allergic to clopidogrel: effect of a drug shortage on selection of dual antiplatelet therapy. Am J Health Syst Pharm. 2013;70:511–3.
38. Lokhandwala J, Best PJ, Henry Y, Berger PB. Allergic reactions to clopidogrel and cross-reactivity to other agents. Curr Allergy Asthma Rep. 2011;11:52–7.
39. Mehta SR, Yusuf S, Peters RJ, et al.; Clopidogrel in Unstable angina to prevent Recurrent Events trial (CURE) Investigators. Effects of pretreatment with clopidogrel and aspirin followed by long-term therapy in patients undergoing percutaneous coronary intervention: the PCI-CURE study. Lancet. 2001;358:527–33.
40. Montalescot G, Wiviott SD, Braunwald E, et al.; TRITON-TIMI 38 investigators. Prasugrel compared with clopidogrel in patients undergoing percutaneous coronary intervention for ST-elevation myocardial infarction (TRITON-TIMI 38): double-blind, randomised controlled trial. Lancet. 2009;373:723–31.
41. Wiviott SD, Braunwald E, Angiolillo DJ, et al.; TRITON-TIMI 38 Investigators. Greater clinical benefit of more intensive oral antiplatelet therapy with prasugrel in patients with diabetes mellitus in the trial to assess improvement in therapeutic outcomes by optimizing platelet inhibition with prasugrel-Thrombolysis in Myocardial Infarction 38. Circulation. 2008;118:1626–36.
42. Cannon CP, Harrington RA, James S, et al.; PLATelet Inhibition and Patient Outcomes Investigators. Comparison of ticagrelor with clopidogrel in patients with a planned invasive strategy for acute coronary syndromes (PLATO): a randomised double-blind study. Lancet. 2010;375:283–93.
43. James S, Budaj A, Aylward P, et al. Ticagrelor versus clopidogrel in acute coronary syndromes in relation to renal function: results from the Platelet Inhibition and Patient Outcomes (PLATO) trial. Circulation. 2010;122:1056–67.
44. Husted S, James S, Becker RC, et al.; PLATO Study Group. Ticagrelor versus clopidogrel in elderly patients with acute coronary syndromes: a substudy from the prospective randomized PLATelet inhibition and patient Outcomes (PLATO) trial. Circ Cardiovasc Qual Outcomes. 2012;5:680–8.
45. Wallentin L, Lindholm D, Siegbahn A, et al.; PLATO Study Group. Biomarkers in relation to the effects of ticagrelor in comparison with clopidogrel in non-ST-elevation acute coronary syndrome patients managed with or without in-hospital revascularization: a substudy from the Prospective Randomized Platelet Inhibition and Patient Outcomes (PLATO) trial. Circulation. 2014;129:293–303.
46. Aradi D, Tornyos A, Pintér T, et al. Optimizing P2Y12 receptor inhibition in patients with acute coronary syndrome on the basis of platelet function testing: impact of prasugrel and high-dose clopidogrel. J Am Coll Cardiol. 2014;63:1061–70.
47. Palmerini T, Calabrò P, Piscione F, et al. Impact of gene polymorphisms, platelet reactivity, and the SYNTAX score on 1-year clinical outcomes in patients with non-ST-segment elevation acute coronary syndrome undergoing percutaneous coronary intervention: the GEPRESS Study. JACC Cardiovasc Interv. 2014;7:1117–27.
48. Hamm CW, Bassand JP, Agewall S, et al.; ESC Committee for Practice Guidelines. ESC Guidelines for the management of acute coronary syndromes in patients presenting without persistent ST-segment elevation: The Task Force for the management of acute coronary syndromes (ACS) in patients presenting without persistent ST-segment elevation of the European Society of Cardiology (ESC). Eur Heart J. 2011;32:2999–3054.
49. Task Force on the management of ST-segment elevation acute myocardial infarction of the European Society of Cardiology (ESC), Steg PG, James SK, Atar D, et al.; ESC guidelines for

the management of acute myocardial infarction in patients presenting with ST-segment elevation. Eur Heart J. 2012;33:2569–619.

50. Alexopoulos D, Xanthopoulou I, Deftereos S, et al. In-hospital switching of oral P2Y12 inhibitor treatment in patients with acute coronary syndrome undergoing percutaneous coronary intervention: prevalence, predictors and short-term outcome. Am Heart J. 2014;167:68–76.

51. Bagai A, Wang Y, Wang TY, et al. In-hospital switching between clopidogrel and prasugrel among patients with acute myocardial infarction treated with percutaneous coronary intervention: insights into contemporary practice from the national cardiovascular data registry. Circ Cardiovasc Interv. 2014;7:585–93.

52. Alexopoulos D, Xanthopoulou I, Deftereos S, et al.; GRAPE Investigators. Contraindications/special warnings and precautions for use of contemporary oral antiplatelet treatment in patients with acute coronary syndrome undergoing percutaneous coronary intervention. Circ J. 2014;78:180–7.

53. Wang TY, presented on behalf of the TRANSLATE-ACS Investigators. Treatment with ADP receptor inhibitorS: longitudinal assessment of treatment patterns and events after acute coronary syndrome. TCT Sept 2014, Washington, DC.

54. Mehran R, Pocock SJ, Nikolsky E, et al. A risk score to predict bleeding in patients 179 with acute coronary syndromes. J Am Coll Cardiol. 2010;55:2556–66.

55. Xanthopoulou I, Deftereos S, Sitafidis G, et al. In-hospital bleeding events in acute coronary syndrome patients undergoing percutaneous coronary intervention in the era of novel P2Y12 inhibitors: insights from the GReek AntiPlatelet rEgistry-GRAPE. Int J Cardiol. 2014;174:160–2.

56. Biondi-Zoccai G, Lotrionte M, Agostoni P, et al. Adjusted indirect comparison meta-analysis of prasugrel versus ticagrelor for patients with acute coronary syndromes. Int J Cardiol. 2011;150:325–31.

57. Chatterjee S, Ghose A, Sharma A, Guha G, Mukherjee D, Frankel R. Comparing newer oral anti-platelets prasugrel and ticagrelor in reduction of ischemic events-evidence from a network meta-analysis. J Thromb Thrombolysis. 2013;36:223–32.

58. Schulz S, Angiolillo DJ, Antoniucci D, et al.; Intracoronary Stenting and Antithrombotic Regimen: Rapid Early Action for Coronary Treatment (ISAR-REACT) 5 Trial Investigators. Randomized comparison of ticagrelor versus prasugrel in patients with acute coronary syndrome and planned invasive strategy--design and rationale of the iNtracoronary Stenting and Antithrombotic Regimen: Rapid Early Action for Coronary Treatment (ISAR-REACT) 5 trial. J Cardiovasc Transl Res. 2014;7:91–100.

59. Alexopoulos D, Galati A, Xanthopoulou I, et al. Ticagrelor versus prasugrel in acute coronary syndrome patients with high on-clopidogrel platelet reactivity following percutaneous coronary intervention: a pharmacodynamic study. J Am Coll Cardiol. 2012;60:193–9.

60. Alexopoulos D, Xanthopoulou I, Mavronasiou E, et al. Randomized assessment of ticagrelor versus prasugrel antiplatelet effects in patients with diabetes. Diabetes Care. 2013;36:2211–6.

61. Alexopoulos D, Stavrou K, Koniari I, et al. Ticagrelor vs prasugrel one-month maintenance therapy: impact on platelet reactivity and bleeding events. Thromb Haemost. 2014;112:551–7.

62. Fournier N, Toesca R, Bessereau J, et al. Ticagrelor or prasugrel for pre-hospital protocols in STEMI? Int J Cardiol. 2013;168:4566–7.

63. Parodi G, Valenti R, Bellandi B, et al. Comparison of prasugrel and ticagrelor loading doses in ST-segment elevation myocardial infarction patients: RAPID (Rapid Activity of Platelet Inhibitor Drugs) primary PCI study. J Am Coll Cardiol. 2013;61:1601–6.

64. Dewilde WJ, Oirbans T, Verheugt FW, et al.; WOEST study investigators. Use of clopidogrel with or without aspirin in patients taking oral anticoagulant therapy and undergoing percutaneous coronary intervention: an open-label, randomised, controlled trial. Lancet. 2013;381:1107–15.

65. Fiedler KA, Maeng M, Mehilli J, et al. Duration of triple therapy in patients requiring oral anticoagulation after drug-eluting stent implantation (ISAR-TRIPLE Trial). TCT Sept 2014, Washington DC.
66. Sarafoff N, Martischnig A, Wealer J, et al. Triple therapy with aspirin, prasugrel, and vitamin K antagonists in patients with drug-eluting stent implantation and an indication for oral anticoagulation. J Am Coll Cardiol. 2013;61:2060–6.

Chapter 19
Invasive Management in CAD Patients with Stage 4 Renal Dysfunction or on Dialysis

Josephine Warren, Usman Baber, and Roxana Mehran

Abstract Chronic kidney disease (CKD) is an independent risk factor for coronary artery disease (CAD), and is associated with more complex coronary pathologies such as multivessel disease and left main involvement. Greater reductions in renal function are associated with increasingly poor outcomes following revascularization therapy. The optimal revascularization approach for obstructive CAD in stable or unstable coronary syndromes in CKD has not been defined as there is a lack of sufficiently powered randomized data in this patient subset. While coronary artery bypass grafting (CABG) appears to be associated with better long-term survival and less long-term ischemic events than percutaneous coronary intervention (PCI), the choice of revascularization therapy should be individualized, taking into account patient co-morbidities, functional status, and preference.

Keywords Dialysis • Renal impairment • Percutaneous coronary intervention • Coronary artery bypass grafting

Introduction

Chronic kidney disease (CKD) is an independent risk factor for the development of coronary artery disease (CAD), and its presence is associated with a higher incidence of complex and diffuse coronary pathology [1–3]. The development of end

Disclosures All authors declare no conflict of interest.

J. Warren, MBBS • R. Mehran, MD (✉)
The Icahn School of Medicine at Mount Sinai, The Zena and Michael A. Wiener Cardiovascular Institute, One Gustave L. Levy Place, Box 1030, New York, NY 10029, USA

Mount Sinai Medical Center, New York, NY, USA
e-mail: josie.warren2@gmail.com; roxana.mehran@mountsinai.org

U. Baber, MD, MS
The Icahn School of Medicine at Mount Sinai, The Zena and Michael A. Wiener Cardiovascular Institute, One Gustave L. Levy Place, Box 1030, New York, NY 10029, USA
e-mail: usman.baber@mountsinai.org

© Springer International Publishing Switzerland 2015
J.A. Ambrose, A.E. Rodríguez (eds.), *Controversies in Cardiology*,
DOI 10.1007/978-3-319-20415-4_19

271

stage renal disease (ESRD, defined as a glomerular filtration rate (GFR) of <15 mL/min/1.73 m^2) further complicates clinical prognosis, conferring increased risk of adverse outcomes following index cardiac events and interventional procedures [4]. Further highlighting the additive and interconnected relationship between these conditions, cardiovascular disease is the greatest driver of mortality in patients with ESRD, responsible for almost 50 % of deaths [5, 6]. These conditions share common risk factors [7], and are projected to rise in prevalence as the population ages, emphasizing the necessity of defining an optimal management strategy.

Several issues remain unresolved in this area. The consensus from the ACCF/AHA/SCAI guidelines indicate an invasive strategy is reasonable (Class IIb) in the management of CAD in patients with chronic renal impairment, and the National Kidney Foundation recommend that the selection of invasive management should be the same for dialyzed as non-dialyzed patients [8]. However, these guidelines were largely formed by randomized clinical trials that excluded patients with severe renal impairment. Current literature pertaining to revascularization in patients with ESRD is limited to observational, retrospective studies with a small sample sizes [9, 10]. Furthermore, despite their worse clinical state, beneficial therapies are paradoxically underutilized in this patient subset for fear of complications or bleeding events, which is referred to as therapeutic nihilism [11].

Further factors contributing to poor outcomes in patients with severe renal impairment undergoing revascularization are the presence of extensive co-morbidities, in particular as diabetes and hypertension, as well as the toxic metabolic environment and the pro-atherosclerotic, prothrombotic state [11]. This chapter will explore the optimal method of revascularization in patients with severe renal disease.

Relationship Between Renal Impairment and Coronary Artery Disease

Delineating the influence of CKD on the pathogenesis of CAD is important in assessing the best invasive technique in this complex patient population. There is a correlation between renal function and the extent of CAD, as CKD is associated with markers of atherosclerotic plaque vulnerability, plaque disruption, accelerated atherosclerosis, and increased blood thrombogenicity and vascular calcification, which renders patients with CKD at a significantly higher risk for myocardial infarction and cardiac death [7, 12, 13]. The interplay between renal impairment and manifestation of CAD is summarized in Fig. 19.1.

Patients with CKD are predisposed towards more complex CAD, with a higher prevalence of multivessel disease, proximal or left main disease and heavy calcification [14, 15]. In addition, renal failure compromises oxygen supply to the myocardium through processes such as anemia, metabolic imbalance and microvascular disease leading to depressed coronary reserve [16].

The oxidative and metabolic processes associated with dialysis, which include renal anemia, uremia, cytokine excess, endothelial dysfunction and accumula-

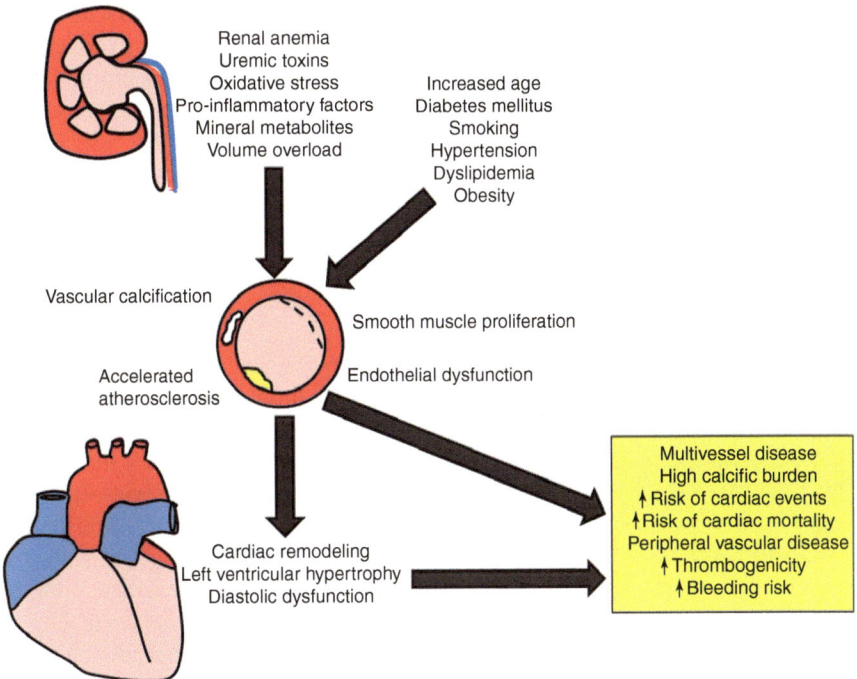

Fig. 19.1 Impact of renal impairment on cardiovascular outcomes

tion of pro-inflammatory products, render the vasculature more vulnerable to accelerated atherosclerosis [12, 13, 17]. Indeed, it is estimated that approximately 40 % of all patients on dialysis suffer CAD, with a recent case series reporting that over 60 % of non-selected dialysis patients had CAD with >75 % stenosis, and an average of 3.3 lesions per patient [18–20]. A significant proportion of patients who start on dialysis already have an extensive risk factor profile for CAD, with large numbers of patients suffering diabetes, dyslipidemia, hypertension and left ventricular dysfunction prior to initiation of therapy [7]. As a result, there is a high rate of de novo CVD development in patients on dialysis, and the co-existence of risk factors also confounds the hazard of poor outcomes following revascularization [21]. Exposure to the dialysis membrane increases the already heightened platelet reactivity seen in patients with severe renal impairment, as well as inflammation and corresponding thrombotic biomarkers [22–24]. Paradoxically, however, platelet reactivity is reduced at the end of dialysis and hemostatic changes are partially corrected for with the reduction of uremic toxins [25].

The risk of myocardial infarction (MI) in patients on dialysis is five-fold higher than that of the general population, and the 1-year mortality rate post-MI approaches 60 % in patients with ESRD [26]. These statistics are compounded by the high rates of silent myocardial infarction in patients with dialysis [27–29]. Symptoms of MI, such as dyspnea and angina, may be mistaken as a manifestation of fluid overload, which is a common complication of dialysis, leading to delayed diagnosis and misidentification or repeat ischemic symptoms. Detection is further complicated by the reduced sensitivity of the ECG for detecting ischemia in patients with ESRD due to a high prevalence of baseline ST-changes and left ventricular hypertrophy [30].

Percutaneous Coronary Intervention Verses Coronary Artery Bypass Grafting

The National Kidney Foundation guidelines indicate that percutaneous coronary intervention (PCI) and coronary artery bypass grafting (CABG) are both viable options for the treatment of obstructive CAD in severe renal impairment, but that CABG should be preferred in the management of triple vessel and left main disease [31]. However, these recommendations are only a Class C level of evidence as they stem from post-hoc observation studies and/or consensus opinion. As in patients without ESRD, the ACCF/AHA/SCAI guidelines indicate that patients with complex multivessel disease or severe disease involving the left main segment should be risk stratified according to the SYNTAX score to determine optimal mode of revascularization [32, 33]. Given these pathologies are more common in ESRD, it is logical that these patients have better survival when undergoing CABG, which has been demonstrated to confer a lower risk of long-term mortality [34].

The Arterial Revascularization Therapies Study (ARTS) trial randomized patients with CKD, defined as creatinine clearance ≤60 mL/min, and multivessel disease to either PCI or CABG. Although survival outcomes at 3 years were similar between patient groups, CABG was associated with a significant reduction in the need for repeat revascularization [35]. However, it is important to note that PCI techniques utilized in ARTS do not reflect contemporary methods and therefore these findings may not be generalizable to contemporary management of PCI patients. Significantly, the risk of poor outcomes conferred by even a mild reduction in renal function persisted at 3 years after intervention. Currently, there is no randomized data on patients with severe renal impairment, but several observational trials have indicated that the long-term benefit of CABG becomes increasingly apparent with greater reductions in renal function [36–40].

PCI and advanced renal disease

The consensus of several meta-analyses comparing invasive management of CAD in patients with severe renal disease has been that PCI is associated with better short-term survival, but confers a higher risk of myocardial infarction, repeat revascularization and long-term mortality compared to CABG. Table 19.1 summarizes the major comparisons between the methods.

Table 19.1 Direct comparison between PCI and CABG for patients with severe renal impairment

	PCI	CABG
Short-term mortality	**Better** [34, 41–43]	Worse
Repeat revascularization	Worse	**Better** [34, 43]
Re-infarction	Worse	**Better** [34, 43]
Long-term mortality	Worse	**Better** [34, 41, 42]
Triple-vessel disease	Worse	**Better** [43]
Diabetics	Worse	**Better** [36, 44, 45]
Length of hospitalization	**Shorter**	Longer [46, 47]
Stroke rate	**Lower** [45, 48]	Higher

Mortality and Ischemic Events

Studies have concluded that PCI is associated with superior short term survival, effectively halving the 30-day mortality rate of CABG [34, 41, 42]. However, this risk reverses at 1-year, with CABG patients experiencing substantially lower long-term mortality rates than those receiving PCI. The survival and adverse event benefit derived from CABG over PCI appears most marked in patients with ESRD [42], and long term mortality rates continue to be superior to 8-year follow-up [38]. It is worth remembering that patients have a poor 1-year survival rate regardless of revascularization strategy, and so choice should be individualized, based on a patient's individual prognosis and baseline profile, as well as operator experience [41]. As well as conferring better long-term survival rates, CABG is associated with an increased duration of vessel patency, with significantly lower rates of repeat revascularization, MI and composite ischemic events [34, 42, 49].

Acute Coronary Syndromes

Among patients with severe renal impairment, mortality following acute myocardial infarction is 16–19 fold higher than that of the general population, approaching 70 % at 1 year following the index event [50, 51]. Both the National Kidney Foundation and European Society of Cardiology guidelines indicate that treatment for dialyzed and ESRD patients should be the same as those without renal impairment, which extends to the use of all drugs and interventional procedures [31, 52]. Emergent PCI is preferred over the use of thrombolysis in patients with STEMI, and care should be given to dose adjustment of drugs with altered clearance in kidney failure [31].

The efficacy of early invasive strategy in patients with severe renal impairment presenting with NSTEACS remains controversial. There is substantial bias presiding over the treatment of this patient group, who are more likely to be treated medically rather than invasively, or undergo revascularization with much greater delay [53]. The current ACC/AHA guidelines for NSTEACS do not specifically define a management protocol for patients with severe renal impairment, but indicate that patients deemed high risk, which generally includes this subset, should undergo an early invasive strategy (Class I) [54].

Several observational trials have attempted to define the role of invasive strategy in NSTEACS with conflicting results. Both the TACTICS-TIMI 18 and SWEDEHEART trials found a reduction in rates of adverse events at 6 months and 1 year, respectively, with an early invasive strategy in patients with mild-moderate renal impairment [55]. However, SWEDEHEART identified that as renal function declined, the survival benefit diminished, and as such patients with ESRD and dialysis derived no benefit from an early invasive strategy [53]. Recently, an analysis pooling data from the FRISC II [56] and ICTUS [57] studies indicated that there was a significant reduction in 5-year rates of cardiac death and MI in patients with moderate-severe renal impairment who underwent early invasive strategy for NSTEACS [58]. However, this subgroup included patients with eGFR <60 and did not conduct a separate analysis on those with ESRD or on dialysis. The risk of stroke and bleeding increases as renal function worsens [59, 60], which is further increased with interventional management. Potentially, the greater bleeding risk coupled with a more modest benefit in ischemic event reduction might favor a more conservative approach in otherwise stable NSTE-ACS patients with advanced renal disease.

The use of early coronary angiography in patients with severe renal function is also an area of contention, as there is an increased risk of cholesterol embolism and AKI in patients with marked reductions in renal function [61]. In patients with more severe (Stage 4–5) renal disease, 1-year mortality is reduced with angiography, but the risk of recurrent MI is higher. Thus, if delaying PCI is feasible, it is recommended to reduce the risk of contrast induced nephropathy [62].

Factors Complicating an Invasive Strategy in Advanced Renal Disease

Percutaneous Coronary Intervention

Studies have demonstrated that there is a dose-dependent increase in peri- and post-procedural cardiac death and ischemic complications with decreasing renal function in patients undergoing PCI [63]. Indeed, in patients with ESRD, PCI may have no benefit over medical management [64]. Factors responsible for complicating PCI in this patient subset are summarized in Table 19.2. Dialysis is an independent predictor of target lesion revascularization, which is driven by the high rates of in-stent restenosis [65–67]. Furthermore, in-stent restenosis is more likely to result in fatality as silent myocardial ischemia is frequent in patients undergoing dialysis in whom fluid overload in common and may mask a timely diagnosis. As a result, some physicians advocate the routine assessment for stent patency using dobutamine stress echocardiography [31, 68]. This modality is preferred as it does not require physical exertion and the sensitivity is not compromised by the presence of left ventricular hypertrophy, which is a limitation of EKG-based assessment in patients with ESRD.

Table 19.2 Factors complicating PCI in ESRD

Factors complicating PCI in ESRD
Co-morbidities e.g. diabetes, hypertension [69]
Increased rates of restenosis due to [70]:
Accelerated atherosclerosis
Poor responsiveness to statin therapy, clopidogrel
Inflammatory processes [71]
Stent hypo-expansion due to calcification [71]
Increased bleeding risk, limiting duration of dual antiplatelet therapy
Peripheral vascular disease complicating access
Problems with stent delivery due to heavy calcification
Increased need for rotablation [66]
Silent ischemia delaying detection of restenosis
Increased risk of acute kidney injury and contrast-induced nephropathy [70, 72]
Reduced efficacy of drug eluting stents

Additional modifications to the PCI procedure must be taken into consideration for ESRD patients. A transradial approach, although shown to reduce bleeding risk, may be contraindicated in patients with ESRD due to the need to preserve the radial artery for the possibility of creating an arteriovenous fistula in the future. Low dose iso-osmolar contrast (such as iodixanol), at a minimum dose, is recommended [31, 32].

A major limitation of PCI is the need for repeat revascularization, which has been partially addressed by the newer generation drug eluting stents (DES). DES have reduced the rates of restenosis and target lesion revascularization in patients on dialysis, but this does not translate to the survival benefit seen in those with normal renal function [67, 73]. Patients on dialysis receiving DES have higher rates of TLR and stent thrombosis than those not on dialysis [74]. A recent analysis comparing stenting with DES to CABG found that in-hospital mortality was lower with DES but the chance of repeat revascularization was still higher [8], indicating that the clinical results still favor CABG [75].

Patients on dialysis are at an increased risk of bleeding and so consideration needs to be made with regards to dual antiplatelet therapy (DAPT) selection and duration [76]. Guidelines indicate that DAPT should be continued for a minimum 12 months but the duration may be reduced under physician guidance if the patient experiences bleeding complications. This additive risk of bleeding may render CABG more attractive for some patients. In addition, anticoagulation medications with complete or substantial renal elimination need to be used with care during PCI, either through down-titration or complete contra-indication. Such medications include low molecular weight heparin, bivalirudin, and small molecule glycoprotein IIb/IIIa inhibitors tirofiban and eptifabtide [52]. Despite this, a recent study indicated that the use of contraindicated antithrombotic agents in patients with severe renal impairment remains unacceptably high [77]. The use of these medications was associated with an increased risk of in-hospital major bleeding in a propensity-matched analysis. Renal insufficiency was found to be an independent predictor of excess dosing of glycoprotein IIb/IIIa inhibitors and unfractionated heparin, which may also contribute to the increased bleeding risk seen in PCI [78].

Coronary Artery Bypass Grafting

The majority of evidence suggests that CABG confers better long-term survival and lower ischemic adverse event rates than PCI in patients with ESRD. However, the procedural complexity and adverse outcomes of CABG are increased significantly in the presence of ESRD.

The short-term mortality of CABG in dialysis patients is higher than the general population [79], as are the rates of stroke, bleeding, and peri-procedural complications [79]. However, the use of the internal mammary artery as the bypass conduit has improved mortality rates markedly in this patient subset [47]. There is a short-term benefit in dialysis patients undergoing off-pump vs. on-pump CABG, but this requires further verification [80–82]. In addition, a greater survival advantage is noted in patients with triple vessel disease, which is a common feature of patients with ESRD and CAD [8, 82]. Factors complicating CABG in ESRD patients are summarized in Table 19.3. Patients undergoing CABG on dialysis have a higher risk of systemic infection, longer duration of surgery, greater need for mechanical ventilation, increased duration of cardiopulmonary bypass and greater need for balloon pump [47, 83, 84].

Generally, it is recommended that patients should be dialyzed prior to surgery in order to establish acceptable fluid and electrolyte balance [84]. Critically, care must be taken to maintain an acceptable blood pressure during dialysis as rapid shifts in intravascular volume can promote significant fluctuations in blood pressure that may not be tolerated by patients with severe obstructive coronary disease.

Another disadvantage of CABG is the potential deleterious impact on renal function. Patients with advanced renal impairment run a greater risk of developing

Table 19.3 Factors complicating CABG in ESRD

Factors complicating CABG in ESRD
Co-morbidities e.g. diabetes, hypertension [69]
Increased risk of infection and sepsis [37, 47]
Left ventricular hypertrophy and conduction abnormalities [85]
Fluid and electrolyte disturbances [86]
Increased medial vascular calcification complicating anastomoses [87] and surgical manipulation of the aorta
Increased O_2 demands from renal anemia, AV fistula
Decreased patency of vein grafts [88]
Altered platelet activity
Complex coronary anatomy: severe distal disease [89], multivessel disease, calcified lesion

ESRD than those undergoing PCI, however the risk of mortality still outweighs the risk of ESRD [47, 90].

Despite the increased risk of morbidity and mortality seen in patients with ESRD, the absolute risk is still considered acceptable among many surgeons. In addition, the excellent symptomatic relief and improvements in functional status provided by CABG make it a very attractive choice for many patients [91]. Finally, a significant benefit of CABG over PCI is its increased efficacy in diabetic patients [36]. Diabetes is a common comorbidity of ESRD and has an additive impact in predicting adverse cardiac outcomes, particularly post-PCI [92]. In addition, CABG reduces long-term mortality in patients with triple vessel and left main disease, an effect that was observed in patients with either one of these pathologies in conjunction with dialysis treatment by Marui et al. [43]. The FREEDOM trial, which examined patients with diabetes and multivessel disease found that CABG reduced the rate of death, MI and stroke as compared to those undergoing PCI with DES [93].

Optimal Medical Management

Not all patients with severe renal impairment are candidates for invasive treatment of treat CAD. Indeed, a considerable proportion of patients with ESRD are still managed pharmacologically. Despite this, studies examining the optimal medical regime for CAD in these patients are limited.

Several randomized trials have indicated that PCI does not confer a survival advantage over medical therapy alone in patients with chronic renal impairment, although symptomatic relief is more marked in those undergoing invasive management [94–96]. Notably, a trend in improved survival begins to arise with greater vessel involvement and more complex disease, which is a common feature of CAD in ESRD [95, 97, 98].

With regards to specific pharamacotherapies, current guidelines indicate that although patients are at an increased risk of bleeding, the medical regime should be the same as in those with preserved renal function [4, 31]. It is important to remember that the data informing these guidelines are largely derived from studies that either exclude those with ESRD or are conducted in small patient groups, usually retrospectively. At present, emergent PCI is preferred over thrombolysis in patients presenting with ACS but there lacks sufficient controlled data to draw a definitive conclusion [31].

Conclusion

1. Ultimately, the optimal revascularization approach for obstructive CAD in stable or unstable coronary syndromes in CKD can only be properly addressed with future randomized trials enrolling large numbers of patients with significant renal impairment.

2. Data incorporating contemporary stenting and surgical techniques, including the use of second generation DES and newer antithrombotic agents, is required to resolve this contentious clinical issue.
3. While CABG appears to be associated with better long-term survival and fewer long-term ischemic events than PCI, the choice of revascularization therapy should be individualized, taking into account patient co-morbidities, functional status, and preference.
4. Current literature regarding invasive management of CAD in ESRD is limited to observational, retrospective trials. Further research is needed incorporating larger patient populations with significant renal impairment.
5. The efficacy of novel stenting techniques and adjunct pharmacotherapy needs to be explored in patients with ESRD.
6. In an effort to overcome therapeutic nihilism, physicians should endeavor to implement evidence based therapies in patients with ESRD.

References

1. Sarnak MJ, Levey AS, Schoolwerth AC, Coresh J, Culleton B, Hamm LL, et al. Kidney disease as a risk factor for development of cardiovascular disease: a statement from the American Heart Association Councils on Kidney in Cardiovascular Disease, High Blood Pressure Research, Clinical Cardiology, and Epidemiology and Prevention. Circulation. 2003;108(17):2154–69.
2. Chen J, Muntner P, Hamm LL, Jones DW, Batuman V, Fonseca V, et al. The metabolic syndrome and chronic kidney disease in U.S. adults. Ann Intern Med. 2004;140(3):167–74.
3. Ix JH, Shlipak MG, Liu HH, Schiller NB, Whooley MA. Association between renal insufficiency and inducible ischemia in patients with coronary artery disease: the heart and soul study. J Am Soc Nephrol: JASN. 2003;14(12):3233–8.
4. Wright RS, Reeder GS, Herzog CA, Albright RC, Williams BA, Dvorak DL, et al. Acute myocardial infarction and renal dysfunction: a high-risk combination. Ann Intern Med. 2002;137(7):563–70.
5. Collins AJ, Foley RN, Chavers B, Gilbertson D, Herzog C, Johansen K, et al. 'United States Renal Data System 2011 Annual Data Report: Atlas of chronic kidney disease & end-stage renal disease in the United States. Am J Kidney Dis Off J Natl Kidney Found. 2012;59(1 Suppl 1): A7. e1–420.
6. Herzog CA. How to manage the renal patient with coronary heart disease: the agony and the ecstasy of opinion-based medicine. J Am Soc Nephrol: JASN. 2003;14(10):2556–72.
7. Longenecker JC, Coresh J, Powe NR, Levey AS, Fink NE, Martin A, et al. Traditional cardiovascular disease risk factors in dialysis patients compared with the general population: the CHOICE Study. J Am Soc Nephrol. 2002;13(7):1918–27.
8. Shroff GR, Solid CA, Herzog CA. Long-term survival and repeat coronary revascularization in dialysis patients after surgical and percutaneous coronary revascularization with drug-eluting and bare metal stents in the United States. Circulation (New York, NY). 2013;127(18):1861–9.
9. Tadros GM, Herzog CA. Percutaneous coronary intervention in chronic kidney disease patients. J Nephrol. 2004;17(3):364–8.
10. Coca SG, Krumholz HM, Garg AX, Parikh CR. Underrepresentation of renal disease in randomized controlled trials of cardiovascular disease. JAMA. 2006;296(11):1377–84.
11. McCullough PA. Cardiorenal risk: an important clinical intersection. Rev Cardiovasc Med. 2002;3(2):71–6.

12. Manjunath G, Tighiouart H, Ibrahim H, MacLeod B, Salem DN, Griffith JL, et al. Level of kidney function as a risk factor for atherosclerotic cardiovascular outcomes in the community. J Am Coll Cardiol. 2003;41(1):47–55.
13. Baber U, Stone GW, Weisz G, Moreno P, Dangas G, Maehara A, et al. Coronary plaque composition, morphology, and outcomes in patients with and without chronic kidney disease presenting with acute coronary syndromes. JACC Cardiovasc Imaging. 2012;5(3 Suppl):S53–61.
14. Charytan D, Kuntz RE, Mauri L, DeFilippi C. Distribution of coronary artery disease and relation to mortality in asymptomatic hemodialysis patients. Am J Kidney Dis. 2007;49(3):409–16.
15. Joki N, Hase H, Takahashi Y, Ishikawa H, Nakamura R, Imamura Y, et al. Angiographical severity of coronary atherosclerosis predicts death in the first year of hemodialysis. Int Urol Nephrol. 2003;35(2):289–97.
16. Wizemann V. Coronary artery disease in dialysis patients. Nephron. 1996;74(4):642–51.
17. Lindner A, Charra B, Sherrard DJ, Scribner BH. Accelerated atherosclerosis in prolonged maintenance hemodialysis. N Engl J Med. 1974;290(13):697–701.
18. Cheung AK, Sarnak MJ, Yan G, Berkoben M, Heyka R, Kaufman A, et al. Cardiac diseases in maintenance hemodialysis patients: results of the HEMO Study. Kidney Int. 2004;65(6):2380–9.
19. Joki N, Hase H, Nakamura R, Yamaguchi T. Onset of coronary artery disease prior to initiation of haemodialysis in patients with end-stage renal disease. Nephrol Dial Transpl Off Publ Eur Dial Transplant Assoc – Eur Renal Assoc. 1997;12(4):718–23.
20. Foley RN, Herzog CA, Collins AJ. Blood pressure and long-term mortality in United States hemodialysis patients: USRDS Waves 3 and 4 Study. Kidney Int. 2002;62(5):1784–90.
21. Di Benedetto A, Marcelli D, D'Andrea A, Cice G, D'Isa S, Cappabianca F, et al. Risk factors and underlying cardiovascular diseases in incident ESRD patients. J Nephrol. 2005;18(5):592–8.
22. Aggarwal A, Kabbani SS, Rimmer JM, Gennari FJ, Taatjes DJ, Sobel BE, et al. Biphasic effects of hemodialysis on platelet reactivity in patients with end-stage renal disease: a potential contributor to cardiovascular risk. Am J Kidney Dis. 2002;40(2):315–22.
23. Sreedhara R, Itagaki I, Lynn B, Hakim RM. Defective platelet aggregation in uremia is transiently worsened by hemodialysis. Am J Kidney Dis Off J Natl Kidney Found. 1995;25(4):555–63.
24. Schindler R, Boenisch O, Fischer C, Frei U. Effect of the hemodialysis membrane on the inflammatory reaction in vivo. Clin Nephrol. 2000;53(6):452–9.
25. Weigert AL, Schafer AI. Uremic bleeding: pathogenesis and therapy. Am J Med Sci. 1998;316(2):94–104.
26. Raine AE, Margreiter R, Brunner FP, Ehrich JH, Geerlings W, Landais P, et al. Report on management of renal failure in Europe, XXII, 1991. Nephrol Dial Transpl Off Publ Eur Dial Transplant Assoc – Eur Renal Assoc. 1992;7 Suppl 2:7–35.
27. Aronow WS, Ahn C, Mercando AD, Epstein S. Prognostic significance of silent ischemia in elderly patients with peripheral arterial disease with and without previous myocardial infarction. Am J Cardiol. 1992;69(1):137–9.
28. Bansal N. Clinically silent myocardial infarctions in the CKD community. Nephrol Dial Transplant. 2012;27(9):3387–91.
29. Nesto RW, Watson FS, Kowalchuk GJ, Zarich SW, Hill T, Lewis SM, et al. Silent myocardial ischemia and infarction in diabetics with peripheral vascular disease: assessment by dipyridamole thallium-201 scintigraphy. Am Heart J. 1990;120(5):1073–7.
30. Surana SP, Riella LV, Keithi-Reddy SR, Charytan DM, Singh AK. Acute coronary syndrome in ESRD patients. Kidney Int. 2009;75(5):558–62.
31. K/DOQI Workgroup. K/DOQI clinical practice guidelines for cardiovascular disease in dialysis patients. Am J Kidney Dis. 2005;45(4 Suppl 3):16–153.
32. Levine GN, Bates ER, Blankenship JC, Bailey SR, Bittl JA, Cercek B, et al. 2011 ACCF/AHA/SCAI Guideline for Percutaneous Coronary Intervention: executive summary: a report of the

American College of Cardiology Foundation/American Heart Association Task Force on Practice Guidelines and the Society for Cardiovascular Angiography and Interventions. Circulation. 2011;124(23):2574–609.

33. Serruys PW, Morice M-C, Kappetein AP, Colombo A, Holmes DR, Mack MJ, et al. Percutaneous coronary intervention versus coronary-artery bypass grafting for severe coronary artery disease. N Engl J Med. 2009;360(10):961–72.

34. Zheng H, Xue S, Lian F, Huang R-t, Z-I H, Wang Y-Y. Meta-analysis of clinical studies comparing coronary artery bypass grafting with percutaneous coronary intervention in patients with end-stage renal disease. Eur J Cardiothorac Surg. 2013;43(3):459–67.

35. Ix JH, Mercado N, Shlipak MG, Lemos PA, Boersma E, Lindeboom W, et al. Association of chronic kidney disease with clinical outcomes after coronary revascularization: the Arterial Revascularization Therapies Study (ARTS). Am Heart J. 2005;149(3):512–9.

36. Herzog CA, Ma JZ, Collins AJ. Comparative survival of dialysis patients in the United States after coronary angioplasty, coronary artery stenting, and coronary artery bypass surgery and impact of diabetes. Circulation. 2002;106(17):2207–11.

37. Agirbasli M, Weintraub WS, Chang GL, King SB, Guyton RA, Thompson TD, et al. Outcome of coronary revascularization in patients on renal dialysis. Am J Cardiol. 2000;86(4):395–9.

38. Hemmelgarn BR. Survival after coronary revascularization among patients with kidney disease. Circulation (New York, NY). 2004;110(14):1890–5.

39. Rinehart AL. A comparison of coronary angioplasty and coronary artery bypass grafting outcomes in chronic dialysis patients. Am J Kidney Dis. 1995;25(2):281–90.

40. Ohmoto Y, Ayabe M, Hara K, Sugimoto T, Tagawa H, Fukuda S, et al. Long-term outcome of percutaneous transluminal coronary angioplasty and coronary artery bypass grafting in patients with end-stage renal disease. Jpn Circ J. 1999;63(12):981–7.

41. Nevis IF, Mathew A, Novick RJ, Parikh CR, Devereaux PJ, Natarajan MK, et al. Optimal method of coronary revascularization in patients receiving dialysis: systematic review. Clin J Am Soc Nephrol. 2009;4(2):369–78.

42. Kannan A, Poongkunran C, Medina R, Ramanujam V, Poongkunran M, Balamuthusamy S. Coronary revascularization in chronic and end-stage renal disease: a systematic review and meta-analysis. Am J Ther. 2014.

43. Marui A, Kimura T, Nishiwaki N, Mitsudo K, Komiya T, Hanyu M, et al. Percutaneous coronary intervention versus coronary artery bypass grafting in patients with end-stage renal disease requiring dialysis (5-year outcomes of the CREDO-Kyoto PCI/CABG Registry Cohort-2). Am J Cardiol. 2014;114(4):555–61.

44. King 3rd SB, Marshall JJ, Tummala PE. Revascularization for coronary artery disease: stents versus bypass surgery. Annu Rev Med. 2010;61:199–213.

45. Kar S, Coats W, Aggarwal K. Percutaneous coronary intervention versus coronary artery bypass graft in chronic kidney disease: optimal treatment options. Hemodial Int Int Symp Home Hemodial. 2011;15 Suppl 1:S30–6.

46. Anderson RJ, O'Brien M, MaWhinney S, VillaNueva CB, Moritz TE, Sethi GK, et al. Renal failure predisposes patients to adverse outcome after coronary artery bypass surgery. VA Cooperative Study #5. Kidney Int. 1999;55(3):1057–62.

47. Cooper WA, O'Brien SM, Thourani VH, Guyton RA, Bridges CR, Szczech LA, et al. Impact of renal dysfunction on outcomes of coronary artery bypass surgery: results from the Society of Thoracic Surgeons National Adult Cardiac Database. Circulation. 2006;113(8):1063–70.

48. Gibbons RJ, Fihn SD. Coronary revascularization: new evidence, new challenges. Ann Intern Med. 2007;147(10):732–4.

49. Deo SV, Shah IK, Dunlay SM, Erwin PJ, Dillon JM, Park SJ. Myocardial revascularisation in renal dysfunction: a systematic review and meta-analysis. Heart Lung Circ. 2013;22(10):827–35.

50. Herzog CA, Ma JZ, Collins AJ. Long-term outcome of dialysis patients in the United States with coronary revascularization procedures. Kidney Int. 1999;56(1):324–32.

51. Herzog CA, Ma JZ, Collins AJ. Poor long-term survival after acute myocardial infarction among patients on long-term dialysis. N Engl J Med. 1998;339(12):799–805.

52. Bassand JP, Hamm CW, Ardissino D, Boersma E, Budaj A, Fernandez-Aviles F, et al. Guidelines for the diagnosis and treatment of non-ST-segment elevation acute coronary syndromes. Eur Heart J. 2007;28(13):1598–660.
53. Szummer K, Lundman P, Jacobson SH, Schon S, Lindback J, Stenestrand U, et al. Influence of renal function on the effects of early revascularization in non-ST-elevation myocardial infarction: data from the Swedish Web-System for Enhancement and Development of Evidence-Based Care in Heart Disease Evaluated According to Recommended Therapies (SWEDEHEART). Circulation. 2009;120(10):851–8.
54. Amsterdam EA, Wenger NK, Brindis RG, Casey DE, Ganiats TG, Holmes DR, et al. 2014 AHA/ACC Guideline for the Management of Patients with Non-ST-Elevation Acute Coronary Syndromes: a report of the American College of Cardiology/American Heart Association Task Force on Practice Guidelines. Circulation. 2014;130(25):2354–94.
55. Januzzi JL, Cannon CP, DiBattiste PM, Murphy S, Weintraub W, Braunwald E. Effects of renal insufficiency on early invasive management in patients with acute coronary syndromes (The TACTICS-TIMI 18 Trial). Am J Cardiol. 2002;90(11):1246–9.
56. Lagerqvist B, Husted S, Kontny F, Stahle E, Swahn E, Wallentin L. 5-year outcomes in the FRISC-II randomised trial of an invasive versus a non-invasive strategy in non-ST-elevation acute coronary syndrome: a follow-up study. Lancet. 2006;368(9540):998–1004.
57. Damman P, Hirsch A, Windhausen F, Tijssen JGP, de Winter RJ. 5-year clinical outcomes in the ICTUS (Invasive versus Conservative Treatment in Unstable coronary Syndromes) Trial a randomized comparison of an early invasive versus selective invasive management in patients with non–ST-segment elevation acute coronary syndrome. J Am Coll Cardiol. 2010;55(9):858–64.
58. Woudstra P, Damman P, Clayton T, Wallentin L, Lagerqvist B, Fox K, et al. Routine invasive versus selective invasive strategy and long-term outcomes in patients with reduced renal function presenting with non-ST-segment elevation acute coronary syndrome. J Am Coll Cardiol. 2012;59(13 Suppl 1):E392–E.
59. Santopinto JJ, Fox KAA, Goldberg RJ, Budaj A, Piñero G, Avezum A, et al. Creatinine clearance and adverse hospital outcomes in patients with acute coronary syndromes: findings from the global registry of acute coronary events (GRACE). Heart. 2003;89(9):1003–8.
60. Anavekar NS, McMurray JJV, Velazquez EJ, Solomon SD, Kober L, Rouleau J-L, et al. Relation between renal dysfunction and cardiovascular outcomes after myocardial infarction. N Engl J Med. 2004;351(13):1285–95.
61. Rihal CS, Textor SC, Grill DE, Berger PB, Ting HH, Best PJ, et al. Incidence and prognostic importance of acute renal failure after percutaneous coronary intervention. Circulation. 2002;105(19):2259–64.
62. Chen Y-Y, Wang J-F, Zhang Y-J, Xie S-L, Nie R-Q. Optimal strategy of coronary revascularization in chronic kidney disease patients: a meta-analysis. Eur J Intern Med. 2013;24(4):354–61.
63. Best PJM, Lennon R, Ting HH, Bell MR, Rihal CS, Holmes Jr DR, et al. The impact of renal insufficiency on clinical outcomes in patients undergoing percutaneous coronary interventions. J Am Coll Cardiol. 2002;39(7):1113–9.
64. Reddan DN, Szczech LA, Tuttle RH, Shaw LK, Jones RH, Schwab SJ, et al. Chronic kidney disease, mortality, and treatment strategies among patients with clinically significant coronary artery disease. J Am Soc Nephrol: JASN. 2003;14(9):2373–80.
65. Best PJ, Berger PB, Davis BR, Grines CL, Sadeghi HM, Williams BA, et al. Impact of mild or moderate chronic kidney disease on the frequency of restenosis: results from the PRESTO trial. J Am Coll Cardiol. 2004;44(9):1786–91.
66. Osten MD, Ivanov J, Eichhofer J, Seidelin PH, Ross JR, Barolet A, et al. Impact of renal insufficiency on angiographic, procedural, and in-hospital outcomes following percutaneous coronary intervention. Am J Cardiol. 2008;101(6):780–5.
67. El-Menyar AA, Al Suwaidi J, Holmes Jr DR. Use of drug-eluting stents in patients with coronary artery disease and renal insufficiency. Mayo Clin Proc. 2010;85(2):165–71.

68. Krotin M, Vukovic D, Stojanovic O, Milovanovic B, Celeketic D, Blagojevic R. Prognostic value of dobutamine stress echocardiography in patients with terminal renal insufficiency undergoing hemodialysis--a 5-year follow up. Med Pregl. 2007;60(7–8):333–7.

69. Francis GS, Sharma B, Collins AL, Helseth HK, Comty CM. Coronary-artery surgery in patients with end-stage renal disease. Ann Intern Med. 1980;92(4):499–503.

70. Gruberg L, Dangas G, Mehran R, Mintz GS, Kent KM, Pichard AD, et al. Clinical outcome following percutaneous coronary interventions in patients with chronic renal failure. Catheter Cardiovasc Interv Off J Soc Card Angiogr Interv. 2002;55(1):66–72.

71. Tsutsui M, Shimokawa H, Tanaka S, Yoshihara S, Higuchi S, Matsuguchi T, et al. Granulocyte activation in restenosis after percutaneous transluminal coronary angioplasty. Jpn Circ J. 1996;60(1):27–34.

72. Mehran R, Aymong ED, Nikolsky E, Lasic Z, Iakovou I, Fahy M, et al. A simple risk score for prediction of contrast-induced nephropathy after percutaneous coronary intervention: development and initial validation. J Am Coll Cardiol. 2004;44(7):1393–9.

73. Athappan G, Ponniah T. Clinical outcomes of dialysis patients after implantation of DES: meta analysis and systematic review of literature. Minerva Cardioangiol. 2009;57(3):291–7.

74. Baber U, Mehran R, Sharma SK, Brar S, Yu J, Suh JW, et al. Impact of the everolimus-eluting stent on stent thrombosis: a meta-analysis of 13 randomized trials. J Am Coll Cardiol. 2011;58(15):1569–77.

75. Manabe S, Shimokawa T, Fukui T, Fumimoto KU, Ozawa N, Seki H, et al. Coronary artery bypass surgery versus percutaneous coronary artery intervention in patients on chronic hemodialysis: does a drug-eluting stent have an impact on clinical outcome? J Card Surg. 2009;24(3):234–9.

76. Hiremath S. Antiplatelet medications in hemodialysis patients: a systematic review of bleeding rates. Clin J Am Soc Nephrol. 2009;4(8):1347–55.

77. Tsai TT, Maddox TM, Roe MT, et al. Contraindicated medication use in dialysis patients undergoing percutaneous coronary intervention. JAMA. 2009;302(22):2458–64.

78. Alexander KP, Chen AY, Roe MT, et al. EXcess dosing of antiplatelet and antithrombin agents in the treatment of non–st-segment elevation acute coronary syndromes. JAMA. 2005;294(24):3108–16.

79. Liu JY, Birkmeyer NJO, Sanders JH, Morton JR, Henriques HF, Lahey SJ, et al. Risks of morbidity and mortality in dialysis patients undergoing coronary artery bypass surgery. Circulation. 2000;102(24):2973–7.

80. Sezai A, Nakata K, Hata M, Yoshitake I, Wakui S, Hata H, et al. Long-term results of dialysis patients with chronic kidney disease undergoing coronary artery bypass grafting. Ann Thoracic Cardiovasc Surg Off J Assoc Thorac Cardiovasc Surg Asia. 2013;19(6):441–8.

81. Beckermann J, Van Camp J, Li S, Wahl SK, Collins A, Herzog CA. On-pump versus off-pump coronary surgery outcomes in patients requiring dialysis: perspectives from a single center and the United States experience. J Thorac Cardiovasc Surg. 2006;131(6):1261–6.

82. Shroff GR, Li S, Herzog CA. Survival of patients on dialysis having off-pump versus on-pump coronary artery bypass surgery in the United States. J Thorac Cardiovasc Surg. 2010;139(5):1333–8.

83. Labrousse L, de Vincentiis C, Madonna F, Deville C, Roques X, Baudet E. Early and long term results of coronary artery bypass grafts in patients with dialysis dependent renal failure. Eur J Cardiothorac Surg Off J Eur Assoc Cardiothorac Surg. 1999;15(5):691–6.

84. Castelli P, Condemi A, Munari M. Immediate and long-term results of coronary revascularization in patients undergoing chronic hemodialysis. Eur J Cardiothorac Surg. 1999;15(1):51–4.

85. Middleton RJ, Parfrey PS, Foley RN. Left ventricular hypertrophy in the renal patient. J Am Soc Nephrol: JASN. 2001;12(5):1079–84.

86. Salem MM, Mujais S. Coronary revascularization in dialysis patients: the need for vigilance. Int J Artif Organs. 1991;14(1):7–9.

87. Lockhart ME, Robbin ML, McNamara MM, Allon M. Association of pelvic arterial calcification with arteriovenous thigh graft failure in haemodialysis patients. Nephrol Dial Transplant Off Publ Eur Dial Transplant Assoc – Eur Renal Assoc. 2004;19(10):2564–9.
88. Crawford FA, Selby JH, Bower JD, Lehan PH. Coronary revascularization in patients maintained on chronic hemodialysis. Circulation. 1977;56(4):684–7.
89. Franga DL, Kratz JM, Crumbley AJ, Zellner JL, Stroud MR, Crawford FA. Early and long-term results of coronary artery bypass grafting in dialysis patients. Ann Thorac Surg. 2000;70(3):813–8. discussion 9.
90. Charytan DM, Li S, Liu J, Herzog CA. Risks of death and end-stage renal disease after surgical compared with percutaneous coronary revascularization in elderly patients with chronic kidney disease. Circulation. 2012;126(11 Suppl 1):S164–9.
91. Owen CH. Coronary artery bypass grafting in patients with dialysis-dependent renal failure. Ann Thorac Surg. 1994;58(6):1729–33.
92. Baber U, Mehran R, Kirtane AJ, Christodoulidis G, Maehara A, Witzenbichler B, et al. TCT-486 additive and independent impact of chronic kidney disease and diabetes mellitus on high platelet reactivity and adverse events following PCI: results from the ADAPT-DES registry. J Am Coll Cardiol. 2014;64(11_S).
93. Farkouh ME, Domanski M, Sleeper LA, Siami FS, Dangas G, Mack M, et al. Strategies for multivessel revascularization in patients with diabetes. N Engl J Med. 2012;367(25):2375–84.
94. Parisi AF, Folland ED, Hartigan P. A comparison of angioplasty with medical therapy in the treatment of single-vessel coronary artery disease. Veterans Affairs ACME Investigators. N Engl J Med. 1992;326(1):10–6.
95. RITA-2 Trial Participants. Coronary angioplasty versus medical therapy for angina: the second Randomised Intervention Treatment of Angina (RITA-2) trial. Lancet. 1997;350(9076):461–8.
96. Hueb WABG, de Oliveira SA, Arie S, de Albuquerque CP, Jatene AD, Pileggi F. The Medicine, Angioplasty or Surgery Study (MASS): a prospective, randomized trial of medical therapy, balloon angioplasty or bypass surgery for single proximal left anterior descending artery stenoses. J Am Coll Cardiol. 1995;26(7):1600–5.
97. Yasuda K, Kasuga H, Aoyama T, Takahashi H, Toriyama T, Kawade Y, et al. Comparison of percutaneous coronary intervention with medication in the treatment of coronary artery disease in hemodialysis patients. J Am Soc Nephrol. 2006;17(8):2322–32.
98. Mark DB, Nelson CL, Califf RM, Harrell Jr FE, Lee KL, Jones RH, Fortin DF, Stack RS, Glower DD, Smith LR, et al. Continuing evolution of therapy for coronary artery disease. Initial results from the era of coronary angioplasty. Circulation. 1994;89(5):2015–25.

Chapter 20
What Is the Optimal Stent Design? – The Pathologist's Opinion

Hiroyoshi Mori, Kazuyuki Yahagi, Renu Virmani, Michael Joner, and Aloke V. Finn

Abstract More than 5 millions stents have been implanted in patients all over the world and it is estimated that the number will increase to 6.6 million by 2020. It has been almost 30 years since the first stent was implanted in man. Initially, stents were mainly used for bail out in patients with acute occlusion due to coronary dissection following balloon angioplasty. The first stents were typically mounted on high profile, rigid delivery platforms and were difficult to deploy, leading to acute/subacute stent thrombosis. Greater understanding of the need for effective antiplatelet therapy and also improvement in delivery and better stent designs helped to overcome early stent thrombosis. The resulting lower rates of restenosis as compared to balloon angioplasty propelled the use of stents in routine practice. However, restenosis was the "Achilles heel" of bare metal stents and the birth of drug eluting stents (DES) helped dramatically reduce restenosis but late stent thrombosis became an issue. Second generation DES have reduced the incidence of late stent thrombosis however, one of the mechanisms of late stent thrombosis is the development of atherosclerosis within the stented segment ("neoatherosclerosis"), which remains an issue because its development is increased in DES compared to BMS. Recently, third generation DES, using bioabsorbable polymer rather than permanent polymer to deliver drug and fully biodegradable vascular scaffolds are available. Many believe that these will overcome the drawback of stenting as no permanent metal or polymer will be left behind. Studies in animals show that when bioabsorbable polymers are used the endothelial lining is far more competent as compared to permanent polymers that have been shown to induce hypersensitivity reaction. Also, clinical studies have shown that bioabsorbable polymers induce less late thrombosis as compared to permanent polymers. Similarly, in fully bioabsorbable scaffolds, the vascular reactivity and lumen enlargement are seen between 1 and 2 years after implantation and

H. Mori, MD • K. Yahagi, MD • R. Virmani, MD (✉) • M. Joner, MD, CEO
CVPath Institute, Inc., 19 Firstfield Road, Gaithersburg, MD 20878, USA
e-mail: hmori@cvpath.org; kyahagi@cvpath.org; rvirmani@cvpath.org; mjoner@cvpath.org

A.V. Finn, MD
Department of Internal Medicine, Emory University School of Medicine,
101 Woodruff Circle, WMB, 319B, Atlanta, GA 30322, USA
e-mail: avfinn@emory.edu

© Springer International Publishing Switzerland 2015
J.A. Ambrose, A.E. Rodríguez (eds.), *Controversies in Cardiology*,
DOI 10.1007/978-3-319-20415-4_20

the polymers get replaced by proteoglycan matrix and collagen over time and that mild to moderate inflammation is associated with vessel enlargement. Overall what remains unclear is that bulky scaffolds ≥150 μm thickness may be associated again with greater late stent thrombosis. Therefore, we have to remain vigilant that we do not implant these fully bioabsorbable polymeric scaffolds in patients presenting with acute myocardial infarction until clearly clinical trials prove their safety.

Keywords Stent • BMS • DES • Neoatherosclerosis • Stent thrombosis • Delayed healing • Hypersensitivity

Introduction

The most frequent cause of death, in the Western World for the last century has remained coronary heart disease. Until the introduction of percutaneous balloon angioplasty in the late 1970s followed by the placement of intracoronary stents to prevent acute closure in the mid 1980s, treatment of coronary artery disease remained medical therapy and surgical coronary bypass grafting usually with the use of saphenous veins as conduits. Now almost 30 years after the first stent technology was reported by Sigwart et al. [1] and especially since the introduction of drug eluting stents (DES) in Europe in 2002, and the USA in 2004, we are now able to claim that the first line of treatment for coronary artery disease is percutaneous coronary intervention procedures [2].

Stenting of coronary arteries was introduced to prevent acute threatened closure from thrombosis and dissection and late restenosis after plain old balloon angioplasty (POBA). Ultimately, randomized trials showed that stent implantation was superior to POBA with a reduction in restenosis [3]. However, early work in coronary stenting when assessed in a core laboratory was associated with a high mortality at 1-year of 7.6 %, subacute thrombosis of 6.7 %, and restenosis of 32 % in patients who received a Wallstent [4]. Nonetheless, it did reduce the incidence of emergent bypass grafting as compared to balloon angioplasty [5]. Similarly, post-procedure bleeding was also an issue, due to the intense combination of anticoagulation (warfarin) and anti-platelet agents used to prevent stent thrombosis. The use of dual antiplatelet therapy with aspirin and ticlopidine [6] reduced not only bleeding complications but also stent associated thrombus [7]. All these difficulties were ultimately overcome with the Belgium Netherland Stent Arterial Revascularization Therapies Study (BENESTENT) and the North American Stent Restenosis Study (STRESS), which demonstrated the superiority of BMS as compared to POBA, and stenting became the standard of care with better, thinner, less visible, and more biocompatible stents being developed [3, 8].

Early reperfusion had been shown in animal models to reduce infarct size and it became the corner stone of treating patients presenting with acute myocardial infarction and STEMI with thrombolytic agents. However, many trails showed that POBA had better results as compared to thrombolysis but achieving TIMI flow >2 remained the "Achilles heel" of POBA along with abrupt closure before hospital discharge as well as high restenosis rates at 6 months [9]. PAMI was the first large randomized study comparing stenting to POBA in patients presenting with AMI and it showed that death, re-infarction, disabling stroke, or target-vessel revascularization occurred in fewer patients in the stent arm than in POBA (7.7 % vs. 17.0 %, p=0.01) [10]. Today emergent stenting of patients presenting with AMI is the standard of care.

During the era of BMS it was appreciated that ease of use, deliverability, strut thickness, stent design (open-cell or closed cell), visibility and restenosis were all important to the success of long-term stenting in patients. Because of the high rate of restenosis in BMS, drug-eluting stents (DES) with antiproliferative coatings were introduced and in randomized trials in stable patients showed dramatic reductions in restenosis rates [2]. This eventually also lead to their application in even more complex lesions [11]. However, recurrent problems of late catch up and stent thrombosis in the first generation DES made us aware that we should be cautious in their use in complex patients [12]. We have shown that the main mechanism by which DES reduced restenosis was by delayed arterial healing [13, 14]. Also, the sirolimus eluting Cypher stent was associated with hypersensitivity reactions to the polymer whereas the paclitaxel eluting DES Taxus stents were associated with excessive fibrin deposition and malapposition with late stent thrombosis. Second generation DES have thinner struts, are more biocompatible and thinner polymer coatings and less drug. These design changes have shown both clinically and pathologically to have less late stent thrombosis and better stent coverage [15, 16]. The third generation of DES uses even thinner struts with bioabsorable polymer to deliver drugs, with the drug and polymer disappearing within 3–6 months leaving behind a bare metal stent. Finally, fully biodegradable vascular scaffolds have emerged to avoid these late adverse effects of metallic stents by fully degrading by 2–4 years and have resulted in the return of vasomotion within 1–2 years as well as vessel remodeling with lumen enlargement [17].

Stent Configuration and Thickness

Stents have been divided in two groups based on the configuration of the stent. These are the coil and the slotted tube stents. Wiktor stent (Medtronic, Minneapolis, MN), Gianturco-Roubin Flex/GR-2 (Cook, Bloomington, IN) stent and GFX (Applied Vascular Engineering, Santa Rosa, CA) were examples of coil stents. Palmaz-Shatz/PS stent (Cordis, Johnson & Johnson, Warren, NJ) and Multi-Link (Advanced Cardiovascular Systems) were slotted tube stents and the Palmaz-Shatz was the first stent that showed superiority to POBA in a randomized trial. Coil stent designs were very flexible and allowed side branch access. But radial force was weak and they had more recoil and more tissue prolapse as compared to the slotted tube. These concerns resulted in inferior outcomes of coil stents compared to slotted tube stents in randomized trials [18]. GR-II stents also had a higher stent thrombosis rate (3.9 % vs. 0.5 %, P<0.001) and higher restenosis rates (47.3 % vs. 20.6 %, P<0.001) compared to the PS stent [18].

A preclinical study showed that artery geometry after stent deployment determined neointimal thickness [19]. In this study, stents designed with 12 struts per cross section had 50–60 % less mural thrombus and two-fold less neointimal area than identical stents with only eight struts per cross section. Thus, it is ideal that polygonal luminal shape post stent implantation be more close to circular as compared to one with eight struts, and therefore will have less neointimal growth. Also, the extent of injury as well as the extent of inflammation determine neointimal thickness and % stenosis following stent placement [20, 21].

Stent configuration can be divided into open-cell and close-cell stent types. In curved vessels, closed-cell stent struts open evenly while open-cell stent open more widely in the outer curvature and are narrower in the inner curvature [22], allowing better configuration at bends of arteries. In other words, when used in a curved situation, open-cell stent are thought to expand more unevenly than closed-cell stents. On the other hand, conformability and deliverability is better in open-cell stents than closed-cell stent. Stent fracture is less in open-cell stents than in closed-cell stents [23]. Side branch access is also easier in open-cell stent than closed-cell stents [24]. Nowadays, open-cell stents are preferred to closed-cell stent in coronary intervention. In peripheral artery disease, closed-cell stents are widely used because they are more likely to prevent plaque protrusion.

Many studies have previously shown superiority of thin strut stents compared to thick strut stents. Thick struts provide more radial force and better arterial support with greater vessel injury inducing more neointimal growth. ISAR-STEREO trial compared thin strut stents to thick strut stents and showed a significant reduction in angiographic and clinical restenosis with the use of the thinner-strut device following coronary artery stenting. They compared thinner stents (strut thickness of 50 μm, ACS RX Multi-Link, Guidant, Santa Clara, CA) with thicker stents (strut thickness of 140 μm, **BX Velocity**, **Cordis Corp**, **Miami**, **Florida**) in 651 patients. The angiographic in-stent restenosis (more than 50 % diameter stenosis at follow-up angiography) rates were 15.0 % in the thin-strut group and 25.8 % in the thick-strut group (P=0.003) [25]. Although strut thickness has been emphasized, configuration of the strut has not been emphasized to be of much importance. Jimenez et al. reported ideal strut design from computational fluid dynamics point of view [26]. They used two different geometries; rectangular 2:1, 4:1, and 8:1, and compared to circular arc 2:1, 4:1, and 8:1. The flatter the strut design the less the shear stress forces and the more circular the strut design, the less the shear stress. They showed that less shear stress prevented stent thrombosis. Contemporary stent designs are mainly square with few like the Driver design being circular.

Pathology

Pathophysiology of Vascular Healing Following BMS Implantation in Man

Before delving into DES it is important to understand the process of vascular healing after BMS implantation. The time course of reendothelialization and neointimal growth following stent deployment is different between animal species (e.g., in pig and rabbit) and human iliac and coronary arteries (Fig. 20.1a). In the human coronary

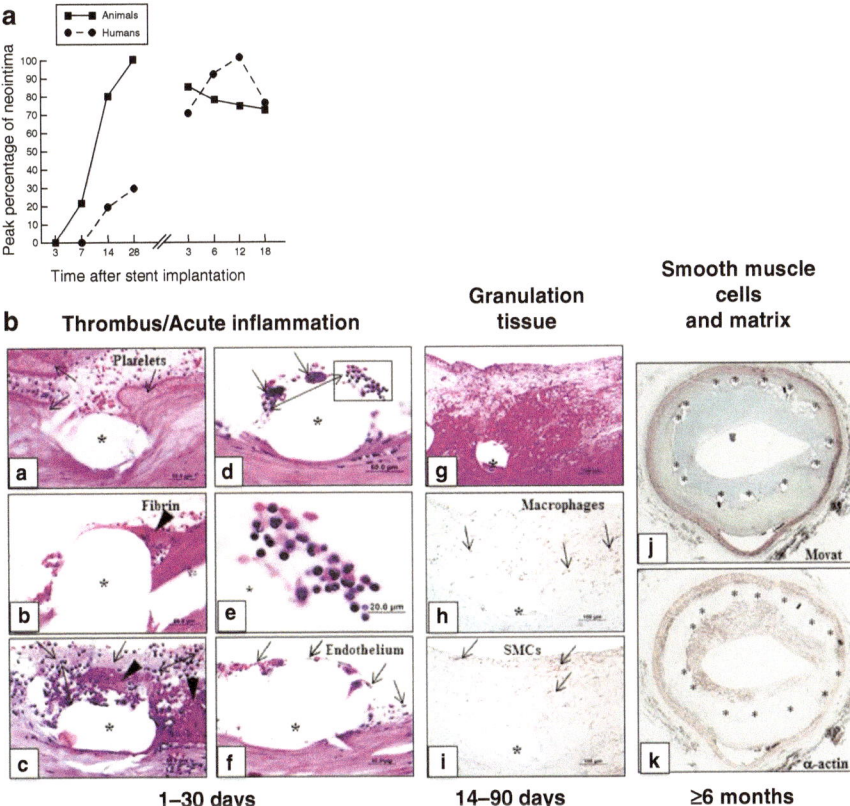

Fig. 20.1 (**a**) BMS healing in animals vs. humans. Line plot showing the temporal relation of peak neointimal growth in animals and humans following the placement of bare stainless steel stent. The plots are predominantly derived from morphometric analysis of pig and human coronary stents. In animals, peak neointimal growth in stainless steel stents is observed at 28 days, compared with 6–12 months in humans (Reproduced from Virmani et al. [31], with permission of BMJ Publishing Group Ltd). (**b**) Arterial healing following balloon expandable BMS implantation in human coronary arteries. (*a*) Platelet-rich thrombus (*arrows*) is identified around a stent strut (*) 1 day after the placement of Driver stent. (*b*) A fibrin-rich thrombus (*arrowhead*) is focally present around a stent strut 1 day after the placement of Express stent. (*c–f*) Platelet- (*arrow*) and fibrin- (*arrowheads*) rich thrombus (*c*) with numerous inflammatory cell infiltration around stent struts (*double arrows*, *c–e*) and focal endothelialization (*f*). Five days after the placement of Multi-Link Vison stent. Giant cells are occasionally observed (*arrows*, *d*). The presence of inflammatory cells consisting of neutrophils and lymphocytes (boxed area in *d*) are highlighted in (*d* and *g–i*). Early neointima presents 23 days after Multi-Link Vision stent placement. (*g*) Intimal cells within extracellular matrix seen above the stent strut. (*h*) KP-1 immunostaining identifying macrophages (*arrows*) adjacent to the strut at base of neointima. (*i*) Actin staining identifying smooth muscle cells close to luminal surface of neointima (*arrows*). (*j, k*). Smooth muscle cell-rich neointima in stented coronary artery (duration .6 months). Actin staining shows smooth muscle cells close to luminal surface of the neointima in (*i*). (*a–g*) are stained with haematoxylin and eosin, while (*j*) is stained with Movat pentachrome (Reproduced from Chaabane et al. [33], with permission of Oxford University Press)

arteries (Fig. 20.1b), platelet /fibrin deposition is the earliest change occurring within the first hours to few days. Up to 11 days, more than 70 % of stent sections show platelet deposition and aggregation [27]. At 12–30 days, platelet deposition and aggregation decreases to 24 % of sections examined, and by 30 days, platelet deposition is rarely observed. On the other hand, fibrin-rich thrombus is also seen around the struts. It was seen in every section until 11 days, and 19 % of sections at 12–30 days. Therefore, it is important and reasonable to provide intensive dual anti platelet therapy especially in the first 30 days following BMS implantation.

Inflammation

Acute and chronic inflammation is observed during the process of vascular healing (Fig. 20.1b). Acute inflammatory cells (neutrophils) are associated with stent struts and were observed in 79 % of sections within 3 days, 83 % of sections in 4–11 days, 72 % of sections in 12–30 days and 0 % after 30 days. Chronic inflammatory cells (lymphocytes and macrophages) around stent struts are also seen in 82 % of sections within 3 days, 67 % of sections in 4–11 days, 97 % of sections at 12–30 days and 85 % of sections after 30 days. Multinucleated giant cells were seen in only 10 % of sections at 12–30 days and 29 % of sections after 30 days. The extent of injury and the underlying plaque morphology were associated with the extent of inflammation. The cases that have medial disruption or necrotic core disruption showed a greater inflammatory response. Overall, the extent of inflammation correlated with neointimal growth [27].

SMC and Matrix

Migration and proliferation of smooth muscle cells promote organization of thrombus. From 12 to 30 days, approximately 50 % of cases showed smooth muscle cells. After 30 days, smooth muscle cells are seen in all cases. Initially, their appearance looks rhomboid in shape that gradually re-differentiate into contractile α-actin positive smooth muscle cells. There are mainly two theories about the source of smooth muscle cells. One is from medial smooth muscle cells, the other is from circulating progenitor cells [28, 29]. Up to 18 month after implantation, the neointima is rich in smooth muscle cells, type 3 collagen, proteoglycans and hyaluronan. Thereafter, smooth muscle cells tend to be more compact and align circularly towards the lumen with little matrix that is mainly type 1 collagen [30].

Endothelialization

The endothelium is denuded by ballooning and stenting. In the process of healing, neointimal coverage occurs gradually with 30 % of the stent surface area covered by endothelial cells at 1 month, and 80–100 % by 3–4 months following BMS deployment [14]. There are mainly two theories regarding the source of neointimal endothelial cells. One is from the proximal and distal non-treated segments and from branch points while the other is from circulating CD 34-positive progenitor cells. Both theories seems to contribute, however, we favor the former theory simply because re-endothelialization is greater in the proximal and distal ends than in the middle. This indicates that avoiding geographic miss (no injury to the non-stented segments) is important for re-endothelializaion to occur early [14].

Vascular Healing in Animal Models

On the other hand in animals, platelet/fibrin deposition is observed up to 3–7 days and granulation tissue is observed by 7 days consisting of smooth muscle cells, macrophages and scattered lymphocytes with luminal endothelial cells. At 14 days fibrin is still present with few chronic inflammatory cells and giant cells seen close to stent struts. At this stage smooth muscle cells within a proteoglycan matrix are observed over and between the struts, by 28-days the neointima contains a large number of smooth muscle cells, proteoglycans and collagen [31].

Mature Endothelial Cell

Mature endothelial cells have a complex set of junction proteins that help maintain the integrity of the endothelium that play a pivotal role in the regulation of its permeability and signal transduction. The endothelium provides vital anti-thrombotic and vasoprotective effects via the production of nitric oxide, prostacyclin, tissue plasminogen activator, thrombomodulin, heparin-like molecules, and tissue factor pathway inhibitor. Therefore, mature endothelial should be the ideal goal of re-endothelialization following stent placement. However, in the real world, this goal may not be achievable as the underlying plaque as well as risk factors in the individual patients may also play an important role [32].

Drug Eluting Stents – First, Second, and Third Generation

Prior to the introduction of DES, the concept of oral drug delivery to alter the neointimal response in the era of balloon angioplasty had failed, likely because our understanding of the mechanisms of neointimal growth was incomplete. We now know that smooth muscle cell proliferation and migration, along with the extent of thrombus, inflammation and injury are all important and that it is vital not to ignore any one of them. Although many cytokines and mediators are involved, the final common route is the entry of smooth muscle cells into the cell cycle pathway. Once activated the smooth muscle cells enter the cycle of cell division (G0, G1, S, G2 and M) where many factors control the rate and extent of proliferation, including cyclins that are required at different steps of the cell cycle along with cytokines and growth factors that control intracellular dependent phosphoinositide-dependent kinases and Akt. The latter is capable of phosphorylating the mammalian target of rapamycin [33] (Fig. 20.2).

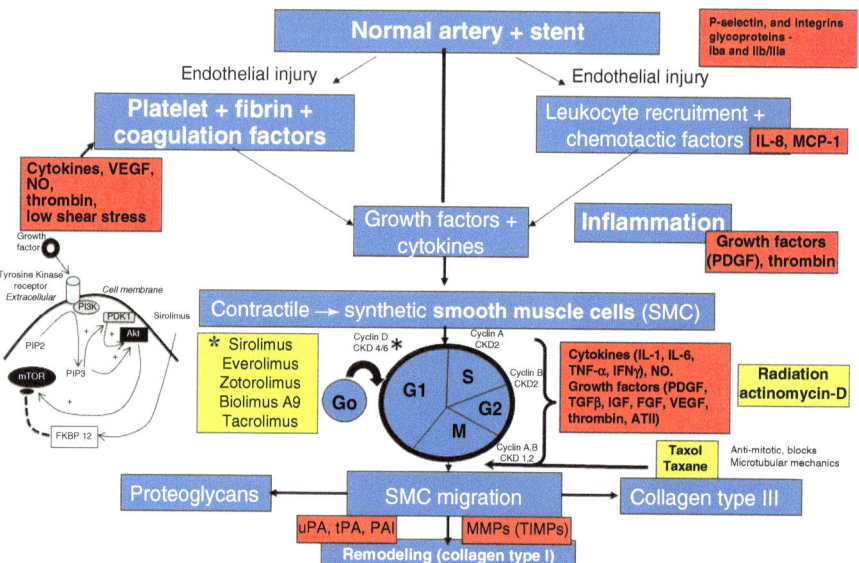

Fig. 20.2 Overview of the molecular mechanisms of restenosis and their inhibitors. The normal coronary artery is injured secondarily from ballooning and stenting resulting in endothelial cells (EC) loss followed by mural thrombus consisting of platelet aggregation with fibrin deposition. The platelets within the thrombus release a number of chemokines essential for the initiation of inflammation. This includes activation of P-selectin and integrins such as b2-integrin Mac-1 and thrombin. Local production of chemokines like interleukin (IL)-1, IL-6, interferon (IFNγ), and tumor necrosis factor-alpha (TNFα) by macrophages result in the induction of inflammation at the injury site. The injury is not only to the endothelium but also to the underlying medial wall. There is an imbalance between stimulatory growth factors (PDGF, FGF, TGF-β, and IGF-1) and chemokines and the inhibitory factors like endothelial-derived nitric oxide and heparin sulfate proteoglycans that result in the activation of smooth muscle cells (SMCs). The SMCs within the media transform from a quiescent contractile to a synthetic cell which not only proliferate but also migrate into the intima. Within the intima they further proliferate but also secrete extracellular matrix. SMC proliferation involves cell division with different cyclins that are required at different steps of the cell cycle. CDK (cyclin-dependent kinase) activity is also regulated by cell-cycle inhibitory proteins called cyclin-dependent kinase inhibitors (CKIs), which counteract CDK activity. SMC membranes are also stimulated by several classes of tyrosine kinase receptors (TKR). One of the intracellular signalling pathways involves the phosphatidylinositol (PI)3-kinase (PI3K) pathway. PI3K is a lipid kinase that phosphorylates PI. The dominant lipid product generated by PI3K—PI 3,4-biphosphate (PIP2) and PI 3,4,5-triphosphate (PIP3), the latter recruits phosphoinositide-dependent kinase-1 and Akt. Akt is then capable of phosphorylating the mammalian target of rapamycin (mTOR). The *yellow squares* show the various inhibitors and at which site of the cell cycle they are involved, especially sirolimus and its analogues which inhibit mTOR, whereas paclitaxel blocks microtubular mechanisms (Chaabane et al. [33], with permission of Oxford University Press, and Charron et al. [49])

The better understanding of the importance of SMC proliferation and migration resulted in the use of the immunosuppressant drug, like sirolimus to not only affect SMC and endothelial cell proliferation but also to decrease inflammation [33]. However, the cytotoxic drug, paclitaxel was also used in the first generation of drug eluting stents. In order to deliver drug, anywhere from 1 to 3 months and longer, it required the use of a polymer coating, which in the first and second generation have been permanent, whereas in the third generation, they are biodegradable polymers as the polymer disappears once the drug is delivered (Fig. 20.2). Clinical studies as well as autopsy studies have shown a marked reduction in neointimal formation with DES, irrespective of strut size, using permanent or bioabsorbable polymers. Most have used sirolimus or its analogs as drugs of choice and the results in both early and long-term clinical trials have been better with sirolimus analogs than with cytotoxic drugs, like paclitaxel [34]. All have shown delayed vascular healing as the mechanism of reduced neointima growth [14].

Delayed Healing in DES

We have shown in both the first and second generation DES that there is delay in vessel healing as compared to BMS (Fig. 20.3). We defined delayed healing as the persistence of fibrin in animal models at 28-days along with poor smooth muscle cell presence and incomplete endothelialization. However, animal models have variability with complete endothelialization observed in the porcine coronary model at 28 days although fibrin deposition persists, whereas there is greater delay in endothelialization in the rabbit iliac artery model with incomplete endothelialization observed even at 28-days. In man, complete endothelialization is observed at 3–4 months in BMS but in DES there is a delay which persists for a long time [14]. In a human autopsy study [14], when comparing first generation DES to BMS stents that had been implanted >30 days (implant duration 223 ± 253 and 229 ± 360 days, respectively) DES showed greater suppression of neointimal growth than BMS (neointimal area 2.8 ± 1.1 vs. 4.9 ± 3.0 mm^2, p<0.0003). On the other hand, covered struts (% strut endothelialized) were significantly delayed in DES than BMS (55.8 ± 26.5 vs. 89.8 ± 20.9 %, p=0.0001, respectively) and fibrin deposition was greater in DES than BMS (fibrin score 2.3 ± 1.1 vs. 0.9 ± 0.8, p<0.0001, respectively). Therefore, it is not surprising in our study that late stent thrombosis in the first generation DES was significantly higher as compared to BMS (61 % vs. 8 %, respectively, p=0.0001) [14]. In a detailed study of examining only DES, 28 with thrombosis and 34 without thrombosis, those with thrombosis had a lower percentage of endothelialization coverage as compared to those without thrombosis (40.5 ± 29.8 vs. 80.0 ± 25.2 %, P<0.0001) [35]. The ratio of uncovered to total stent struts (RUTSS) per section was also significantly greater in thrombosed DES lesion than non-thrombosed DES lesion (0.50 ± 0.23 vs. 0.19 ± 0.25, P<0.0001). What is interesting is that the distance between individual stent struts (inter-strut distance) was significantly less in thrombosed DES lesions than non-thrombosed DES lesions (0.52 ± 0.24 vs. 0.70 ± 0.25 mm) suggesting that regional drug concentrations determine strut coverage and vessel

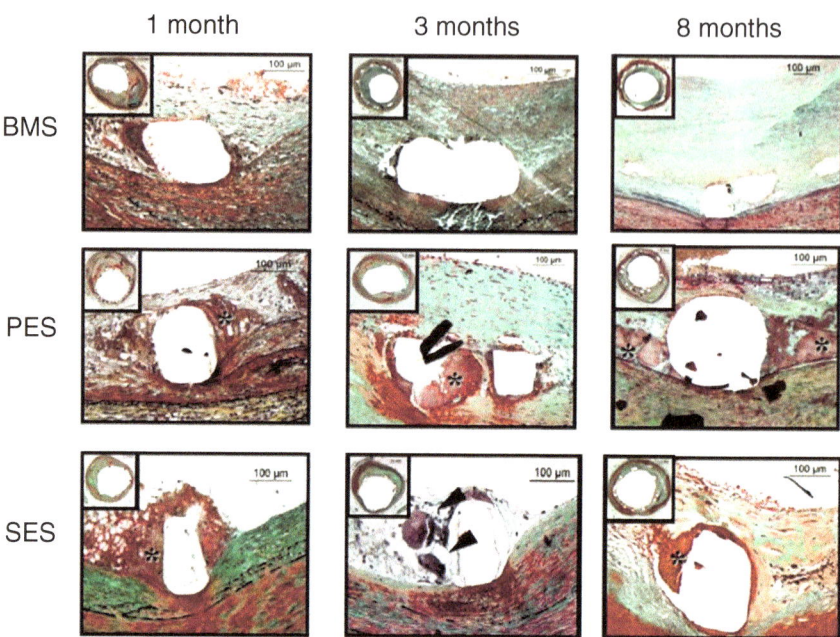

Fig. 20.3 Delayed arterial healing following drug-eluting stent (DES) versus bare metal stent (BMS) implantation. Time course of arterial healing in BMS, paclitaxel-eluting stents (PES: Taxus DES), and sirolimus-eluting stents (SES: Cypher DES) from 1 to 8 months after stent implantation. Although some peristrut inflammation is observed in BMS at 1 month, complete arterial healing, including a well-established neointimal layer, is seen at 3 and 8 months' duration. PES shows early fibrin deposition surrounding stent struts (*), which persists up to 8 months, as a sign of delayed healing. In contrast, *SES* shows predominance of inflammatory cells, including giant cell formation (*black arrowheads*), at early time points (1 and 3 months), whereas fibrin deposition is stronger at 8 months (Reproduced from Lüscher et al. [50], with permission of Wolters-Kluwer Health)

healing rates. Endothelialization was the best predictor of late stent thrombosis by multivariate logistic analysis. The odds ratio for thrombosis was nine times greater when >30 % uncoverd struts were present as compared to those with <30 % [35]. Recently introduced intravascular imaging technologies such as optical coherence tomography (OCT) and optical frequency domain imaging (OFDI) can recognize uncovered struts and have been shown to correlate with stent thrombosis [36].

Acute Myocardial Infarction

Underlying plaque morphology also plays an important role in the process of vascular healing after DES implantation. Ruptured plaque and strut penetration into a necrotic core have been reported to trigger restenosis in BMS and delayed vascular healing in DES (Fig. 20.4). The culprit site of acute myocardial infarction (AMI) showed delayed healing compared to the non-culprit site within the same lesion [37]. The culprit site showed greater RUTSS (49 % vs. 9 %, P=0.01), greater fibrin deposition

(63±28 % vs. 36±27 %, P=0.008) and a greater inflammation score (35 % vs. 17 %, P=0.003) than the non-culprit site. What is interesting is that neointimal thickness at the culprit site was significantly less than at the non-culprit site (0.04 vs. 0.07, P=0.008). Current DESs (-limus and paclitaxel) are highly lipophilic drugs and therefore it is possible that these drugs have a high affinity for lipidic necrotic core and dwell within these areas for a longer period. It is likely that culprit sites with necrotic core and persistent drug show greater delayed healing than non-culprit sites with less drug persistence because of underlying fibrous or calcific plaques.

Another feature that is associated with BMS is restenosis that has been reported to correlate with severe injury. Although DES reduce restenosis, restenosis has been reported in randomized clinical trials **in diabetics** to occur in 26.6 % at 4 years [38]. We have shown in a recent publication that the regional gradient of drug concentration which is dependent on uneven distribution of struts is the likely cause of excessive neointimal overgrowth. The presence of calcification and/or necrotic core and plaque eccentricity affects non-uniform strut distribution and the extent of vessel injury [39].

Difference Between Sirolimus and Paclitaxel-Eluting in First Generation DES

The prevalence of stent thrombosis and restenosis is different between the sirolimus-eluting stent (SES) and paclitaxel-eluting stent (PES) in clinical trials [40]. Pathological responses are also likely different (Fig. 20.3). A human autopsy study [41] showed a similar rate of early stent thrombosis (implant duration <1 month) for SES and PES (44 % vs. 38 % P=0.79). Similarly, no difference in the extent of inflammation and fibrin deposition was observed in SES and PES. In the same study, severe medial injury, necrotic core prolapse and strut mal-apposition were the main factors responsible for early thrombosis in both DESs, suggesting that early stent thrombosis is procedure-related rather than stent type [39].

Nevertheless, clear differences in pathologic findings were observed at later time-points (implant duration >1 month). Fibrin accumulation was significantly greater in PES than SES (Fibrin score: 1.8 vs. 1.0, P=0.007) while eosinophils and giant cells were consistently observed in SES, whereas eosinophils were absent and giant cells were fewer in PES. Mechanisms of thrombosis are different and depend on DES type although the incidence of late thrombosis between SES and PES is not different (21 % vs. 27 %, P=0.47). In both stents, poor endothelialization is the underlying mechanism of late stent thrombosis. However, a hypersensitivity reaction consisting of eosinophils, and T-lymphocytes is the feature of SES while excessive fibrin deposition behind and around the struts is the main cause of malapposition in PES. Drugs and polymer are thought to contribute to the phenomenon of hypersensitivity observed in SES. In SES, the polymer may be the main factor responsible for the hypersensitivity reaction because the drug (sirolimus) is completely eluted by 3 months following implantation and hypersensitivity to sirolimus is rarely observed in patients receiving this drug for kidney transplantation. The excessive fibrin deposition seen in PES is likely because the drug is cytotoxic [42].

Second Generation DES

First generation DES showed dramatic reductions in in-stent restenosis, however, problems with late stent thrombosis became apparent. Human autopsy studies showed that delayed healing with poor endothelialization either from excessive drug or from polymer usage may be the main mechanism of thrombosis. Therefore second generation DESs everolimus-eluting stents (EES) and zotalimus-eluting stents (ZES), were introduced with the hope that reducing the drug dose and/or decreasing the polymer as well as better polymers will have beneficial effects and therefore reduce late stent thrombosis. These stent struts were thinner, causing less vessel injury and less inflammation when they were deployed in preclinical animals models. Because of reduced drug dose it was expected to promote early re-endothelialization and faster healing. Polymers were also different and had a reduced thickness, which should result in more biocompatibility than the first generation DES. In a recent autopsy study following implantation of EES (duration >1 month) [16], the frequency of late and very late stent thrombosis in the specimens examined was significantly less in EES (4 %) compared to first

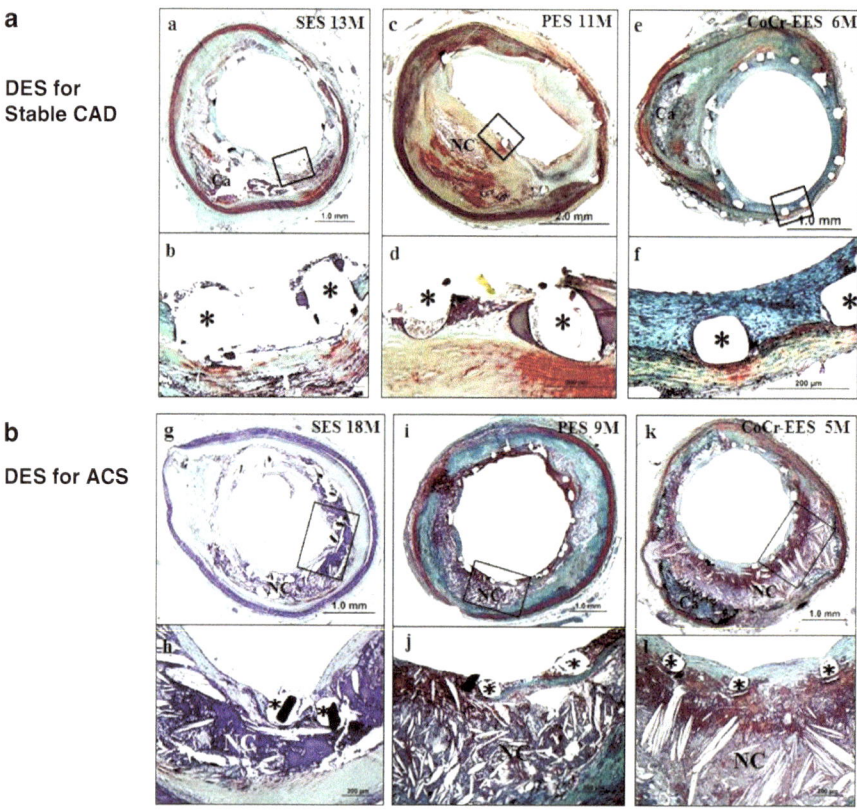

generation SES (21 %, P=0.029) and PES (26 %, P=0.008). RUTSS was less in EES (2.6 %) than SES (18.0 %, P<0.0005) and PES (18.7 %, P<0.0005) whereas neointimal thickness was comparable among the groups, at all time-points. Inflammation was also less in EES (0.26) than SES (1.00, P<0.0005) and PES (1.00, P<0.0005). The percentage of struts with fibrin was similarly less in EES (8.5, P<0.0005 than SES (29.9 %, P=0.0001) and PES (51.1 %, P<0.0005). Thus, these findings showed that second generation DESs were better than the first generation of DES. However, recently we have reported a patient with a hypersensitivity reaction (Fig. 20.5) to both EES and ZES at 238 days following Xience and Resolute stent implantation [43]. Although EES have shown better healing than SES and PES, nevertheless the prevalence of neoatherosclerosis is also observed following EES (29 %) implantation and the prevalence is comparable to that observed with SES (35 %, P=0.91) and PES (19 %, P=0.19). To date we have not observed any case of plaque rupture with EES, which may be related to the fact that the mean duration of implants in our autopsy study was only 200 [IQR, 121–360] days.

Fig. 20.4 DES for stable ACS and DES for ACS. Representative images of sirolimus-eluting stent (*SES*), paclitaxel-eluting stent (*PES*), and cobalt-chromium everolimus-eluting stent (*CoCr-EES*) implanted for stable coronary artery disease (*CAD*; **a**: *a–f*) and for acute coronary syndromes (*ACS*; **b**: *g–l*). *a* and *b*, Histological sections from a 53-year-old-man with SES implanted in the proximal left anterior descending coronary artery for 13 months. A low-power image (*a*) shows mild neointimal growth and underlying fibrocalcific plaque. Focal uncovered struts are highlighted in a high-power image in *b*.*Stent strut. *c*, *d* histological sections from a 71-year-old man with PES implanted in the right coronary artery 11 months antemortem. A low-power image (*c*) shows mild to moderate neointimal proliferation and underlying fibroatheroma. Note uncovered struts with persistent peri-strut fibrin deposition shown at high-power image in *d*. *e*, *f* histological sections from a 60-year-old man who received CoCr-EES in the mid left circumflex artery 6 months antemortem. A low-power image (*e*) shows mild neointimal proliferation and underlying fibrocalcific plaque. All struts are covered with proteoglycan-rich neointima with absence of fibrin, which is highlighted in a high-power image in *f*. *g*, *h* histological sections from a 74-year-old woman who received SES in the proximal left anterior descending coronary artery for acute myocardial infarction 18 months antemortem, who died of diffuse severe coronary artery disease. A low-power image (*g*) shows mild neointimal proliferation. Note focal uncovered struts and strut penetration into the necrotic core (NC; *h*). *i* and *j*, Histological sections from a 64-year-old woman with PES implanted in the right coronary artery for acute myocardial infarction 9 months antemortem, who died of congestive heart failure. A low-power image (*i*) shows patent lumen with stent struts surrounded by fibrin and an underlying NC. Note uncovered struts with fibrin deposition that overlie the NC (*j*). *k* and *l*, Histological sections from a 67-year-old man who received CoCr-EES in the proximal left anterior descending coronary artery for non–ST segment elevation acute myocardial infarction 5 months antemortem, who died of noncardiac causes. A low-power image (*k*) shows mild neointimal proliferation and an underlying large NC. All struts are covered with a thin neointima overlying the NC, which is highlighted in the high-power image in *l*. All histological sections are stained with Movat pentachrome. DES indicates drug-eluting stents (Reproduced from Otsuka et al. [16], with permission of Wolters-Kluwer Health)

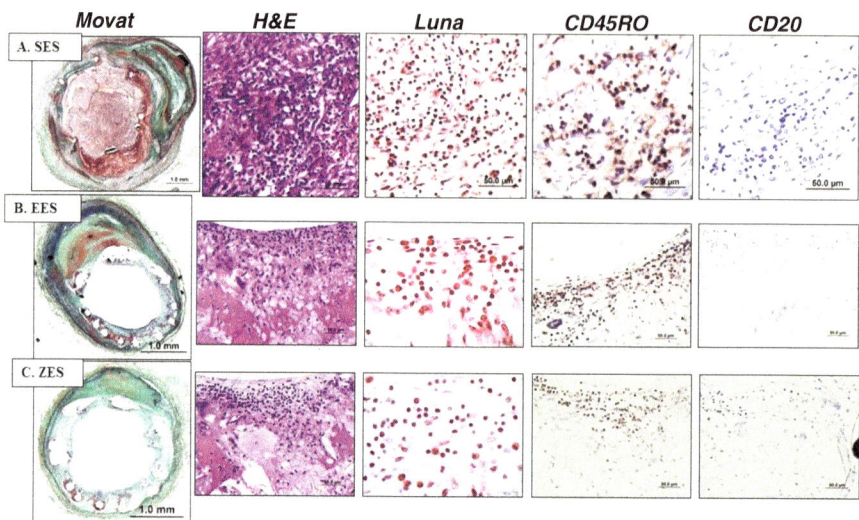

Fig. 20.5 (**a**) Hypersensitivity reaction to SES. A low-power histology image in Movat shows occlusive platelet-rich thrombus with transmural inflammation and extensive malapposition of stent struts with fibrin deposition. High-power images show extensive inflammation predominantly consisting of eosinophils (Luna stain, *red areas*) and T lymphocytes (CD45RO, *brown areas*) but rare B lymphocytes (CD20, *brown areas*) (Reproduced from Otsuka et al. [16], with permission of Wolters-Kluwer Health). (**b**, **c**) Hypersensitivity reaction to EES and ZES. HE images of histological sections show persitent fibrin deposition and extensive chronic inflammation with prominent palsading macrophages and giant cells. High power images show the presence of eosino phils (Luna stain), and Tl lymphocytes (CD45RO, brown areas) and absence of B-lymphocytes (CD20) (Reproduced from Otsuka et al. [43], with permission of Wolters Kluwer Health)

Neoatherosclerosis

Atherosclerosis progression usually takes decades from early lesion to advanced fibroatheromas, progressing to thin cap fibroatheroma (TCFA), with eventual rupture of the plaque with luminal thrombosis. However, newly developed atherosclerosis within the neointima following BMS and DES implantation (what we call "neoatherosclerosis") progresses within months to a few years (Fig. 20.6) [44]. Accumulation of lipid-containing foamy macrophages which are often observed around struts or near the lumen has been described as the first neoatherosclerotic change [44]. The time when foamy macrophage accumulation was observed following stent implantation was 70 days for PES, 120 days for SES, and 900 days for BMS. Unstable plaques of neoatherosclerosis i.e., in-stent TCFA and plaque rupture were observed at 6.2 ± 1.5 years in BMS and 3.4 ± 1.7 years in DES. DES showed a greater incidence of neoatherosclerosis than BMS (31 % vs. 16 %, P<0.001) in spite of longer duration of implant for BMS (721 days [271–1801] than DES (361 days [172–540]). Thus, neoatherosclerosis in DES is earlier and more frequent than in BMS [16].

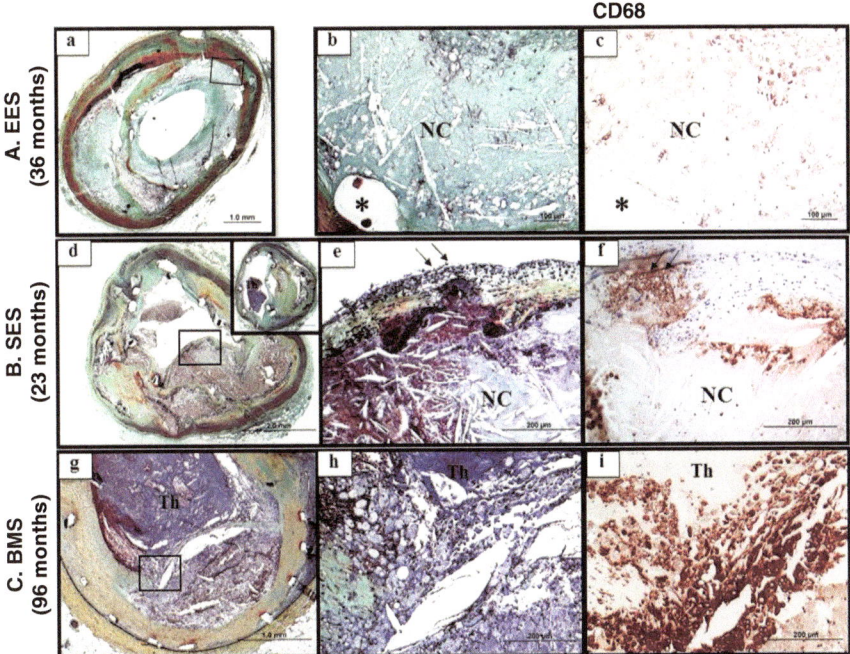

Fig. 20.6 Neoatherosclerosis. Representative cases showing atherosclerotic change following implantation of EES, SES, and BMS. (**a**) EES: Histological sections from a 73-year-old man with CoCr-EES implanted in the mid left anterior descending coronary artery for 3 years. A low-power image (*a*) (Movat) shows moderate luminal narrowing with moderate neointimal growth (69 % stenosis) and underlying fibroatheroma. A high-power image (*b*) of the boxed area in (*a*) shows necrotic core (NC) formation within the neointima where CD68-positive macrophages are identified (*c*) (Reproduced from Otsuka et al. [16], with permission of Wolters-Kluwer Health). (**b**) SES: Histological sections from a 59-year old man with SES implanted for 23 months, who died of stent thrombosis. (*d*) The thrombus (Th) was more apparent in the distal section taken 3-mm apart. (*e*) Note thin-cap fibroatheroma with fibrous cap disruption (*arrows*), from boxed area in D. (*f*) The CD68-positive macrophages are seen in the fibrous cap and in the underlying necrotic core (*arrows*). (**c**) BMS; Histologic section from a 47-year-old man who had a BMS implanted 8 years before death. Note occlusive thrombus (Th) in the lumen and ruptured plaque (*g*) (boxed area), which is shown at higher magnification in (*h*) with large number of macrophages within the lumen as well as at the ruptured cap. (*i*) Note large number of CD68-positive macrophages at the site of rupture ((**b**) and (**c**) are reproduced from Nakazawa et al. [44], with permission of Elsevier)

Incomplete endothelialization or impaired endothelial function is thought to be the primary cause of early neoatherosclerosis. Cell-cell junctions within the neo-intima following DES implantation are poorly formed, with less expression of PECAM1 as compared to BMS [32]. The immature endothelium is unable to protect insudation of circulating lipid and monocyte/macrophage infiltration into the vessel wall. Accumulation of extracellular matrix (ECM) proteoglycan is another factor that may promote neoatherosclerosis through ionic interaction between gly-cosamineoglycans and lipoproteins. We have shown that the presence of proteogly-can is greater in DES than in BMS [39]. The presence of poor endothelial junctions and excessive proteoglycan deposition may be either secondary to the drugs and or polymers used on DES.

Bioabsorbable Polymer Coated Stents

In preclinical studies it has been shown that bioabsorbable polymer usage to deliver drugs may be the ideal mechanism as the polymer disappears and leaves behind a BMS that is covered by a thin neointimal tissue without any significant inflammation-a finding reported with permanent polymer coated stents [14]. Currently in the USA no bioabsorbable metallic stents have been approved by the FDA. However, the Synergy (Boston Scientific Corp., Boston, MA) with poly (lactic-co- glycolic acid) or PLGA and everolimus eluting stent has a lower profile than the current second generation DES and abluminal PLGA coating of 4 μm thickness and 1.0 μg/mm^2 of drug. As of yet clinical trial results show similar MACE rate to that of Promus element (similar to Xience however the metallic stent design is different) and long-term data in larger studies will be needed to show greater efficacy [45]. Preclinical animal studies show much less inflammation as compared to permanent polymer; the neointima is similar as is the extent of fibrin deposition [46]. Although we will not discuss here in detail the totally bioabsorbable scaffold, they may be the future as over-time they leave behind no trace of the scaffold and it is possible that with the return of vasomotion, they may prevent the progression of "neoatheroslcerois" within the scaffolds. However, what remains unclear is that bulky scaffolds $\geq$150 μm thickness such as is present with bioabsorbable scaffolds may be associated again with greater late stent thrombosis [47]. Therefore, we have to remain vigilant that we do not implant these fully bioabsorbable polymeric scaffolds in patients presenting with acute myocardial infarction until clearly clinical trials prove their safety.

Conclusions

1-Pathologic studies have clearly shown that optimal stent design is a stent that promotes endothelialization within a short period, without inducing inflammation and excessive neotinimal growth but enough to cover all struts. The presence of mature endothelium should prevent thrombosis.

2-BMS reduced acute closure and reduced restenosis as compared to balloon angioplasty.

3-DES were instrumental in reducing restenosis which was the "Achilles heal" of BMS. However, the first generation DES had the drawback of inducing late stent thrombosis and also neoatherosclerosis. Late stent thrombosis was related to delayed healing and poor endothelialization with >30 % uncovered stent struts being predictive of thrombosis. Also, neoatherosclerosis was observed with greater frequency and at earlier time points as compared to BMS.

4-Second generation DES that have lower strut thickness, less polymers thickness and better polymer, along with lower drug concentration have resulted in reducing late stent thrombosis. However, "neoatherosclerosis" prevalence remains high in the second generation of DES.

5-Bioabsorbable polymer usage to deliver drugs may be the ideal mechanism as the polymer disappears and leaves behind a BMS that is covered by a thin neointimal tissue without any significant inflammation [48]. It is possible that the totally bioabsorbable scaffold may be the future since normal vessel vasomotion returns following scaffold disappearance and this might prevent neoatherosclerosis from developing. More data, however, are needed.

References

1. Sigwart U, Puel J, Mirkovitch V, et al. Intravascular stents to prevent occlusion and restenosis after transluminal angioplasty. N Engl J Med. 1987;316:701–6. doi:10.1056/NEJM198703193161201.
2. Morice M-C, Serruys PW, Sousa JE, et al. A randomized comparison of a sirolimus-eluting stent with a standard stent for coronary revascularization. N Engl J Med. 2002;346:1773–80. doi:10.1056/NEJMoa012843.
3. Serruys PW, de Jaegere P, Kiemeneij F, et al. A comparison of balloon-expandable-stent implantation with balloon angioplasty in patients with coronary artery disease. Benestent Study Group. N Engl J Med. 1994;331:489–95. doi:10.1056/NEJM199408253310801.
4. Serruys PW, Strauss BH, Beatt KJ, et al. Angiographic follow-up after placement of a self-expanding coronary-artery stent. N Engl J Med. 1991;324:13–7. doi:10.1056/NEJM199101033240103.
5. Roubin GS, Cannon AD, Agrawal SK, et al. Intracoronary stenting for acute and threatened closure complicating percutaneous transluminal coronary angioplasty. Circulation. 1992;85:916–27.
6. Shömig A, Neumann FJ, Kastrati A, et al. A randomized comparison of antiplatelet and anticoagulant therapy after the placement of coronary-artery stents. N Engl J Med. 1996;334:1084–9.
7. Serruys PW, Kutryk MJB, Ong ATL. Coronary-artery stents. N Engl J Med. 2006;354:483–95. doi:10.1056/NEJMra051091.
8. Schatz RA, Baim DS, Leon M, et al. Clinical experience with the Palmaz-Schatz coronary stent. Initial results of a multicenter study. Circulation. 1991;83(1):148–61.
9. Mehta RH, Harjai KJ, Cox D, et al. Clinical and angiographic correlates and outcomes of suboptimal coronary flow inpatients with acute myocardial infarction undergoing primary percutaneous coronary intervention. J Am Coll Cardiol. 2003;42:1739–46.
10. Grines CL, Cox DA, Stone GW, et al. Coronary angioplasty with or without stent implantation for acute myocardial infarction. Stent Primary Angioplasty in Myocardial Infarction Study Group. N Engl J Med. 1999;341:1949–56. doi:10.1056/NEJM199912233412601.
11. Moses JW, Leon MB, Popma JJ, et al. Sirolimus-eluting stents versus standard stents in patients with stenosis in a native coronary artery. N Engl J Med. 2003;349:1315–23. doi:10.1056/NEJMoa035071.
12. Kerner A, Gruberg L, Kapeliovich M, Grenadier E. Late stent thrombosis after implantation of a sirolimus-eluting stent. Catheter Cardiovasc Interv. 2003;60:505–8. doi:10.1002/ccd.10712.
13. Virmani R, Guagliumi G, Farb A, et al. Localized hypersensitivity and late coronary thrombosis secondary to a sirolimus-eluting stent: should we be cautious? Circulation. 2004;109:701–5. doi:10.1161/01.CIR.0000116202.41966.D4.

14. Joner M, Finn AV, Farb A, et al. Pathology of drug-eluting stents in humans: delayed healing and late thrombotic risk. J Am Coll Cardiol. 2006;48:193–202. doi:10.1016/j.jacc.2006.03.042.
15. Dangas GD, Serruys PW, Kereiakes DJ, et al. Meta-analysis of everolimus-eluting versus paclitaxel-eluting stents in coronary artery disease: final 3-year results of the SPIRIT clinical trials program (Clinical Evaluation of the Xience V Everolimus Eluting Coronary Stent System in the Treatment of Patients with De Novo Native Coronary Artery Lesions). JACC Cardiovasc Interv. 2013;6:914–22. doi:10.1016/j.jcin.2013.05.005.
16. Otsuka F, Vorpahl M, Nakano M, et al. Pathology of second-generation everolimus-eluting stents versus first-generation sirolimus- and paclitaxel-eluting stents in humans. Circulation. 2014;129:211–23. doi:10.1161/CIRCULATIONAHA.113.001790.
17. Brugaletta S, Garcia-Garcia HM, Serruys PW, Maehara A, Farooq V, Mintz GS, de Bruyne B, Marso SP, Verheye S, Dudek D, Hamm CW, Farhat N, Schiele F, McPherson J, Lerman A, Moreno PR, Wennerblom B, Fahy M, Templin B, Morel MA, van Es GA, Stone GW. Relationship between palpography and virtual histology in patients with acute coronary syndromes. JACC Cardiovasc Imaging. 2012;5(3 Suppl):S19–27.
18. Lansky AJ, Roubin GS, O'Shaughnessy CD, et al. Randomized comparison of GR-II stent and Palmaz-Schatz stent for elective treatment of coronary stenoses. Circulation. 2000; 102:1364–8.
19. Garasic JM, Edelman ER, Squire JC, et al. Stent and artery geometry determine intimal thickening independent of arterial injury. Circulation. 2000;101:812–8. doi:10.1161/01. CIR.101.7.812.
20. Schwartz RS, Huber KC, Murphy JG, et al. Restenosis and the proportional neointimal response to coronary artery injury: results in a porcine model. J Am Coll Cardiol. 1992;19:267–74.
21. Kornowski R, Hong MK, Tio FO, et al. In-stent restenosis: contributions of inflammatory responses and arterial injury to neointimal hyperplasia. J Am Coll Cardiol. 1998;31:224–30.
22. Siewiorek GM, Finol EA, Wholey MH. Clinical significance and technical assessment of stent cell geometry in carotid artery stenting. J Endovasc Ther. 2009;16:178–88. doi:10.1583/08-2583.1.
23. Canan T, Lee MS. Drug-eluting stent fracture: incidence, contributing factors, and clinical implications. Catheter Cardiovasc Interv. 2010;75:237–45. doi:10.1002/ccd.22212.
24. Murasato Y, Hikichi Y, Horiuchi M. Examination of stent deformation and gap formation after complex stenting of left main coronary artery bifurcations using microfocus computed tomography. J Interv Cardiol. 2009;22:135–44. doi:10.1111/j.1540-8183.2009.00436.x.
25. Kastrati A, Mehilli J, Dirschinger J, et al. Intracoronary stenting and angiographic results: strut thickness effect on restenosis outcome (ISAR-STEREO) trial. Circulation. 2001; 103:2816–21.
26. Jiménez JM, Davies PF. Hemodynamically driven stent strut design. Ann Biomed Eng. 2009;37:1483–94. doi:10.1007/s10439-009-9719-9.
27. Farb A, Sangiorgi G, Carter AJ, et al. Pathology of acute and chronic coronary stenting in humans. Circulation. 1999;99:44–52. doi:10.1161/01.CIR.99.1.44.
28. Sata M, Saiura A, Kunisato A, et al. Hematopoietic stem cells differentiate into vascular cells that participate in the pathogenesis of atherosclerosis. Nat Med. 2002;8:403–9. doi:10.1038/nm0402-403.
29. Ross R. Atherosclerosis–an inflammatory disease. N Engl J Med. 1999;340:115–26. doi:10.1056/NEJM199901143400207.
30. Farb A, Kolodgie FD, Hwang JY, et al. Extracellular matrix changes in stented human coronary arteries. Circulation. 2004;110:940–7. doi:10.1161/01.CIR.0000139337.56084.30.
31. Virmani R, Kolodgie FD, Farb A, Lafont A. Drug eluting stents: are human and animal studies comparable? Heart. 2003;89:133–8.
32. Otsuka F, Finn AV, Yazdani SK, et al. The importance of the endothelium in atherothrombosis and coronary stenting. Nat Rev Cardiol. 2012;9:439–53. doi:10.1038/nrcardio.2012.64.
33. Chaabane C, Otsuka F, Virmani R, Bochaton-Piallat ML. Biological responses in stented arteries. Cardiovasc Res. 2013;99:353–63. doi:10.1093/cvr/cvt115.

34. Dibra A, Kastrati A, Mehilli J, et al. Paclitaxel-eluting or sirolimus-eluting stents to prevent restenosis in diabetic patients. N Engl J Med. 2005;353:663–70. doi:10.1056/NEJMoa044372.
35. Finn AV, Joner M, Nakazawa G, et al. Pathological correlates of late drug-eluting stent thrombosis: strut coverage as a marker of endothelialization. Circulation. 2007;115:2435–41. doi:10.1161/CIRCULATIONAHA.107.693739.
36. Guagliumi G, Sirbu V, Musumeci G, et al. Examination of the in vivo mechanisms of late drug-eluting stent thrombosis: findings from optical coherence tomography and intravascular ultrasound imaging. JACC Cardiovasc Interv. 2012;5:12–20. doi:10.1016/j.jcin.2011.09.018.
37. Nakazawa G, Finn AV, Joner M, et al. Delayed arterial healing and increased late stent thrombosis at culprit sites after drug-eluting stent placement for acute myocardial infarction patients: an autopsy study. Circulation. 2008;118:1138–45. doi:10.1161/CIRCULATIONAHA.107.762047.
38. De Waha A, Stefanini GG, King LA, et al. Long-term outcomes of biodegradable polymer versus durable polymer drug-eluting stents in patients with diabetes a pooled analysis of individual patient data from 3 randomized trials. Int J Cardiol. 2013;168:5162–6. doi:10.1016/j.ijcard.2013.07.263.
39. Nakano M, Otsuka F, Yahagi K, et al. Human autopsy study of drug-eluting stents restenosis: histomorphological predictors and neointimal characteristics. Eur Heart J. 2013;34:3304–13. doi:10.1093/eurheartj/eht241.
40. Windecker S, Remondino A, Eberli FR, et al. Sirolimus-eluting and paclitaxel-eluting stents for coronary revascularization. N Engl J Med. 2005;353:653–62. doi:10.1056/NEJMoa051175.
41. Nakazawa G, Finn AV, Vorpahl M, et al. Coronary responses and differential mechanisms of late stent thrombosis attributed to first-generation sirolimus- and paclitaxel-eluting stents. J Am Coll Cardiol. 2011;57:390–8. doi:10.1016/j.jacc.2010.05.066.
42. Farb A, Heller PF, Shroff S, et al. Pathological analysis of local delivery of paclitaxel via a polymer-coated stent. Circulation. 2001;104:473–9.
43. Otsuka F, Yahagi K, Ladich E, Kutys R, Alexander R, Fowler D, Virmani R, Joner M. Images in cardiovascular medicine hypersensitivity reaction in the US Food and Drug Administration-approved second-generation drug-eluting stents: histopathological assessment with ex vivo optical coherence tomography. Circulation. 2015;131(3):322–4. doi:10.3904/kjim.2013.28.1.108.4.
44. Nakazawa G, Otsuka F, Nakano M, et al. The pathology of neoatherosclerosis in human coronary implants bare-metal and drug-eluting stents. J Am Coll Cardiol. 2011;57:1314–22. doi:10.1016/j.jacc.2011.01.011.
45. Meredith IT, Verheye S, Dubois CL, et al. Primary endpoint results of the EVOLVE trial: a randomized evaluation of a novel bioabsorbable polymer-coated, everolimus-eluting coronary stent. J Am Coll Cardiol. 2012;59:1362–70. doi:10.1016/j.jacc.2011.12.016.
46. Koppara T, Wittchow E, Byrne RA, et al. Permanent and biodegradable polymer coatings in the absence of antiproliferative drugs in a porcine model of coronary artery stenting. EuroIntervention. 2014. doi:10.4244/EIJY14M10_08.
47. Otsuka F, Pacheco E, Perkins LEL, et al. Long-term safety of an everolimus-eluting bioresorbable vascular scaffold and the cobalt-chromium XIENCE V stent in a porcine coronary artery model. CircCardiovascInterv.2014;7:330–42.doi:10.1161/CIRCINTERVENTIONS.113.000990.
48. Nakazawa G, Finn AV, Kolodgie FD, Virmani R. A review of current devices and a look at new technology: drug-eluting stents. Expert Rev Med Devices. 2009;6:33–42. doi:10.1586/17434440.6.1.33.
49. Charron T, Nili N, Straus BH. The cell cycle: a critical therapeutic target to prevent vascular proliferative disease. Can J Cardiol. 2006;22:41B–55B.
50. Lüscher TF, Steffel J, Eberli FR, Joner M, Nakazawa G, Tanner FC, Virmani R. Drug-eluting stent and coronary thrombosis: biological mechanisms and clinical implications. Circulation. 2007;115(8):1051–8.

Chapter 21
What Is the Optimal Stent Design Interventionalist's View

Scot Garg and Patrick W. Serruys

Abstract There are three main components to a coronary stent, and modifications to either the stent platform, stent polymer or drug coating can affect procedural success and influence clinical outcomes. This chapter discusses the pros and cons of modifying these parts of a coronary stent in an attempt to produce the ideal device.

Keywords Drug-eluting stent • Bare metal stent • Biodegradable polymer • Polymer free stent • Bioresorbable scaffolds

Introduction

Coronary stents have evolved exponentially since Puel and Sigwart first deployed the Wallstent in March 1986 [1]. Stents are used in a majority of percutaneous coronary interventions (PCI), and globally represent a multi-billion dollar industry. In the ensuing years they have undergone numerous modifications with the ambition of creating the ultimate stent which can be deployed in any lesion, in any patient, with minimal subsequent risk of restenosis, stent thrombosis (ST), cardiovascular morbidity and cardiovascular mortality, all without hindering further percutaneous or surgical revascularization. This chapter will discuss some of the unresolved issues in developing this ideal stent including:

1. Whether the device should elute an anti-proliferative drug?
2. If so, which drug?

S. Garg, MBChB, MRCP, PhD, FESC
Department of Cardiology, Royal Blackburn Hospital, East Lancashire Hospitals NHS Trust, Blackburn, Lancashire BB2 3HH, UK
e-mail: scot.garg@elht.nhs.uk

P.W. Serruys, MD, PhD, FESC (✉)
Department of Cardiology, Erasmus Medical Centre, Rotterdam, The Netherlands

International Centre for Cardiovascular Health, Imperial College, London, UK
e-mail: patrick.w.j.c.serruys@gmail.com

© Springer International Publishing Switzerland 2015

J.A. Ambrose, A.E. Rodríguez (eds.), *Controversies in Cardiology*,
DOI 10.1007/978-3-319-20415-4_21

3. How should this anti-proliferative drug be eluted from the stent?
4. Should the device platform be made from a permanent metal or a bioresorbable material?

Drug-Eluting Stent Versus Bare Metal Stent

There is little debate that the introduction of first generation drug-eluting stents (DES, Table 21.1) in 2002 transformed PCI by significantly reducing rates of restenosis compared to bare metal stents (BMS) [2]. Shortly after their introduction, however, concerns were raised as to whether the price to pay for this improved efficacy was justified following reports of increased rates of death and myocardial infarction (MI) due to ST occurring many months after DES implantation [3–5]. In response to these fears, numerous patient level meta-analyses were performed all of which failed to identify any significant increased risk of death and/or MI with the use of first generation DES compared to BMS [6–10]. More contemporary analyses, which include data from the newer generations of DES (Table 21.1) which were developed on the background of the prior safety concerns, and have access to many more years of patient follow-up data, have helped dispell once and for all the concerns regarding the risks of adverse events with DES (Table 21.2) [11–16]. Reassuringly, these studies also endorse the superior efficacy of DES over BMS, with results consistent in all lesion and patient subsets including small vessels, large vessels, long lesions, diabetic patients and those with acute MI.

Despite the above data, BMS continue to have a role, albeit limited, in clinical practice. Some of the cited reasons for using BMS [17] can be refuted with contemporary data, which have failed to demonstrate similar efficacy between BMS and DES for large vessel intervention, [18] or an increased risk of ST with DES compared to BMS in primary PCI for ST-elevation MI [15]. Other factors influencing the decision include patient age, and cost/reimbursement. Overall, however, the commonest cited reason to use a BMS appears to be conflict related to the use of dual anti-platelet therapy (DAPT) be it the risk of bleeding from prolonged use due to co-morbidities, or its anticipated premature interruption due to suspected poor compliance or planned non-cardiac surgery. Use of a BMS in these scenarios may be considered more appropriate as premature interruption of DAPT is an important risk for ST, [19, 20] and implantation of a BMS mandates only 1 month of DAPT, as opposed to 6–12 months for DES [21]. As a caveat however, there are emerging data, which confirm the safety of using shorter durations of DAPT with DES, [22–25]. More information will be available in the future. The currently recruiting Global Leaders Study includes one arm where patients treated with a DES receive only 1 month of DAPT.

Which Anti-proliferative Agent?

The previous discussions have established the clear clinical benefits of DES compared to BMS, however which anti-proliferative drug should be eluted? The role of this agent is ultimately to limit neointimal proliferation, and consequently its ideal

Table 21.1 Specifications of the first and second generation DES

	Stent	Drug (concentration)	Polymer	Polymer thickness (µm)	Release kinetics (days)	Metal	Geometry	Strut thickness (µm)
First generation stents	CYPHER	Sirolimus (140 µg/cm²)	Polyethelyne co-vinyl acetate & PBMA	12.6	80 % (28)	SS	Closed cell	140
	TAXUS express	Paclitaxel (100 µg/cm²)	Poly(styrene-b-isobutylene-b-styrene)	16	<10 % (28)	SS	Open cell	132
	TAXUS liberté	Paclitaxel (100 µg/cm²)	Poly(styrene-b-isobutylene-b-styrene)	16	<10 % (28)	SS	Hybrid	97
Second generation stents	TAXUS element	Paclitaxel (100 µg/cm²)	Poly(styrene-b-isobutylene-b-styrene)	15	<10 % (90)	PtCr	Open cell	81
	Endeavor	Zotarolimus (100 µg/cm²)	Phosphorylcholine	4.1	95 % (14)	CoCr	Open cell	91
	Endeavor RESOLUTE	Zotarolimus (10 µg/mm)	Biolinx	4.1	85 % (60)	CoCr	Open cell	91
	Xience V	Everolimus (100 µg/cm²)	PBMA & PVDF-HFP	7	80 % (90)	CoCr	Open cell	81
	PROMUS element	Everolimus (100 µg/cm²)	PBMA & PVDF-HFP	7	80 % (90)	PtCr	Open cell	81

SS stainless steel, *CoCr* cobalt chromium, *PtCr* platinum chromium, *PBMA* poly (n-butyl methacrylate) (PBMA), *PVDF-HFP* poly (vinylidene fluoride-co-hexafluoropropylene)

Table 21.2 Rates of death, myocardial infarction, target lesion revascularization and stent thrombosis from meta-analyses of drug eluting stents compared to bare metal stents

Reference	Type of meta-analysis	Number of patients (DES/BMS)	Longest follow-up (years)	Death (DES vs. BMS)	MI (DES vs. BMS)	TLR (DES vs. BMS)	Definite ST (DES vs. BMS)
Stettler et al. [10][a]	Collaborative network	18,023 (13,102/4921)	4	HR 0.96	HR 0.83*	HR 0.70*	[c]HR 0.95 to HR 1.02
							[d]HR 1.14 to HR 1.61
							[e]HR 1.43 to HR 3.57
Kirtane et al. [9] [on-label]	Comprehensive	9470 (4867/4603)	5	HR 1.05	HR 1.03	HR 0.54*	
Kirtane et al. [9] [off-label]				HR 0.84	HR 0.83	HR 0.42*	
Kang [11][a,b]	Bayesian approach network	90,584 (80,744/9844)	5	HR 0.62 to HR 0.87	HR 0.42* to HR 0.85	HR 0.19* to HR 0.43*	[c,d]HR 0.25* to HR 0.84
							[e]HR 0.23* to HR 2.13*
Bangalore [12][b]	Mixed treatment comparison	106,427	5	RR 0.69 to RR 0.89	RR 0.61* to RR 0.98	RR 0.30* to RR 0.57*	[c,d,e]RR 0.35* to RR 1.17

Differences non-significant unless indicated. Results from final follow-up unless indicated
BMS bare metal stent, *DES* drug eluting stent, *MI* myocardial infarction, *TLR* target lesion revascularization, *ST* stent thrombosis, *HR* hazard ratio, *RR* risk ratio
*p < 0.05
[a]Results at 1-year follow-up
[b]Multiple DES tested against BMS – worst and best results reported
[c]Early ST
[d]Late ST
[e]Very late ST

properties should include the following: a wide therapeutic window, a low inflammatory potential, a select ability to suppress smooth muscle cell proliferation without being toxic to the medial and adventitial cell layers and an ability to promote re-endothelialization.

Throughout the DES era two main classess of drugs have been used (Fig. 21.1): (1) immuosupressant limus analogues which function by inhibiting the mammalian target of rapamycin (mTOR), thereby reversibly inhibiting growth factor and cytokine stimulated cell proliferation in the G_1 phase of the cell cycle, and (2) antiproliferative paclitaxel which inhibits cell replication predominantly in the G_0/G_1 and G_2/M phases of the cell cycle. The demonstrated superiority of limus-eluting DES compared to paclitaxel in randomized studies and subsequent meta-analyses in terms of significantly lower late lumen loss, repeat revascularizations, and ST [11,

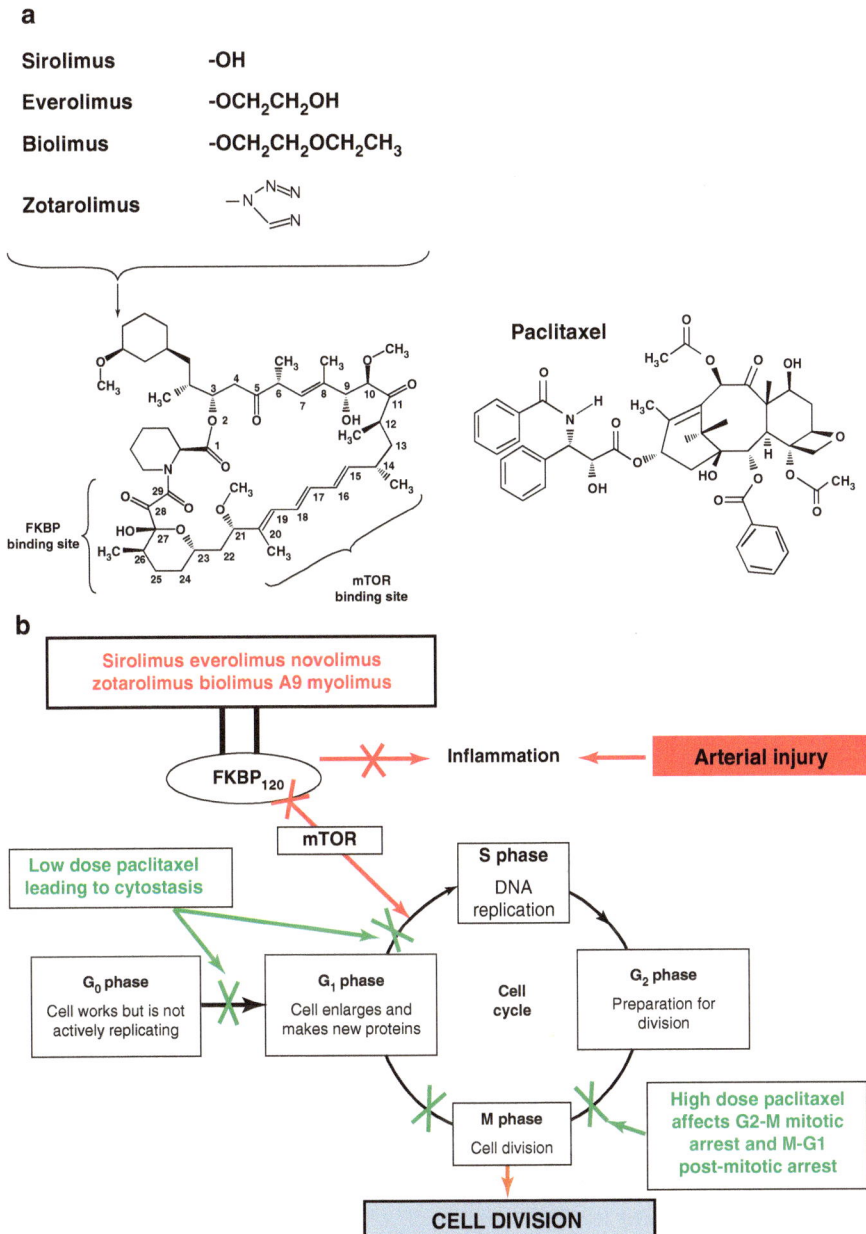

Fig. 21.1 The chemical structure (**a**) and mechanism of action (**b**) of the macrocyclic lactone group of anti-proliferative drugs and paclitaxel

12, 26] has largely led to paclitaxel losing its role in contemporary DES. However, its properties have resulted in it being the anti-proliferative agent of choice to be released from drug-coated balloons [27].

It follows that contemporary DES elute macrocyclic lactones, which are similar to sirolimus. However, modifications on the carbon atom 40 of the macrocyclic ring have lead to the development of zotarolimus, everolimus, and biolimus. Other agents such as novolimus have been produced through removal of a methyl group from carbon atom 16, and myolimus through replacement of the oxygen on carbon atom 32 of the macrocyclic ring. These agents all offer subtle differences in degrees of immunosuppression and liphophilicity, with the latter influencing the rate of drug absorption into the arterial wall. The direct influence of these different agents on stent performance is impossible to evaluate in isolation, as concurrent modifications to other aspects of stent design have also been made. Pre-clinical data comparing stents with identical platforms, polymers, drug loads and drug release kinetics but releasing everolimus, sirolimus, or zotarolimus—demonstrate that all three limus drugs have comparable effects on neointimal suppression [28]. Clinical data are available from numerous randomized studies and their subsequent meta-analyses, comparing sirolimus-, everolimus-, zotarolimus- and biolimus- eluting stents individually with either BMS or other DES, with additional data obtained from indirect comparisons between these DES from network meta-analyses [10–12, 14, 16].

Conclusions from the largest network meta-analysis by Bangalore et al. [12] which included data from 126 trials and 258,544 patient years of follow-up suggest that the thin-strut, fluoro-polymer coated everolimus-eluting stent (EES, Table 21.1) has the best combination of efficacy and safety as evidenced by:

1. EES being the only DES to show a significant reduction in mortality compared to BMS (HR 0.72, 95 % CI 0.58–0.90). No significant differences in mortality were seen in comparisons between different DES.
2. EES having the greatest reduction in the risk of MI compared to BMS (HR 0.61, 95 % CI 0.44–0.87). In comparison, other limus DES reduce the risk of MI versus BMS with hazard ratios of 0.71–0.83. No significant differences in mortality were seen in comparisons between different DES.
3. EES being the only DES to significantly reduce the rate of definite ST compared to BMS (HR 0.35, 95 % CI 0.21–0.53). A subsequent analysis demonstrated, with an 81 % probability, that EES was associated with the lowest rate of definite ST compared to other DES.
4. EES has the greatest reduction in target vessel revascularization compared to BMS (HR 0.37, 95 % CI 0.26–0.52). In comparison, other limus DES reduce the risk of target vessel revascularization versus BMS with hazard ratios of 0.38–0.59. No significant differences in mortality were seen in comparisons between different DES.

The cobalt chromium EES stent has a strut thickness of 81 μm, and is coated with a 7.6 μm thick, non-erodable, co-polymer of poly vinylidene fluoride co-hexafluoropropylene (PVDF-HFP), and poly n-butyl methacrylate (PBMA), which facilitates elution of everolimus over 120-days. *Everolimus* ($C_{53}H_{83}NO_{14}$, molecular weight 958 Da) is a sirolimus derivative, in which the hydroxyl group at position

C40 of sirolimus has been alkylated with a 2-hydroxy-ethyl group. It is slightly more lipophilic than sirolimus, and therefore, it is more rapidly absorbed into the arterial wall. Although binding of everolimus to the FKBP-12 domain is three-fold and immunosuppressive activity *in vitro* two to five-fold lower than with sirolimus, oral everolimus proved at least as potent as sirolimus in models of autoimmune disease and heart transplantation. The EES platform is potentially associated with less inflammation than SES and PES [29]. The thin-strut structure of the stent platform, the thromboresistant properties of the fluoro-polymer, and the reduced polymer and drug load may contribute to the low rate of ST with EES [30]. The notion of a DES being safer than a BMS represents a paradigm shift in the evolution of PCI.

Stent Polymer

The role of the stent polymer is to facilitate controlled elution of anti-proliferative drugs over a specified period of time, with their presence obsolete once drug elution has been completed. This latter fact, together with evidence identifying polymers, particularly the non-biocompatible polymers found on first generation DES as a nidus for chronic inflammation within the arterial wall leading to hypersensitivity reactions, endothelial dysfunction and subsequent delayed healing, has led to accusations that they are central to triggering late and very late ST [29, 31–33]. Valid questions have therefore been raised regarding whether the polymer should be permanent or biodegradable, (i.e. biodegrade once drug elution has been completed), or whether they are needed at all.

Permanent Versus Biodegradable Polymer

In theory, stents with biodegradable polymers offer the anti-restenotic benefits of conventional DES during vascular healing. However, once drug elution has been completed and the polymer has broken down, the stent should offer the safety benefits of a BMS. While this concept is attractive, there remain several challenges including (1) establishing the optimal biocompatibility, composition, formulation, and degradation time of the polymer; (2) identifying the optimal pharmacokinetics of the anti-proliferative agent released by the degradation of the polymer; (3) managing variations in polymer degradation time which can be affected by production factors such as the use of long polymer chains, decreased polymer hydrophobicity and greater polymer crystalinization and biological environmental factors; [34] (4) dealing with the potential complications of an inflammatory and immune reaction to polymer breakdown [35].

Despite these conceptual challenges, numerous DES utilizing biodegradable polymers, such as poly-lactic acid, poly-L-lactic acid (PLLA), and poly(D,L-lactide-co-glycolide), have been developed and undergone clinical evaluation in first-in-man studies, and randomized clinical studies with BMS and/or permanent polymer DES as the comparator arm (Table 21.3) [18, 36–58]. Reassuringly,

Table 21.3 Metallic stents with a biodegradable polymer which are either currently available or undergoing clinical evaluation

Stent (manufacturer) (Ref)	Drug (dosage)	Drug release (%) release/ time	Stent platform	Strut/max coating thickness (μm)	Polymer type (duration of biodegradation, months)	In-stent late loss (mm)
Supralimus (Sahajanand Medical) [43]	Sirolimus (125 μg/19 mm)	50 % 9–11 days	SS	80/4–5	PLLA, PLGA, PLC, PVP (7)	0.09*
Excel stent (JW Medical System) [44]	Sirolimus (195–376 μg)	NA	SS	119/15	PLA (6–9)	0.21*
FIREHAWK (MicroPort) [45]	Sirolimus (55 μg/18 mm)	75 % 30 days	CoCr with grooves	NA	Abluminal groove filled PLA (9)	0.13§
MiStent (Micell) [46]	Crystalline Sirolimus (9–11 μg/mm)	100 % 60 days	CoCr	64/15	PLGA (3)	0.03§
BioMatrix (Biosensors) [36, 47]	Biolimus A9 (15.6 μg/mm)	45 % 30 days	SS	112/10ª	Abluminal PLA (6–9)	0.13†
NOBORI (Terumo) [48]	Biolimus A9 (15.6 μg/mm)	45 % 30 days	SS	112/10ª	Abluminal PLA (6–9)	0.11†
Axxess (Biosensors) [49]	Biolimus A9 (22 μg/ mm)	45 % 30 days	Nitinol	152/15ª	Abluminal PLA (6–9)	0.29 MB† 0.29SB†
SYNERGY (Boston Scientific) [37]	Everolimus (LD 56 μg/20 mm) (SD 113 μg/20 mm)	50 % 60 days	PtCr	71/3 (LD) 4 (SD)	PLGA Rollcoat Abluminal (3)	0.13 (LD)* 0.10 (SD)*
Combo (OrbusNeich) [50]	EPC + Sirolimus (5 μg/mm)	95 % 35 days	SS	100/3–5ª	Abluminal PLA, PLGA, CAP(<3)	0.39†
DESyne BD (Elixir Medical) [51]	Novolimus (5 μg/ mm)	90 % 90 days	CoCr	81/<3	PLA (6–9)	0.16*
Elixir Myolimus (Elixir Medical) [52]	Myolimus (3 μg/ mm)	90 % 90 days	CoCr	81/<3	PLA (6–9)	0.08*
Svelte (Svelte Medical) [53]	Sirolimus (220 μg/ cm²)	80 % 28 days	CoCr	81/6	PLGA (12)	0.22*
BioMime (Meril Life Sciences) [54]	Sirolimus (1.25 μg/ mm²)	NA	CoCr	65/2	PLGA + PLLA	0.15^

(continued)

Table 21.3 (continued)

Stent (manufacturer) (Ref)	Drug (dosage)	Drug release (%) release/ time	Stent platform	Strut/max coating thickness (μm)	Polymer type (duration of biodegradation, months)	In-stent late loss (mm)
Orsiro (Biotronik) [55]	Sirolimus (1.4 μg/ mm²)	100 % 100 days	CoCr	71/11	PLLA (15)	0.05†
Inspiron DES (Scitech) [56]	Sirolimus (56 μg/13 mm)	NA	CoCr	75/5ᵃ	PLA + PLGA (6–8)	0.22*
Infinnium (Sahajanand) [57, 58]	Paclitaxel (122 μg/19 mm)	50 % 9–11 days	SS	80/4–5	PLLA, PLGA, PLC PVP (7)	0.54†

All differences are not significant unless stated
Angiographic follow-up at 4(§), 6 (*), 8 (^) and 9 (†) months
PLC 75/25 poly L-lactide-*co*-caprolactone, *CAP* ε-caprolactone, *CoCr* cobalt chromium, *EPC* endothelial progenitor capture, *LD* low dose, *NA* not available, *PES* paclitaxel eluting stent, *PLGA* 50/50 Poly DL-Lactide-co-Glycolide, *PLLA* poly-L-lactic acid, *PtCr* platinum chromium, *PVP* polyvinyl pyrrolidone, *SD* standard dose, *SES* sirolimus eluting stent, *SS* stainless steel
ᵃAbluminal polymer

porcine studies have shown less inflammation, [59] and clinical studies, improved vasomotion, [60, 61] and fewer uncovered struts as assessed by optical coherency tomography at 6–8 months follow-up [62] with biodegradable versus permanent polymer DES. Unfortunately however, proof-of-concept remains to be reliably established as only few studies are available with sufficiently long enough follow-up to examine whether these devices truly offer an advantage in terms of long-term clinical safety [63]. One such study is the LEADERS study, which showed a significantly lower rate of very late definite ST between 1- and 5-years follow-up with the BioMatrix (Biosensor, Morges, Switzerland), biodegradable polymer biolimus-eluting stent (BES) compared to Cypher permanent polymer SES (Fig. 21.2) [63].

Several meta-analyses have been conducted to compare the outcomes from the use of permanent versus biodegradable polymer DES. However, it must be noted that these are unable to overcome the absence of long-term follow-up data [11, 12, 14, 64, 65]. Stefanini et al. performed [64] a patient-level meta-analysis of the LEADERS, ISAR TEST 3 and ISAR TEST 4 studies reporting outcomes from 2358 patients treated with biodegradable polymer DES, and 1704 patients treated with permanent polymer first generation DES. In support of the benefits of biodegradable polymer DES were the significantly lower rates of overall definite ST (HR 0.56, p=0.02), and very-late (>1 year after stent deployment) ST (HR 0.22, p=0.004) observed with their use at 4-years follow-up. Efficacy as assessed by target lesion revascularization (TLR, HR 0.82, p=0.03) was also in shown to be in their favor. Similar positive signals in favor of biodegradable polymer DES were identified by

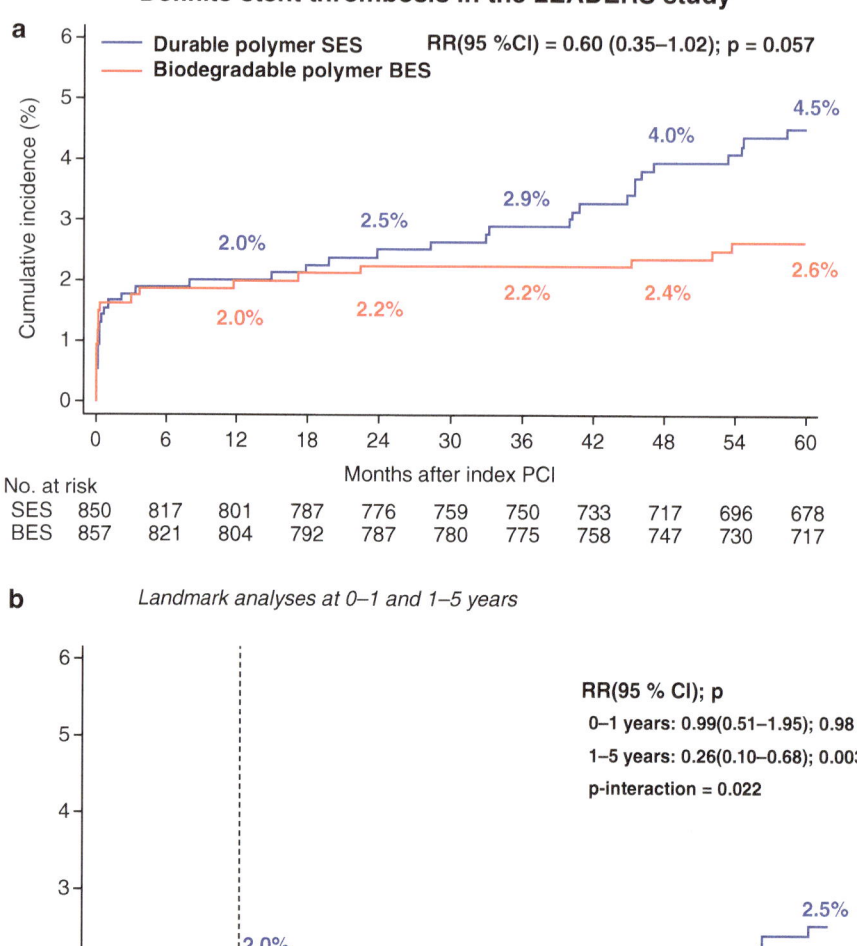

Fig. 21.2 The cumulative incidence (**a**) and landmark analyses (**b**) of definite stent thrombosis for patients receiving the biodegradable polymer biolimus-eluting stent versus the permanent polymer sirolimus-eluting stent in the all-comers randomized LEADERS study [63]. The rates of stent thrombosis were comparable for both stents at 1-year, and significantly lower with the biodegradable polymer stent between 1 and 5 years follow-up

Navarese et al. [65] who reported a significantly lower in-stent late loss (p=0.004), and late/very late ST (OR 0.60, p=0.02) among patients at a median of 9-months follow-up who were randomized to biodegradable polymer stents eluting paclitaxel, sirolimus or biolimus (n=3977) or permanent polymer first generation SES or PES (n=3487).

Larger network meta-analyses, which have included results from studies of newer generation DES, have failed to identify any significant differences in safety and efficacy between biodegradable and permanent polymer DES [11, 12, 14]. Notably, significantly higher rates of definite ST have been reported with biodegradable polymer DES compared to EES at 1-year (OR 2.44, 95 % CI 1.30–4.76), which was largely driven by early events [14]. Long-term, albeit in the presence of limited data, no significant differences have been seen between biodegradable polymer and newer generation DES with regards to the risk of very late ST. It is noteworthy that recent large randomized studies of the biodegradable polymer BES which have shown non-inferiority with EES in terms of major adverse cardiovascular events (MACE), (COMPARE 2 study) [38] and TLR (NEXT study) [40] at 12-months follow-up are absent, as is the SORT OUT VI study which showed that the Resolute ZES was non-inferior to BES in terms of 12-months MACE [41].

Ultimately, robust data to support the improvements in long-term safety with biodegradable polymer DES remain absent. Furthermore, their ability to show the hypothesized improvement in safety has been made more arduous in light of the concurrent development and advances in the biocompatibility of the permanent polymers on newer generation DES such as EES and ZES.

Polymer Versus Polymer-Free DES

Building on the principal that the polymer is a trigger for adverse safety is the development of DES which elute anti-proliferative drugs without any polymeric coating. Drug elution, which is completed between 50 h and 90 days for current devices, is achieved through either physical modifications to the stent's surface or using a non-polymeric biodegradable carrier. Eliminating the polymer avoids any potential long-term adverse effects from their presence. It also improves the integrity of the stent's surface owing to the absence of potential polymer cracking, webbing and peeling off – which have been observed *in vitro* with polymeric DES [66, 67]. In theory, these devices should offer the safety of BMS, and the efficacy of a DES from the time of deployment. Pre-clinical studies provide evidence of support with improved healing and reduced inflammation seen at 180 days in the porcine model when a polymer-free BES was compared to permanent polymer SES [68]. Clinical studies remain largely limited to first-in-man studies or randomized studies of select patient/lesion groups with first generation DES (mainly PES) as the control stent [69–72]. Powered for angiographic outcomes, results have been mixed, especially for early iterations, which had late loss values of up to 0.48 mm [69]. This was

Polymer free DES

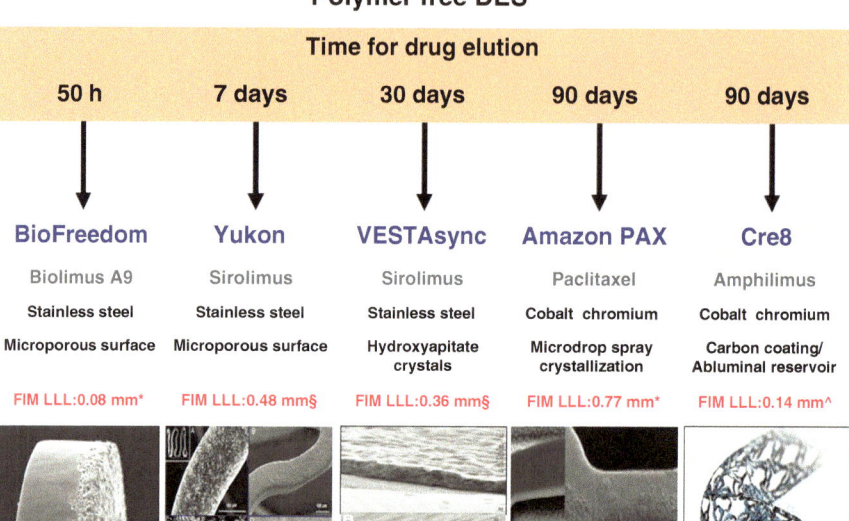

Time for drug elution				
50 h	**7 days**	**30 days**	**90 days**	**90 days**
BioFreedom	**Yukon**	**VESTAsync**	**Amazon PAX**	**Cre8**
Biolimus A9	Sirolimus	Sirolimus	Paclitaxel	Amphilimus
Stainless steel	Stainless steel	Stainless steel	Cobalt chromium	Cobalt chromium
Microporous surface	Microporous surface	Hydroxyapitate crystals	Microdrop spray crystallization	Carbon coating/ Abluminal reservoir
FIM LLL:0.08 mm*	FIM LLL:0.48 mm§	FIM LLL:0.36 mm§	FIM LLL:0.77 mm*	FIM LLL:0.14 mm^

Fig. 21.3 Key features of the five main polymer-free stents. Stent surfaces have been modified in a variety of ways to facilitate elution of the anti-proliferative agent over a different time periods ranging from 50 h to 90-days. Late loss values shown are from 4-(*), 6-(^) or 9-(§) months angiographic follow-up

thought to be due to rapid drug elution, however, contemporary devices eluting biolimus (over 50 h) [72] and amphilimus (over 3 months) [70] have restored some confidence in the devices with late loss values of 0.08 mm and 0.14 mm, respectively which are comparable to controls (Fig. 21.3).

In the presence of limited data, the utility of these devices is yet to be established. An attractive potential role is in those patients who require the efficacy of a DES, but are unable to take DAPT for a prolonged period. This scenario which is being assessed in the LEADER FREE study which is enrolling 2500 patients who, owing to comorbidity or a high-risk of bleeding, are unable to receive DAPT for longer than 1 month [73]. As with biodegradable polymer devices, the concurrent improvements in permanent polymer DES, together with the shortened mandatory period for DAPT may limit the ability of these devices to enter mainstream practice, particularly considering the cost premium that is currently attached with their use.

Stent Platform

The stent platform is the skeleton of the stent, which provides sufficient radial force at the time of deployment to prevent acute vessel closure following balloon-induced plaque dissection. Long-term its role is to provide a scaffold to facilitate vessel healing and prevent plaque prolapse. Presently, most stent platforms are made of permanent metals. However, similar to the polymer, the effective role of the stent is complete once the vessel has healed and endothelialization has occurred, paving the way for bioresorbable scaffolds.

Permanent Stent Platform

Permanent stent platforms have undergone numerous modifications, which have been fuelled by the observed relationship between stent strut geometry and the degree of vessel wall injury and subsequent restenosis [74, 75]. Coupled with this is the evolution in the complexity of coronary anatomy treated with PCI and the desire to improve procedural success and clinical outcomes.

The early stents were made of stainless steel, however this has been replaced on contemporary devices, other than the BES, with cobalt or platinum chromium. Beside improved radio-opacity, these alloys have a greater tensile strength allowing sufficient radial strength to be generated from struts of less than 100 μm—the Orsiro (Biotronik, Germany) stent has a strut thickness of only 60 μm—compared to 140 μm with the Cypher SES.

Thinner struts improve deliverability and side branch accessibility, and in theory lead to better outcomes through superior re-endothelialization, reduced peri-stent inflammation and fibirin deposition, a smaller obstacle for blood flow with less shear disturbances and a lower risk of vascular trauma to the elastic lamina and medial wall [74–79]. It is important to acknowledge that some of these postulated benefits may only be applicable to BMS devices, as studies comparing thick strut DES to thin strut BMS have shown that drug elution influences outcomes more than strut thickness [80]. Data from OCT performed 6–8 months after implantation of DES with thin or thick struts demonstrated improved strut coverage with thinner strut DES, however no differences in neointimal hyperplasia were seen. In the PERSUS study, comparable angiographic and clinical outcomes were seen among patients receiving a PES, which had either a thin strut platinum chromium or thick strut stainless steel platform [81].

In addition to altering stent strut thickness, stent flexibility and deliverability have been optimized by modifications to the cell design and connectors between cells. The Cypher SES had a closed cell design, which activated fewer platelets and reduced tissue prolapsed. However, this design limited its flexibility and subsequently increased its risk of fracture [82, 83]. In contrast, greater flexibility and its related lower degree of arterial injury can be achieved with open cell designs with fewer cell connectors.

While the reductions in strut thickness and number of connectors have been welcomed, case reports of longitudinal stent deformation and its subsequent clinical sequellae have raised anxieties [84]. Re-evaluation in prospective studies has alleviated some of these worries, [85] which have also been overcome with education and subtle design modifications, such as the introduction of additional connectors.

In summary, the optimal permanent stent platform is one that has adequate tensile strength to allow thin stent struts with high radio-opacity, and a cell configuration, which balances the need for deliverability and flexibility against minimizing the unsupported circumferential sectional area, stent deformity, and risk of tissue prolapse.

Bioresorbable Scaffolds

Interest in bioresorbable scaffolds has grown in an attempt to overcome the perceived disadvantages of permanent metallic stents, which include the absence of any functionality once vessel healing has taken place, the risk of neoatherosclerosis and adverse events, allergic reaction to metals, hypersensitivity to polymers and the inability to anastomose a stented segment with a bypass graft. In essence, these bioresorbable scaffolds help maintain vessel patency and prevent acute vessel closure at the time of balloon angioplasty. Over time, they biodegrade into inert substances allowing vessel physiology to be restored removing any residual intra-vascular foreign material [86–89]. Numerous bioresorbable scaffolds have been developed, with clinical data confined for the most to first-in-man studies (Table 21.4) [90–100]. The results of these, together with data from the extensively studied ABSORB EES (ABBOTT Vascular, Santa Clara, CA) scaffold, [89, 101–103] which includes registries and a randomized study versus a permanent metallic DES, have helped bring the theoretical advantages into reality. Notwithstanding, several challenges remain.

Numerous different materials have been used as the backbone of these scaffolds ranging from magnesium, salicylic acid, tyrosine-derived polycarbonate, and most-commonly PLLA (Table 21.4, Fig. 21.4) [86, 104]. As a consequence of the tensile strength of these bioresorbable materials being at least ten times less than the alloys used in metallic stents (PLLA 40–65 Mpa vs. Cobalt chromium >1000 Mpa), thicker stent struts are required to provide sufficient radial support, and prevent acute vessel recoil during vessel healing. Current devices have strut thickness' ranging from 100 to 200 μm. Understandably, this can affect many aspects of stent deployment not least the need to use larger guiding catheters (with the resultant increased risks of vascular access site complications) and difficulties with delivering stents particularly in challenging coronary anatomy. Reassuringly, despite this, real world data of the ABSORB EES show that it can be used in bifurcation lesions, ostial lesions, chronic total occlusions and can be overlapped [105–109].

Other issues related to thick struts are their greater neointimal area, while struts abutting into the lumen can interfere with blood flow dynamics, potentially adding to the risk of ST [110–113]. The earlier discussion indicates a clear advantage for thinner struts with permanent metallic devices. However, there are no data to confirm whether this is also applicable to bioresorbable scaffolds, not least because the healing response to these devices is different with continuing positive remodeling which can negate the effects of neointimal hyperplasia [89, 101, 112]. Of note, data from

Table 21.4 Specifications of bioresorbable scaffolds

Company	Strut material	Coating	Eluted drug	Radio-opacity	Strut thickness (μm)	Duration of radial support	Resorption time (months)	Angiographic late loss, (mm)
Igaki–Tamai (Kyoto medical)	PLLA	Nil	Nil	Gold marker	170	6 months	24–36	0.48*
AMS (Biotronik)	Mg alloy	Nil	Nil	Nil	165	Days or months	<4	1.08§
DREAMS I (Biotronik)	Mg alloy	PLGA	Paclitaxel	Nil	125		9	0.64*
DREAMS II (Biotronik)	Mg alloy	PLA	Sirolimus	Marker	120–150	NA	NA	NA
BVS 1.0 (Abbott Vascular)	PLLA	PDLLA	Everolimus	Platinum marker	156	Weeks	24	0.44*
Absorb BVS 1.1 (Abbott Vascular)	PLLA	PDLLA	Everolimus	Platinum marker	156	6 months	24	0.19*
REVA (REVA Medical)	Tyrosine-derived polycarbonate polymer	Nil	None	Scaffold	200	3–6 months	24	1.81*
ReZolve (REVA Medical)	Tyrosine-derived polycarbonate polymer	Nil	Sirolimus	Scaffold	114–228	4–6 months	24	NA
Fantom (REVA Medical)	Des-aminotyrosine-Derived Polycarbonate	NA	Sirolimus	Scaffold	<127	NA	36	NA

(continued)

Table 21.4 (continued)

Company	Strut material	Coating	Eluted drug	Radio-opacity	Strut thickness (μm)	Duration of radial support	Resorption time (months)	Angiographic late loss, (mm)
IDEAL BioStent (Xenogenics)	Polylactide anhydride mixed with a polymer of salicylic acid with a sebacic acid linker	Salicilate linged with adipic acid	Sirolimus	Scaffold	160–175	3 months	6	NA
DESolve (Elixir)	PLLA	PLLA	Novolimus	Marker	150	NA	12–24	0.19†
DESolve100 (Elixir)	PLLA	PLLA	Novolimus	Marker	100	NA	12–24	NA
ART18Z (ART)	PLLA	Nil	Nil	Nil	170	3–6 months	18	NA
Amaranth PLLA (Amaranth)	PLLA	Nil	Nil	None	150–200	3–6 months	12	0.9*
Fortitude (Amaranth)	PLLA	NA	NA	NA	120	NA	NA	NA
Xinsorb (Huaan)	PLLA, PCL, PLGA	N/A	Sirolimus	Marker	160		N/A	0.17*
On-ABS (OrbusNeich)	PLLA, PDLLA, PCL	EPC	Sirolimus	None	150		N/A	NA

Angiographic follow-up at 4(§), 6 (*), and 8 (†) months

PCL poly-L-lactide-co-ε-caprolactone, *Mg* magnesium, *PDLLA* poly-D, L-lactide, *PLGA* poly-lactide-co-glycolide, *PLLA* poly-L-lactic acid, *PLGA* poly-lactide-co-glycolide, *N/A* not applicable, *EPC* endothelial progenitor capture

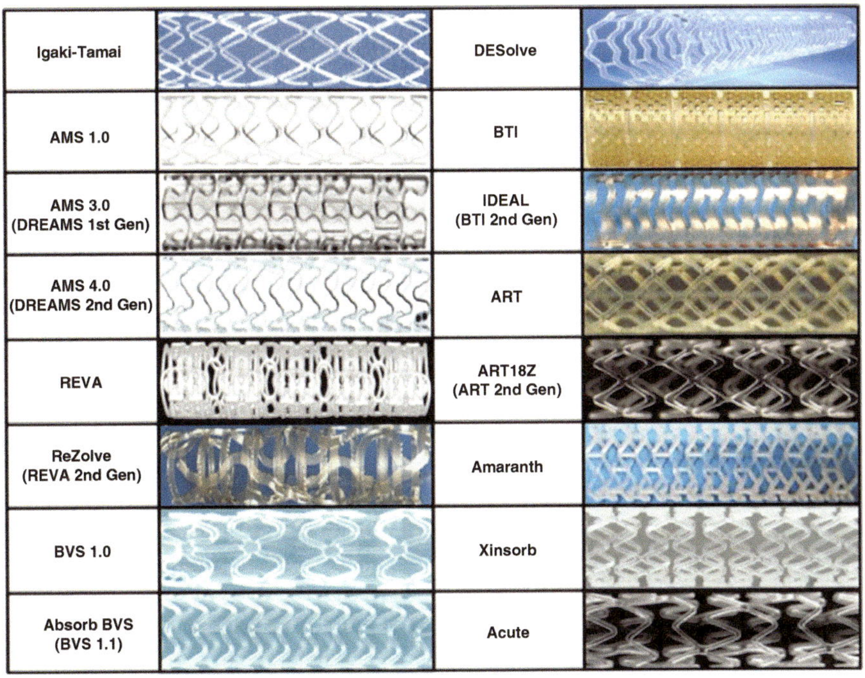

Fig. 21.4 Bioresorbable scaffolds undergoing pre-clinical and clinical evaluation

initial first-in-man studies showed unacceptable late loss, with values of up to 1.81 mm at 6-months follow-up of the REVA stent [93]. This poor efficacy was related to a failure to establish the optimal properties of the scaffold material, and the absence of anti-proliferative drugs on early scaffolds. Like the permanent metal DES, the absence of drug elution appears to lead to unacceptable rates of neointimal hyperplasia with scaffolds. Fortunately, contemporary scaffolds, which elute macro-cyclic lactones, have been able to dispel the theoretical concerns of inferior efficacy with thick struts as evidenced by late loss values from first-in-man studies of 0.19 mm with the ABSORB EES (strut thickness 157 µm) [114] and DESolve nyolimus-eluting scaffold (strut thickness 150 µm, Elixir Medical, Sunnyvale, CA) [94]. Furthermore, there are comparable rates of TLR in the ABSORB II study which randomized the ABSORB EES to the Xience V EES (strut thickness 81 µm) [103].

Emerging data have shown that bioresorbable scaffolds are not immune to the risk of thrombotic events. In the ABSORB II study there were two definite scaffold thromboses (one acute, one sub-acute) versus zero for EES. One of these involved overlapping scaffolds with the other treatment of a bifurcation lesion. Other examples of definite scaffold thrombosis have been reported with one reported event as late as 22 months following scaffold implantation (very late) [115]. While these events are scarce, they serve to increase vigilance, and indicate that no intra-coronary implant is exempt from thrombosis.

Conclusions

The following conclusions can be made regarding the optimal coronary stent design:

1. It is desirable to implant coronary stents that elute an anti-proliferative drug, with macrocyclic lactone inhibitors the preferred agents of choice.
2. Paclitaxel should not be used in DES, and its current use should be limited to drug-eluting balloons.
3. Contemporary data have not found any increased risk of adverse safety events with the newer generation DES compared with BMS.
4. Data from large contemporary meta-analyses confirm that the everolimus-eluting stent currently has the best combined efficacy and safety attributable to its thin-struts, and biocompatible fluoro-polymer which elutes 80 % of its everolimus in the first month after deployment
5. The absence of long-term follow-up data makes definitive conclusions difficult regarding the durable safety benefits of biodegradable polymer DES compared with newer generation permanent polymer DES.
6. The clinical utility of polymer free DES remains to be established in light of limited clinical data.
7. The optimal permanent stent platform is one that has adequate tensile strength to allow thin stent struts with high radio-opacity, and a cell configuration, which balances the need for deliverability and flexibility against minimizing the unsupported circumferential sectional area and the risk of stent deformity and tissue prolapse.
8. Bioresorbable scaffolds offer the potential to overcome some of the inherent problems of permanent metallic stents and emerging clinical trial data support their comparable performance in simple lesion types.
9. Bioresorbable scaffolds are not immune to the problems of acute, late or very late scaffold thrombosis.

References

1. Sigwart U, Puel J, Mirkovitch V, Joffre F, Kappenberger L. Intravascular stents to prevent occlusion and restenosis after transluminal angioplasty. N Engl J Med. 1987;316:701–6.
2. Morice MC, Serruys PW, Sousa JE, Fajadet J, Ban Hayashi E, Perin M, et al. A randomized comparison of a sirolimus-eluting stent with a standard stent for coronary revascularization. N Engl J Med. 2002;346:1773–80.
3. Nordmann AJ, Briel M, Bucher HC. Mortality in randomized controlled trials comparing drug-eluting vs. bare metal stents in coronary artery disease: a meta-analysis. Eur Heart J. 2006;27:2784–814.
4. Camenzind E, Steg PG, Wijns W. Stent thrombosis late after implantation of first-generation drug-eluting stents: a cause for concern. Circulation. 2007;115:1440–55; discussion 1455.
5. Pfisterer M, Brunner-La Rocca HP, Buser PT, Rickenbacher P, Hunziker P, Mueller C, et al. Late clinical events after clopidogrel discontinuation may limit the benefit of drug-eluting

stents: an observational study of drug-eluting versus bare-metal stents. J Am Coll Cardiol. 2006;48:2584–91.

6. Stone GW, Moses JW, Ellis SG, Schofer J, Dawkins KD, Morice M-C, et al. Safety and efficacy of sirolimus- and paclitaxel-eluting coronary stents. N Engl J Med. 2007;356: 998–1008.

7. Spaulding C, Daemen J, Boersma E, Cutlip DE, Serruys PW. A pooled analysis of data comparing sirolimus-eluting stents with bare-metal stents. N Engl J Med. 2007;356:989–97.

8. Mauri L, Hsieh WH, Massaro JM, Ho KK, D'Agostino R, Cutlip DE. Stent thrombosis in randomized clinical trials of drug-eluting stents. N Engl J Med. 2007;356:1020–9.

9. Kirtane AJ, Gupta A, Iyengar S, Moses JW, Leon MB, Applegate R, et al. Safety and efficacy of drug-eluting and bare metal stents: comprehensive meta-analysis of randomized trials and observational studies. Circulation. 2009;119:3198–206.

10. Stettler C, Wandel S, Allemann S, Kastrati A, Morice MC, Schomig A, et al. Outcomes associated with drug-eluting and bare-metal stents: a collaborative network meta-analysis. Lancet. 2007;370:937–48.

11. Kang SH, Park KW, Kang DY, Lim WH, Park KT, Han JK, et al. Biodegradable-polymer drug-eluting stents vs. bare metal stents vs. durable-polymer drug-eluting stents: a systematic review and Bayesian approach network meta-analysis. Eur Heart J. 2014;35:1147–58.

12. Bangalore S, Toklu B, Amoroso N, Fusaro M, Kumar S, Hannan EL, et al. Bare metal stents, durable polymer drug eluting stents, and biodegradable polymer drug eluting stents for coronary artery disease: mixed treatment comparison meta-analysis. BMJ. 2013;347:f6625.

13. Valgimigli M, Sabate M, Kaiser C, Brugaletta S, de la Torre Hernandez JM, Galatius S, et al. Effects of cobalt-chromium everolimus eluting stents or bare metal stent on fatal and nonfatal cardiovascular events: patient level meta-analysis. BMJ. 2014;349:g6427.

14. Palmerini T, Biondi-Zoccai G, Della Riva D, Mariani A, Sabate M, Smits PC, et al. Clinical outcomes with bioabsorbable polymer- versus durable polymer-based drug-eluting and bare-metal stents: evidence from a comprehensive network meta-analysis. J Am Coll Cardiol. 2014;63:299–307.

15. Sabate M, Raber L, Heg D, Brugaletta S, Kelbaek H, Cequier A, et al. Comparison of newer-generation drug-eluting with bare-metal stents in patients with acute ST-segment elevation myocardial infarction: a pooled analysis of the EXAMINATION (clinical Evaluation of the Xience-V stent in Acute Myocardial INfArcTION) and COMFORTABLE-AMI (Comparison of Biolimus Eluted From an Erodible Stent Coating With Bare Metal Stents in Acute ST-Elevation Myocardial Infarction) trials. JACC Cardiovasc Interv. 2014;7:55–63.

16. Palmerini T, Biondi-Zoccai G, Della Riva D, Stettler C, Sangiorgi D, D'Ascenzo F, et al. Stent thrombosis with drug-eluting and bare-metal stents: evidence from a comprehensive network meta-analysis. Lancet. 2012;379:1393–402.

17. Morice MC, Urban P, Greene S, Schuler G, Chevalier B. Why are we still using coronary bare-metal stents? J Am Coll Cardiol. 2013;61:1122–3.

18. Kaiser C, Galatius S, Jeger R, Gilgen N, Jensen JS, Naber C, et al. Long-term efficacy and safety of biodegradable-polymer biolimus-eluting stents: main results of the Basel Stent Kosten-Effektivitats Trial-PROspective Validation Examination II (BASKET-PROVE II), a randomized, controlled noninferiority 2-year outcome trial. Circulation. 2015;131:74–81.

19. Garg S, Serruys P. Benefits of and safety concerns associated with drug-eluting coronary stents. Expert Rev Cardiovasc Ther. 2010;8:449–70.

20. van Werkum JW, Heestermans AA, Zomer AC, Kelder JC, Suttorp MJ, Rensing BJ, et al. Predictors of coronary stent thrombosis: the Dutch Stent Thrombosis Registry. J Am Coll Cardiol. 2009;53:1399–409.

21. Wijns W, Kolh P, Danchin N, Di Mario C, Falk V, Folliguet T, et al. Guidelines on myocardial revascularization. Eur Heart J. 2010;31:2501–55.

22. Valgimigli M, Campo G, Monti M, Vranckx P, Percoco G, Tumscitz C, et al. Short- versus long-term duration of dual-antiplatelet therapy after coronary stenting: a randomized multi-center trial. Circulation. 2012;125:2015–26.

23. Kim BK, Hong MK, Shin DH, Nam CM, Kim JS, Ko YG, et al. A new strategy for discontinuation of dual antiplatelet therapy: the RESET Trial (REal Safety and Efficacy of 3-month dual antiplatelet Therapy following Endeavor zotarolimus-eluting stent implantation). J Am Coll Cardiol. 2012;60:1340–8.

24. Valgimigli M, Patialiakas A, Thury A, McFadden E, Colangelo S, Campo G, et al. Zotarolimus-eluting versus bare-metal stents in uncertain drug-eluting stent candidates. J Am Coll Cardiol. 2015;65:805–15.

25. Gilard M, Barragan P, Noryani AA, Noor HA, Majwal T, Hovasse T, et al. 6- versus 24-month dual antiplatelet therapy after implantation of drug-eluting stents in patients nonresistant to aspirin: the randomized, multicenter ITALIC trial. J Am Coll Cardiol. 2015;65:777–86.

26. Schomig A, Dibra A, Windecker S, Mehilli J, Suarez de Lezo J, Kaiser C, et al. A meta-analysis of 16 randomized trials of sirolimus-eluting stents versus paclitaxel-eluting stents in patients with coronary artery disease. J Am Coll Cardiol. 2007;50:1373–80.

27. Scheller B, Hehrlein C, Bocksch W, Rutsch W, Haghi D, Dietz U, et al. Treatment of coronary in-stent restenosis with a paclitaxel-coated balloon catheter. N Engl J Med. 2006;355: 2113–24.

28. Steigerwald K, Ballke S, Quee SC, Byrne RA, Vorpahl M, Vogeser M, et al. Vascular healing in drug-eluting stents: differential drug-associated response of limus-eluting stents in a pre-clinical model of stent implantation. EuroIntervention. 2012;8:752–9.

29. Joner M, Nakazawa G, Finn AV, Quee SC, Coleman L, Acampado E, et al. Endothelial cell recovery between comparator polymer-based drug-eluting stents. J Am Coll Cardiol. 2008;52:333–42.

30. Kolandaivelu K, Swaminathan R, Gibson WJ, Kolachalama VB, Nguyen-Ehrenreich KL, Giddings VL, et al. Stent thrombogenicity early in high-risk interventional settings is driven by stent design and deployment and protected by polymer-drug coatings. Circulation. 2011;123:1400–9.

31. Joner M, Finn AV, Farb A, Mont EK, Kolodgie FD, Ladich E, et al. Pathology of drug-eluting stents in humans: delayed healing and late thrombotic risk. J Am Coll Cardiol. 2006;48:193–202.

32. Cook S, Ladich E, Nakazawa G, Eshtehardi P, Neidhart M, Vogel R, et al. Correlation of intravascular ultrasound findings with histopathological analysis of thrombus aspirates in patients with very late drug-eluting stent thrombosis. Circulation. 2009;120:391–9.

33. Holmes Jr DR, Kereiakes DJ, Garg S, Serruys PW, Dehmer GJ, Ellis SG, et al. Stent thrombosis. J Am Coll Cardiol. 2010;56:1357–65.

34. Waksman R, Pakala R. Coating bioabsorption and chronic bare metal scaffolding versus fully bioabsorbable stent. EuroIntervention. 2009;5(Suppl F):F36–42.

35. De Jong WH, Eelco Bergsma J, Robinson JE, Bos RR. Tissue response to partially in vitro predegraded poly-L-lactide implants. Biomaterials. 2005;26:1781–91.

36. Windecker S, Serruys PW, Wandel S, Buszman P, Trznadel S, Linke A, et al. Biolimus-eluting stent with biodegradable polymer versus sirolimus-eluting stent with durable polymer for coronary revascularisation (LEADERS): a randomised non-inferiority trial. Lancet. 2008;372:1163–73.

37. Meredith IT, Verheye S, Dubois CL, Dens J, Fajadet J, Carrie D, et al. Primary endpoint results of the EVOLVE trial: a randomized evaluation of a novel bioabsorbable polymer-coated, everolimus-eluting coronary stent. J Am Coll Cardiol. 2012;59:1362–70.

38. Smits PC, Hofma S, Togni M, Vazquez N, Valdes M, Voudris V, et al. Abluminal biodegradable polymer biolimus-eluting stent versus durable polymer everolimus-eluting stent (COMPARE II): a randomised, controlled, non-inferiority trial. Lancet. 2013;381:651–60.

39. Christiansen EH, Jensen LO, Thayssen P, Tilsted HH, Krusell LR, Hansen KN, et al. Biolimus-eluting biodegradable polymer-coated stent versus durable polymer-coated sirolimus-eluting stent in unselected patients receiving percutaneous coronary intervention (SORT OUT V): a randomised non-inferiority trial. Lancet. 2013;381:661–9.

40. Natsuaki M, Kozuma K, Morimoto T, Kadota K, Muramatsu T, Nakagawa Y, et al. Biodegradable polymer biolimus-eluting stent versus durable polymer everolimus-eluting stent: a randomized, controlled, noninferiority trial. J Am Coll Cardiol. 2013;62:181–90.

41. Raungaard B, Jensen LO, Tilsted HH, Christiansen EH, Maeng M, Terkelsen CJ, et al. Zotarolimus-eluting durable-polymer-coated stent versus a biolimus-eluting biodegradable-polymer-coated stent in unselected patients undergoing percutaneous coronary intervention (SORT OUT VI): a randomised non-inferiority trial. Lancet. 2015;385(9977):1527–35.

42. Raber L, Kelbaek H, Ostojic M, Baumbach A, Heg D, Tuller D, et al. Effect of biolimus-eluting stents with biodegradable polymer vs bare-metal stents on cardiovascular events among patients with acute myocardial infarction: the COMFORTABLE AMI randomized trial. JAMA. 2012;308:777–87.

43. Dani S, Kukreja N, Parikh P, Joshi H, Prajapati J, Jain S, et al. Biodegradable-polymer-based, sirolimus-eluting Supralimus stent: 6-month angiographic and 30-month clinical follow-up results from the series I prospective study. EuroIntervention. 2008;4:59–63.

44. Han Y, Jing Q, Xu B, Yang L, Liu H, Shang X, et al. Safety and efficacy of biodegradable polymer-coated sirolimus-eluting stents in "real-world" practice: 18-month clinical and 9-month angiographic outcomes. J Am Coll Cardiol Intv. 2009;2:303–9.

45. Firehawk GR. Abluminal groove filled bioabsorbable polymer sirolimus eluting stent: Update on the first in man TARGET I and TARGET II studies. Presentation at Transcatheter Cardiovascular Therapeutics, San Francisco, 10th Nov 2011.

46. Ormiston J, Webster M, Stewart J, Vrolix M, Whitbourn R, Donohoe D, et al. First-in-human evaluation of a bioabsorbable polymer-coated sirolimus-eluting stent: imaging and clinical results of the DESSOLVE I Trial (DES with sirolimus and a bioabsorbable polymer for the treatment of patients with de novo lesion in the native coronary arteries). JACC Cardiovasc Interv. 2013;6:1026–34.

47. Garg S, Sarno G, Serruys PW, de Vries T, Buszman P, Linke A, et al. The twelve-month outcomes of a biolimus eluting stent with a biodegradable polymer compared with a sirolimus eluting stent with a durable polymer. EuroIntervention. 2010;6:233–9.

48. Chevalier B, Silber S, Park S-J, Garcia E, Schuler G, Suryapranata H, et al. Randomized comparison of the Nobori Biolimus A9-eluting coronary stent with the Taxus Liberte paclitaxel-eluting coronary stent in patients with stenosis in native coronary arteries: the NOBORI 1 trial--Phase 2. Circ Cardiovasc Interv. 2009;2:188–95.

49. Verheye S, Agostoni P, Dubois CL, Dens J, Ormiston J, Worthley S, et al. 9-month clinical, angiographic, and intravascular ultrasound results of a prospective evaluation of the Axxess self-expanding biolimus A9-eluting stent in coronary bifurcation lesions: the DIVERGE (Drug-Eluting Stent Intervention for Treating Side Branches Effectively) study. J Am Coll Cardiol. 2009;53:1031–9.

50. Haude M, Lee SW, Worthley SG, Silber S, Verheye S, Erbs S, et al. The REMEDEE trial: a randomized comparison of a combination sirolimus-eluting endothelial progenitor cell capture stent with a paclitaxel-eluting stent. JACC Cardiovasc Interv. 2013;6:334–43.

51. Verheye S. Overview of novolimus eluting and myolimus elution from durable and bioabsorbable polymers. Presentation at Transcatheter Cardiovascular Interventions, Washington, USA, 22nd Sept 2010.

52. Schofer J. Multicentre, first-in-man study on the Elixir Myolimus-eluting coronary stent system with bioabsorbable polymer: 12-month clinical and angiographic/IVUS results. Presentation EuroPCR, 25th–28th May 2010, Paris, France. Available [online] http://www.pcronline.com/Lectures/2010/Multicentre-first-in-man-study-on-the-Elixir-Myolimus-eluting-coronary-stent-system-with-bioabsorbable-polymer-12-month-clinical-and-angiographic-IVUS-results. Accessed 29 May 2010.

53. Webster M, Harding S, McClean D, Jaffe W, Ormiston J, Aitken A, et al. First-in-human evaluation of a sirolimus-eluting coronary stent on an integrated delivery system: the DIRECT study. EuroIntervention. 2013;9:46–53.

54. Dani S, Costa RA, Joshi H, Shah J, Pandya R, Virmani R, et al. First-in-human evaluation of the novel BioMime sirolimus-eluting coronary stent with bioabsorbable polymer for the treatment of single de novo lesions located in native coronary vessels - results from the meriT-1 trial. EuroIntervention. 2013;9:493–500.
55. Hamon M, Niculescu R, Deleanu D, Dorobantu M, Weissman NJ, Waksman R. Clinical and angiographic experience with a third-generation drug-eluting Orsiro stent in the treatment of single de novo coronary artery lesions (BIOFLOW-I): a prospective, first-in-man study. EuroIntervention. 2013;8:1006–11.
56. Lemos PA. Inspiron sirolimus eluting stent. Clinical Research Program Update. Presentation at Transcatheter Therapeutics, Miami. Oct 2012. Available http://www.tctmd.com.
57. Lemos PA, Moulin B, Perin MA, Oliveira LA, Arruda JA, Lima VC, et al. Randomized evaluation of two drug-eluting stents with identical metallic platform and biodegradable polymer but different agents (paclitaxel or sirolimus) compared against bare stents: 1-Year results of the PAINT trial. Catheter Cardiovasc Interv. 2009;74(5):665–73.
58. Vranckx P, Serruys PW, Gambhir S, Sousa E, Abizaid A, Lemos P, et al. Biodegradable-polymer-based, paclitaxel-eluting Infinnium stent: 9-Month clinical and angiographic follow-up results from the SIMPLE II prospective multi-centre registry study. EuroIntervention. 2006;2:310–7.
59. Koppara T, Joner M, Bayer G, Steigerwald K, Diener T, Wittchow E. Histopathological comparison of biodegradable polymer and permanent polymer based sirolimus eluting stents in a porcine model of coronary stent implantation. Thromb Haemost. 2012;107:1161–71.
60. Hamilos M, Sarma J, Ostojic M, Cuisset T, Sarno G, Melikian N, et al. Interference of drug-eluting stents with endothelium-dependent coronary vasomotion: evidence for device-specific responses. Circ Cardiovasc Interv. 2008;1:193–200.
61. Tada T, Kastrati A, Byrne RA, Schuster T, Cuni R, King LA, et al. Randomized comparison of biolimus-eluting stents with biodegradable polymer versus everolimus-eluting stents with permanent polymer coatings assessed by optical coherence tomography. Int J Cardiovasc Imaging. 2014;30:495–504.
62. Barlis P, Regar E, Serruys PW, Dimopoulos K, van der Giessen WJ, van Geuns RJ, et al. An optical coherence tomography study of a biodegradable vs. durable polymer-coated limus-eluting stent: a LEADERS trial sub-study. Eur Heart J. 2010;31:165–76.
63. Serruys PW, Farooq V, Kalesan B, de Vries T, Buszman P, Linke A, et al. Improved Safety and Reduction in Stent Thrombosis Associated With Biodegradable Polymer-Based Biolimus-Eluting Stents Versus Durable Polymer-Based Sirolimus-Eluting Stents in Patients With Coronary Artery Disease: Final 5-Year Report of the LEADERS (Limus Eluted From A Durable Versus ERodable Stent Coating) Randomized Noninferiority Trial. JACC Cardiovasc Interv. 2013;6:777–89.
64. Stefanini GG, Byrne RA, Serruys PW, de Waha A, Meier B, Massberg S, et al. Biodegradable polymer drug-eluting stents reduce the risk of stent thrombosis at 4 years in patients undergoing percutaneous coronary intervention: a pooled analysis of individual patient data from the ISAR-TEST 3, ISAR-TEST 4, and LEADERS randomized trials. Eur Heart J. 2012; 33:1214–22.
65. Navarese EP, Tandjung K, Claessen B, Andreotti F, Kowalewski M, Kandzari DE, et al. Safety and efficacy outcomes of first and second generation durable polymer drug eluting stents and biodegradable polymer biolimus eluting stents in clinical practice: comprehensive network meta-analysis. BMJ. 2013;347:f6530.
66. Basalus MW, Ankone MJ, van Houwelingen GK, de Man FH, von Birgelen C. Coating irregularities of durable polymer-based drug-eluting stents as assessed by scanning electron microscopy. EuroIntervention. 2009;5:157–65.
67. Basalus MW, van Houwelingen KG, Ankone M, de Man FH, von Birgelen C. Scanning electron microscopic assessment of the biodegradable coating on expanded biolimus-eluting stents. EuroIntervention. 2009;5:505–10.

68. Tada N, Virmani R, Grant G, Bartlett L, Black A, Clavijo C, et al. Polymer-free biolimus a9-coated stent demonstrates more sustained intimal inhibition, improved healing, and reduced inflammation compared with a polymer-coated sirolimus-eluting cypher stent in a porcine model. Circ Cardiovasc Interv. 2010;3:174–83.

69. Mehilli J, Kastrati A, Wessely R, Dibra A, Hausleiter J, Jaschke B, et al. Randomized trial of a nonpolymer-based rapamycin-eluting stent versus a polymer-based paclitaxel-eluting stent for the reduction of late lumen loss. Circulation. 2006;113:273–9.

70. Carrie D, Berland J, Verheye S, Hauptmann KE, Vrolix M, Violini R, et al. A multicenter randomized trial comparing amphilimus- with paclitaxel-eluting stents in de novo native coronary artery lesions. J Am Coll Cardiol. 2012;59:1371–6.

71. Costa Jr JR, Abizaid A, Costa R, Feres F, Tanajura LF, Abizaid A, et al. 1-year results of the hydroxyapatite polymer-free sirolimus-eluting stent for the treatment of single de novo coronary lesions: the VESTASYNC I trial. J Am Coll Cardiol Intv. 2009;2:422–7.

72. Grube E. Biofreedom: polymer-free drug-eluting stent – 3 year results. Presentation at Transcatheter Cardiovascular Therapeutics. October 2012. Available http://www.tctmd.com.

73. Urban P, Abizaid A, Chevalier B, Greene S, Meredith I, Morice MC, et al. Rationale and design of the LEADERS FREE trial: a randomized double-blind comparison of the BioFreedom drug-coated stent vs the Gazelle bare metal stent in patients at high bleeding risk using a short (1 month) course of dual antiplatelet therapy. Am Heart J. 2013;165:704–9.

74. Garasic JM, Edelman ER, Squire JC, Seifert P, Williams MS, Rogers C. Stent and artery geometry determine intimal thickening independent of arterial injury. Circulation. 2000;101:812–8.

75. Sullivan TM, Ainsworth SD, Langan EM, Taylor S, Snyder B, Cull D, et al. Effect of endovascular stent strut geometry on vascular injury, myointimal hyperplasia, and restenosis. J Vasc Surg. 2002;36:143–9.

76. Kastrati A, Mehilli J, Dirschinger J, Dotzer F, Schuhlen H, Neumann FJ, et al. Intracoronary stenting and angiographic results: strut thickness effect on restenosis outcome (ISAR-STEREO) trial. Circulation. 2001;103:2816–21.

77. Pache J, Kastrati A, Mehilli J, Schuhlen H, Dotzer F, Hausleiter J, et al. Intracoronary stenting and angiographic results: strut thickness effect on restenosis outcome (ISAR-STEREO-2) trial. J Am Coll Cardiol. 2003;41:1283–8.

78. Briguori C, Sarais C, Pagnotta P, Liistro F, Montorfano M, Chieffo A, et al. In-stent restenosis in small coronary arteries: impact of strut thickness. J Am Coll Cardiol. 2002;40:403–9.

79. Timmins LH, Miller MW, Clubb Jr FJ, Moore Jr JE. Increased artery wall stress post-stenting leads to greater intimal thickening. Lab Invest. 2011;91:955–67.

80. Pache J, Dibra A, Mehilli J, Dirschinger J, Schomig A, Kastrati A. Drug-eluting stents compared with thin-strut bare stents for the reduction of restenosis: a prospective, randomized trial. Eur Heart J. 2005;26:1262–8.

81. Kereiakes DJ, Cannon LA, Feldman RL, Popma JJ, Magorien R, Whitbourn R, et al. Clinical and angiographic outcomes after treatment of de novo coronary stenoses with a novel platinum chromium thin-strut stent: primary results of the PERSEUS (Prospective Evaluation in a Randomized Trial of the Safety and Efficacy of the Use of the TAXUS Element Paclitaxel-Eluting Coronary Stent System) trial. J Am Coll Cardiol. 2010;56:264–71.

82. Aoki J, Nakazawa G, Tanabe K, Hoye A, Yamamoto H, Nakayama T, et al. Incidence and clinical impact of coronary stent fracture after sirolimus-eluting stent implantation. Catheter Cardiovasc Interv. 2007;69:380–6.

83. Park MW, Chang K, Her SH, Lee JM, Choi YS, Kim DB, et al. Incidence and clinical impact of fracture of drug-eluting stents widely used in current clinical practice: comparison with initial platform of sirolimus-eluting stent. J Cardiol. 2012;60:215–21.

84. Mamas MA, Williams PD. Longitudinal stent deformation: insights on mechanisms, treatments and outcomes from the Food and Drug Administration Manufacturer and User Facility Device Experience database. EuroIntervention. 2012;8:196–204.

85. von Birgelen C, Sen H, Lam MK, Danse PW, Jessurun GA, Hautvast RW, et al. Third-generation zotarolimus-eluting and everolimus-eluting stents in all-comer patients requiring a percutaneous coronary intervention (DUTCH PEERS): a randomised, single-blind, multi-centre, non-inferiority trial. Lancet. 2014;383:413–23.

86. Garg S, Serruys PW. Coronary stents: looking forward. J Am Coll Cardiol. 2010; 56:S43–78.

87. Serruys PW, Onuma Y, Lafont A, Abizaid A, Waksman R, Ormiston J. Bioresorable Scaffolds. In: Eeckhout E, Serruys PW, Wijns W, Vahanian A, van Sambeek M, editors. Percutaneous interventional cardiovascular medicine. Paris: Europa Edition Publishing; 2012. p. 145–77. Part III, Chapter 4.

88. Serruys PW, Onuma Y, Dudek D, Smits PC, Koolen J, Chevalier B, et al. Evaluation of the second generation of a bioresorbable everolimus-eluting vascular scaffold for the treatment of de novo coronary artery stenosis: 12-month clinical and imaging outcomes. J Am Coll Cardiol. 2011;58:1578–88.

89. Serruys PW, Ormiston JA, Onuma Y, Regar E, Gonzalo N, Garcia-Garcia HM, et al. A bioabsorbable everolimus-eluting coronary stent system (ABSORB): 2-year outcomes and results from multiple imaging methods. Lancet. 2009;373:897–910.

90. Erbel R, Di Mario C, Bartunek J, Bonnier J, de Bruyne B, Eberli FR, et al. Temporary scaffolding of coronary arteries with bioabsorbable magnesium stents: a prospective, non-randomised multicentre trial. Lancet. 2007;369:1869–75.

91. Haude M, Erbel R, Erne P, Verheye S, Degen H, Bose D, et al. Safety and performance of the drug-eluting absorbable metal scaffold (DREAMS) in patients with de-novo coronary lesions: 12 month results of the prospective, multicentre, first-in-man BIOSOLVE-I trial. Lancet. 2013;381:836–44.

92. Abizaid A. The REVA tyrosine polycarbonate bioabsorbable stent: lessons learned and future directions. Presentation at Transcatheter Therapeutics, San Francisco, 22nd Sept 2009. Available online: http://www.tctmd.com/txshow.aspx?tid=939090&id=84050&trid=938634. Accessed 14 Oct 2009.

93. Abizaid A, Brachnam JC, Coste J, et al. 12 Morth Angiographic and clinical results of the REZOLVE sirolimos eluting bioresorbable coronary scaffold: the restore trial. J Am Coll Cardiol 2013;62(18–51):B13.

94. Yan J, Bhat VD. Elixir Medical's bioresorbable drug eluting stent (BDES) programme: an overview. EuroIntervention. 2009;5:F80–2.

95. Chammie D, Abizaid A, Webste M, et al. Evaluation of the novel desolve myolimus-eluting bioresorbable coronary scaffold system for theatment of de novo coronary arteries: six months optical coherence tomography results from de solve FIM. Trial J Am Coll Cardiol 2012;60(17–5)

96. Jabara R, Chronos N, Robinson K. Novel bioabsorbable salicylate-based polymer as a drug-eluting stent coating. Catheter Cardiovasc Interv. 2008;72:186–94.

97. Jabara R, Pendyala L, Geva S, Chen J, Chronos N, Robinson K. Novel fully bioabsorbable salicylate-based sirolimus-eluting stent. EuroIntervention. 2009;5(Suppl F):F58–64.

98. Fajadet J. The ART stent: design and early first-in-man experiences. Miami: Transcatheter Cardiovascular Therapeutics; October 15, 2012.

99. Shen L, Wang Q, Wu Y, Xie J, Zhang F, Ge L, et al. Preliminary evaluation of fully bioabsorbable PLLA sirolimus eluting stents in a porcine model. Chin J Interv Cardiol. 2009;19:301–5.

100. Shen L, Wang Q, Wu Y, Xie J, Ge J. Short-term effects of sirolimus eluting fully bioabsorbable polymeric coronary stents in a porcine model. Transcatheter Cardiovascular Therapeutics, 2011.

101. Ormiston JA, Serruys PW, Regar E, Dudek D, Thuesen L, Webster MW, et al. A bioabsorbable everolimus-eluting coronary stent system for patients with single de-novo coronary artery lesions (ABSORB): a prospective open-label trial. Lancet. 2008;371:899–907.

102. Abizaid A, Costa Jr JR, Bartorelli AL, Whitbourn R, van Geuns RJ, Chevalier B, et al. The ABSORB EXTEND study: preliminary report of the twelve-month clinical outcomes in the first 512 patients enrolled. EuroIntervention. 2014;10(12):1396–401.
103. Serruys PW, Chevalier B, Dudek D, Cequier A, Carrie D, Iniguez A, et al. A bioresorbable everolimus-eluting scaffold versus a metallic everolimus-eluting stent for ischaemic heart disease caused by de-novo native coronary artery lesions (ABSORB II): an interim 1-year analysis of clinical and procedural secondary outcomes from a randomised controlled trial. Lancet. 2015;385:43–54.
104. Muramatsu T, Onuma Y, Zhang YJ, Bourantas CV, Kharlamov A, Diletti R, et al. Progress in treatment by percutaneous coronary intervention: the stent of the future. Rev Esp Cardiol (Engl Ed). 2013;66:483–96.
105. Costopoulos C, Latib A, Naganuma T, Miyazaki T, Sato K, Figini F, et al. Comparison of early clinical outcomes between ABSORB bioresorbable vascular scaffold and everolimus-eluting stent implantation in a real-world population. Catheter Cardiovasc Interv. 2015;85:E10–5.
106. Capranzano P, Gargiulo G, Capodanno D, Longo G, Tamburino C, Ohno Y, et al. Treatment of coronary bifurcation lesions with bioresorbable vascular scaffolds. Minerva Cardioangiol. 2014;62:229–34.
107. Grundeken MJ, Hassell ME, Kraak RP, de Bruin DM, Koch KT, Henriques JP, et al. Treatment of coronary bifurcation lesions with the Absorb bioresorbable vascular scaffold in combination with the Tryton dedicated coronary bifurcation stent: evaluation using two- and three-dimensional optical coherence tomography. Eurointervention 2014: pii 20130806. doi:104244 (Epud ahead of print).
108. Mattesini A, Secco GG, Dall'Ara G, Ghione M, Rama-Merchan JC, Lupi A, et al. ABSORB biodegradable stents versus second-generation metal stents: a comparison study of 100 complex lesions treated under OCT guidance. JACC Cardiovasc Interv. 2014;7:741–50.
109. Kraak RP, Hassell ME, Grundeken MJ, Koch KT, Henriques JP, Piek JJ, et al. Initial experience and clinical evaluation of the Absorb bioresorbable vascular scaffold (BVS) in real-world practice: the AMC Single Centre Real World PCI Registry. EuroIntervention. 2015;10:1160–8.
110. Ormiston JA, Serruys PW, Onuma Y, van Geuns RJ, de Bruyne B, Dudek D, et al. First serial assessment at 6 months and 2 years of the second generation of absorb everolimus-eluting bioresorbable vascular scaffold: a multi-imaging modality study. Circ Cardiovasc Interv. 2012;5:620–32.
111. Bourantas CV, Papafaklis MI, Kotsia A, Farooq V, Muramatsu T, Gomez-Lara J, et al. Effect of the endothelial shear stress patterns on neointimal proliferation following drug-eluting bioresorbable vascular scaffold implantation: an optical coherence tomography study. JACC Cardiovasc Interv. 2014;7:315–24.
112. Serruys PW, Onuma Y, Garcia-Garcia HM, Muramatsu T, van Geuns RJ, de Bruyne B, et al. Dynamics of vessel wall changes following the implantation of the absorb everolimus-eluting bioresorbable vascular scaffold: a multi-imaging modality study at 6, 12, 24 and 36 months. EuroIntervention. 2014;9:1271–84.
113. Farooq V, Serruys PW, Heo JH, Gogas BD, Onuma Y, Perkins LE, et al. Intracoronary optical coherence tomography and histology of overlapping everolimus-eluting bioresorbable vascular scaffolds in a porcine coronary artery model: the potential implications for clinical practice. JACC Cardiovasc Interv. 2013;6:523–32.
114. Serruys PW, Onuma Y, Ormiston JA, de Bruyne B, Regar E, Dudek D, et al. Evaluation of the second generation of a bioresorbable everolimus drug-eluting vascular scaffold for treatment of de novo coronary artery stenosis: six-month clinical and imaging outcomes. Circulation. 2010;122:2301–12.
115. Sato T, Abdel-Wahab M, Richardt G. Very late thrombosis observed on optical coherence tomography 22 months after the implantation of a polymer-based bioresorbable vascular scaffold. Eur Heart J. 2015;36(20):1273.

Chapter 22
Role of Oral Therapies in the Prevention of Coronary Restenosis: Insights from Randomized Clinical Trials

A. Matías Rodríguez-Granillo, Omar Santaera, and Alfredo E. Rodríguez

Abstract Neo intimal hyperplasia after implantation of a bare metal stent (BMS) has become the main pathophysiology mechanism of coronary restenosis and stent failure during percutaneous coronary interventions (PCI). The use of drug eluting stents (DES) with local immunosuppressive drugs minimized the high frequency of in stent restenosis (ISR) observed after PCI with BMS and significantly reduced the risk of re-intervention. However, in spite of the world wide penetration of DES, in the USA, a quarter of PCI-patients still receive BMS and according to recent data, the market for BMS globally contributed around 40–45 % of the global coronary stent market in 2010 and it is expected to grow at a rate of 2 % between 2011 and 2016. BMS use is particularly high (over 50 %) in certain geographic areas with socioeconomic issues. Thus, many contemporary PCI-patients do not receive DES and are at a higher risk of restenosis. In the last decade, simultaneous with the introduction of DES, oral immunosuppressive or anti-inflammatory drugs given after BMS implantation have been used to reduce neo-intimal hyperplasia and ISR. From anti-inflammatory drugs such as prednisone or colchicine to immunosuppressive drugs like sirolimus, data are now

A.M. Rodríguez-Granillo, MD
Cardiovascular Research Center (CECI), Capital Federal, Ciudad de Buenos Aires, Argentina
e-mail: mrodriguezgranillo@centroceci.com.ar

O. Santaera, MD
Interventional Cardiology Department, Sanatorio Las Lomas,
Avda Diego Carman 555, San Isidro, Buenos Aires B 555, Argentina
e-mail: osantaera@gmail.com

A.E. Rodríguez, MD, PhD, FACC, FSCAI (✉)
Cardiac Unit, Department of Interventional Cardiology, Revista Argentina de Cardioagiologia Intervencionista (RACI), Otamendi Hospital, Buenos Aires, Argentina

Director, Cardiovascular Research Center (CECI), Buenos Aires, Argentina

Interventional Cardiology Unit, Department of Interventional Cardiology, Otamendi Hospital, Buenos Aires, Argentina

University of Buenos Aires, Post-Graduate Buenos Aires School of Medicine,
Buenos Aires, Argentina
e-mail: arodriguez@centroceci.com.ar

© Springer International Publishing Switzerland 2015
J.A. Ambrose, A.E. Rodríguez (eds.), *Controversies in Cardiology*,
DOI 10.1007/978-3-319-20415-4_22

available and several randomized studies had been conducted and reported their results, some of them at long term. However, in spite of these positive reports, none of these agents are included within revascularization guidelines. In this chapter, we review all randomized data in an attempt to find a clinical indication for these oral agents.

Keywords Coronary restenosis • Oral immunosuppressive therapy • Stents • Sirolimus • Prednisone • Cilostazol • Drug eluting stents

Introduction

Ever since the beginning of percutaneous coronary interventions (PCI) for the treatment of coronary artery disease (CAD) with balloon angioplasty, restenosis was the main limitation of this revascularization strategy. Acute vessel recoil, chronic remodeling and intimal hyperplasia were involved in the progression of this process [1–3]. The introduction of bare metal stents (BMS) in clinical practice mostly avoided the first two mechanisms but the inflammatory reaction at the stented site resulted in intimal proliferation and it became the main mechanism for in-stent restenosis (ISR) [4]. The use of drug eluting stents (DES) with local immunosuppressive drugs minimized the high frequency of restenosis observed after PCI with BMS [5, 6] reducing the relative risk of re-intervention by 50–70 % [7]. However, DES is associated with a higher risk of stent thrombosis particularly with first-generation platforms [8, 9]. Concerns with a higher risk of bleeding or noncompliance with the mandatory dual antiplatelet therapy (DAPT) became relative contraindications to DES in PCI-patients with specific clinical conditions [10–12] or certain socioeconomic issues which are more relevant in certain geographic areas where BMS are still used to a great extent. In the USA, a quarter of PCI-patients still receive BMS. According to recent data, the market for BMS globally contributed around 40–45 % of the global coronary stent market in 2010 and it is expected to grow at a rate of 2 % between 2011 and 2016 [13]. Thus, many contemporary PCI-patients do not receive DES and are at a higher risk of restenosis.

Given these disparities, another possible alternative arose. Would the immunosuppressive drugs delivered locally at the stented site with a DES have a similar efficacy and safety if administered systemically? To answer this question, another line of research developed – the use of oral immunosuppressive or anti-inflammatory (OI) drugs with balloon angioplasty or bare metal stents [14–19]. Data from pre-clinical research suggested that neointimal proliferation after stent implantation occurred during the first 2 weeks after initial vascular injury due to the initial procedure [20] and that this inflammatory response after coronary stenting was deeply involved in ISR [21]. Therefore, OI agents given for a short period of time after PCI might result in a reduction in angiographic and clinical restenosis. From anti-inflammatory drugs such as prednisone or colchicine to immunosuppressive drugs like sirolimus, data are available to show benefit although the results in some studies were conflicting [22, 23]. On the other hand, several randomized clinical trials

(RCT) (Table 22.1) have been conducted with positive outcomes utilizing various agents [15, 17, 23–32]. In spite of a great deal of positive data, the role of OI in patients treated with coronary stents still remains a matter of controversy. None of these agents are included in any revascularization guidelines. In this chapter, we sought to review the possible options for oral therapy with these agents in the prevention of restenosis after stent implantation.

Corticosteriods

The effects of corticosteroids are numerous and of importance is their ability to alter the immune response [33]. The known inhibition of inflammatory cells activation, an essential player in the process of neointimal proliferation and restenosis after stent implantation [33–35], was the basis to evaluate corticosteroids for the reduction of restenosis. Experimental studies showed a reduction in neointimal hyperplasia after a 2-week period of continuous hydrocortisone infusion after an aortic balloon injury, although the initial clinical trials in humans failed to achieve equivalent results. Possible reasons for failure were that they were performed in the pre-stent era or the steroids were given intravenously for a short period of time [14, 36].

Two clinical trials comparing oral prednisone with BMS vs. controls showed positive clinical results [15, 37]. The first one [15], evaluated a selected group of non-diabetic patients with CAD and an elevated C reactive protein (CRP) 72 h after successful PCI with a BMS who were randomized either to high and decremental doses of oral prednisone (n = 41) or placebo (n = 42) for 45 days. The primary clinical endpoint was 12 months event-free survival rate, defined as freedom from death, myocardial infarction (MI) or revascularization; angiographic endpoints were late loss and the restenosis rate at 6 months. Event-free survival at 12 months, was significantly lower with placebo (p = 0.006) due to a higher rate of repeat procedures for restenosis. Angiographic restenosis and late loss were also less with prednisone (p = 0.001 for both).

The IMPRESS II/MVD registry [37], included patients with multi vessel disease and showed an event-free survival rate at 12 months of 93 % with prednisone group and 69.8 % with control (p = 0.006) and a significant TVR favorable to the prednisone group (p = 0.01). The pooled data of both studies [38] revealed that, at a mean follow-up of 6.5 ± 1.4 years, event-free survival was significantly better with prednisone (87.8 vs. 47.6 %, p < 0.001). The same investigators went further and presented in 2011 and 2012 the CEREA-DES trial [24, 39], where they randomized a larger population to three arms: BMS plus placebo (n = 125), BMS plus prednisone (n = 122) and DES alone (n = 127) groups. Prednisone was given orally for 40 days, 1 mg/Kg the first 15 days after baseline PCI, 0.5 mg/kg/days 16–30 days and 0.25 mg/kg for the last 31–40 days. The primary endpoint was major adverse cardiac events (MACE) at 12 months (death, MI and target vessel revascularization [TVR]). The authors found that patients receiving BMS alone had lower event-free survival versus those treated with prednisone or DES; 80.8 % in controls compared

Table 22.1 Randomized clinical trials evaluating oral treatment for the prevention of restenosis

RCT	N° patients	Active treatment	Comparator	Time of active treatment	Time to FU angiography (if mandatory)	Max period FU	Primary endpoint
IMPRESS [15]	83	Prednisone	Placebo	45 days	6 months	12 months	Death, myocardial infarction and TVR
OSIRIS [17]	300	Usual-dose of sirolimus High-dose of sirolimus	Placebo	10 days	6 months	4 years	Angiographic restenosis
CEREA-DES [39]	375	Prednisone	BMS (control) DES (control)	40 days	NA	4 years	Cardiovascular death, myocardial infarction and TVR
ORAR II [25]	100	Sirolimus	BMS	14 days	9 months	12 months	Angiographic restenosis and late loss
Stojkovic et al. [26]	80	Sirolimus	BMS	30 days	6 months	6 months	Angiographic restenosis and late loss
Cernigliaro et al. [27]	108	Sirolimus	BMS	30 days	6 months	5 years	In-stent restenosis
CREST [29]	705	Cilostazol	DAPT + Placebo	6 months	6 months	6 months	Minimal luminal diameter
DECLARE-long [30]	500	Cilostazol	DAPT	6 months	6 months	9 months	In-stent late loss
DECLARE-diabetes [31]	400	Cilostazol	DAPT	6 months	6 months	9 months	In-stent late loss
ORAR III [32]	200	Sirolimus	Cypher, Taxus, Endeavour	14 days	NA	5 years	Cost-effectiveness

RCT randomized clinical trial, *FU* follow-up, *BMS* bare metal stent, *DES* drug eluting stent, *DAPT* dual antiplatelet therapy, *NA* not applicable, *TVR* Target vessel revascularization to 88.0 % with prednisone and 88.8 % in DES groups, respectively (P = 0.04 and 0.006). At long term follow-up, patients receiving a BMS alone had significantly lower event-free survival (75.3 %) compared with 84.1 % with prednisone (p = 0.007) and 80.6 % with DES (p = 0.03). DES patients suffered more very late stent thrombosis and MI. The need for TVR remained lower in the prednisone and DES groups (13.6 and 15.2 %, respectively), compared with BMS (23.2 %).

Therefore, in this non-diabetic population, prednisone therapy compared to BMS improved event-free survival at 1 and 4 years. While nearly 15 % of patients suffered minor drug-related side effects, such as facial edema (7 %) and transient hyperglycemia (5 %) none of them discontinued the treatment. A recent pooled data also suggested that prednisone had a significant reduction in restenosis when associated with BMS implantation [40] and may represent a clinical option in non-diabetic patients who are poor candidates for DES.

Cilostazol

Cilostazol is used for the treatment of intermittent claudication. It is a pleiotropic molecule that selectively inhibits the subtype phosphodiesterase 3 (PDE III) that degrades cAMP, causing an accumulation of cAMP within the cell [41], resulting in a direct dilatation of the vascular smooth muscular cell (VSMC). It also acts directly on inhibiting platelet aggregation and VSMC proliferation by inhibiting the mitogen-activated protein kinase (MAPK) and inducing apoptosis via the anti-oncogene p53. There is evidence suggesting that the molecule determines the up-regulation of hepatocyte growth factor (HGF), an endothelial grow factor that accelerates re-endothelization . Also, cilostazol exerts an anti-inflammatory effect by inhibiting leukocyte integrin (MAC-1), which was linked to neointimal thickening and restenosis when its expression and activation during coronary interventions is increased [42]. In summary, its multiple mechanisms of action make it promising for both reducing restenosis and as an antithrombotic agent.

Approved by the FDA, the safety profile of the drug is well established and its pleiotropic characteristics centered attention to its use in CAD, particularly for the prevention of ISR. Data showed a significant reduction in restenosis after PCI in the pre-stent era [18, 19]. With BMS, the CREST trial [29] evaluated cilostazol as a component of triple antiplatelet therapy (TAPT), including aspirin and ADP-receptors antagonists vs. DAPT alone. 705 patients were enrolled and randomized to receive either placebo or cilostazol for 6 months. At follow up angiography, late loss was significantly less with TAPT (p = 0.01) and there was a 52 % reduction in the risk of restenosis.

Subsequently, the DECLARE trials [30, 31] designed to compare DAPT with TAPT in special patient subgroups using DES, also showed favorable results. One of these, the DECLARE-Long Trial, evaluated the impact of 6 months of cilostazol after PCI with DES in patients with lesions >25 mm. The authors randomly assigned 500 patients to DAPT and TAPT groups. At 6 months the primary endpoint of in-stent and in-segment late loss was significantly lower in the TAPT group (p=0.031 and p=0.001, respectively). TLR (2.8 % vs. 6.8 %, respectively p=0.03), and MACE (2.8 % vs. 7.6 %, p=0.01) were also in favor of TAPT, with a similar incidence of stent thrombosis at 6 months (0.99). In the DECLARE-Diabetes trial [31] they compared TAPT (n=200) with DAPT (n=200) for 6 months in diabetics receiving DES and the results again were in favor of TAPT, with significant differences in in-stent and in-segment late loss (p=0.02 and p=0.031, respectively). These findings were consistent with the results of a meta-analysis recently published [43] that evaluated 7670 patients from ten controlled clinical trials comparing DAPT with TAPT; they found a significant reduction in ISR using TAPT for 6 months without differences in mortality, MI, TVR and stent thrombosis. In summary, there appears to be an important role for cilostazol in high risk patients, such as diabetics and patients with long lesions and long stents [44].

Sirolimus (Rapamycin)

A macrolide derived from the *Streptomyces hygroscopicus*, sirolimus is a potent immunosuppressive and antimitotic agent first approved in 1999 to prevent acute rejection of renal transplants [45] and now used in major heart transplant centers to mitigate transplant allograft vasculopathy [46]. It acts by inhibiting the mammalian target of rapamycin (mTOR), blocking cell division in G1 to S1 phases of the mitotic cell cycle thus reducing VSMC proliferation and migration as well as inhibiting extracellular matrix formation [47, 48].

In 1999, the first preclinical data evaluating the use of oral sirolimus after PCI with BMS for the reduction of neointimal thickening in animal restenosis models showed positive results [48]. This lead to studies evaluating the safety and feasibility in pilot trials [49, 50] where patients with de-novo coronary lesions received sirolimus for short periods immediately after BMS. These trials used doses from 2 to 5 mg per day for 14–30 days and both evaluated the incidence of TLR and late loss by angiography at 6 months. The results showed a significant reduction in binary restenosis and the ORAR pilot studies were the first ones that established a significant reduction in both parameters versus BMS alone, when sirolimus serum levels were >8 ng/ml [16, 50]. Subsequently, three RCTs in de-novo coronary lesions confirmed these positive results [25–27].

In 2004, the OSIRIS randomized trial [17] evaluated this approach for the treatment of in-stent restenosis, comparing placebo versus two different loading doses; usual loading dose (8 mg) and high loading dose (24 mg) of sirolimus, both followed by 2 mg per day during 7 days. In accordance with other publications, TVR and restenosis were significantly reduced, with a significant correlation in blood concentration levels on the day of the procedure with late lumen loss reduction at follow-up (p<0.001).

The Oral Rapamacyn in ARgentina (ORAR) III trial was a randomized comparison between BMS implantation followed by 14 days of rapamycin versus a DES strategy without rapamycin. The DEStents used were Taxus (Boston Scientific Corporation, Natick, MA, USA), Endeavour (Medtronic Vascular, Santa Rosa, CA,

USA) and Cypher, (Cordis, Warren, NJ, USA) in 98 % of cases. Patients were followed at 1, 3 and 5 years after PCI [28, 32, 51]. The primary objectives were costs and TVR. Safety was defined as the composite of death, MI and stroke. In the OR arm, patients received a sirolimus-loading dose of 10 mg the day before stent implantation followed by 3 mg per day for 13 days. OR patients received clopidogrel 75 mg a day for 1 month, and DES patients for at least 1 year. Briefly, at 1 and 3 years DES and OR groups had similar safety and efficacy although the OR strategy was cost saving [28, 51]. At 5 years [32], major differences in clinical adverse events between both groups were seen. The incidence of death was 6 % with OR and 16 % with DES (p=0.02), the composite of death, MI and stroke was 12 % with OR and 25 % with DES (p=0.01), TLR was 10 % with OR and 17.6 % with DES (p=0.05) and target vessel revascularization, the composite of cardiac death, MI and target vessel revascularization, 26 % with OR and 36 with DES (p=0.08) (Fig. 22.1). These differences were driven by poor outcomes with DES in the elderly sub-group of patients. At 5 years, stent thrombosis (definitive/probable/possible) was significantly greater with DES versus OR (9 % vs. 2 %, respectively, p=0.03). Cumulative cost was higher in the DES group. In conclusion, at 5 years follow-up, the initial DES strategy failed to be cost effective compared to OR plus BMS [32] and this later strategy had a significant reduction in mortality and in the combined

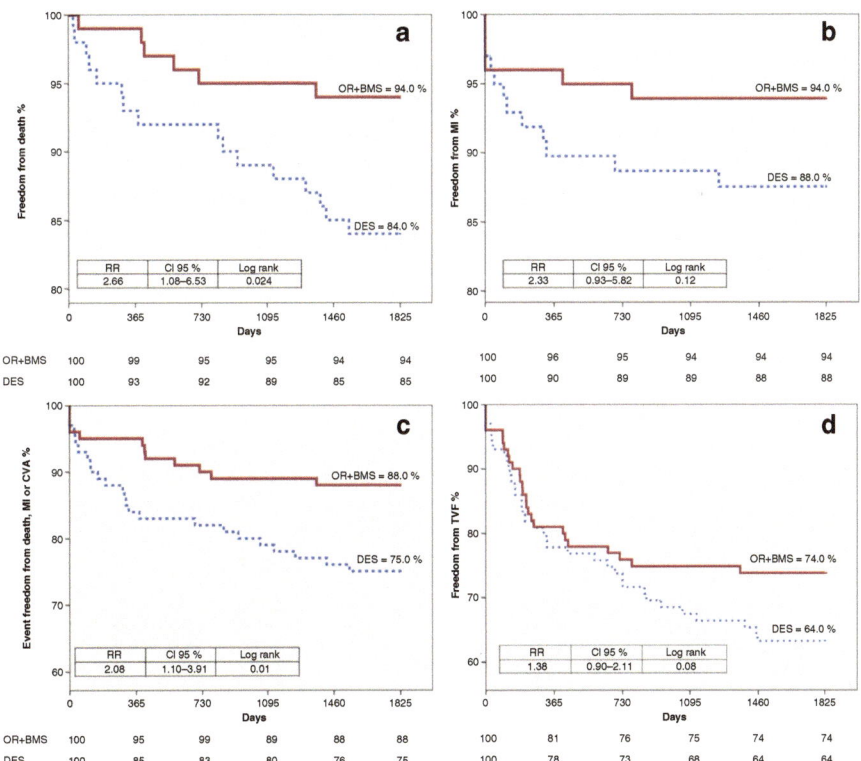

Fig. 22.1 Survival curves for clinical outcomes from 5 years of follow-up from ORAR III randomized clinical trial (OR + BMS vs. first generation DES) (Modified from Rodriguez et al. [32])

end point of death, MI and stroke. The slow progressive deterioration of results with these first generation DES beyond 3 years was observed in other studies. This was in agreement with the findings of ORAR III at 5 years [52–55].

Most studies using short treatment protocols of sirolimus (10–14 days) reported low side effects with low rates of discontinuation, around 3 or 4 % [51]. Platelet counts declined transiently with OR therapy but there was no clinical sequellae and they returned to normal after the drug was stopped. A systematic review evaluating the effectiveness of OR after BMS implantation for the prevention of restenosis was published in 2013 [56] including four RCTs in patients with de-novo coronary artery lesions. Three studies were versus BMS alone and the fourth vs. first generation DES. Follow-up duration ranged from 7 months to 5 years and they demonstrated that, compared to BMS alone, early short-term systemic use of OR after BMS led to a significant reduction in both TLR and any adverse cardiac events.

Meta-Analysis

In 2014 a meta-analysis was published [57] using patient level data from all eligible RCTs, using OI therapy with either sirolimus or prednisone for the prevention of restenosis. A total of 1246 patients (608 randomized to BMS plus OI and 638 randomized to BMS/DES and no OI) and 1456 lesions (711 randomized to BMS plus OI and 745 randomized to BMS/DES) were included. In two trials [24, 39], 1 mg/kg/day of prednisone was administered after PCI for 10–15 days with subsequent tapering until complete drug withdrawal after 40–45 days. Five OR RCTs were included [17, 25–28]; in four of them, the loading dose range was 4–24 mg; the other one [26] didn't use a loading dose. All five RCTs used a daily maintenance dose of 2–3 mg for a period of time lasting from 7 to 30 days after PCI. The primary efficacy outcome was TLR/TVR and the primary safety outcome was the composite of death and MI. Every RCT reported that an independent committee adjudicated clinical endpoints. The meta-analysis found that there was a decrease in the risk of TLR/TVR compared with control arms and, in patients with follow-up angiography,

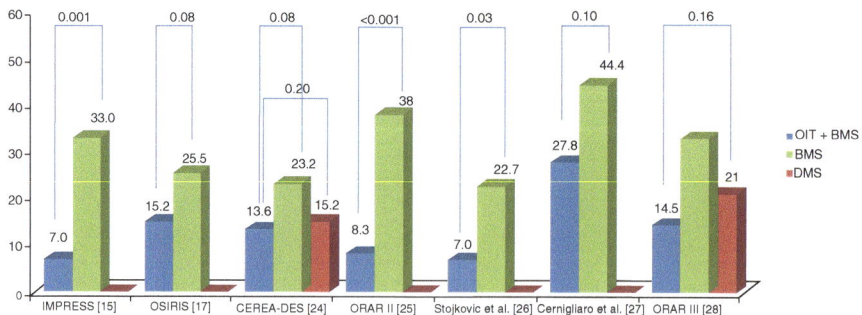

Fig. 22.2 Target vessel revascularization rates from all RCTs included in RAMSES cooperation comparing OIT + BMS vs. BMS/DES [64]

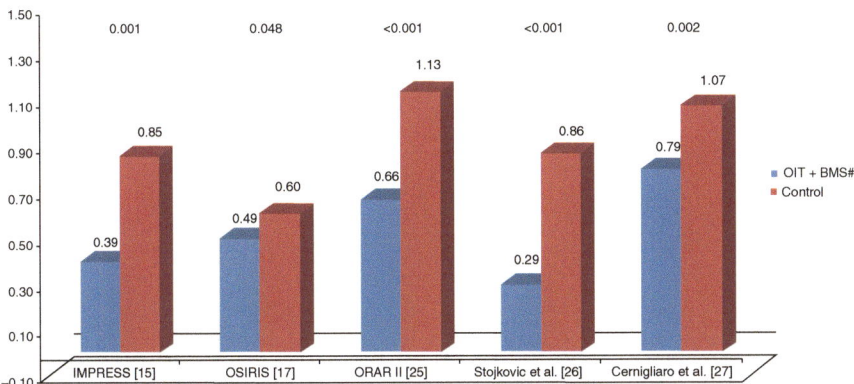

Fig. 22.3 Late luminal loss (mean) from all RCT included in RAMSES cooperation comparing OIT + BMS vs. control (either BMS/DES) at 6 months of follow-up measured by quantitative coronary angiography [64]

the oral therapy reduced late loss providing a biologic explanation for these results (Figs. 22.2 and 22.3). Moreover, oral treatment didn't affect the incidence of death and MI compared to controls.

The authors of the manuscript stated that in patients undergoing PCI, the addition of OI therapy to BMS reduced the risk of TLR as compared with BMS alone but not when the comparison was with DES. There were no differences in the composite of death/MI between these therapies (Figs. 22.4 and 22.5). The advantage of adding OI therapy to BMS was related to a lower risk of vessel re-narrowing as compared with BMS alone. Both drugs showed similar efficacy with a low rate of side effects. This strategy could be a valuable alternative for PCI-patients with a relative contraindication to DES.

Other Drugs

Colchicine

Originally indicated for the treatment of gout, colchicine is an old and well known drug that inhibits the mitotic spindle acting over the microtubules assembly [58] affecting the expression of cytokines and other components of the immune system with proven safety in cardiac patients [59]. It has been evaluated for the prevention of restenosis due to its capacity to inhibit cellular hyperplasia. Similarly to other oral agents, initial studies during the pre-stent era failed to show efficacy [60, 61]. Following the introduction of BMS, it was anticipated that it might reduce restenosis given its effects on limiting intimal hyperplasia. To prove this hypothesis, Defteros et al. in a double-blind, prospective, placebo-controlled RCT [62] assessed colchicine's effect as an anti-restenotic agent in a high risk population of diabetic patients with CAD and contraindications for DES. ISR was measured by angiography and with intravascular ultrasound (IVUS) immediately after BMS implantation and at

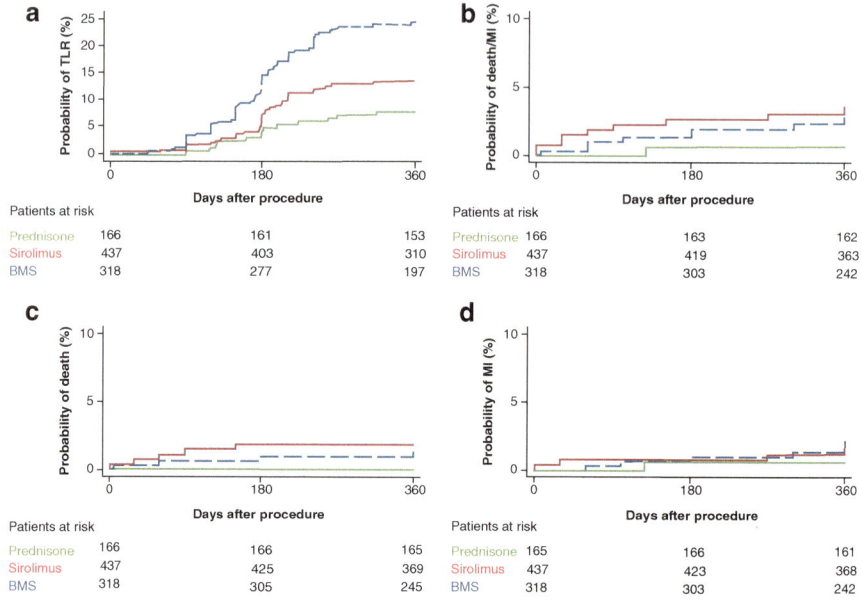

Fig. 22.4 Survival curves for primary and secondary endpoints according to the treatment received (BMS + OI [prednisone or sirolimus] or BMS) (With permission from Atherosclerosis Cassese et al. [57]). *BMS* bare metal stents, *OI* oral immunosuppressive, *MI* myocardial infarction

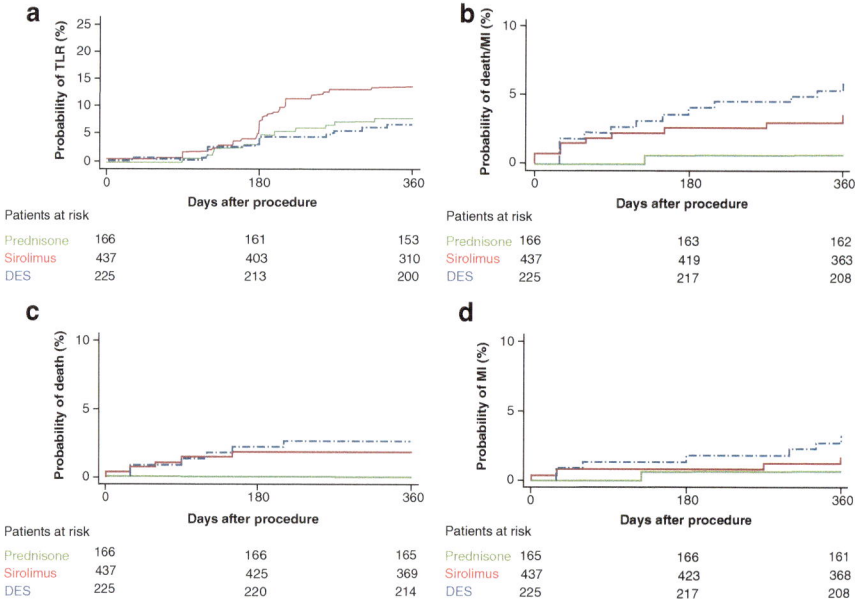

Fig. 22.5 Survival curves for primary and secondary endpoints according to the treatment received (BMS + OI [prednisone or sirolimus] or DES) (With permission from Atherosclerosis Cassese et al. [57]). *BMS* bare metal stents, *OI* oral immunosuppressive, *DES* drug eluting stents, *MI* myocardial infarction

6 months of follow-up. Both colchicine and placebo were administrated orally for 6 months. No serious adverse events were reported, although 17 % of patients in the colchicine group discontinued treatment. Colchicine reduced 6 month angiographic ISR rate by 52 % compared to control (p = 0.007) and, similarly, the IVUS-ISR rate was also reduced (p = 0.006). Thus, low dose colchicine was efficacious in terms of diminishing neointimal hyperplasia leading to restenosis in a high risk population.

Probucol

This drug is an anti-oxidant that reduces the adhesion of inflammatory cells and promotes growth of endothelial cells [63]. It was used as a lipid lowering agent before statins. In the pre-stent era, RCTs showed benefits when the drug was administrated for 1 month before PCI and continued for 6 months [64]. Another trial using probucol in non-acute coronary syndrome patients and started on the day before PCI didn't showed differences with placebo [65]. The CART-1 RCT tested probucol with BMS and the results failed to demonstrate benefits over placebo [66]; a later trial had similar results [67]. The pathophysiology of restenosis may explain these negative results. Probucol affects vascular remodeling after balloon PCI but has no effect on neointimal hyperplasia. Another main limitation of this drug was Q-T interval prolongation which was found in 22 % of treated patients [68].

Tranilast

It has an immunomodulatory action over mast cells and an antiproliferative effect in fibroblasts. It inhibits VSMC proliferation in animal models [69] and it was hypothesized that it might reduce restenosis based on a combination of these effects. Initial trials in humans showed good results when compared to placebo [70, 71]. However, as a result of these preliminary studies, a large RCT was performed in the United States, the PRESTO trial. It enrolled over 11,000 patients and didn't show significant differences between transilast and placebo in terms of reducing clinical events or ISR [72].

Pioglitazone

Aside from its antidiabetic properties, the drug acts by reducing VSMC proliferation and cell migration [73]. Several studies evaluated its efficacy to prevent restenosis but results were inconclusive [74, 75]. Only one that selected a population of insulin-resistant diabetics showed a significant reduction in ISR (p = 0.005) [76]. These conflicting results and the presence of important side effects [77] limit the use of pioglitazone for the prevention of restenosis.

Conclusions

1. *Oral Immunosuppressive therapy after BMS implantation significantly reduced restenosis rates compared to BMS alone. The reduction was driven by less late lumen loss with OI.*
2. *Taking into consideration the randomized data, rapamycin and prednisone appear to be the most promising in this setting. However, prednisone cannot be used in diabetics which limits its use.*
3. *Cilostazol has also shown benefit in reducing restenosis particularly in patients at high risk. However, its value in patients at low or intermediate risk of restenosis needs further assessment.*
4. *The use of oral agents to reduce restenosis should be considered in all patients with relative contraindications for DES implantation as outlined in this chapter. We believe that the guidelines should be amended to include these agents in certain specific situations.*

References

1. Rodríguez AE, et al. Early decrease in minimal luminal diameter after successful percutaneous transluminal coronary angioplasty predicts late restenosis. Am J Cardiol. 1993;71:1391–5.
2. Rodríguez AE, et al. Time course and mechanism of early luminal diameter loss after percutaneous transluminal coronary angioplasty. Am J Cardiol. 1995;76:1131–4.
3. Mintz G, et al. Arterial remodeling after coronay angioplasty. A serial intravascular ultrasound study. Circulation. 1996;94:35–44.
4. Serruys PW, et al. A comparison of balloon expandable stent implantation with balloon angioplasty in patients with coronary artery disease. N Engl J Med. 1994;331:489–95.
5. Kastrati A, et al. Analysis of 14 trials comparing sirolimus-eluting stents with bare-metal stents. N Engl J Med. 2007;356(10):1030–9.
6. Dangas GD, et al. In-stent restenosis in the drug-eluting stent era. J Am Coll Cardiol. 2010;56(23):1897–907.
7. Bangalore S, et al. Short- and long-term outcomes with drug-eluting and bare-metal coronary stents: a mixed treatment comparison analysis of 117,762 patient-years of follow-up from randomized trials. Circulation. 2012;125(23):2873–91.
8. MacFadden EP, et al. Late stent trombosis in drug-eluting coronary stent after discontinuation of antiplatelet therapy. Lancet. 2004;364:1419–21.
9. Rodriguez A, et al. Late stent thrombosis the Damocles sword of drug eluting stents. EuroIntervention. 2007;2:512–7.
10. Task Force on Myocardial Revascularization of the European Society of Cardiology and the European Association for Cardio-Thoracic Surgery; European Association for Percutaneous Cardiovascular Interventions. Guidelines on myocardial revascularization. Eur Heart J. 2010;31(20):2501–55.
11. Levine GN, et al. 2011 ACCF/AHA/SCAI Guideline for Percutaneous Coronary Intervention: a report of the American College of Cardiology Foundation/American Heart Association Task Force on Practice Guidelines and the Society for Cardiovascular Angiography and Interventions. Circulation. 2011;124(23):e574–651.
12. Dehmer GJ, et al. A contemporary view of diagnostic cardiac catheterization and percutaneous coronary intervention in the United States: a report from the CathPCI Registry of the National

Cardiovascular Data Registry, 2010 through June 2011. J Am Coll Cardiol. 2012;60(20): 2017–31.

13. PRWeb. Global coronary stents market (drug eluting & bare metal) is expected to reach USD 8.3 billion by 2016: transparency market. 2013. http://www.prweb.com/releases/2013/9/prweb11112353.htm. Accessed 30 Oct 2014.

14. Lee CW, et al. Prospective randomized trial of corticosteroids for the prevention of restenosis after intracoronary stent implantation. Am Heart J. 1999;138:60–3.

15. Versaci F, et al. Immunosuppressive Therapy for the Prevention of Restenosis after Coronary Artery Stent Implantation Study. Immunosuppressive Therapy for the Prevention of Restenosis after Coronary Artery Stent Implantation (IMPRESS Study). J Am Coll Cardiol 2002;40(11):1935–42.

16. Rodriguez AE, et al. Pilot study of oral rapamycin to prevent restenosis in patients undergoing coronary stent therapy: Argentina Single-Center Study (ORAR Trial). J Invasive Cardiol. 2003;15(10):581–4.

17. Hausleiter J, et al. Randomized, double-blind, placebo-controlled trial of oral sirolimus for restenosis prevention in patients with in-stent restenosis: the Oral Sirolimus to Inhibit Recurrent In-stent Stenosis (OSIRIS) trial. Circulation. 2004;110(7):790–5.

18. Tsuchikane E, et al. Impact of cilostazol on restenosis after percutaneous coronary balloon angioplasty. Circulation. 1999;100:21–6.

19. Nagaoka N, et al. Comparison of ticlopidine and cilostazol for the prevention of restenosis after percutaneous transluminal coronary angioplasty. Jpn Heart J. 2001;42:43–54.

20. Kornowski R, et al. In-stent restenosis: contributions of inflammatory responses and arterial injury to neointimal hyperplasia. J Am Coll Cardiol. 1998;31(1):224–30.

21. Farb A, et al. Pathology of acute and chronic coronary stenting in humans. Circulation. 1999;99(1):44–52.

22. Brara PS, et al. Pilot trial of oral rapamycin for recalcitrant restenosis. Circulation. 2003;107:1722–4.

23. Guarda E, et al. Oral rapamycin to prevent human coronary stent restenosis: a pilot study. Am Heart J. 2004;148(2):e9.

24. Ribichini F, et al. Immunosuppressive therapy with oral prednisone to prevent restenosis after PCI. A multicenter randomized trial. Am J Med. 2011;124(5):434–43.

25. Rodriguez AE, et al. Oral rapamycin after coronary bare-metal stent implantation to prevent restenosis: the Prospective, Randomized Oral Rapamycin in Argentina (ORAR II) Study. J Am Coll Cardiol. 2006;47:1522–9.

26. Stojkovic S, et al. Systemic rapamycin without loading dose for restenosis prevention after coronary bare metal stent implantation. Catheter Cardiovasc Interv. 2010;75:317–25.

27. Cernigliaro C, et al. Preventing restenosis after implantation of bare stents with oral rapamycin: a randomized angiographic and intravascular ultrasound study with a 5-year clinical follow-up. Cardiology. 2010;115:77–86.

28. Rodriguez AE, et al. Randomized comparison of cost-saving and effectiveness of oral rapamycin plus bare-metal stents with drug-eluting stents: three-year outcome from the randomized oral rapamycin in Argentina (ORAR) III trial. Catheter Cardiovasc Interv. 2012;80:385–94.

29. Douglas JS, et al. Cilostazol for Restenosis Trial (CREST) Investigators. Coronary stent restenosis in patient treated with cilostazol. Circulation. 2005;112(18):2826–32.

30. Lee SW, et al. Comparison of triple versus dual antiplatelet therapy after drug-eluting stent implantation (from the DECLARE-Long trial). Am J Cardiol. 2007;100(7):1103–8.

31. Lee SW, Lee SW, et al. Drug-eluting stenting followed by cilostazol treatment reduces late restenosis in patients with diabetes mellitus the DECLARE-DIABETES Trial (A Randomized Comparison of Triple Antiplatelet Therapy with Dual Antiplatelet Therapy After Drug-Eluting Stent Implantation in Diabetic Patients). J Am Coll Cardiol. 2008;51(12):1181–7.

32. Rodriguez AE, et al. Comparison of cost-effectiveness of oral rapamycin plus bare-metal stents versus first generation of drug-eluting stents (from the Randomized Oral Rapamycin in Argentina [ORAR] 3 trial). Am J Cardiol. 2014;113(5):815–21.

33. Rhen T, Cidlowski JA. Antiinflammatory action of glucocorticoids — new mechanisms for old drugs. N Engl J Med. 2005;353:1711–23.
34. Buffon A, et al. Preprocedural serum levels of C-reactive protein predict early complications and late restenosis after coronary angioplasty. J Am Coll Cardiol. 1999;34:1512–21.
35. Kornowoski R, et al. In-stent restenosis: contributions of inflammatory responses and arterial injury to neointimal hyperplasia. J Am Coll Cardiol. 1998;31:224–30.
36. Stone GW, et al. A randomized trial of corticosteroids for the prevention of restenosis in 102 patients undergoing repeat coronary angioplasty. Cathet Cardiovasc Diagn. 1989;18:227–31.
37. Ribichini F, et al. Immunosuppressive oral prednisone after percutaneous interventions in patients with multi-vessel coronary artery disease. The IMPRESS-2/MVD study. EuroIntervention. 2005;2:173–80.
38. Ferrero V, et al. Long term results of immunosuppressive oral prednisone after coronary angioplasty in non-diabetic patients with elevated C- reactive protein levels. EuroIntervention. 2009;5:250–4.
39. Ribichini F, et al. Long-term clinical follow-up of the multicentre, randomized study to test immunosuppressive therapy with oral prednisone for the prevention of restenosis after percutaneous coronary interventions: Cortisone plus BMS or DES veRsus BMS alone to EliminAte Restenosis (CEREA-DES). Eur Heart J. 2013;34(23):1740–8.
40. Sardar P, et al. Steroids for the prevention of restenosis in bare-metal stents–a systematic review and meta-analysis. J Invasive Cardiol. 2012;24(3):98–103.
41. Goto S. Cilostazol: potential mechanism of action for antithrombotic effects accompanied by a low rate of bleeding. Atheroscler Suppl. 2005;6(4):3–11.
42. Inoue T, et al. Cilostazol inhibits leukocyte integrin Mac-1, leading to a potential reduction in restenosis after coronary stent implantation. J Am Coll Cardiol. 2004;44:1408–14.
43. Zhou H, et al. Triple versus dual antiplatelet therapy for coronary heart disease patients undergoing percutaneous coronary intervention: a meta-analysis. Exp Ther Med. 2013;6(4):1034–40.
44. Lee SW, et al. Comparison of dual versus triple antiplatelet therapy after drug-eluting stent according to stent length (from the pooled analysis of DECLARE trials). Am J Cardiol. 2013;112:1738–44.
45. Groth CG, et al. Sirolimus (rapamycin)-based therapy in human renal transplantation. Transplantation. 1997;67:1036–42.
46. Mancini D, et al. Use of rapamycin slows progression of cardiac transplantation vasculopathy. Circulation. 2003;108:48–53.
47. Poon M, et al. Rapamycin inhibits vascular smooth muscle cell migration. J Clin Invest. 1996;98:2277–83.
48. Gallo R, et al. Inhibition of intimal thickening after balloon angioplasty in porcine coronary arteries by targeting regulators of the cell cycle. Circulation. 1999;99:2164–70.
49. Waksman R, et al. Oral rapamycin to inhibit restenosis after stenting of de novo coronary lesions: the Oral Rapamune to Inhibit Restenosis (ORBIT) study. J Am Coll Cardiol. 2004;44:1386–92.
50. Rodriguez AE, et al. Role of oral rapamycin to prevent restenosis in patients with de novo lesions undergoing coronary stenting: results of the Argentina single centre study (ORAR trial). Heart. 2005;91:1433–7.
51. Rodriguez AE, et al. Percutaneous coronary intervention with oral sirolimus and bare metal stents has comparable safety and efficacy to treatment with drug eluting stents, but with significant cost saving: long-term follow-up results from the randomised, controlled ORAR III (Oral Rapamycin in ARgentina) study. EuroIntervention. 2009;5:255–64.
52. Dangas GD, et al. Long-term outcome of PCI versus CABG in insulin and non-insulin-treated diabetic patients: results from the FREEDOM trial. J Am Coll Cardiol. 2014;64(12):1189–97.
53. Mohr FW, et al. Coronary artery bypass graft surgery versus percutaneous coronary intervention in patients with three-vessel disease and left main coronary disease: 5-year follow-up of the randomised, clinical SYNTAX trial. Lancet. 2013;381(9867):629–38.
54. Wijns W, et al. Endeavour zotarolimus-eluting stent reduces stent thrombosis and improves clinical outcomes compared with cypher sirolimus-eluting stent: 4-year results of the PROTECT randomized trial. Eur Heart J. 2014;35(40):2812–20.

55. Gada H, et al. 5-year results of a randomized comparison of XIENCE V everolimus-eluting and TAXUS paclitaxel-eluting stents: final results from the SPIRIT III trial (clinical evaluation of the XIENCE V everolimus eluting coronary stent system in the treatment of patients with de novo native coronary artery lesions). JACC Cardiovasc Interv. 2013;6(12):1263–6.
56. Dasari TW, et al. Systematic review of effectiveness of oral sirolimus after bare-metal stenting of coronary arteries for prevention of in-stent restenosis. Am J Cardiol. 2013;112(9):1322–7.
57. Cassese S, et al. ORAl iMmunosuppressive therapy to prevent in-stent rEstenosiS (RAMSES) cooperation: a patient-level meta-analysis of randomized trials. Atherosclerosis. 2014. http://dx.doi.org/10.1016/j.atherosclerosis.2014.09.021.
58. Molad Y. Update on colchicine and its mechanism of action. Curr Rheumatol Rep. 2002;4:252–6.
59. Imazio M, et al. COlchicine for the Prevention of the Post-pericardiotomy Syndrome (COPPS): a multicentre, randomized, double-blind, placebocontrolled trial. Eur Heart J. 2010; 31:2749–54.
60. O'Keefe Jr JH, et al. Ineffectiveness of colchicine for the prevention of restenosis after coronary angioplasty. J Am Coll Cardiol. 1992;19:1597–600.
61. Gradus-Pizlo I, et al. Local delivery of biodegradable microparticles containing colchicine or a colchicine analogue: effects on restenosis and implications for catheter-based drug delivery. J Am Coll Cardiol. 1995;26:1549–57.
62. Deftereos S, et al. Colchicine treatment for the prevention of bare-metal stent restenosis in diabetic patients. J Am Coll Cardiol. 2013;61(16):1679–85.
63. Ferns GA, et al. Probucol inhibits mononuclear cell adhesion to vascular endothelium in the cholesterol-fed rabbit. Atherosclerosis. 1993;100:171–81.
64. Tardif JC, et al. Probucol and multivitamins in the prevention of restenosis after coronary angioplasty. Multivitamins and Probucol Study Group. N Engl J Med. 1997;337:365–72.
65. Tardif JC, et al. Effects of succinobucol (AGI- 1067) after an acute coronary syndrome: a randomised, double-blind, placebo-controlled trial. Lancet. 2008;371:1761–8.
66. Tardif JC, et al. Effects of AGI-1067 and probucol after percutaneous coronary interventions. Circulation. 2003;107:552–8.
67. Nunes GL, et al. Role of probucol in inhibiting intimal hyperplasia after coronary stent implantation: a randomized study. Am Heart J. 2006;152(914):e1–7.
68. Reinoehl J, et al. Probucol-associated tachyarrhythmic events and QT prolongation: importance of gender. Am Heart J. 1996;131:1184–91.
69. Takahashi A, et al. Tranilast inhibits vascular smooth muscle cell growth and intimal hyperplasia by induction of p21(waf1/cip1/sdi1) and p53. Circ Res. 1999;84:543–50.
70. Tamai H, et al. Impact of tranilast on restenosis after coronary angioplasty: tranilast restenosis following angioplasty trial (TREAT). Am Heart J. 1999;138:968–75.
71. Tamai H, et al. The impact of tranilast on restenosis after coronary angioplasty: the Second Tranilast Restenosis Following Angioplasty Trial (TREAT-2). Am Heart J. 2002;143:506–13.
72. Holmes Jr DR, et al. Results of Prevention of REStenosis with Tranilast and its Outcomes (PRESTO) trial. Circulation. 2002;106:1243–50.
73. Kasai T, et al. Pioglitazone attenuates neointimal thickening via suppression of the early inflammatory response in a porcine coronary after stenting. Atherosclerosis. 2008;197:612–9.
74. Marx N, et al. Pioglitazone reduces neointima volume after coronary stent implantation: a randomized, placebo-controlled, double-blind trial in nondiabetic patients. Circulation. 2005;112:2792–8.
75. Takagi T, et al. A prospective, multicenter, randomized trial to assess efficacy of pioglitazone on in-stent neointimal suppression in type 2 diabetes: POPPS (Prevention of In-Stent Neointimal Proliferation by Pioglitazone Study). JACC Cardiovasc Interv. 2009;2:524–31.
76. Nishio K, et al. A randomized comparison of pioglitazone to inhibit restenosis after coronary stenting in patients with type 2 diabetes. Diabetes Care. 2006;29:101–6.
77. Nesto RW, et al. Thiazolidinedione use, fluid retention, and congestive heart failure: a consensus statement from the American Heart Association and American Diabetes Association. Circulation. 2003;108:2941–8.

Chapter 23
When Should Ablation Be Considered in the Treatment of Atrial Fibrillation – A Clinician's View

Ralph J. Wessel

Abstract Catheter ablation is a relatively recent and evolving modality for the maintenance of sinus rhythm in patients with atrial fibrillation. What its role is in the management of the general patient population with atrial fibrillation remains unclear. In order to understand the role of catheter ablation for treatment of atrial fibrillation, an overview of the problem of atrial fibrillation will be discussed. Management strategies will be considered. The mechanisms of atrial fibrillation along with a history of ablation and a rationale for atrial fibrillation ablation will be presented. Data on the outcomes, efficacy and complications of catheter ablation will be reviewed. Finally, patient selection will be discussed.

Keywords Atrial Fibrillation • Radio-frequency Ablation of Atrial Fibrillation • Pulmonary Vein Isolation • Efficacy of Catheter Ablation of Atrial Fibrillation • RAFFT-2 Trial • SARA Study • Patient Selection for Atrial Fibrillation Ablation

Introduction

Catheter ablation is a relatively recent and evolving modality for the maintenance of sinus rhythm in patients with atrial fibrillation (AF). What its role is in the management of the general population with AF remains unclear. The general population with AF is elderly with multiple comorbidities and concomitant cardiac disorders. Studies demonstrating catheter ablation's superiority over antiarrhythmic drug therapy for maintaining sinus rhythm have involved a significantly younger population with fewer comorbidities and concomitant cardiac disorders than the general

R.J. Wessel, MD, FACC (✉)
Division of Cardiology, UCSF – Fresno, Fresno, CA, USA

Department of Cardiology, Medicine UCSF, Community Regional Medical Center—Fresno, Fresno, CA, USA
e-mail: ralphjwessel@gmail.com

© Springer International Publishing Switzerland 2015
J.A. Ambrose, A.E. Rodríguez (eds.), *Controversies in Cardiology*,
DOI 10.1007/978-3-319-20415-4_23

population with AF. This chapter discusses the role of catheter ablation in the management of the different presentations of AF in the general population.

Overview of the Problem

AF is the most common significant arrhythmia encountered in clinical practice. The estimated prevalence is 2–2.5 % of the adult population, which is likely an underestimation of the true prevalence [1, 2]. The incidence increases with age. The aging of our population and the increasing prevalence of hypertension, diabetes mellitus, and obesity are leading to its increasing prevalence. The average AF patient is 73 years old and AF is unusual prior to the age of 55 years [2]. Men are slightly more likely than women to develop AF. However, because women live longer than men, there are more women than men with AF. The lifetime risk of developing AF after the age of 40 was found to be approximately 25 % in the Framingham Heart Study [3]. This was confirmed in the Rotterdam Study where the lifetime risk of AF at age 55 years old was 23.8 % in men and 22.2 % in women [4].

Patients with AF have a high likelihood of having significant co-morbidities. In a large population study of 176,891 patients with AF, 87.4 % had hypertension, 43.3 % had diabetes mellitus, 42.1 % had heart failure, 33.8 % had asthma/COPD, and 20.4 % had vascular disease [2]. The average CHA2DS2-VASc was 4.2 making this population at high risk of stroke requiring chronic anticoagulation therapy to decrease thromboembolic events [2].

In order to more specifically classify the overall population with AF, the following classification of AF has been adopted by HRS/EHRA/ECAS in collaboration with the ACC, AHA, APHRS, and STS in 2012 [5]:

- AF Episode – AF documented by ECG monitoring with a duration of $\geq$30 s., or if <30 s. is present continuously throughout the ECG monitoring.
- Paroxysmal AF – Recurrent AF ($\geq$2 episodes) terminating spontaneously within 7 days or $\leq$48 h with electrical or medical cardioversion.
- Persistent AF – Continuous AF >7 days or cardioverted after >48 h and $\leq$12 months.
- Long-standing persistent AF – Continuous AF for >12 months.
- Permanent AF – AF patients where the decision is not to restore or maintain sinus rhythm (NSR) by any means, including catheter or surgical ablation.

Management Strategies

The three strategies related to AF are prevention of thromboembolic events, control of ventricular rate, and maintenance of NSR. Prevention of thromboembolism applies to all types of AF and to all patients. Control of ventricular rate is referred to as "rate control" and maintenance of NSR is "rhythm control". These are the two competing approaches in AF management.

Use of the CHA2DS2-VASc score is the recommended tool to evaluate thrombo-embolic risk and to aid in the selection of the appropriate therapeutic intervention to reduce the risk of an event by all the major cardiac societies [6] (See Table 23.1). For patients with a CHA2DS2-VASc score of ≥2 oral anticoagulant therapy is rec-ommended. This includes the vast majority with AF. In patients who have under-gone catheter ablation, the continuation of long-term oral anticoagulant therapy post-ablation is recommended for all with a CHA2DS2-VASc score of ≥2, irrespec-tive of procedural success [7]. Only patients with a CHA2DS2-VASc score of 0 or possibly 1 should be considered for discontinuation of long-term oral anticoagula-tion therapy after successful ablation [7].

The role of the competing strategies of rate control versus rhythm control remains an unsettled issue. In the perfect world, most practitioners would opt for rhythm control. The publication of the AFFIRM [8] and RACE [9] trials in 2002 demon-strated that rate control was not inferior to rhythm control with medication and that rate control may be advantageous to rhythm control. As a result, rate control became the preferred strategy in the majority of AF cases. With the advent of catheter abla-tion of AF the pendulum appears to be shifting back toward rhythm control. However, due to a lack of a well-designed large randomized study related to abla-tion with long term follow-up and hard clinical end points of morbidity and mortal-ity to establish its clinical benefit, its benefit for rhythm control remains unsettled.

Mechanisms of Atrial Fibrillation

There are two main mechanisms involved in the genesis and maintenance of AF: 1-the multiple wavelet hypothesis with large and small reentrant wavelets, 2- the focal trigger hypothesis with enhanced automaticity of 1 or several rapidly depolar-izing foci [5]. In most cases, it is the combination that results in the development of AF with focal triggers leading to the initiation of reentry that eventually leads to atrial remodeling causing additional focal triggers and perpetuation of reentry.

	Condition	Points
C	CHF	1
H	HTN	1
A2	Age ≥75 years	2
D	Diabetes mellitus	1
S2	Prior stroke or TIA or TE	2
V	Vascular disease	1
A	Age 65–74 years	1
SC	Sex (female gender)	1

Table 23.1 CHA2DS2VASC Score

Until the 1980's, the multiple wavelet hypothesis was widely accepted as the dominant mechanism. The development of the surgical Cox-Maze procedure, first performed in 1987, was predicated on this AF model and the concept that maintenance of AF needs a critical number of circulating wavelets, each of which requires a critical mass of atrial tissue [5]. The multiple thru and thru surgical atrial incisions were designed to interrupt all macro-reentry circuits preventing the ability of the atrium to fibrillate. Procedural success contributed to development of catheter ablation with creation of multiple ablation lines to interrupt reentry.

The focal trigger hypothesis became a major factor for the initiation of AF in the 1990's with identification of rapidly depolarizing ectopic foci in the atrium and pulmonary veins that would trigger AF or act as a rapid driver to maintain AF. These ectopic foci usually originated from myocardial muscle tissue found in the proximal 1–3 cm of the pulmonary (PVs) veins [5] and became the target of catheter ablation.

History and Rationale of AF Catheter Ablation

In 1994, Michel Haissaguerre presented the first successful catheter ablations of AF in three patients [10]. He found rapidly firing foci in the right atrium and successfully treated them with RF catheter ablation. These results supported the concept of a focal mechanism for AF that can be treated by ablation.

The concept of focal triggers was further supported in 1998 in another study by Haissaguerre et al. [11]. They found that the vast majority of the focal triggers of AF were in the proximal portion of the PVs. In the 45 patients studied, a total of 69 triggering foci were found of which 64 (94 %) were found in the proximal few centimeter of the PVs: 31 foci in the left superior, 17 in the right superior, 11 in the left inferior and 6 in the right inferior PV. 4 foci were found in the atrium: 3 in the right atrium and 1 in the posterior left atrium. RF catheter ablation of the triggering foci was undertaken. A single session resulted in successful ablation of the foci in 14 patients, 25 patients required two sessions, and 6 patients required three. At a mean follow-up 8 ± 6 months AF was completely eliminated in 28 patients (62 %) without drug therapy.

As a result, an initial strategy for catheter ablation was to induce AF triggers, map, and ablate the triggers within the PVs. This strategy was limited by the inability to induce AF triggers in up to 1/3 and a high recurrence rate after ablation. Freedom from recurrence of AF at 14 months without drugs was 33 %. An additional 13 % had no AF, but remained on drugs. PV ablation led to PV stenosis in up to 38 %. While treatment of PV stenosis with stenting was possible, a better approach was needed to improve success and decrease complications.

To avoid the need to induce, map and ablate the individual PV triggers, Pappone et al. in 2000, described the technique of PV isolation [12]. This technique was performed using a circular catheter with multiple electrodes on it that was positioned outside each of the PVs which isolated the triggers from the left atrium preventing any triggers inside the PVs from starting AF. Since 2001, the location of the

PV isolation has moved more proximally into the left atrium, resulting in PV antral isolation [13]. PV antral isolation is now the standard for most patients with paroxysmal AF. A search for AF triggers outside the PV may be needed in other patients.

In patients with persistent and especially in long-standing AF, atrial remodeling becomes an important mechanistic factor for maintenance of AF [14] resulting in a high recurrence rate with PV antral isolation alone [14]. To achieve success, these patients often require a more complex ablation strategy which includes lines of linear ablation, ablation of non-PV triggers, ablation of complex fractionated atrial electrograms, extensive ablation of left atrial posterior wall, and/or ablation of the ganglionated plexi [14]. The resultant extensive scar formation can lead to possible adverse consequences in the left atrium [14].

Outcomes and Efficacy of Catheter Ablation

Well-designed large randomized multicenter trails have been the mainstay of cardiovascular research to evaluate outcomes and efficacy for cardiovascular disease for over 30 years. These data are presently lacking for AF ablation. The available data for AF ablation is largely limited to a small number of randomized studies with small sample sizes of <100 in each arm that studied younger patients (<60 years old) with few comorbidities and predominately paroxysmal AF with a short follow-up of a year or two. The end points were usually suppression of AF compared to antiarrhythmic drug therapy rather than the harder clinical end points of morbidity and mortality outcomes. Although the available data are less than ideal, catheter ablation is superior to antiarrhythmic drug therapy in maintaining NSR. Prior studies (AFFIRM [8] and RACE [9]) comparing rate control to rhythm control failed to show the superiority of rhythm control with antiarrhythmic drugs over rate control in most AF cases. Whether a strategy of rhythm control using catheter ablation will be the superior strategy remains unknown.

The most important predictor for success of catheter ablation is the type of AF being treated [12]. Paroxysmal AF has a significantly higher success rate for NSR maintenance than persistent AF which has a higher success rate than long-standing persistent AF. Similarly, variables such as age, concomitant cardiac disease, obesity, sleep apnea, and LA size impact outcome [12].

The 5 year follow up results of catheter ablation for maintaining NSR has been reported by Weerasooriya et al. [15]. The average age at inclusion was 55.7 ± 9.6 years, 64 % had paroxysmal AF, 22 % had persistent AF, and 14 % had long-standing persistent AF. Structural heart disease was present in only 36 %, with 16 % having LVH, and the LVEF was normal at 70 ± 11 %. The CHADS2 score was 0 in 48 %, 1 in 32 % and ≥ 2 in 20 % of the subjects. For this group of younger, generally healthier patients than the general AF population, freedom from recurrent AF at 5 years was 63 %. However, 51 % required repeat interventions. The 5 year results for freedom from recurrent AF with a single procedure was disappointing at only 29 % (Fig. 23.1). There was an 8.9 % gradual straight line annual recurrence rate of AF after the last ablation attempt over the 5 year follow-up period (Fig. 23.2). The 8.9 % annual recurrence rate after the last ablation attempt is consistent with results from other studies with "long-term" follow-up of 2–3 years. Based on these results, it appears that catheter ablation is not a cure but a treatment for AF that requires continued long term follow-up.

In a recently reported randomized trail comparing radiofrequency ablation vs antiarrhythmic drugs as first-line treatment of paroxysmal AF (RAFFT-2), 61 patients in the antiarrhythmic drug group and 66 patients in the radiofrequency ablation group were followed for 2 years for recurrence and quality of life measures [16]. The patients had an average age of 55 years old, little comorbidity, an average LVEF of 61 %, a normal or mildly increased LA size, and a median CHADS2 score of 0. These patients do not represent the typical AF population. Recurrence of AF occurred in 72.1 % with antiarrhythmics and 54.5 % with ablation at 2 years follow-up. There was no difference in the quality of life measures between the groups at baseline and during the study at the 1 year follow-up. There was a 9 % rate of serious adverse events with ablation, with pericardial effusion and tamponade occurring in 6 % [16] (Table 23.2).

In the above study, ablation was superior to antiarrhythmics; however, 54.5 % with ablation experienced recurrent AF at 2 year follow-up and quality of life measures were similar [16]. If the follow-up would be extended to 5 years and the 8.9 % annual recurrence rate of AF observed in other long term studies occurred in this population, 81.2 % of the ablation patients would be predicted to have experienced recurrence.

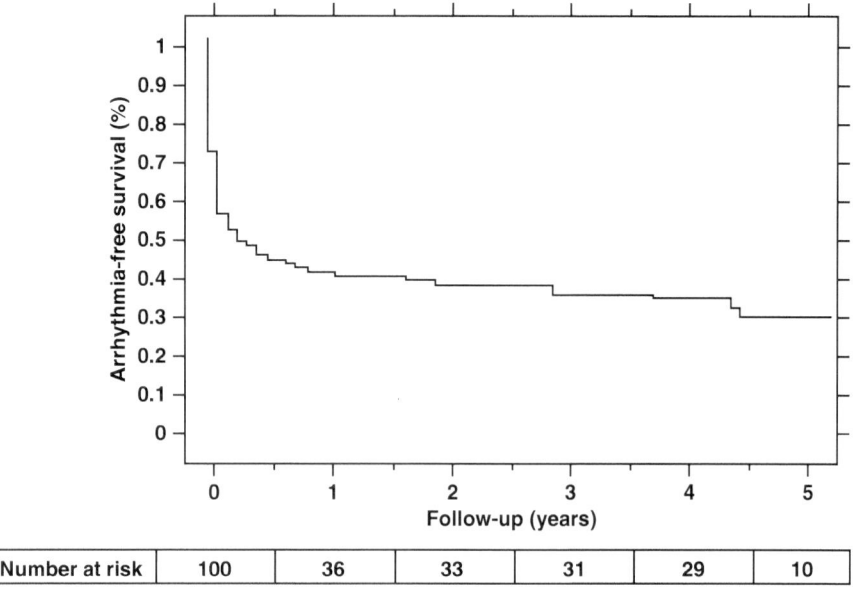

Fig. 23.1 Single Procedure Success. Kaplan-Meier event-free survival curve after a single catheter ablation attempt (Reproduced from Weerasooriya et al. [15], with permission of Elsevier)

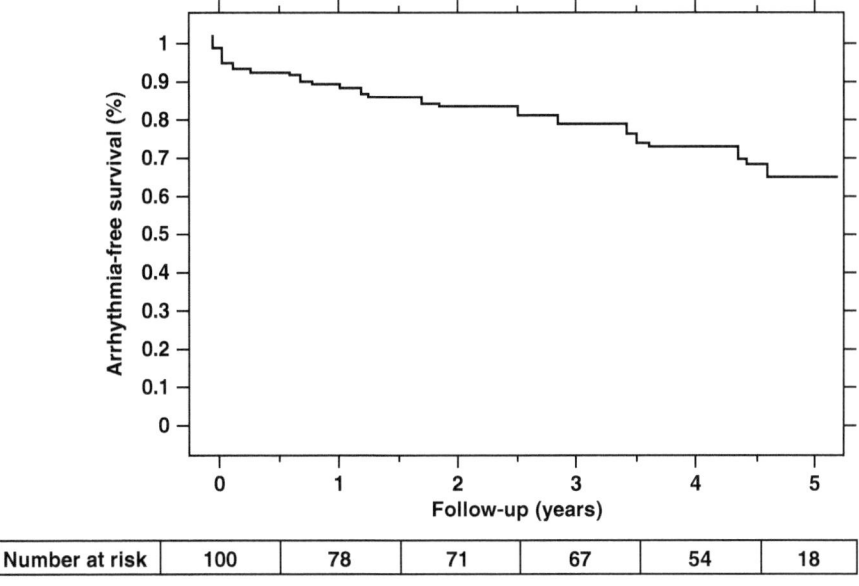

Fig. 23.2 Multiple Procedure Success. Kaplan-Meier event-free survival curve after the last catheter ablation attempt (Reproduced from Weerasooriya et al. [15], with permission of Elsevier)

Table 23.2 Randomized trials of catheter ablation

RAAFT-2 (paroxysmal AF)

RX	#	Age (mean)	LA Size (cm)	LVEF %	HTN %	DM %	CHADS2 (mean)	Recurrent AF >30 s @ 2 years	QOL score baseline	QOL score @ 1 year
AAD	61	54.3 years	4.3	60.8	41.0	6.6	0.7	72.1 %	0.84	1
CA	66	56.3 years	4.0	61.4	42.4	1.5	0.5	54.5 %	0.86	1
P value		.30	.09	.65	.87	.14	.48	.02	>.99	.25

SARA study (persistent AF)

RX	#	Age (mean)	LA Size (cm)	LVEF %	Free from AF>24 h @ 1 year	Free from any recurrent AF>30 s @ 1 year	QOL score baseline	QOL score @ 1 year
AAD	48	55 years	4.27	60.8	43.7 %	29.2 %	49.3	53.0
CA	98	55 years	4.13	61.1	70.4 %	60.2 %	42.0	56.8
P value					.002	<0.001		.41

AAD antiarrhythmic drug treatment, *CA* catheter ablation, *QOL* score quality of life score: EQ5D Tariff score in RAAFT-2 and AF-QoL score in SARA Study

When it comes to persistent AF, the available data on outcome and efficacy are very limited. The only randomized, multicenter, controlled trail that has been published to date is the SARA study [17]. This compared catheter ablation to antiarrhythmic drug in persistent AF – 146 were randomized 2:1 to ablation (98 patients) or antiarrhythmic drug therapy with a Class III or IC drug (48 patients). The patients were again young with an average age of 55 years and had few comorbidities and concomitant cardiac disorders. Their LA sizes were only mildly enlarged and an average LVEF was 61 %. The follow-up was only for 1 year. The primary outcome was defined as freedom from an episode of AF or flutter lasting >24 h or requiring cardioversion after a 3 months blanking period. Secondary outcomes included freedom from any recurrence of AF or flutter lasting ≥30 s after the 3 month blanking period, hospitalization related to arrhythmia, cardioversion, therapeutic crossover, AV node ablation, quality of life questionnaire at baseline and 6 and 12 months, and complications. In the ablation arm, 36 % received antiarrhythmic drug therapy thruout the follow-up period and 8.2 % underwent a second ablation procedure. No patients in the antiarrhythmic drug group underwent an ablation prior to completing the study or having a primary outcome event.

The results of the SARA study [17] for the primary outcome were that 70.4 % in the ablation group and 43.7 % in the antiarrhythmic drug group had freedom from sustained episodes of AF at 12 months (p=0.002). The secondary end point of freedom from any AF or atrial flutter lasting >30 s were 60.2 % in the ablation group and 29.2 % in the antiarrhythmic drug group during the 12 month follow-up (p<0.001). The need for cardioversion was higher with antiarrhythmics (50 % vs 34.7 %, respectively). Hospitalizations due to arrhythmia recurrence were similar. There were no significant differences in AF quality of life scores between groups. There was a 6.1 % periprocedural complication rate during the ablation procedure and one patient developed symptomatic PV requiring stenting (Table 23.2).

The results of the SARA study [17] provide evidence that radiofrequency ablation is superior to antiarrhythmic drug therapy for maintaining NSR in a select group followed only 12 months. The subjects were relatively young (average age 55 years) without significant comorbidities or concomitant cardiac disease. Despite the improvement in maintaining NSR with ablation, there was no benefit in decreasing hospitalization or improving quality of life scores and there was a 7 % complication rate related to ablation.

There are no randomized trials comparing catheter ablation to antiarrhythmic drug therapy in long-standing AF [18]. As mentioned above, the changes in the left atrium that occur with long-standing AF usually require a more extensive and complex ablation strategy. These more extensive ablation strategies result in more extensive scar formation in the left atrium [14].

The 5 year results of a study using a sequential catheter ablation strategy for long-standing persistent AF has been reported [18]. These subjects had an average age of 61 years, only 16 % had structural heart disease, LA size was moderately enlarged, and LVEF was 60±7 %. After the first ablation procedure, NSR was maintained at 5 years in 20.3 %. After multiple procedures (up to 5 procedures), sinus rhythm was maintained at 5 years in 45 %, including 26 % who were receiving antiarrhythmic drugs. Patients with a duration of long-standing persistent of >2 years were 2.81 times more likely to relapse to AF. In those who underwent >1 redo, the incidence of atrial tachycardia as a clinical arrhythmia increased. The arrhythmia was felt to be related to scar formation in the LA [19].

Catheter ablation for long-standing persistent AF is a challenging procedure for the electrophysiologist. The more extensive ablation approach requires a careful evaluation of the risk/benefit ratio. Longer procedure and fluoroscopy times along with an increased risk of complications including atrial tachycardia need to be considered [5, 19]. Randomized trials are needed to evaluate to outcomes of various ablation strategies.

Patient Selection for Ablation

The role of catheter ablation for AF in the overall patient population is unclear. The available studies related to its efficacy, as mentioned earlier, have largely been limited to a small group with predominately paroxysmal AF and are significantly younger with fewer comorbidities than the general population with AF. In this select group, ablation is superior to antiarrhythmic drug therapy in maintaining NSR. Catheter ablation still has a significant recurrence rate of AF over time and frequently requires repeat ablation procedures to maintain NSR. In patients who are not significantly symptomatic in AF while on medical therapy, studies have failed to show an improvement in quality of life measures with ablation [16, 17]. At the present time there is insufficient evidence to support the use of catheter ablation to reduce all-cause mortality, stroke, or heart failure. Serious complications related to an AF ablation procedure are not uncommon, reported in ~6 % of procedures [5]. The present guidelines for the management of AF recommend the chronic continuation of anticoagulation therapy based on the CHA2DS2-VASc score irrespective of the results of ablation [7, 20].

The patient selection for ablation needs to be individualized depending on numerous factors including age, sex, type and duration of AF, presence of structural heart disease, LA size, presence of comorbidities, response to rate control therapy, failure or intolerance of antiarrhythmic drug therapy, and provision of patient-informed consent. The primary indication for AF ablation is for significantly symptomatic paroxysmal AF that is refractory or intolerant to at least one Class I or III antiarrhythmic medication when a rhythm control strategy is desired (Class I, EOL:A) [5, 6]. Prior to consideration for ablation, assessment of the procedural risk and outcomes is recommended (Class I, EOL:C) [5, 6]. These two are the only Class I recommendations according to the 2014 ACA/AHA guidelines [6].

The 2014 guidelines consider catheter ablation as a reasonable initial strategy for the management of recurrent symptomatic paroxysmal AF when a rhythm control strategy is warranted prior to therapeutic trials of antiarrhythmic drug therapy, after weighing risks and outcomes of drug and ablation therapy (Class IIa, EOL:B) [6]. They also consider ablation as a reasonable option for selected patients with symptomatic persistent AF refractory or intolerant to at least 1 class I or III antiarrhythmic medication (Class IIa, EOL: A) [6].

A weaker recommendation is considered for symptomatic persistent AF prior to a trial of antiarrhythmic drug therapy (Class IIb, EOL:C) or for symptomatic long-standing AF refractory or intolerant to antiarrhythmics, when a rhythm control strategy is warranted (Class IIb, EOL:B) [6]. AF ablation is not warranted and is considered harmful for the restoration of NSR with the sole intent of avoiding anticoagulation (Class III, EOL:C) [6].

There are ongoing clinical trials that are assessing the role of ablation for reducing mortality, stroke, or heart failure compared to standard care with rate and/or rhythm control drugs. Their results will not be available for a few years. These are the CABANA (Catheter Ablation Versus Antiarrhythmic Drug Therapy for Atrial Fibrillation) and the EAST (Early Therapy of Atrial Fibrillation for Stroke Prevention Trial) studies. We should proceed cautiously in widening the indications for AF catheter ablation until the results of these and other future studies are available.

Conclusions

1. The general population with AF is usually elderly with multiple comorbidities and concomitant cardiac disorders, and high CHA2DS2-VASc scores.
2. Anticoagulation is recommended for AF patients with a CHA2DS2-VASc score ≥ 2.
3. A rate control strategy is not inferior to rhythm control with medication and rate control may be advantageous to rhythm control.
4. Focal triggers predominantly in the proximal PVs and altered atrial myocardial substrate resulting in multiple reentry wavelets that are the underlying mechanisms for AF are potentially amenable to catheter ablation.
5. Catheter ablation of AF is superior to antiarrhythmic drug therapy for maintaining NSR.
6. There is a high recurrence rate of AF after ablation over the long term that frequently requires repeat ablation.
7. There is a significant complication rate related to each ablation procedure.
8. The role of ablation compared to a rate or rhythm control strategy with medication in managing the general population with AF is unsettled.
9. Chronic anticoagulation therapy based on the CHA2DS2-VASc score is still required despite the apparent success of ablation.
10. The published trials of ablation almost exclusively involve significantly younger patients with fewer comorbidities or concomitant cardiac disease than the general population with AF and the trials have a short follow up. Therefore, these cannot be necessarily applied to the general AF population.
11. At the present time catheter ablation should be limited to younger patients with paroxysmal or persistent AF who are significantly symptomatic despite standard medical therapy.
12. Broader application of ablation should await results of on-going long term trials.

References

1. Miyasaka Y, et al. Secular trends in incidence of atrial fibrillation in Olmsted County, Minnesota, 1980 to 2000, and implications on the projections for future prevalence. Circulation. 2006;114:119–25.
2. Wilke T, et al. Incidence and prevalence of atrial fibrillation: an analysis based on 8.3 million patients. Europace. 2013;15:486–93.
3. Lloyd-Jones DM, et al. Lifetime risk for development of atrial fibrillation – the Framingham Heart Study. Circulation. 2004;110:1042–6.
4. Heeringa J, et al. Prevalence, incidence and lifetime risk of atrial fibrillation: the Rotterdam study. Eur Heart J. 2006;27:949–53.
5. Calkins H, et al. 2012 HRS/EHRA/ECAS expert consensus statement on catheter and surgical ablation of atrial fibrillation: recommendations for patient selection, procedural techniques, patient management and follow-up, definitions, endpoints and research trial design. Heart Rhythm. 2012;9:632–96.
6. January CT, et al. 2014 AHA/ACC/HRS guideline for the management of patients with atrial fibrillation. J Am Coll Cardiol. 2014. doi:10.1016/j.jacc.2014.03.022.
7. Camm AJ, et al. 2012 focused update of the ESC Guidelines for the management of atrial fibrillation: an update of the 2010 ESC guidelines for the management of atrial fibrillation. Eur Heart J. 2012;33:2719–47.
8. Wyse DG, et al. A comparison of rate control and rhythm control in patients with atrial fibrillation. N Engl J Med. 2002;347:1825–33.
9. Gelder V, et al. A comparison of rate control and rhythm control in patients with recurrent persistent atrial fibrillation. N Engl J Med. 2002;347:1834–40.
10. Haissaguerre M, et al. Radiofrequency catheter ablation in unusual mechanisms of atrial fibrillation: report of three cases. J Cardiovasc Electrophysiol. 1994;5:743–51.
11. Haissaguerre M, et al. Spontaneous initiation of atrial fibrillation by ectopic beats originating in the pulmonary veins. N Engl J Med. 1998;339:659–66.
12. Pappone C, et al. Circumferential radiofrequency ablation of pulmonary vein ostia: a new anatomic approach for curing atrial fibrillation. Circulation. 2000;102:2619–28.
13. Oral H, et al. Circumferential pulmonary-vein ablation for chronic atrial fibrillation. N Engl J Med. 2006;354:934–41.
14. Letsas KP, et al. Current ablation strategies for persistent and long-standing persistent atrial fibrillation. Cardiol Res Pract. 2011. doi:10.4061/2011/376969.
15. Weerasooriya R, et al. Catheter ablation for atrial fibrillation: are results maintained at 5 years of follow-up? J Am Coll Cardiol. 2011;57:160–6.
16. Morillo CA, et al. Radiofrequency ablation vs antiarrhythmic drugs as first-line treatment of paroxysmal atrial fibrillation (RAAFT-2). JAMA. 2014;311:692–9.
17. Mont L, et al. Catheter ablation vs. antiarrhythmic drug treatment of persistent atrial fibrillation: a multicenter, randomized, controlled trial (SARA study). Eur Heart J. 2014;35:501–7.
18. Tilz RR, et al. Catheter ablation of long-standing persistent atrial fibrillation: 5-year outcomes of the Hamburg Sequential Ablation Strategy. J Am Coll Cardiol. 2012;60:1921–9.
19. Castrejon-Castrejon S, et al. Organized atrial tachycardias after atrial fibrillation ablation. Cardiol Res Pract. 2011. doi:10.4061/2011/957538.
20. Camm AJ, et al. Guidelines for the management of atrial fibrillation: the Task Force for the management of Atrial Fibrillation of the European Society of Cardiology (ESC). Europace. 2010;12:1360–420.

Chapter 24
Radial and Femoral Access in Percutaneous Intervention

Francesco Costa and Marco Valgimigli

Abstract Femoral and radial accesses are the most commonly used approaches in interventional cardiology. Femoral access-site has been implemented for many years in percutaneous coronary intervention and still today is the most used approach in several countries. Radial access, more recently introduced, guarantees a less invasive procedure and a reduced incidence of vascular access site complications.

The purpose of this chapter is to review critically the most recent evidence comparing radial and femoral approaches for percutaneous coronary intervention. Advantages and limitations of each technique will be evaluated with respect to the most recent interventional procedures.

Keywords Percutaneous coronary intervention • PCI • Radial access • Femoral access • Bleeding • Vascular access site complications • STEMI • Non-ST elevated myocardial infarction • Myocardial infarction • Coronary artery disease

Introduction

Femoral and radial access sites are the most commonly used approaches in current interventional cardiology. However, it is interesting to mention that at the inception of invasive cardiology, the brachial access, introduced by Sones in the early 50's, [1] was the default access for left cardiac catheterization. The brachial artery, first

F. Costa, MD
Department of Interventional Cardiology, Thoraxcenter, Erasmus Medical Center, Rotterdam 3015 CE, The Netherlands

Department of Clinical and Experimental Medicine, Policlinico "G. Martino", University of Messina, Messina, Italy

M. Valgimigli, MD, PhD, FESC (✉)
Thoraxcenter, Erasmus Medical Center, Rotterdam 3015 CE, The Netherlands

Erasmus MC, Department of Interventional Cardiology, Thoraxcenter, Rotterdam, The Netherlands
e-mail: m.valgimigli@erasmusmc.nl

© Springer International Publishing Switzerland 2015
J.A. Ambrose, A.E. Rodríguez (eds.), *Controversies in Cardiology*,
DOI 10.1007/978-3-319-20415-4_24

approached with a surgical cutdown and later percutaneously with the Seldinger's technique [2], was extensively used until the late 60's when Amplatz and Judkins demonstrated the feasibility of the percutaneous femoral access in a large case series [3]. Afterwards, interventional cardiology made huge progress in the techniques and devices used and femoral access became the default approach for almost all of them.

In the last 20 years, after Campeau's report of a transradial approach (TRA) for coronary angiography, the radial artery has been increasingly employed as an alternative access site for both diagnostic and therapeutic procedures [4].

The main advantage of the radial artery use is a reduced invasiveness, given by its superficial position, the smaller caliber and the high predictability of its compression. The lack of important adjacent structures decreases the hazard during the puncture. However, these benefits come at the cost of an increased complexity in the maneuverability of the catheters, with an increased procedure time and radiation exposure, especially in non-experienced operators [5]. Moreover, its anatomical limitations do not permit the use of bulky devices or bigger catheters, occasionally needed for more complex procedures.

Discussion

The Bleeding Issue: Access Site and Non-access Site Bleeding During Percutaneous Coronary Intervention (PCI) and Their Impact on Patients' Outcome

Bleeding is a frequent complication during PCI and 30–70 % of these events are related to the access site. This broad variability depends mostly on the patient's clinical presentation. In fact, acute patients are more prone to access site bleeding, whereas in stable patients two-thirds are not access site related [6].

The radial approach brings a 65 % reduction of major vascular access site complications, 49 % of non–CABG-related major bleeding, and 35 % reduction of the transfusion rate compared with the femoral approach [7]. Interestingly, radial access benefit persisted when vascular closure devices were used in the femoral cohort [8].

The reduction of bleeding events is of paramount importance considering the strong correlation between major bleeding and mortality [9, 10]. In a study of over 26,000 patients with non–ST-segment elevation ACS, there was a significant interaction between bleeding severity and the rate of death at 30-days, death at 6 months or the composite of death and MI [11].

A sub-analysis of the TRITON-TIMI 38 trial [12] showed that serious spontaneous bleeding tended to have a sustained impact on mortality for approximately 1 month, as it was shown by an elevated hazard ratio within the first 30 days after PCI followed by a non-significant trend thereafter. Similarly, a recent analysis from the PLATO trial also demonstrated that procedure-related bleeding is strongly associated with short-term mortality [13].

To further corroborate these findings, the application of bleeding prevention strategies demonstrated a better survival during an acute coronary syndrome. The OASIS-5 trial compared fondaparinux with enoxaparin in a court of 20,078 patients with non-ST-segment elevation ACS. This study showed that fondaparinux was not inferior to enoxaparin with respect to 9 day composite ischemic endpoints, and superior with respect to major bleeding at 9 days (fondaparinux 2.2 % vs. enoxaparin 4.1 %, $p < 0.001$) [14] eventually resulting in a significant reduction of death from all causes at 1 month (deaths in fondaparinux arm 574 vs. deaths in enoxaparin arm 638, $p = 0.05$).

Similarly, in HORIZONS AMI, the implementation of the direct thrombin inhibitor bivalirudin, compared with unfractionated heparin plus glycoprotein IIb/IIIa inhibitors in patients undergoing primary PCI, resulted in both a reduction of major bleeding (4.9 % vs. 8.3 %, $p < 0.001$) and mortality at 30 days (2.1 % vs. 3.1 %, $p = 0.047$) [15].

However, it is worth mentioning that patients with a higher bleeding risk usually carry also a higher ischemic risk. In fact, bleeding more frequently occurs in sicker patients, and a possible lack of cause-effect between the two events could be argued, being this correlation driven by host or putative mechanisms [16]. On the other hand, discontinuation of antithrombotic therapy, transfusions and severe anemia after bleeding are likely to be important prognostic modifiers and all need to be prevented [17].

Finally, it has been demonstrated that non-access site related bleeding carries a relatively higher risk of death compared with access site bleeding (HR 2.2) [18, 19]. Access site selection hardly affects non-access-site bleeding, on the other hand, the application of a modern antithrombotic regimen and optimal anti platelet therapy could mitigate the excess bleeding risk and improve the outcome [15, 20].

Is Radial Access Effective as Femoral?

The limits of the radial technique have been pushed far forward since its first introduction. The advances in experience and technology allow today the treatment of complex PCI cases like bifurcations, unprotected left main coronary artery [21] and chronic total occlusions [22] from the radial access. Importantly, the rates of procedural success are similar to the femoral approach [23] but only for experienced radial operators.

Many studies tried to delineate the learning curve of the radial technique. Ball et al. prospectively collected from 1999 to 2008 a total of 1672 patients with non-urgent, single vessel disease, underwent TR-PCI by 28 operators. The outcomes were stratified into chronological groups of cases for operators starting transracial technique in their institution: the first group from case 1 to case 50 and so on 51–100, 101–150, 151–300. The control group consisted of experienced radial operators with more than 300 TR-PCI. The study found that the PCI failure rate was inversely related with the case volume, with a 32 % decrease in PCI failure every additional 50 PCIs performed. The author's eventually concluded that a case volume of at least 50 PCI is needed to achieve an outcome comparable with an expert radial operator.

However, considering that this study included non-urgent, single vessel disease, the learning curve for more complex PCI is likely to be steeper [24]. Similarly, Looi et al. showed how after 6 months of practice in diagnostic radial angiography, fellows reached results comparable with senior operators [25].

Interestingly, another single study about the radial approach learning curve showed that the left radial approach had a shorter learning curve compared to right radial access [26]. These results could be explained by a lower impact of subclavian tortuosity in the left radial artery (OR 2,7) and by an easier maneuverability of the catheters that, originally designed for the femoral route, adapt better to the left radial anatomy [26].

Certainly, the more complex is the radial anatomy, the more difficult and longer is the procedure with consequences on procedural times and radiation exposure. This is particularly true for the diagnostic angiograms whereas the impact on PCI is milder. As could be expected, procedural times and radiation dose decrease with operator's expertise [5].

Radial vs. Femoral: The Evidence

In the past few years an important burden of evidence has been collected for the comparison of femoral and radial access approaches.

The MORTAL registry, published in 2008 by Chase et al. retrospectively analyzed 38,872 patients treated with PCI either via TRA (7,972 patients) or TFA (30,900 patients). The results showed that TRA reduced the need for blood transfusion (1.4 % vs. 2.8 %) and 1-year mortality (3.9 % vs. 2.8 %). Importantly, the patient population mainly consisted of ACS treated on an urgent basis [27]. Other observational studies demonstrated afterwards the same conclusions.

The lack of a randomized trial comparing the two strategies was finally overcome with the presentation of the pivotal radial versus femoral access for coronary angiography and intervention in patients with acute coronary syndromes (RIVAL) trial. RIVAL recruited 7,021 patients in 32 countries, of which 3,507 patients were randomly assigned to radial access and 3,514 to femoral access. The primary outcome was the composite of death, myocardial infarction, stroke, or non- coronary artery bypass graft (non-CABG)-related major bleeding at 30 days. The trial ultimately failed to demonstrate a significant superiority of the radial access with respect to the primary endpoint (3.7 % vs. 4.0 %, [HR] 0.92, 95 %CI 0.72–1.17; p=0.50). Major vascular access site complications were significantly reduced in the radial arm (1.4 % vs. 3.7 % P<0.0001), whereas non-CABG-related TIMI major bleeding (0.5 % vs. 0.5 % P=1.00) and access site major bleeding (0.2 % vs. 0.3 % P=NS) were similar in the two groups [7].

Importantly, it has been shown that, in patients with STEMI, there was a benefit with radial access for the composite of death, MI and stroke ($P_{int}=0.011$), and death for all causes (interaction $P_{int}=0.001$). A significant interaction for the primary outcome was finally noted in the highest tertile volume radial centers (HR 0.49, 95 %CI

0.28–0.87; p = 0.015). These findings strongly questioned the previous results suggested by the observational studies. However, at a deeper analysis some of the reasons of such a divergence could be identified.

First, a post-hoc analysis that evaluated the actual location of the access-site major bleeding showed that all the six reported events found in the radial group did not consist of real radial-related complications but of consequences of IABP or radial-to-femoral cross-over confounded by the intention-to-treat design of the study. Thus, after reallocating the bleeding events in the pertinent group, a significant relation between access-site major bleeding and femoral access (0 vs. 18 events) was present also in RIVAL [7].

Second, the bleeding definition used to adjudicate the events is of paramount importance. In fact, the use Acute Catheterization and Urgent Intervention strategy (ACUITY) trial bleeding criteria showed a significant reduction of major bleeding in the radial cohort (p < 0.0001).

Third, the number of bleeding events was unusually low in the RIVAL population compared with previous ACS trials and only 32 % were access site related. Therefore, the trial may have been underpowered to detect a difference in non–CABG-related major bleeding and consequently to demonstrate a superiority of radial access on the primary endpoint [7].

The RIVAL result left many perplexities, and further evidence was needed. The Radial versus Femoral Randomized Investigation in ST- Elevation Acute Coronary Syndrome (RIFLE-STEACS) trial, presented in 2011, randomized 1,001 patients undergoing primary PCI to radial or femoral access. The aim of the study was to demonstrate a benefit on hard endpoints of the radial access in the STEMI population [28]. The trial used the new Bleeding Academic Research Consortium (BARC) definition and was powered to assess the superiority over the primary endpoint of death, MI, TLR, stroke or non–CABG-related major bleeding at 30 days. RIFLE-STEACS demonstrated a net reduction of the primary endpoint (13.6 % vs. 21 %; P = 0.003), of the non–CABG-related major bleeding (7.8 % vs. 12.2 %; P = 0.026) and of mortality (5.2 % vs. 9.2 % P = 0.02) in the radial arm at 30 days.

This apparently striking results need to be critically analyzed.

Firstly, the operators in the RIFLE-STEACS were all expert radialists performing more than 300 PCI/year. Notwithstanding, the crossover rate from radial to femoral was 9.6 %, mainly due to shock, peripheral vascular disease and previous thrombolysis.

Secondly, the total mortality and the bleeding rates of the RIFLE-STEACS population were particularly high compared to previous STEMI trials, probably because the population included higher risk patients with cardiogenic shock and rescue PCIs, and the treatment frequently included GP inhibitors (70 %).

Finally, even if the access-site bleeding was reduced by the radial access in the main study, at a post-hoc analysis this benefit was no longer present when the TIMI bleeding definition was used [28].

Another recent randomized trial evaluated the effect of the access-site in patients undergoing PCI. The STEMI-RADIAL randomized 707 patients with STEMI to radial and femoral approach before the primary PCI [29]. The primary endpoint, consisting of a composite of major bleeding and vascular access site complications at 30 days, occurred significantly more in the femoral access group (1.4 % vs. 7.2 %; P<0.0001). The rate of net adverse clinical events (NACE) defined as a composite of death, MI, stroke, and major bleeding/vascular complications was also reduced by the radial access strategy (4.6 % vs. 11 %; P=0.0028). In contrast with the RIFLE-STEACS, mortality at 30 days in the STEMI-RADIAL was similar in the two groups (2.3 % vs. 3.1 %; P=0.64), result probably driven by the exclusion of very high-risk patients.

Mortality: Does the Access Site Matter?

The impact of access-site on mortality has been tested by numerous randomized trials, observational studies and metanalysis.

Before the RIVAL publication many observational studies including the already mentioned MORTAL registry showed a mortality reduction with the radial approach. The PREVAIL, a non randomized prospective study, also showed a benefit of radial on hard endpoints including death (1.1 % vs. 4.9 %) [30]. Similarly, a systematic review of the literature involving 2,808 STEMI patients, who were largely recruited in a non-randomized fashion, showed that trans-radial intervention was associated with almost 50 % decrease of overall mortality [31].

The RIVAL overturned these data, not showing a significant mortality difference between the two groups. However, the subgroup analysis of patients with STEMI showed an impressive 54 % mortality reduction after the trans-radial treatment. Conversely, patients with NSTEACS showed a worrisome trend towards a 66 % increase in mortality (P=0.082) [7].

Finally in the RIFLE-STEACS trial a 50 % mortality reduction was found in the radial group [28]. Consistent with these findings, an observational region-wide study compared the medium-term outcomes of trans-radial versus trans-femoral intervention in 12,407 patients who underwent PCI for STEMI. This study showed a 30 % mortality reduction at 2 years in favor of the trans-radial intervention reflecting an early significant mortality benefit within 30 days after treatment [32].

From all the data collected so far, radial access emerged as the most important single mortality reducer during primary PCI. However, the reason of such an impressive impact on survival is not completely clear. The reduction in access site major bleeding is a clear benefit of the radial access but can hardly explain these massive differences. Furthermore, non-access site bleeding affects mortality two times more than access site bleeding and reasonably cannot be influenced by the access selection [6].

Analyzing the detailed cause of death in the RIFLE-STEACS trial, most of the patients died early after PCI and frequently from acute heart failure. Accordingly, it is difficult to speculate why the radial approach provides such a significant benefit.

Potential beneficial mechanisms of the radial approach could be related to the earlier ambulation (lower risk of venous thromboembolism) and earlier hospital discharge (lower risk of nosocomial infection) but these hypotheses have yet to be tested [33].

Although the impact of the radial approach on mortality remains elusive, this should not underestimate the growing evidence showing a sensible benefit from the radial approach.

Cost and Hospitality stay:

Radial access sensibly reduces the hospital costs. Safley et al. examined costs among 61,509 procedures and observed a reduction of expenses in radial procedures, mostly driven by a reduced in hospital length of stay [34]. This benefit was consistent in the RIFLE-STEACS and in the STEMI-RADIAL trials.

Limitations of the Radial Artery

Trans-radial approach carries several limitations.

First of all radial artery anatomy is still a technical limitation, being 50–70 % smaller than the femoral artery, it does not allow the same flexibility in the device and procedure strategy selection as compared to the femoral approach. In fact, the rate of vascular access site failure in the RIVAL study was higher in the radial group (7 % vs. 0.9 %). Access site failure was mostly related to radial spasm (5 %) and vessel tortuosity in the radial (1.3 %) and in the subclavian segment (1.9 %).

Part of the technical complexity of the radial approach is obtaining an optimal support of the guiding catheter, especially during left coronary artery intervention [35]. This could be challenging for the imperfect compatibility of the standard catheters, designed for the femoral route, with the radial anatomy [36]. Even if some of these technical difficulties could be overcome with left radial access, [37] more than 90 % of operators use the right approach [36] and dedicated radial catheter are not commonly utilized.

Noteworthy, the radial approach reduces dramatically access-site complication but it cannot be considered a complication-free procedure. Compartmental syndrome or catheter entrapment with radial avulsion are rare, but must be carefully prevented. More frequent is the radial artery patency loss that occurs in up to 12 % of patients at 24 h after radial catheterization [38]. This should not be considered a minor complication because it might hinder the potential future use of the radial artery (arterial fistula for dialysis, arterial harvesting for CABG, further catheterizations), and could eventually be prevented with the systematic use of the patent hemostasis technique [38].

Lastly, the radiation dose appears to be higher with the radial approach [5]. This is true especially during the first part of the learning curve, and it is reduced with operator experience.

When Femoral Artery Is Necessary

Given the strong relationship between radial access and reduced vascular complications, the American College of Cardiology Foundation, American Heart Association, Society for Cardiovascular Angiography and Interventions PCI practice guidelines now give a strong recommendation to the radial approach [39], and the European Association of Percutaneous Cardiovascular Interventions group has recently stated in a position paper that it should be the default access site for PCI [40].

Nevertheless, in many situations the femoral approach is still essential. Not mentioning the imperative necessity of the femoral access for all structural heart disease procedures, the use of bulky devices such as intra-aortic balloon pump, Impella device or ECMO require a large diameter arterial access. Moreover, femoral access is still the first choice during complex PCI's when better control and flexibility are needed.

Conclusion

The benefit of the radial use in clinical practice has been shown in many different randomized trials. Although the mechanism of benefit for some end points remains unclear, a continuous effort should be made to improve proficiency in the radial approach without loosing expertise in the femoral technique.

Furthermore, the implementation of strategies to prevent non-access site related bleeding, such as the use of bivalirudin and the optimal adjustment of anti-platelet therapy, are likely to be important steps to improve the prognosis of ACS patients.

In the near future ongoing trials such as SAFARI-STEMI (NCT01398254) and MATRIX (NCT01433627) will give useful information about the role of vascular access in the context of a modern anticoagulant therapy.

References

1. Sones FSE, Shirey E, Proudfit W, Wescott R. Cine coronary arteriography. Circulation. 1959;20:773–4.
2. Seldinger SI. Catheter replacement of the needle in percutaneous arteriography. A new technique. Acta Radiol Suppl. 2008;434:47–52.
3. Judkins MP. Selective coronary arteriography. I. A percutaneous transfemoral technic. Radiology. 1967;89(5):815–24.
4. Campeau L. Percutaneous radial artery approach for coronary angiography. Cathet Cardiovasc Diagn. 1989;16(1):3–7.
5. Neill J, Douglas H, Richardson G, Chew EW, Walsh S, Hanratty C, et al. Comparison of radiation dose and the effect of operator experience in femoral and radial arterial access for coronary procedures. Am J Cardiol. 2010;106(7):936–40.
6. Verheugt FW, Steinhubl SR, Hamon M, Darius H, Steg PG, Valgimigli M, et al. Incidence, prognostic impact, and influence of antithrombotic therapy on access and nonaccess site bleeding in percutaneous coronary intervention. JACC Cardiovasc Interv. 2011;4(2): 191–7.

7. Jolly SS, Yusuf S, Cairns J, Niemela K, Xavier D, Widimsky P, et al. Radial versus femoral access for coronary angiography and intervention in patients with acute coronary syndromes (RIVAL): a randomised, parallel group, multicentre trial. Lancet. 2011;377(9775):1409–20.
8. Mann T, Cowper PA, Peterson ED, Cubeddu G, Bowen J, Giron L, et al. Transradial coronary stenting: comparison with femoral access closed with an arterial suture device. Catheter Cardiovasc Interv. 2000;49(2):150–6.
9. Doyle BJ, Rihal CS, Gastineau DA, Holmes Jr DR. Bleeding, blood transfusion, and increased mortality after percutaneous coronary intervention: implications for contemporary practice. J Am Coll Cardiol. 2009;53(22):2019–27.
10. Vranckx P, Leonardi S, Tebaldi M, Biscaglia S, Parrinello G, Rao SV, et al. Prospective validation of the Bleeding Academic Research Consortium classification in the all-comer prodigy trial. Eur Heart J. 2014;35(37):2524–9. doi:10.1093/eurheartj/ehu161.
11. Rao SV, O'Grady K, Pieper KS, Granger CB, Newby LK, Van de Werf F, et al. Impact of bleeding severity on clinical outcomes among patients with acute coronary syndromes. Am J Cardiol. 2005;96(9):1200–6.
12. Hochholzer W, Wiviott SD, Antman EM, Contant CF, Guo J, Giugliano RP, et al. Predictors of bleeding and time dependence of association of bleeding with mortality: insights from the Trial to Assess Improvement in Therapeutic Outcomes by Optimizing Platelet Inhibition With Prasugrel--Thrombolysis in Myocardial Infarction 38 (TRITON-TIMI 38). Circulation. 2011;123(23):2681–9.
13. Ducrocq G, Schulte PJ, Becker RC, Cannon CP, Harrington RA, Held C, et al. Association of spontaneous and procedure-related bleeds with short- and long-term mortality after acute coronary syndromes: an analysis from the PLATO trial. EuroIntervention. 2014. doi:10.4244/EIJY14M09_11.
14. Fifth Organization to Assess Strategies in Acute Ischemic Syndromes Investigators, Yusuf S, Mehta SR, Chrolavicius S, Afzal R, Pogue J, et al. Comparison of fondaparinux and enoxaparin in acute coronary syndromes. N Engl J Med. 2006;354(14):1464–76.
15. Stone GW, Witzenbichler B, Guagliumi G, Peruga JZ, Brodie BR, Dudek D, et al. Bivalirudin during primary PCI in acute myocardial infarction. N Engl J Med. 2008;358(21):2218–30.
16. Lopes RD, Subherwal S, Holmes DN, Thomas L, Wang TY, Rao SV, et al. The association of in-hospital major bleeding with short-, intermediate-, and long-term mortality among older patients with non-ST-segment elevation myocardial infarction. Eur Heart J. 2012;33(16):2044–53.
17. Rao SV, Jollis JG, Harrington RA, Granger CB, Newby LK, Armstrong PW, et al. Relationship of blood transfusion and clinical outcomes in patients with acute coronary syndromes. JAMA. 2004;292(13):1555–62.
18. Mehran R, Pocock S, Nikolsky E, Dangas GD, Clayton T, Claessen BE, et al. Impact of bleeding on mortality after percutaneous coronary intervention results from a patient-level pooled analysis of the REPLACE-2 (randomized evaluation of PCI linking angiomax to reduced clinical events), ACUITY (acute catheterization and urgent intervention triage strategy), and HORIZONS-AMI (harmonizing outcomes with revascularization and stents in acute myocardial infarction) trials. JACC Cardiovasc Interv. 2011;4(6):654–64.
19. Chhatriwalla AK, Amin AP, Kennedy KF, House JA, Cohen DJ, Rao SV, et al. Association between bleeding events and in-hospital mortality after percutaneous coronary intervention. JAMA. 2013;309(10):1022–9.
20. Valgimigli M, Campo G, Percoco G, Monti M, Ferrari F, Tumscitz C, et al. Randomized comparison of 6- versus 24-month clopidogrel therapy after balancing anti-intimal hyperplasia stent potency in all-comer patients undergoing percutaneous coronary intervention Design and rationale for the PROlonging Dual-antiplatelet treatment after Grading stent-induced Intimal hyperplasia study (PRODIGY). Am Heart J. 2010;160(5):804–11.
21. Yang YJ, Kandzari DE, Gao Z, Xu B, Chen JL, Qiao SB, et al. Transradial versus transfemoral method of percutaneous coronary revascularization for unprotected left main coronary artery disease: comparison of procedural and late-term outcomes. JACC Cardiovasc Interv. 2010;3(10):1035–42.

22. Rathore S, Hakeem A, Pauriah M, Roberts E, Beaumont A, Morris JL. A comparison of the transradial and the transfemoral approach in chronic total occlusion percutaneous coronary intervention. Catheter Cardiovasc Interv. 2009;73(7):883–7.

23. Rao SV, Ou FS, Wang TY, Roe MT, Brindis R, Rumsfeld JS, et al. Trends in the prevalence and outcomes of radial and femoral approaches to percutaneous coronary intervention: a report from the National Cardiovascular Data Registry. JACC Cardiovasc Interv. 2008;1(4):379–86.

24. Ball WT, Sharieff W, Jolly SS, Hong T, Kutryk MJ, Graham JJ, et al. Characterization of operator learning curve for transradial coronary interventions. Circ Cardiovasc Interv. 2011;4(4):336–41.

25. Looi JL, Cave A, El-Jack S. Learning curve in transradial coronary angiography. Am J Cardiol. 2011;108(8):1092–5.

26. Sciahbasi A, Romagnoli E, Trani C, Burzotta F, Pendenza G, Tommasino A, et al. Evaluation of the "learning curve" for left and right radial approach during percutaneous coronary procedures. Am J Cardiol. 2011;108(2):185–8.

27. Chase AJ, Fretz EB, Warburton WP, Klinke WP, Carere RG, Pi D, et al. Association of the arterial access site at angioplasty with transfusion and mortality: the M.O.R.T.A.L study (Mortality benefit Of Reduced Transfusion after percutaneous coronary intervention via the Arm or Leg). Heart. 2008;94(8):1019–25.

28. Romagnoli E, Biondi-Zoccai G, Sciahbasi A, Politi L, Rigattieri S, Pendenza G, et al. Radial versus femoral randomized investigation in ST-segment elevation acute coronary syndrome: the RIFLE-STEACS (Radial Versus Femoral Randomized Investigation in ST-Elevation Acute Coronary Syndrome) study. J Am Coll Cardiol. 2012;60(24):2481–9.

29. Bernat I, Horak D, Stasek J, Mates M, Pesek J, Ostadal P, et al. ST-segment elevation myocardial infarction treated by radial or femoral approach in a multicenter randomized clinical trial: the STEMI-RADIAL trial. J Am Coll Cardiol. 2014;63(10):964–72.

30. Pristipino C, Trani C, Nazzaro MS, Berni A, Patti G, Patrizi R, et al. Major improvement of percutaneous cardiovascular procedure outcomes with radial artery catheterisation: results from the PREVAIL study. Heart. 2009;95(6):476–82.

31. Vorobcsuk A, Konyi A, Aradi D, Horvath IG, Ungi I, Louvard Y, et al. Transradial versus transfemoral percutaneous coronary intervention in acute myocardial infarction Systematic overview and meta-analysis. Am Heart J. 2009;158(5):814–21.

32. Valgimigli M, Saia F, Guastaroba P, Menozzi A, Magnavacchi P, Santarelli A, et al. Transradial versus transfemoral intervention for acute myocardial infarction: a propensity score-adjusted and -matched analysis from the REAL (REgistro regionale AngiopLastiche dell'Emilia-Romagna) multicenter registry. JACC Cardiovasc Interv. 2012;5(1):23–35.

33. Vuurmans T, Byrne J, Fretz E, Janssen C, Hilton JD, Klinke WP, et al. Chronic kidney injury in patients after cardiac catheterisation or percutaneous coronary intervention: a comparison of radial and femoral approaches (from the British Columbia Cardiac and Renal Registries). Heart. 2010;96(19):1538–42.

34. Safley DM, Amin AP, House JA, Baklanov D, Mills R, Giersiefen H, et al. Comparison of costs between transradial and transfemoral percutaneous coronary intervention: a cohort analysis from the Premier research database. Am Heart J. 2013;165(3):303–9 e2.

35. Ikari Y, Nagaoka M, Kim JY, Morino Y, Tanabe T. The physics of guiding catheters for the left coronary artery in transfemoral and transradial interventions. J Invasive Cardiol. 2005;17(12):636–41.

36. Bertrand OF, Rao SV, Pancholy S, Jolly SS, Rodes-Cabau J, Larose E, et al. Transradial approach for coronary angiography and interventions: results of the first international transradial practice survey. JACC Cardiovasc Interv. 2010;3(10):1022–31.

37. Sciahbasi A, Romagnoli E, Burzotta F, Trani C, Sarandrea A, Summaria F, et al. Transradial approach (left vs right) and procedural times during percutaneous coronary procedures: TALENT study. Am Heart J. 2011;161(1):172–9.

38. Pancholy S, Coppola J, Patel T, Roke-Thomas M. Prevention of radial artery occlusion-patent hemostasis evaluation trial (PROPHET study): a randomized comparison of traditional versus

patency documented hemostasis after transradial catheterization. Catheter Cardiovasc Interv. 2008;72(3):335–40.

39. Levine GN, Bates ER, Blankenship JC, Bailey SR, Bittl JA, Cercek B, et al. 2011 ACCF/AHA/ SCAI Guideline for Percutaneous Coronary Intervention. A report of the American College of Cardiology Foundation/American Heart Association Task Force on Practice Guidelines and the Society for Cardiovascular Angiography and Interventions. J Am Coll Cardiol. 2011;58(24):e44–122.

40. Hamon M, Pristipino C, Di Mario C, Nolan J, Ludwig J, Tubaro M, et al. Consensus document on the radial approach in percutaneous cardiovascular interventions: position paper by the European Association of Percutaneous Cardiovascular Interventions and Working Groups on Acute Cardiac Care** and Thrombosis of the European Society of Cardiology. EuroIntervention. 2013;8(11):1242–51.

Chapter 25
Advanced and Expensive Cardiovascular Procedures in the Very Elderly–Can We or Should We Limit Access?

Pranav Kansara, Konstantinos Kossidas, Sandra Weiss, and William S. Weintraub

Abstract With the increasing proportion of elderly patients in the population, physicians are often faced with challenging treatment decisions for the management of coronary artery diseases, valvular heart diseases, advanced heart failure and prevention of sudden cardiac death in the elderly patient population. Comprehensive review of the literature and available evidence is summarized in this chapter to guide such complex clinical decisions. Elderly patients presenting with an acute coronary syndrome (ACS) appear to benefit from percutaneous coronary intervention (PCI) with the use of drug eluting stents (DES). Though current guidelines do not consider age as a prohibitive factor, the risk of major bleeding complications and stroke should be carefully considered. For elderly patients with severe aortic stenosis, trans-catheter aortic valve replacement (TAVR) is superior compared to medical therapy for inoperable patients. TAVR, when performed via the transfemoral approach, remains non inferior and cost effective compared to surgical aortic valve replacement (SAVR). Trans-catheter mitral valve repair (TMVR) using MitraClip appears to be beneficial for inoperable patients with degenerative severe mitral regurgitation but more data are needed. Implantable cardioverter defibrillator (ICD) implantation in the elderly population remains a controversial topic especially for secondary prevention. The current evidence suggests that age should not be the sole withholding factor but the decision for ICD implantation should account for comorbidities and patient preference. On the other hand, cardiac resynchronization therapy (CRT) has definitely a mortality and morbidity benefit in the management of elderly patients with advanced heart failure.

Keywords Elderly • Percutaneous coronary intervention • Trans-catheter aortic valve replacement • Trans-catheter mitral valve repair • Implantable cardioverter defibrillator • Cardiac resynchronization therapy

P. Kansara, MD, MS • K. Kossidas, MD • S. Weiss, MD, FACC
W.S. Weintraub, MD, MACC (✉)
Department of Cardiology, Christiana Care Health System, Newark, DE, USA
e-mail: pkansara@christianacare.org

© Springer International Publishing Switzerland 2015
J.A. Ambrose, A.E. Rodríguez (eds.), *Controversies in Cardiology*,
DOI 10.1007/978-3-319-20415-4_25

Abbreviations

ASSENT	Assessment of the Safety and Efficacy of a New Thrombolytic
AVID	The Antiarrhythmic vs Implantable Defibrillators
CARE-HF	Cardiac Resynchronization in Heart Failure study
CASH	Cardiac Arrest Study Hamburg
CIDS	Canadian Implantable Defibrillator Study
COMPANION	The Comparison of Medical Pacing and Defibrillator Therapies in Heart Failure Trial
EVEREST	Endovascular Valve Edge-to-Edge Repair Study
GUSTO	Global Utilization of Streptokinase and Tissue Plasminogen Activator for Occluded Coronary Arteries
HERO	Hirulog Early Reperfusion or Occlusion
MADIT–CRT	Multicenter Automatic Defibrillator Implantation trial with Cardiac Resynchronization Therapy
MADITT-II	Multicenter Automatic Defibrillator Implantation Trial-II
MIRACLE	Multicenter InSync ICD Randomized Clinical Evaluation
PAMI	Primary Angioplasty in Myocardial Infarction
PARAGON	The Platelet IIb/IIIa Antagonist for the Reduction of Acute coronary syndrome events in a Global Organization Network
PARTNER	Placement of Aortic Transcatheter Valve
PURSUIT	The Platelet Glycoprotein IIb/IIIa in Unstable Angina: Receptor Suppression Using Integrilin Therapy
TACTICS-TIMI 18	Treat angina with Aggrastat and determine Cost of Therapy with an Invasive or Conservative Strategy--Thrombolysis in Myocardial Infarction 18

Introduction

With an improved overall survival at the population level, the number of geriatric patients has significantly increased. With that comes more complex coronary and valvular heart disease, management of which has been revolutionized over the last decade with advances in interventional cardiology. There are several unresolved issues related to what is the appropriate therapy in this population. Along with the advent of catheter-based treatment of valvular heart diseases such as transcatheter aortic valve replacement (TAVR) and transcatheter mitral valve repair (TMVR) using the MitraClip system (Abbott vascular, CA), there have been remarkable improvements in stent technology and stent delivery systems for percutaneous coronary intervention (PCI). At the same time, physicians, patients and their families are increasingly faced with decisions about device–based therapies, especially implantable cardioverter defibrillator (ICD) and cardiac resynchronization (CRT) in elderly patients who meet conventional criteria for device implantation. As one can imagine, such procedures have substantially increased the cost of care. The available evidence with respect to clinical efficacy, quality of life improvement and cost effectiveness with respect to PCI for acute coronary syndrome, TAVR, TMVR, ICD and CRT for the elderly population (age ≥75 years) is reviewed here.

Catheter Based Therapies

Percutaneous Coronary Intervention

There has been a limited representation of patients ≥75 years of age in the early clinical trials for non ST segment elevation acute coronary syndrome (NSTE ACS) ranging from 17 to 22 % (pooled data from GUSTO IIb, Paragon A, Paragon B, PURSUIT, GUSTO-IV ACS) and for ST segment elevation ACS (STE ACS) ranging from 12 to 18 % (pooled data from GUSTO I, GUSTO IIb, GUSTO III, ASSENT-2, ASSENT-3, HERO-2). Furthermore, there was only 2 % representation for patients age ≥85 years for both NSTE and STE ACS [1, 2]. TACTICS-TIMI 18 provided the initial evidence of a reduction in death or myocardial infarction (MI) at 6 months with an early invasive (EI) strategy compared to initial conservative (IC) management for high risk NSTE ACS in patients with age ≥75 years (21.6 vs 10.8, OR 0.44, total n = 278) [3]. With an accepted societal threshold of $50,000/death or MI prevented, cost effectiveness analysis (CEA) suggested that the incremental cost effectiveness ratio (ICER) for death or MI prevented was $25,478 with an EI approach, and therefore cost effective [4]. However, CEA was not stratified based on age. Due to this under representation and limited evidence, the 2007 AHA scientific statement for the management of NSTE ACS patients of age ≥75 years underscored the need for prospective randomized outcomes data in elderly patients for definite treatment recommendations [1]. Since the writing of these statement guideline, a contemporary randomized control trial of 313 patients (age ≥75 years, mean age 82) comparing the EI approach (88 % angiography, 55 % revascularization) to IC therapy for patients presenting with NSTE ACS (29 % angiography, 23 % revascularization) demonstrated comparable rates of mortality and MI between the two strategies at 1 year [5]. However, the primary endpoint (composite of death, MI, stroke, rehospitalization or severe bleeding at 1 year) was significantly lower in patients managed with an EI approach who presented with elevated troponin (HR 0.43, 95 % CI: 0.23–0.80) but not with normal troponin (HR 1.67, 95 % CI: 0.75–3.17) [5].

For elderly patients with STE ACS, primary PCI (PPCI) was demonstrated to be superior compared to fibrinolysis (FL) in the earlier trials. The senior PAMI trial (n = 481, age >70 years) demonstrated a 55 % reduction in death, non-fatal stroke or reinfarction in the PPCI group compared to FL (11.6 % vs 18 %, p = 0.05) at 30-days but it was not significant for patients >80 years of age [6]. In a pooled analysis of 11 randomized clinical trials of PPCI versus FL therapy for STE ACS conducted between 1989 and 1996 (n = 2635), PPCI lowered 30-day mortality compared to FL

(13.3 vs 23.6, p<0.05) for elderly patients (age ≥70 years, n=641) [7]. Balloon angioplasty was the PPCI modality among these earlier clinical trials. As such, the 2007 AHA statement for the management of STE ACS indicated superior efficacy of PPCI in STE ACS in elderly patients but underscored the need for additional evidence in elderly patients with age >80 years of age [2].

Again, since the writing of the AHA statement, a contemporary meta-analysis of 22 randomized trials (n=6763) compared 30-day mortality, MI and stoke between FL and PPCI across various age groups (<50, 50–60, 60–70, 70–80, >80 years) [8]. Mortality increased with age but the treatment effect demonstrated mortality reduction with PPCI compared to FL in all age groups except age <50 (overall OR 0.65, 95 % CI: 0.52–0.79) [8]. Further, mortality benefit of PCI persists in elderly patients presenting with acute MI complicated by cardiogenic shock at 1-year [9].

Trends in PCI volume over the last 25 years demonstrate that the proportion of patients undergoing PCI in the age range between 75 and 84 years has doubled and has increased by 5 fold for patients with age >85 years [10]. The angiographic success rates and clinical benefits are not different in the elderly patients compared to younger patients [11] In a prospective randomized trial of 800 octogenarian patients (age >80 years), drug eluting stent use (DES-Xience) was compared to bare metal stent use (BMS-Vision) for the 1-year composite of death, MI, stroke, target vessel revascularization (TVR) and major hemorrhage [12]. Rate of dual antiplatelet therapy at 1-year for the BMS group was 32 % and for the DES group was 94 % [12]. There was a trend towards a lower primary endpoint for DES compared to BMS (14.3 % vs 18.7 %, p=0.09) with comparable 1-year rates of mortality, major hemorrhage and stroke [12]. TVR (2 % vs 7 %, p=0.001) and MI (4.3 % vs 8.7 %, p=0.01) were significantly lower in the DES group compared to BMS at 1-year [12]. Therefore, the available evidence suggests that elderly patients requiring PCI benefit from PCI with use of DES, similar to younger populations. The 2011 ACCF/AHA/SCAI PCI guidelines do not consider age as a prohibitive factor but warrant careful consideration of risk compared to benefit due to the increased risk of bleeding complications and stroke in elderly patients undergoing PCI [13–15].

Transcatheter Aortic Valve Replacement

The prevalence of aortic stenosis is 12.4 % and severe aortic stenosis is 3.4 % among elderly patients (age >75 years) [16]. Among patients with severe aortic stenosis, approximately 75 % are symptomatic and 40 % do not receive aortic valve surgery [16]. Patients with severe aortic stenosis and prohibitive operative mortality (inoperable) or high operative risk utilize tremendous amounts of medical resources. Clinical and economic outcomes analysis of medically managed patients with severe aortic stenosis demonstrated approximately 88 % mortality over 5-years with 1.8 years of mean survival [17]. During a 5-year follow up period, an average patient experienced 4–5 hospitalization, with a total 5-year health care cost of $63,844/patient and annual follow up cost of $29,278/year alive [17]. The estimated cost of providing care to medically managed patients with severe aortic stenosis among the Medicare population is $1.3 billion/year [17]. TAVR is an attractive treatment strategy for such patients.

Efficacy and safety of TAVR was compared to standard therapy for patients with prohibitively higher operative mortality in the PARTNER trial (Inoperable-cohort B, mean age 83 years, total n = 358) [18]. Compared to standard therapy, TAVR resulted in a 20 % reduction in mortality, improved functional status and reduced hospitalization rates at 1 year [18]. Long term outcomes up to 5 years have demonstrated significantly lower all cause mortality (71.8 % vs 93.6 %, p < 0.0001) and lower re-hospitalization (47.6 % vs 87.3 %, p < 0.0001) with TAVR compared to standard therapy [19]. The total cost of care at 12-months was higher in the TAVR group compared to standard therapy driven mainly by the cost of the initial procedure and longer length of rehabilitation and skilled nursing [20]. The cost effectiveness analysis, accounting for improved survival and quality of life, demonstrated TAVR to be superior than standard therapy for inoperable severe aortic stenosis patients [20]. TAVR for patients with inoperable severe aortic stenosis appears to be either comparable or favorable to many other advanced procedures frequently performed in the elderly patients such as use of defibrillators in the primary prevention of sudden cardiac death, PCI, atrial fibrillation ablation, hemodialysis and destination left ventricular assist devices [20].

The PARTNER trial (cohort A) compared TAVR (mean age 84 years, total n = 699) in patients considered high, but not prohibitive, risk for perioperative mortality, with surgical aortic valve replacement (SAVR) [21]. One-year and subsequently reported 2-year outcomes demonstrated comparable rates of mortality and stroke [21]. Quality of life with TAVR was comparable to SAVR at 1-year [22]. TAVR can be performed via transfemoral (TF-TAV) or transapical (TA-TAVR) approaches for high risk severe aortic stenosis patients [21]. TA-TAVR is performed in patients who do not have favorable femoral artery anatomy [21]. Cost effectiveness analysis suggested that, compared to SAVR, TF-TAVR and not the TA-TAVR remains an economically attractive strategy due to reduced ICU stay and reduced length of hospitalization [22].

In summary, for elderly patients with severe aortic stenosis, available evidence suggests that TAVR is superior compared to standard therapy for inoperable patients. For high-risk patients, TAVR performed via the transfemoral route remains non-inferior and cost effective compared to SAVR.

Transcatheter Mitral Valve Repair

Among patients with symptomatic severe mitral regurgitation (SMR), functional disease (74 %) from dilation of the left ventricle and primary degenerative disease (21 %) represent the predominant mechanisms [23]. Approximately, 64 % of patients with functional and 16 % of patients with degenerative SMR do not undergo surgery due to increased operative risk [23]. Among unoperated patients, 1 and 5-year mortality remain high at 20 % and 50 %, respectively, and among survivors, heart failure admissions increase from 41 % at 1 year to 90 % at 5-years [23]. Percutaneous catheter based edge-to-edge mitral valve repair with the MitraClip system has emerged as a potential option for patients with prohibitive operative risk for degenerative SMR. The EVEREST II trial evaluated safety and efficacy of TMVR (MitraClip) in 121 patients with degenerative SMR and prohibitive operative risk with a median follow up of 1.47 years [24]. Mean age was 82 years and 87 % of the population had New York Heart Association (NYHA) class III/IV symptoms. Thirty-day mortality was 6.3 %, MI was 0.8 % and stroke was 2.4 %. One-year mortality was 23.6 % [24]. Among patients alive at 1-year; 83 % had MR ≤ 2+; 87 % had NYHA class I or II symptoms, heart failure rehospitalization were significantly reduced and there was significant improvement in quality of life (measured by SF-36 quality of life scores) [24]. Although the mean age in this study was 82 years and suggested meaningful improvements on multiple levels for this age group, larger studies would be required to evaluate the impact of TMVR on mortality and its cost effectiveness compared to standard therapy before it can be widely recommended for elderly patients. MitraClip currently remains investigational for patients with functional SMR.

Device Based Therapies

In real world practice, more than 40 % of ICDs are implanted in patients >70 years of age; however, elderly patients have not been adequately represented in clinical trials, and the trial definition of "elderly" has been quite variable. Therefore conclusions about the benefit of device-based therapy in this group are largely uncertain. In order to critically review the evidence for implantation of ICDs in the elderly, we note that the main indications for implantation are primary and secondary prevention of sudden cardiac arrhythmia-mediated death. In contrast, CRT can be performed both for prolongation of life and improvement in functional status [25].

Primary Prevention ICD

A large observational study of Medicare beneficiaries >65 who received primary prevention ICDs from 2003 to 2005 demonstrated a significant mortality benefit from ICD implantation. Although the additional health care costs of ICD implantation were substantial in this study, the procedure was deemed cost effective with similar risk of complications compared to younger age groups [26]. However, as with all observational studies, there is the potential for residual confounding due to treatment selection bias. The randomized MADITT-II study responded to these concerns. In this trial, patients post myocardial infarction with an ejection fraction ≤30 % were randomized to primary prevention ICD or standard care and were followed for a mean period of 17.2 months. The trial included 204 patients ≥75 years of age (16.5 % of the total population), among whom there was a 44 % relative reduction in mortality with ICD implantation. Although these finding in this relatively small population were underpowered to reach statistical significance (P=0.08), the hazard ratio was more significant than even that for younger patients. The authors therefore concluded that ICD implantation was beneficial in patients ≥75 years of age [27]. Although the threshold defining elderly was reduced to 65 years of age, a subsequent meta-analysis incorporating data from three major primary prevention trials including MADIT-II confirmed a small reduction in mortality in the elderly patient population [28]. When evaluating survival post ICD implantation, octogenarians were noted to live on average more than 4 years [29]; hence, concerns surrounding abbreviated life expectancy in this population were not supported as an adequate factor to preclude this procedure.

On the other hand, there is evidence against the use of ICD for primary prevention in elderly patients. One retrospective analysis of primary prevention ICD implantation in octogenarians did not demonstrate a reduction in mortality after adjusting for age, GFR and other comorbidities [30]. This was further supported by a retrospective study looking at primary prevention ICD implantation in octogenarians with an ejection fraction below 20 %. One year mortality was found to be markedly elevated in this population and without additional survival benefit from the ICD [31]. One must look at these data critically as these analyses were retrospective, non-randomized and confounded by treatment selection bias. However, taking into consideration that ICDs deliver therapy only for life-threatening arrhythmias, their benefit may be less prominent in elderly patients with reduced EF and renal dysfunction as this population has been noted to die more commonly of non arrhythmogenic causes compared to younger age groups [32].

Consistent with the above disparate findings, the 2012 AHA/HRS/ACC guidelines note the equivocal survival evidence in the existing literature for primary prevention in the elderly. This is in part, due to the non-standardized age definition. The guidelines further recognize that the average patient hospitalized with heart failure with reduced ejection fraction (HFrEF) >75 years of age carries two or more comorbidities, being quite different from the typical patient in the randomized ICD trials (age <65 with little comorbidity), more closely resembling the retrospective analyses noted above. The 1 year mortality rate for this real-world population is 30–50 % with a two fold increase in death in patients with estimated creatinine clearance less than 60 ml. Therefore, the guidelines state that age should not be used as a sole criterion to withhold device-based therapy, but the importance of assessing comorbidities as well as the higher complication rate and importantly the patients' preference is emphasized. Further investigation with a randomized control trial including patients with an average age >75 years could be beneficial to clarify this issue.

Secondary Prevention ICD

The issue of ICD implantation in elderly patients with a history of aborted VT/VF is even murkier. A widely cited meta-analysis by Healey incorporated data from all three major secondary prevention trials (CASH, AVID and CIDS) and failed to demonstrate a survival benefit in patients >75 years of age. Although potentially underpowered because of the relative small number of patients (n = 253), it was suggested that elderly patients may derive less benefit from defibrillators for secondary prevention of sudden arrhythmogenic death compared to younger ones [33]. On the other hand, a recent publication using data from an inclusive ICD registry (5399 patients) in Ontario Canada, that included 453 patients >80 years (275 primary and 157 secondary prevention indications) demonstrated that there was no difference in the rate of appropriate shocks among different age groups. Thus, it showed that benefit from device therapy was still derived despite older age, and decisions regarding ICD implantation should not be based on the grounds of age alone [34].

The guidelines currently offer little direction regarding ICD implantation for secondary prevention in elderly patients; therefore, it comes down to the physician-patient level when an elderly patient is evaluated for secondary-prevention ICD implantation. Physician should attempt to risk stratify patients based on all factors predisposing to mortality and not just age, as those with moderate mortality risk are likely to derive the most benefit.

Cardiac Resynchronization Therapy

Progression of left ventricular systolic dysfunction is frequently accompanied by impaired electromechanical coupling, which may further diminish effective ventricular contractility and lead to adverse remodeling. It has been established that modification of ventricular delay with multisite pacing and re-establishment of coordinated ventricular contraction can potentially reverse the above effect and even induce favorable remodeling with reduction of cardiac chamber dimensions.

Despite the encouraging results from CRT in recent trials, patient clinical responses vary significantly as up to 30 % are non-responders. Concerns about cost have prompted the search for patient subgroups not likely to benefit from CRT therapy. The elderly population has been suggested as such a potential group. Unfortunately and similar to the data on primary and secondary prevention ICD, we again see that prospective randomized trials for CRT have not specifically focused on elderly patients.

In the two major CRT trials, CARE-HF and COMPANION, the mean age was 65 years and the benefit from CRT was the same above and below that threshold [35]. MIRACLE and MIRACLE ICD included 839 patients with class III or IV symptoms that were implanted with CRT or CRT-D (CRT with defibrillator) devices. Importantly among the participants, 174 (21 %) were >75 years. After implantation, patients underwent randomization turning the CRT feature on or off for 6 months. Post hoc analysis that divided patients into age groups demonstrated that at 6 months, improvement in NYHA class and in LVEF was similar across all ages. Adverse events were also found not to be different among younger versus older patients [36].

MADIT–CRT trial was the first study to assess the efficacy of CRT in patients with mild or no symptoms. In a sub-study examining the effect of CRT in different age groups, CRT was associated with a significant clinical benefit in older patients (>60 years) during an average follow-up of 2.4 years. Beneficial effects were preserved for patients >75 years and somewhat surprisingly attenuated for age <60. There was no significant effect >80 years of age, but this could be attributed to the small sample size, as it comprised only 6 % of the study population. This analysis showed that patients >75 continue to derive a significant clinical and echocardiographic benefit from CRT. Risk reduction was found to be less pronounced and nonsignificant in the younger population (perhaps because of the lower event rate). Consistent with the previous reports, complication rates were not higher in older patients [37].

In a study presented at the American College of Cardiology annual meeting in 2012, 164 patients eligible for CRT >80 years of age were compared to 338 CRT-eligible patients aged 70–79. Follow-up for 43 (± 23) months demonstrated similar survival benefit and reverse remodeling in both groups. It was important to note that 19 octogenarians with unsuccessful left ventricle lead placement had statistically significant decreased survival compared to similar octogenarian patients with CRT [38].

The available data indicate that older patients even with comorbidities but with a good life expectancy can benefit from CRT. The lack of definite benefit in elderly patients for ICD therapy can probably be explained by the marked increase of non-arrhythmic death in this group. On the other hand, CRT, which predominately seems to reduce non–arrhythmic mortality, seems to have a consistently positive effect across the age spectrum.

The question regarding the benefit of the defibrillator feature of CRT remains. In selected elderly patients with severe comorbidities and frequent hospitalizations, CRT without ICD back up may be a good choice to improve quality of life, irrespective of impact on mortality.

Conclusions

1. Elderly patients presenting with acute coronary syndrome (ACS) appear to benefit from percutaneous coronary intervention (PCI) with the use of drug eluting stent (DES). Though current guidelines do not consider age as a prohibitive factor, the risk of major bleeding complications and stroke should be carefully considered.
2. For elderly patients with severe aortic stenosis, trans-catheter aortic valve replacement (TAVR) is superior compared to medical therapy for inoperable patients. TAVR, when performed via the transfemoral approach, remains non inferior and cost effective compared to surgical aortic valve replacement (SAVR).
3. Trans-catheter mitral valve repair (TMVR) using MitraClip appears to be beneficial for inoperable patients with degenerative severe mitral regurgitation but more data are needed.
4. ICD implantation in the elderly population remains a controversial topic especially for secondary prevention. The current evidence suggests that age should

not be the sole withholding factor but the decision for ICD implantation should account for comorbidities and patient preference.

5. On the other hand, cardiac resynchronization therapy (CRT) has definitely a mortality and morbidity benefit in the management of elderly patients with advanced heart failure.

References

1. Alexander KP, Newby LK, Cannon CP, et al. Acute coronary care in the elderly, part I: non-ST-segment-elevation acute coronary syndromes: a scientific statement for healthcare professionals from the American Heart Association Council on Clinical Cardiology: in collaboration with the Society of Ger. Circulation. 2007;115(19):2549–69. doi:10.1161/CIRCULATIONAHA.107.182615.
2. Alexander KP, Newby LK, Armstrong PW, et al. Acute coronary care in the elderly, part II: ST-segment-elevation myocardial infarction: a scientific statement for healthcare professionals from the American Heart Association Council on Clinical Cardiology: in collaboration with the Society of Geriatric. Circulation. 2007;115(19):2570–89. doi:10.1161/CIRCULATIONAHA.107.182616.
3. Cannon CP, Weintraub WS, Demopoulos L, et al. Comparison of early invasive and conservative strategies in patients with unstable coronary syndromes treated with the glycoprotein IIb/IIIa inhibitor Tirofiban. N Engl J Med. 2001;344(25):1879–87.
4. Mahoney EM, Jurkovitz CT, Becker ER, et al. Invasive vs conservative strategy for the ST-segment elevation myocardial infarction. JAMA. 2002;288(15):1851–8.
5. Savonitto S, Cavallini C, Petronio AS, et al. Early aggressive versus initially conservative treatment in elderly patients with non-ST-segment elevation acute coronary syndrome: a randomized controlled trial. JACC Cardiovasc Interv. 2012;5(9):906–16. doi:10.1016/j.jcin.2012.06.008.
6. Grines CL. SENIOR PAMI: a prospective randomized trial of primary angioplasty and thrombolytic therapy in elderly patients with acute myocardial infarction. In: Presented at: Transcatheter Cardiovascular Therapeutics 2005; October 19, 2005; Washington, DC.
7. Grines C, Patel A, Zijlstra F, Weaver WD, Granger C, Simes RJ. Primary coronary angioplasty compared with intravenous thrombolytic therapy for acute myocardial infarction: six-month follow up and analysis of individual patient data from randomized trials. Am Heart J. 2003;145(1):47–57. doi:10.1067/mhj.2003.40.
8. De Boer SPM, Westerhout CM, Simes RJ, Granger CB, Zijlstra F, Boersma E. Mortality and morbidity reduction by primary percutaneous coronary intervention is independent of the patient's age. JACC Cardiovasc Interv. 2010;3(3):324–31. doi:10.1016/j.jcin.2009.11.022.
9. Lim HS, Farouque O, Andrianopoulos N, et al. Survival of elderly patients undergoing percutaneous coronary intervention for acute myocardial infarction complicated by cardiogenic shock. JACC Cardiovasc Interv. 2009;2(2):146–52. doi:10.1016/j.jcin.2008.11.006.
10. Singh M, Rihal CS, Gersh BJ, et al. Twenty-five-year trends in in-hospital and long-term outcome after percutaneous coronary intervention: a single-institution experience. Circulation. 2007;115:2835–41. doi:10.1161/CIRCULATIONAHA.106.632679.
11. Moonen LAA, van't Veer M, Pijls NHJ. Procedural and long-term outcome of primary percutaneous coronary intervention in octogenarians. Neth Heart J. 2010;18:129–34.
12. De Belder A, de la Torre Hernandez JM, Lopez-Palop R, et al. A prospective randomized trial of everolimus-eluting stents versus bare-metal stents in octogenarians: the XIMA Trial (Xience or Vision Stents for the Management of Angina in the Elderly). J Am Coll Cardiol. 2014;63(14):1371–5. doi:10.1016/j.jacc.2013.10.053.

13. Guagliumi G, Stone GW, Cox DA, et al. Outcome in elderly patients undergoing primary coronary intervention for acute myocardial infarction: results from the controlled abciximab and device investigation to lower late angioplasty complications (CADILLAC) trial. Circulation. 2004;110:1598–604. doi:10.1161/01.CIR.0000142862.98817.1F.
14. Levine GN, Bates ER, Blankenship JC, et al. 2011 ACCF/AHA/SCAI Guideline for Percutaneous Coronary Intervention. A report of the American College of Cardiology Foundation/American Heart Association Task Force on Practice Guidelines and the Society for Cardiovascular Angiography and Interventions. J Am Coll Cardiol. 2011;58(24):e44–122. doi:10.1016/j.jacc.2011.08.007.
15. Thomas MP, Moscucci M, Smith DE, et al. Outcome of contemporary percutaneous coronary intervention in the elderly and the very elderly: insights from the Blue Cross Blue Shield of Michigan Cardiovascular Consortium. Clin Cardiol. 2011;34(9):549–54. doi:10.1002/clc.20926.
16. Osnabrugge RLJ, Mylotte D, Head SJ, et al. Aortic stenosis in the elderly: disease prevalence and number of candidates for transcatheter aortic valve replacement: a meta-analysis and modeling study. J Am Coll Cardiol. 2013;62(11):1002–12. doi:10.1016/j.jacc.2013.05.015.
17. Clark MA, Arnold SV, Duhay FG, et al. Five-year clinical and economic outcomes among patients with medically managed severe aortic stenosis: results from a Medicare claims analysis. Circ Cardiovasc Qual Outcomes. 2012;5(5):697–704. doi:10.1161/CIRCOUTCOMES.112.966002.
18. Leon MB, Smith CR, Mack M, et al. Transcatheter aortic-valve implantation for aortic stenosis in patients who cannot undergo surgery. N Engl J Med. 2010;363:1597–607. doi:10.1056/NEJMoa1008232.
19. Kapadia SR. Five-year data from clinical trial studying transcatheter aortic valve replacement in patients with severe aortic stenosis demonstrates persistent mortality benefit and lower rate of repeat hospitalizations compared to standard therapy. In: 26th Annual Transcatheter Cardiovascular Therapeutics (TCT) Scientific Symposium, October 2014, Washington; 2014.
20. Reynolds MR, Magnuson EA, Wang K, et al. Cost-effectiveness of transcatheter aortic valve replacement compared with standard care among inoperable patients with severe aortic stenosis: results from the placement of aortic transcatheter valves (PARTNER) trial (Cohort B). Circulation. 2012;125(9):1102–9. doi:10.1161/CIRCULATIONAHA.111.054072.
21. Smith CR, Leon MB, Mack MJ, et al. Transcatheter versus surgical aortic-valve replacement in high-risk patients. N Engl J Med. 2011;364:2187–98. doi:10.1097/01.SA.0000410147.99581.d4.
22. Reynolds MR, Magnuson EA, Lei Y, et al. Cost-effectiveness of transcatheter aortic valve replacement compared with surgical aortic valve replacement in high-risk patients with severe aortic stenosis: results of the PARTNER (Placement of Aortic Transcatheter Valves) trial (Cohort A). J Am Coll Cardiol. 2012;60(25):2683–92. doi:10.1016/j.jacc.2012.09.018.
23. Goel SS, Bajaj N, Aggarwal B, et al. Prevalence and outcomes of unoperated patients with severe symptomatic mitral regurgitation and heart failure: comprehensive analysis to determine the potential role of MitraClip for this unmet need. J Am Coll Cardiol. 2014;63(2):185–6. doi:10.1016/j.jacc.2013.08.723.
24. Lim DS, Reynolds MR, Feldman T, et al. Improved functional status and quality of life in prohibitive surgical risk patients with degenerative mitral regurgitation after transcatheter mitral valve repair. J Am Coll Cardiol. 2014;64(2):182–92. doi:10.1016/j.jacc.2013.10.021.
25. Epstein AE, DiMarco JP, Ellenbogen KA, et al. 2012 ACCF/AHA/HRS focused update incorporated into the ACCF/AHA/HRS 2008 guidelines for device-based therapy of cardiac rhythm abnormalities: a report of the American College of Cardiology Foundation/American Heart Association Task Force on Practice Guidelines and the Heart Rhythm Society. J Am Coll Cardiol. 2013;61(3):e6–75. doi:10.1016/j.jacc.2012.11.007.
26. Groeneveld PW, Farmer SA, Suh JJ, Matta MA, Yang F. Outcomes and costs of implantable cardioverter-defibrillators for primary prevention of sudden cardiac death among the elderly. Heart Rhythm. 2008;5(5):646–53. doi:10.1016/j.hrthm.2008.01.038.

27. Huang DT, Sesselberg HW, McNitt S, et al. Improved survival associated with prophylactic implantable defibrillators in elderly patients with prior myocardial infarction and depressed ventricular function: a MADIT-II substudy. J Cardiovasc Electrophysiol. 2007;18(8):833–8. doi:10.1111/j.1540-8167.2007.00857.x.
28. Santangeli P, Di Biase L, Dello Russo A, et al. Review annals of internal medicine meta-analysis: age and effectiveness of prophylactic implantable. Ann Intern Med. 2010; 153:592–9.
29. Koplan BA, Epstein LM, Albert CM, Stevenson WG. Survival in octogenarians receiving implantable defibrillators. Am Heart J. 2006;152(4):714–9. doi:10.1016/j.ahj.2006.06.008.
30. Mezu U, Adelstein E, Jain S, Saba S. Effectiveness of implantable defibrillators in octogenarians and nonagenarians for primary prevention of sudden cardiac death. Am J Cardiol. 2011;108(5):718–22.
31. Ertel D, Phatak K, Makati K, et al. Predictors of early mortality in patients age 80 and older receiving implantable defibrillators. Pacing Clin Electrophysiol. 2010;33(8):981–7. doi:10.1111/j.1540-8159.2010.02729.x.
32. Krahn AD, Connolly SJ, Roberts RS, Gent M. Diminishing proportional risk of sudden death with advancing age: implications for prevention of sudden death. Am Heart J. 2004;147(5):837–40. doi:10.1016/j.ahj.2003.12.017.
33. Healey JS, Hallstrom AP, Kuck K-H, et al. Role of the implantable defibrillator among elderly patients with a history of life-threatening ventricular arrhythmias. Eur Heart J. 2007;28 (14):1746–9. doi:10.1093/eurheartj/ehl438.
34. Yung D, Birnie D, Dorian P, et al. Survival after implantable cardioverter-defibrillator implantation in the elderly. Circulation. 2013;127(24):2383–92. doi:10.1161/CIRCULATIONAHA.113.001442.
35. António N, Elvas L, Gonçalves L, Providência L. a. Cardiac resynchronization therapy in the elderly: a realistic option for an increasing population? Int J Cardiol. 2012;155(1):49–51. doi:10.1016/j.ijcard.2011.01.079.
36. Kron J, Aranda JM, Miles WM, et al. Benefit of cardiac resynchronization in elderly patients: results from the Multicenter InSync Randomized Clinical Evaluation (MIRACLE) and Multicenter InSync ICD Randomized Clinical Evaluation (MIRACLE-ICD) trials. J Interv Card Electrophysiol. 2009;25(2):91–6. doi:10.1007/s10840-008-9330-2.
37. Penn J, Goldenberg I, Moss AJ, et al. Improved outcome with preventive cardiac resynchronization therapy in the elderly: a MADIT-CRT substudy. J Cardiovasc Electrophysiol. 2011;22(8):892–7. doi:10.1111/j.1540-8167.2011.02011.x.
38. Adelstein EC, Gorcsan J, Jain S, Saba S. Cardiac resynchronization therapy benefits patients eighty years of age or older. J Am Coll Cardiol. 2012;59(13):E869. doi:10.1016/S0735-1097 (12)60870-5.

Chapter 26
Cost-Benefit of TAVR: Should Indications Be Expanded?

Alec Vahanian, Dominique Himbert, and Bernard Iung

Abstract The current recommendations state that transcatheter aortic valve replacement (TAVR) is indicated in inoperable patients and should be considered in high-risk patients with severe aortic stenosis. Both sets of recommendations concur to state that TAVR should not be performed in patients at intermediate risk for surgery.

The main ways of expanding the indications of TAVR are as follows:

A better implementation of the Guidelines will lead to the referral of all patients with severe AS and symptoms to heart teams for further management in order to decrease the still present under-treatment of these high-risk patients. An extended Heart Team will help to avoid performing TAVR in patients where it is more futile than utile.

In the future the indications for TAVR will no doubt increase towards lower risk patients given the improvement in risk stratification, careful evaluation of the results and refinement in technology.

We also need better evidence before using TAVR in subgroups which are currently under-represented or even not represented in large trials such as bicuspid or regurgitant valve disease or patients with bioprosthetic valve failure.

Finally, the logistical and economic problems resulting from an increase in the number of TAVR procedures performed should be addressed. Then, it is likely that TAVR will become the preferred way of treating patients with aortic stenosis but it will always remain complementary to surgery and this, in the end, will allow more patients to be treated.

Keywords Aortic stenosis • Transcatheter aortic valve replacement • Valvular heart disease • Valve prostheses

A. Vahanian, MD, FESC, FRCP (Edin.) (✉) • B. Iung, MD
Department of Cardiology, Bichat Hospital, Paris, France
e-mail: alec.vahanian@bch.aphp.fr

D. Himbert, MD
Department of Cardiology, Bichat-Claude Bernard Hospital, Paris, France

© Springer International Publishing Switzerland 2015
J.A. Ambrose, A.E. Rodríguez (eds.), *Controversies in Cardiology*,
DOI 10.1007/978-3-319-20415-4_26

Introduction

Transcatheter aortic valve replacement (TAVR) was introduced 12 years ago for the treatment of severe aortic stenosis (AS) [1] and is now extensively used worldwide. The efficacy and safety of the technique has been proven in multiple registries as well as randomised trials comparing TAVR with optimal medical management in inoperable patients and with surgical aortic valve replacement (SAVR) in high-risk patients [2–11]. As a result the technique now has clear recommendations in both the 2012 European Society of Cardiology/ the European Association for Cardiothoracic Surgery guidelines in Europe [12] and the 2014 American College of Cardiology/American Heart Association guidelines [13]. Both documents are concordant in stating that TAVR is indicated in patients with severe symptomatic AS who are inoperable and who are likely to gain improvement in their quality of life and have life expectancy of more than 1 year. TAVR should be considered in high-risk patients with severe symptomatic AS who may be suitable for surgery but in whom TAVR is favoured by a Heart Team based on the individual risk profile and anatomic suitability.

In this chapter we shall review the main ways of expanding the indications of TAVR, including to other risk groups, after critically discussing the difficulties of risk stratification, specific patient sub-groups, and finally examining the potential organisational consequences of such an expansion of indications.

Other Risk Groups

The Challenge of Risk Stratification in TAVR

Before considering the possible extension of TAVR indications it is necessary to discuss the issue of risk stratification in patients for TAVR.

The first step in risk stratification is to evaluate the risk of SAVR in the given patient. This was originally based on the use of surgical risk scores such as the EuroScore or STS PROM. However, these scores have been shown to be sub-optimal for stratification of the risk of surgery in these high-risk patients. There are several reasons for this: firstly these scores were elaborated mostly from patients undergoing coronary bypass surgery – the patients in the development cohort were mostly at low or intermediate risk which is not the case for TAVR candidates. Overall, these scores were shown to over-predict surgical mortality in TAVR candidates [14]. Secondly, these scores don't take into account many other factors which make surgery very high-risk or even contraindicated such as anatomical factors: hostile chest, presence of coronary bypass grafts crossing the midline, the porcelain aorta, and finally frailty [15] which is a strong predictor of outcome in this elderly population.

Besides the evaluation of the risk of the surgical alternative the second step is to evaluate the risk of TAVR. There have been very few attempts to develop and validate a risk score for TAVR. The first one was performed from the FRANCE 2 registry with the aim of predicting 30-day mortality. The score was developed from 9 variables, mostly pre-procedural and 1 procedural variable. It showed good prediction but only moderate discrimination [16]. This may be due to an insufficient number of patients, the lack of inclusion of parameters such as frailty, the absence of inclusion of peri and post-procedural complications which play an important role in immediate mortality and the fact that this population is extremely heterogeneous and it may be that one score would not be able to capture all of them. Another interesting attempt was carried out from the PARTNER trial where a risk score included both mortality and quality of life at 6 months. Once again the calibration was good but the discrimination was only moderate [17]. Although discrimination was only moderate with both scores, they may help guide treatment choice and advise physicians and patients about the expectation of outcomes based on their presenting characteristics.

Expanding the Indications to All High-Risk Patients

The Euro heart survey, as well as other studies in the early 2000's, has shown that high risk patients with severe AS were undertreated [18]. Following the emergence of TAVR, the referral of high-risk patients with severe symptomatic AS increased whether they were referred to TAVR or SAVR [19]. This is encouraging, however, a recent prospective registry from Spain showed that as many as 47 % of patients over 80 years of age with severe symptomatic aortic stenosis do not receive any intervention suggesting the need to reinforce the implementation of the guidelines in this population subset [20].

All data sets including mid-term/long-term outcomes after TAVR showed an attrition of survival [3, 4, 6, 7, 21–23] due in large part to non-cardiac deaths related to co-morbidities. Thus it seems reasonable to avoid performing TAVR in patients in whom it would be more "futile than utile", that's to say in those who are unlikely to gain improvement in their quality of life and have a "too short" life expectancy mostly due to their non-cardiac comorbidities [24]. In this respect, recent studies provided useful insight in identifying patients who have very poor outcomes after TAVR and should probably not be considered as candidates for this technique such as those who are not ambulatory or oxygen-dependant [25], as well as patients on dialysis who also had atrial fibrillation, [26]. To better select the most appropriate therapy in these patients, risk stratification should be performed, when necessary, by a Heart Team including cardiologists, cardiac surgeons and anaesthesiologists, but also other specialists such as geriatricians and specialists such as pulmonologists, nephrologists, neurologists and oncologists, in order to make the most appropriate decision.

Besides non-cardiac comorbidities, a too advanced cardiac stage could be a contraindication for TAVR. As an illustration, the indication for TAVR in patients with very low ejection fraction ($\leq$20 %) is challenging. These patients were excluded from the existing randomised trials and evidence is very limited. The first question to ask is whether aortic stenosis is severe. This requires careful echocardiographic examination taking into account an integrative evaluation of the severity of the valve stenosis [27] as well as an evaluation of myocardial viability. Dobutamine testing [28] and quantitative evaluation of calcification by MSCT [29] are also useful for identifying "true aortic stenosis". The clinical context is also helpful and recovery of LV function is likely if the decrease in ejection fraction is recent while it is very unlikely if myocardial dysfunction is due to a large scar after extended myocardial infarction. In these patients balloon aortic valvuloplasty may be of interest. TAVR can be performed after a couple of weeks in case of improvement in left ventricular function [30].

Expanding Indications to Lower Risk Patients

Both sets of guidelines [12, 13] clearly state that TAVR should not be performed in patients at intermediate risk for surgery. However, the favourable results of TAVR in terms of survival, quality of life and functional status have already led to a shift in the indications towards lower risk patients in clinical practice as shown in Table 26.1.

Table 26.1 Evolution of risk scores in patients treated by transcatheter aortic valve replacement

	STS PROM (%)
PARTNER A [3]	11.8
PARTNER B [4]	11.2
PARTNER TF continuous access	10.5
Corevalve extreme risk [9]	10.3
Corevalve extreme risk continuous access	9
Corevalve high risk [5]	7.3
TVT inoperable [10]	7
CHOICE trial	6
TVT high risk [10]	5

	Logistic Euro Score (%)
FRANCE 2 [7]	
2009	25
2011	21.9
SOURCE [22]	
2007–2009	25.8
2010–2011	20.5
ADVANCE [11] (2010–11)	19.2

The shift towards performing TAVR in lower risk patients is due to the indication posed by the physician but also to the strong demand from patients to avoid surgery. It should be stressed that a classification as "low-risk" according to the score thresholds does not always parallel the evaluation of the risk by the Heart Team. As an example almost half of the patients classified as low-risk (STS <3 %) in the study by Wenawasser were in fact judged to be either inoperable or at high risk by the Heart Team due to the presence of comorbidities which were not caught in the STS calculation [31].

Before considering the expansion of indications to lower risk patients we should consider what the evidence is if the risk should decrease, and the durability of the prosthetic valves should be proven.

What Is the Evidence?

Several recent observational registries have suggested that patients with low risk scores had good clinical outcome after TAVR. Going one step further, three studies used propensity score analysis to match pairs of TAVR and SAVR patients with STS scores between 3 and 8 % [32–34], (Table 26.2) and showed similar mortality at 30 days and 1 year. However, even a careful propensity score adjustment analysis can only compensate partially for the imbalance in characteristics between groups and the only way to perform an accurate comparison is randomised studies between SAVR and TAVR in patients at intermediate risk. Acknowledging all the limitations previously described in the definition of this group, several trials have been designed to provide such an evidence-based comparison in intermediate risk patients: PARTNER 2a cohort A in the USA, which has completed enrolment; SURTAVI, the UK TAVI trial and finally the Nordic aortic valve intervention trial, which are still enrolling patients in Europe.

The Risk of TAVR Should Decrease

Tables 26.3 and 26.4 show the current clinical outcomes at 30 days in recent registries. The most recent trials and registries show a decrease in mortality form 15–20 % to 5–7 % [5, 7–11]. This is in large part due to a decrease in complications

Table 26.2 Comparison of SAVR and TAVR in intermediate risk patients

	Piazza et al. [32]		OBSERVANT [33]		Latib et al. [34]	
	TAVI (n=255)	SAVR (n=255)	TAVI (n=133)	SAVR (n=133)	TAVI (n=111)	SAVR (n=111)
STS (%, mean)	3–8	3–8	NA	NA	4.6	4.6
Log EuroSCORE (%, mean)	17.3	17.6	8.9	9.4	23.2	24.4
30 day mortality (%)	7.8	7.1	3.8	3.8	1.8	1.8

Table 26.3 Early mortality of TAVR

	STS/ACC TVT Registry [10]			PARTNER trial			France 2	SOURCE [2]		UK SATIRE [6]
	Inoperable	High-risk		Inoperable [3]	High risk [4]					
	TF	TF	TA	TF	TF	TA		TF	TA	
30-day mortality (%)	6.1	4.6	9.8	5.0	3.7	8.7	9.2	6.3	10.3	7.1

TA transapical approach, *TF* transfemoral approach

with improved case selection, device and procedural refinements and increased operator experience [35]. Rare but dramatic complications such as annular rupture or coronary occlusion may occur during the procedure in less than 0.5 %. The incidence of such complications will decrease if not disappear due to very careful pre-procedural screening and their consequences could be limited by an efficient surgical back-up [36, 37]. Paravalvular leaks remain a concern and a comprehensive multiparametric evaluation is key during the procedure. Moderate to severe paravalvular leak carries a poor prognosis while the prognostic impact of mild paravalvular leak is still debated [38]. In the future paravalvular leaks will decrease due to better sizing using 3D imaging and new valve technology. In this respect the results obtained by the new devices are very promising with moderate to severe paravalvular leaks occurring in less than 5 % [39, 40]. Strokes remain an issue. TAVR-associated strokes are multifactorial in origin. Over time it seems that stroke frequency after TAVR has been declining. A recent randomised comparison, including a neurologic assessment, showed that the incidence of major stroke after TAVR is not higher than that of surgery [5]. In the future the incidence of stroke is likely to decrease due to the use of protection devices for which there are promising signs of efficacy, and better pharmacology and prevention of arteriosclerosis. Major vascular complications and bleeds still occur in around 10 % of cases [41]. The reduction of sheath size, which is now down to 14 French, and refinement of the percutaneous suture device technique will improve these figures. Careful patient selection using an integrative approach, including MSCT and angiography, and heart team discussion as regards the use of an alternative approach, will no doubt further decrease these complications. The need for a permanent pacemaker varies considerably and is significantly higher with a self-expandable prosthesis than with a balloon-expandable prosthesis. The negative influence on outcome is still debated in the elderly population currently treated [42] but could be significant when dealing with younger patients. The incidence of renal failure is also an important predictor of poor outcome and should decrease by lowering the use of contrast media and better patient selection.

Overall, the incidence of TAVR-related complications is most likely to further decrease over time thanks to better patient selection and also better management by the Heart Team as well as the availability of more refined devices.

Table 26.4 Clinical outcome at 30 days in recent registries

	ADVANCE [11] transfemoral N = 1015	SOURCE[a] transfemoral N = 1694
All-cause mortality (%)	4.5	4.2
Any stroke (%)	3	3.4
Aortic regurgitation; moderate to severe (%)	15.7	5.8
Myocardial infarction (%)	0.2	0.5
New pacemaker (%)	26.3	8.7
Major bleeding (%)	9.7	7.7
Major vascular complication (%)	10.9	7.9
Renal failure with temporary dialysis (%)	0.4	1.2

[a]Schymick: submitted

What Is the Durability of TAVR?

Durability is a very important issue. It is important to know when and how the prosthetic valves are going to fail. TAVR prostheses and surgical bioprostheses have similar features and the same major causes of failure are expected: calcification and tears in the valve cusp resulting in regurgitation or stenosis. However, transcatheter heart valves are prepared and placed into a delivery system and long-term effect on the longevity of valve leaflet is unknown and may only become apparent on long-term follow-up. TAVR is a relatively new therapy and long-term data over 5–6 years are scarce [21]. However, the studies currently available don't show an alarming incidence of structural degeneration, leaflet thickening, calcification, thrombus formation, or endocarditis over time [43]. A larger number of patients together with longer follow-up is needed for an accurate assessment of durability. It will be difficult to extrapolate data obtained in the current patient population, that's to say elderly patients (over 80 years old), to younger patients where the deterioration of bioprostheses occurs earlier. In the event of accelerated valve failure low-risk patients would remain candidates for surgery or valve-in-a-valve TAVR could be an option. The positive results obtained so far with valve-in-valve in failing bioprostheses are encouraging but the experience in valve-in-valve after TAVR is very limited.

Finally, the specific problem of the feasibility of subsequent percutaneous coronary intervention in patients who have a TAVR prosthesis in place could be an issue and data are very limited.

Specific Groups

Bicuspid Valves

Bicuspid valves are the most common congenital cardiac abnormality. They will be observed more and more as the indication shifts towards lower risk patients of younger age, [44]. TAVR experience in patients with bicuspid valves is still limited

[45] and shows that the technique is feasible with satisfactory short-term results. However, there is a higher incidence of paravalvular regurgitation which deserves attention. Further studies are clearly needed to identify which patients can be safely treated by TAVR. Currently, the indications should be proposed on a case-by-case basis. TAVR may be proposed if there is a strong clinical incentive in patients who do not have too large an annulus or very asymmetric calcification and, above all, in the absence of independent aortopathy which requires, per se, surgery.

Native Aortic Valve Regurgitation

Severe aortic regurgitation is still considered a contraindication due to the risk of embolization and of residual aortic regurgitation. The results available so far are very limited and suggest that the procedure is feasible. However, the incidence of moderate to severe aortic regurgitation seems to be high and a second valve is frequently needed [46]. The results are likely to be improved with second generation TAVR devices [47]. Indications are likely to be limited in industrialised countries where aortic regurgitation is mostly of degenerative origin and where dilatation/aneurysm of the ascending aorta requires treatment.

TAVR in Degenerated Bioprostheses

The data on TAVR in degenerated bioprostheses are encouraging even if they are only observational (Fig. 26.1). They suggest that the procedure is feasible with a high success rate and that it leads to haemodynamic and clinical improvement. The

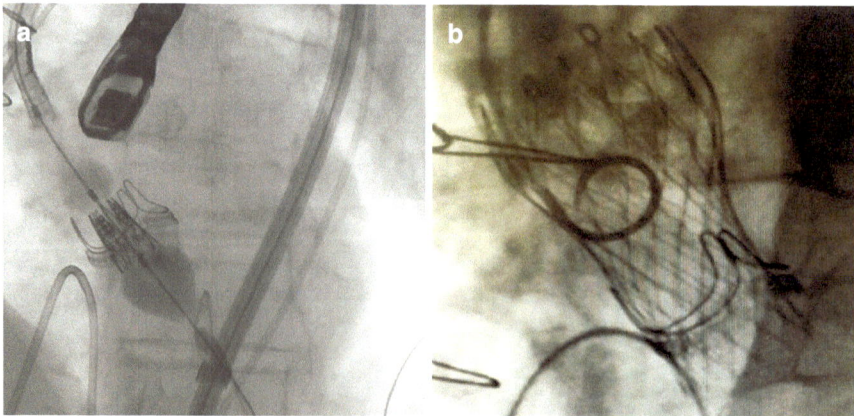

Fig. 26.1 Transcatheter valve implantation in surgically implanted failed bioprosthesis. (**a**) Deployment of a balloon-expandable prosthesis. (**b**) Self-expandable prosthesis after deployment

risk of coronary occlusion and sub-optimal haemodynamic results with a small valve size remains a concern and should be addressed by very careful patient selection by the heart team [48]. A limitation in the number of possible valve-in-valve procedures could occur due to valve size.

In the future, the results should be confirmed by larger series and longer follow-up. Expanded valve sizes are needed and probably specific valve designs. If medium and long-term outcomes remain favourable, the TAVR valve-in-valve option may have important clinical implications as a treatment strategy in patients requiring valvular intervention further increasing the percentage of bioprostheses used for SAVR.

Potential Organisational Consequences of an Expansion of Indications

Cost-Effectiveness and Reimbursement

Recent studies using different modelling approaches concur that TAVR is a cost-effective intervention in patients ineligible for SAVR and is likely to be cost-effective for high-risk patients at least when a transfemoral approach is performed [49–52]. However, uncertainty persists due to the lack of long-term evaluation which could have a substantial impact on estimates of cost-effectiveness. In Europe TAVR use is largely influenced by the proportion of the nation's global product spent on healthcare and the net healthcare expenditure per capita [53]. The largest part of the cost is due to the cost of the device [54] which hopefully is likely to decrease with the introduction of new devices.

Logistics

The expected expansion of the number of TAVR procedures performed will require, besides the economic problems quoted above, the resolution of a number of logistical problems.

It seems undesirable to expand the performance of TAVR to centres without cardiac surgery. The presence of cardiac surgery on-site is the guarantee of having a Heart Team with experience in the management of patients with aortic stenosis and in particular high-risk patients. Such a setting optimises patient selection, performance of the procedure, management of potential complications and post-interventional care. The reorientation of a large number of patients from SAVR to TAVR should be considered in terms of the number of catheterisation laboratories available and the type of catheterisation laboratory [55].

The procedure will become simpler. The use of general anaesthesia will be limited to some approaches specifically surgical approaches and won't be needed in the majority of cases where transfemoral approach will be the default approach. The comparisons between general and local anaesthesia in the field of TAVR are limited but suggest that the results are comparable with a trend towards shorter hospital stays [56]. In experienced centres the simplified or so-called "minimalist" approach to TAVR has proven to be as safe and effective as the more standard traditionalist approach [57]. This should not be interpreted as a dismantling of the Heart Team but a collective move towards a more efficient utilisation of resources. This "minimalist" approach will result in lower procedure-related costs and shorter hospital stays [58].

More physicians should be trained for TAVR. Here again the Heart Team concept remains essential. TAVR will be carried out by dedicated physicians, cardiologists and/or cardiac surgeons, the arrangement in a given institution depending on the local heart team.

Conclusions

The current recommendations on both sides of the ocean are consistent and state that (1) TAVR is indicated in inoperable patients and should be considered in high-risk patients. (2) TAVR should not be performed in patients at intermediate risk for surgery. In patient selection, as well as performance of the procedure, the importance of the Heart Team should be stressed.

A better implementation of the Guidelines will hopefully lead to the referral of all patients with severe AS and symptoms to heart teams for further management in order to decrease the still present under-treatment of these high-risk patients. An extended Heart Team will help to avoid performing TAVR in patients where it is more futile than utile. In the future the indications for TAVR will no doubt increase towards lower risk patients given the improvement in risk stratification, careful evaluation of the results and refinement in technology.

Globally, TAVR will become the preferred way of treating patients with AS but it will always remain complementary to SAVR and this, in the end, will allow more patients with AS to be treated.

References

1. Cribier A, Eltchaninoff H, Bash A, et al. Percutaneous transcatheter implantation of an aortic valve prosthesis for calcific aortic stenosis: first human case description. Circulation. 2002;106:3006–8.
2. Leon MB, Smith CR, Mack M, et al.; PARTNER Trial Investigators. Transcatheter aortic valve implantation for aortic stenosis in patients who cannot undergo surgery. N Engl J Med. 2010;363:1597–607.
3. Kodali SK, Williams MR, Smith CR, et al.; PARTNER Trial Investigators. Two-year outcomes after transcatheter or surgical aortic valve replacement. N Engl J Med. 2012;366:1686–95.
4. Makkar RR, Fontana GP, Jilaihawi H, et al.; PARTNER Trial Investigators. Transcatheter aortic valve replacement for inoperable severe aortic stenosis. N Engl J Med. 2012;366:1696–704.

5. Adams DH, Popma JJ, Reardon MJ, et al. Transcatheter aortic-valve replacement with a self-expanding prosthesis. N Engl J Med. 2014;370:1790–8.
6. Moat NE, Ludman P, de Belder MA, et al. Long-term outcomes after transcatheter aortic valve implantation in high-risk patients with severe aortic stenosis: the UK TAVI (United Kingdom Transcatheter Aortic Valve Implantation) Registry. J Am Coll Cardiol. 2011;58:2130–8.
7. Gilard M, Eltchaninoff H, Iung B, et al.; FRANCE 2 Investigators. Registry of transcatheter aortic valve implantation in high-risk patients. N Engl J Med. 2012;366:1705–15.
8. Hamm CW, Möllmann H, Holzhey D, et al. The German aortic valve registry (GARY): in-hospital outcome. Eur Heart J. 2014;35:1588–98.
9. Popma JJ, Adams DH, Reardon MJ, et al. Transcatheter aortic valve replacement using a self-expandable bioprosthesis in patients with severe aortic stenosis at extreme risk for surgery. J Am Coll Cardiol. 2014;63:1972–81.
10. Mack MJ, Brennan J, Brindis R, et al. Outcomes following transcatheter aortic valve replacement in the United States. JAMA. 2013;310:2069–77.
11. Linke A, Wenaweser P, Gerckens U, et al. Treatment of aortic stenosis with a self-expanding transcatheter valve: the International Multi-centre ADVANCE Study. Eur Heart J. 2014;35:2672–84.
12. Vahanian A, Alfieri O, Andreotti F, et al. Guidelines on the management of valvular heart disease (version 2012). Eur Heart J. 2012;33:2451–96.
13. Nishimura RA, Otto CM, Bonow RO, et al. 2014 AHA/ACC guideline for the management of patients with valvular heart disease: a report of the American College of Cardiology/American Heart Association Task Force on Practice Guidelines. J Am Coll Cardiol. 2014;63:e57–185.
14. Osnabrugge RL, Speir AM, Head SJ, et al. Performance of EuroSCORE II in a large US database: implications for transcatheter aortic valve implantation. Eur J Cardiothorac Surg. 2014;46:400–8.
15. Afilalo J, Eisenberg MJ, Morin JF, et al. Gait speed as an incremental predictor of mortality and major morbidity in elderly patients undergoing cardiac surgery. J Am Coll Cardiol. 2010;56:1668–76.
16. Iung B, Laouénan C, Himbert D, et al. Predictive factors of early mortality after transcatheter aortic valve implantation: individual risk assessment using a simple score. Heart. 2014;100:1016–23.
17. Arnold SV, Reynolds MR, Lei Y, et al. Predictors of poor outcomes after transcatheter aortic valve replacement: results from the PARTNER (Placement of Aortic Transcatheter Valve) trial. Circulation. 2014;129:2682–90.
18. Iung B, Baron G, Butchart EG, et al. A prospective survey of patients with valvular heart disease in Europe: The Euro Heart Survey on Valvular Heart Disease. Eur Heart J. 2003;24:1231–43.
19. Malaisrie SC, Tuday E, Lapin B, et al. Transcatheter aortic valve implantation decreases the rate of unoperated aortic stenosis. Eur J Cardiothorac Surg. 2011;40:43–8.
20. Martinez-Selles M, Gomez Doblas JJ, Carro Hevia A, et al. Prospective registry of symptomatic severe aortic stenosis in octogenarians: a need for intervention. J Intern Med. 2014;275:608–20.
21. Toggweiler S, Humphries KH, Lee M, et al. Long-term outcomes after transcatheter aortic valve implantation: insights on prognostic factors and valve durability from the Canadian multicenter experience. J Am Coll Cardiol. 2012;60(19):1864–75.
22. Thomas M, Schymik G, Walther T, et al. One-year outcomes of cohort 1 in the Edwards SAPIEN Aortic Bioprosthesis European Outcome (SOURCE) registry: the European registry of transcatheter aortic valve implantation using the Edwards SAPIEN valve. Circulation. 2011;124:425–33.
23. Rodés-Cabau J, Webb JG, Cheung A, et al. Long-term outcomes after transcatheter aortic valve implantation: insights on prognostic factors and valve durability from the Canadian multicenter experience. J Am Coll Cardiol. 2012;60:1864–75.
24. Makkar RR, Jilaihawi H, Mack M, et al. Stratification of outcomes after transcatheter aortic valve replacement according to surgical inoperability for technical versus clinical reasons. J Am Coll Cardiol. 2014;63:901–11.

25. Dvir D, Waksman R, Barbash IM, et al. Outcomes of patients with chronic lung disease and severe aortic stenosis treated with transcatheter versus surgical aortic valve replacement or standard therapy: insights from the PARTNER trial (Placement of AoRTic TraNscathetER Valve). J Am Coll Cardiol. 2014;63:269–79.
26. Allende R, Webb JG, Munoz-Garcia AJ, et al. Advanced chronic kidney disease in patients undergoing transcatheter aortic valve implantation: insights on clinical outcomes and prognostic markers from a large cohort of patients. Eur Heart J. 2014;35:2685–96.
27. Clavel MA, Pibarot P. Assessment of low-flow, low-gradient aortic stenosis: multimodality imaging is the key to success. EuroIntervention. 2014;10:U52–60.
28. Monin JL, Quere JP, Monchi M, et al. Low-gradient aortic stenosis: operative risk stratification and predictors for long-term outcome: a multicenter study using dobutamine stress hemodynamics. Circulation. 2003;108:319–24.
29. Clavel MA, Messika-Zeitoun D, Pibarot P, et al. The complex nature of discordant severe calcified aortic valve disease grading: new insights from combined Doppler echocardiographic and computed tomographic study. J Am Coll Cardiol. 2013;62:2329–38.
30. Tissot CM, Attias D, Himbert D, et al. Reappraisal of percutaneous aortic balloon valvuloplasty as a preliminary treatment strategy in the transcatheter aortic valve implantation era. EuroIntervention. 2011;7:49–56.
31. Wenaweser P, Stortecky S, Schwander S, et al. Clinical outcomes of patients with estimated low or intermediate surgical risk undergoing transcatheter aortic valve implantation. Eur Heart J. 2013;34:1894–905.
32. Piazza N, Kalesan B, van Mieghem N, et al. A 3-center comparison of 1-year mortality outcomes between transcatheter aortic valve implantation and surgical aortic valve replacement on the basis of propensity score matching among intermediate-risk surgical patients. JACC Cardiovasc Interv. 2013;6:443–51.
33. D'Errigo P, Barbanti M, Ranucci M, et al.; OBSERVANT Research Group. Transcatheter aortic valve implantation versus surgical aortic valve replacement for severe aortic stenosis: results from an intermediate risk propensity-matched population of the Italian OBSERVANT study. Int J Cardiol. 2013;167:1945–52.
34. Latib A, Maisano F, Bertoldi L, et al. Transcatheter vs surgical aortic valve replacement in intermediate-surgical-risk patients with aortic stenosis: a propensity score-matched case–control study. Am Heart J. 2012;164:910–7.
35. Van Mieghem NM, Chieffo A, Dumonteil N, et al. Trends in outcome after transfemoral transcatheter aortic valve implantation. Am Heart J. 2013;165:183–92.
36. Barbanti M, Yang TH, Rodès Cabau J, et al. Anatomical and procedural features associated with aortic root rupture during balloon-expandable transcatheter aortic valve replacement. Circulation. 2013;128:244–53.
37. Ribeiro HB, Webb JG, Makkar RR, et al. Predictive factors, management, and clinical outcomes of coronary obstruction following transcatheter aortic valve implantation: insights from a large multicenter registry. J Am Coll Cardiol. 2013;62:1552–62.
38. Kodali S, Pibarot P, Douglas PS, et al. Paravalvular regurgitation after transcatheter aortic valve replacement with the Edwards sapien valve in the PARTNER trial: characterizing patients and impact on outcomes. Eur Heart J. 2015;36:449–56. pii: ehu384.
39. Binder RK, Rodés-Cabau J, Wood DA, et al. Transcatheter aortic valve replacement with the SAPIEN 3: a new balloon-expandable transcatheter heart valve. JACC Cardiovasc Interv. 2013;6:293–300. 41.
40. Meredith IT, Walters DL, Dumonteil N, et al. Transcatheter aortic valve replacement for severe symptomatic aortic stenosis using a repositionable valve system: 30-day primary endpoint results from the REPRISE II study. J Am Coll Cardiol. 2014;64:1339–48.
41. Genereux P, Webb JG, Svensson LG, et al. Vascular complications after transcatheter aortic valve replacements: insights from the PARTNER (Placement of AoRTic TraNscathetER Valve) trial. J Am Coll Cardiol. 2012;60:1043–52.

42. Biner S, Michowitz Y, Leshem-Rubinow E, et al. Hemodynamic impact and outcome of permanent pacemaker implantation following transcatheter aortic valve implantation. Am J Cardiol. 2014;113:132–7.
43. Mylotte D, Andalib A, Thériault-Lauzier P, et al. Transcatheter heart valve failure: a systematic review. Eur Heart J. 2015;36:1306–27. pii: ehu388.
44. Roberts WC, Ko JM. Frequency by decades of unicuspid, bicuspid, and tricuspid aortic valves in adults having isolated aortic valve replacement for aortic stenosis, with or without associated aortic regurgitation. Circulation. 2005;111:920–5.
45. O'Sullivan CJ, Windecker S. Implications of bicuspid aortic valves for transcatheter aortic valve implantation. Circ Cardiovasc Interv. 2013;6:204–6.
46. Roy DA, Schaefer U, Guetta V, et al. Transcatheter aortic valve implantation for pure severe native aortic valve regurgitation. J Am Coll Cardiol. 2013;61:1577–84.
47. Seiffert M, Diemert P, Koschyk D, et al. Transapical implantation of a second-generation transcatheter heart valve in patients with noncalcified aortic regurgitation. JACC Cardiovasc Interv. 2013;6:590–7.
48. Dvir D, Webb JG, Bleiziffer S, et al. Transcatheter aortic valve implantation in failed bioprosthetic surgical valves. JAMA. 2014;312:162–70.
49. Osnabrugge RL, Kappetein AP, Reynolds MR, Cohen DJ. Cost-effectiveness of transcatheter valvular interventions: economic challenges. EuroIntervention. 2013;9(Suppl):S48–54.
50. Reynolds MR, Magnuson EA, Lei Y, et al.; PARTNER Investigators. Cost-effectiveness of transcatheter aortic valve replacement compared with surgical aortic valve replacement in high-risk patients with severe aortic stenosis: results of the PARTNER (Placement of Aortic Transcatheter Valves) trial (Cohort A). J Am Coll Cardiol. 2012;60:2683–92.
51. Fairbairn TA, Meads DM, Hulme C, et al. The cost-effectiveness of transcatheter aortic valve implantation versus surgical aortic valve replacement in patients with severe aortic stenosis at high operative risk. Heart. 2013;99:914–20.
52. Eaton J, Mealing S, Thompson J, et al. Is transcatheter aortic valve implantation (TAVI) a cost-effective treatment in patients who are ineligible for surgical aortic valve replacement? A systematic review of economic evaluations. J Med Econ. 2014;17:365–75.
53. Mylotte D, Osnabrugge RLJ, Windecker S, et al. Transcatheter aortic valve replacement in Europe: adoption trends and factors influencing device utilization. J Am Coll Cardiol. 2013;62:210–9.
54. Osnabrugge RL, Head SJ, Genders TS, et al. Costs of transcatheter versus surgical aortic valve replacement in intermediate-risk patients. Ann Thorac Surg. 2012;94:1954–60.
55. Holmes Jr DR, Mack MJ, Kaul S, et al. 2012 ACCF/AATS/SCAI/STS expert consensus document on transcatheter aortic valve replacement. J Am Coll Cardiol. 2012;59:1200–54.
56. Durand E, Borz B, Godin M, et al. Transfemoral aortic valve replacement with the Edwards SAPIEN and Edwards SAPIEN XT prosthesis using exclusively local anesthesia and fluoroscopic guidance: feasibility and 30-day outcomes. JACC Cardiovasc Interv. 2012;5:461–7.
57. Wood DA, Poulter RS, Cook R, et al. A multidisciplinary, multimodality, but minimalist (3M) approach to transfemoral transcatheter aortic valve replacement facilitates safe next day discharge in high-risk patients. J Am Coll Cardiol. 2013;62:B38–9.
58. Meduri C, Potter B, Osnabrugge RL, et al. Reducing the cost of TAVR: an evaluation of the impact of length of stay on the cost of transcatheter aortic valve replacement. J Am Coll Cardiol. 2014;63(12_S).

Chapter 27
Editorial Comments on the Chapters

John A. Ambrose and Alfredo E. Rodríguez

Abstract In reviewing the chapters, we realize that no chapter can be completely up to date given the time delay to publication. As cardiology continues to evolve and new therapies/procedures/techniques are developed, new studies often in the form of randomized trials may provide insight into some of the unresolved issues contained in the book. Furthermore, there might be, in a few cases, information that the editors believe relevant to the reader that may have been omitted. This chapter reviews new or pertinent studies in CT angiography, EECP, dual antiplatelet therapy, thrombectomy prior to STEMI, 2nd generation drug-eluting stents in multivessel disease, radial vs femoral access and contrast-induced nephropathy.

Keywords CT angiography • Thrombectomy • Contrast-induced nephropathy • Radial access • Dual antiplatelet therapy • 2nd generation drug-eluting stents

The editors are extremely grateful to all the authors who contributed to the book for their excellent discussions in their assigned chapters. In reviewing the chapters, we realize that no chapter can be completely up to date given the time delay to publication. As cardiology continues to evolve and more data become available, new studies often in the form of randomized trials may provide insight into some of the unresolved issues contained in the book. Furthermore, there might be, in a

J.A. Ambrose, MD (✉)
Chief of Cardiology, UCSF Fresno, Fresno, CA, USA

Department of Medicine, UCSF Community Regional Medical Center, Fresno, CA, USA
e-mail: jamambrose@yahoo.com

A.E. Rodríguez, MD, PhD, FACC, FSCAI (✉)
Cardiac Unit, Department of Interventional Cardiology, Revista Argentina de Cardioagiologia Intervencionista (RACI), Otamendi Hospital, Buenos Aires, Argentina

Interventional Cardiology Unit, Department of Interventional Cardiology, Otamendi Hospital, Buenos Aires, Argentina

Otamendi Hospital, Post Graduate Buenos Aires School of Medicine, Buenos Aires, Argentina

Director, Cardiovascular Research Center (CECI), Buenos Aires, Argentina

© Springer International Publishing Switzerland 2015
J.A. Ambrose, A.E. Rodríguez (eds.), *Controversies in Cardiology*,
DOI 10.1007/978-3-319-20415-4_27

few cases, information that the editors believe relevant to the reader that may have been omitted. The following are several editor-related comments that we think are relevant:

1. CT angiography versus functional testing for a diagnosis of coronary disease.

    While Chap. 7 considered CT angiography to facilitate ER discharge in patients with chest discomfort, a recent paper compared CT to functional testing in stable out patients with chest pain. Douglas et al. randomized 10,003 symptomatic patients with suspected CAD (pretest probability >50 %) to CT versus functional testing (stress test±echocardiography or nuclear stress test) [1]. Clinical outcomes over a 2 year follow up including death from any cause, myocardial infarction or hospitalization for unstable angina were not improved with CT angiography compared to functional testing.

2. Practically speaking, how should the clinician manage a patient with refractory angina as discussed in Chap. 11 who is not a candidate for any type of intervention? In addition to prescribing the maximum tolerated doses of anti-anginal medications including ranolazine and long acting nitrates, we believe that enhanced external counter pulsation (EECP) should be considered in appropriate patients. In a patient with refractory angina who is otherwise a candidate for this therapy, it can reduce anginal episodes and improve quality of life.

3. In the management of intracoronary thrombus in the cath lab, the final "nail in the coffin" for routine manual thrombectomy during primary PCI for STEMI was recently published by Jolly et al. [2]. In that trial, 10,732 patients were randomized to upfront manual thrombectomy versus no thrombectomy during primary PCI. More than 90 % had definite thrombus present in the culprit vessel. The primary endpoint was a composite of CV death, recurrent MI, cardiogenic shock or Class IV heart failure at 180 days. The rates were 6.9 vs 7.0 % respectively between thrombectomy and no thrombectomy groups. Stroke at 30 days was surprisingly higher with thrombectomy, 0.7 % vs 0.3 % with PCI alone, p=0.02.

    There is another method for dealing with large thrombus burdens during PCI that occasionally can be very helpful. It is never a good idea to stent or even balloon when the thrombus burden is very large. In certain situations where there is antegrade flow in the culprit vessel but either the wire or thrombectomy device cannot be passed distally that intracoronary thrombolytic therapy can help melt away thrombus. This is empiric but one editor (JA) has used, in several cases, a small doses of t-PA (10–15 mg) directly injected slowly into the coronary artery over 15–30 min [3]. If the thrombus dissolves, the procedure can then continue or the patient, if stable, can be heparinized and returned on the following day. As t-PA can activate platelets, potent antiplatelet inhibition should be instituted which, of course, increases the risk of bleeding. Nevertheless, the results are often striking with resolution of thrombus. This benefit is due to the fact that with large amounts of thrombus, there is always fibrin-rich thrombus present that responds nicely to thrombolytics particularly when there is an acute presentation.

4. The first randomized study utilizing everolimus-eluting stents vs CABG for multivessel disease was published by Park et al. [4]. As this was a second generation stent, it was hoped that the results of PCI would be comparable to CABG in multivessel disease. The primary end point was a composite of death, myocar-

dial infarction and target vessel revascularization at 2 years and also at longer follow up. Because of slow enrollment, only 880 patients were randomized which represented about 50 % of the proposed enrollment. Major coronary events at 2 years were higher with PCI (11.0 %) vs 7.9 % for CABG. At long term follow up (average 4.6 years), the event rates were 15.3 % for PCI and 10.6 % for CABG, p=.04 and this was mainly driven by the need for repeat revascularization. There was no significant difference in the rate of death or myocardial infarction between the two treatment strategies. Like in the SYNTAX trial, those with a score ≤22 had equivalent results between strategies. In diabetics, there was a trend to better results with CABG, p=.06.

In the above trial, the total stent length was a mean of 85.3 mm with an average SYNTAX score of 24.2 and stent length was similar to that from the SYNTAX study (86.1 mm) This was a more aggressive strategy than that performed by Rodriguey et al. who assessed the use of 2nd generation stents from the multicenter ERACI 4 registry [4]. This was an open label study in 225 patients with multivessel disease. They employed a more conservative approach than that of Park et al. with a total stent length on average of 40.8 mm and a mean SYNTAX score of 27.7. One year major adverse cardiac events (MACCE) were only 2.4 %. Whether this more conservative strategy will result in low 5 year MACCE rates is presently unknown.

5. There have been several recent trials assessing the long term use of dual antiplatelet therapy in secondary prevention. The DAPT (Dual Anti Platelet Therapy) study randomly assigned 9961 patients to continued DAPT for 30 months following a drug eluting stent vs those who discontinued DAPT at 12 months [5]. The co-primary efficacy end points were stent thrombosis and a composite of death, MI or stroke after the 12 month window. The primary safety end point was moderate or severe bleeding. There was an absolute 1–2 % improvement in efficacy end points with prolonged DAPT which was statistically significant but essentially the same percentage increase in bleeding with prolonged therapy. There were also 24 more deaths in the prolonged therapy arm that was not statistically significant versus 12 months of therapy.

In another study recently published, Bonaca et al. randomly assigned in a double blind fashion, 21,162 patients with a myocardial infarction 1–3 years earlier to either ticagrelor 90 mg twice daily, ticagrelor 60 mg twice daily or placebo [6]. All received low dose aspirin and were followed for a median of 33 months. The primary efficacy end point was CV death, MI or stroke. The primary safety end point was TIMI bleeding. There was an absolute improvement of about 1.2 % in efficacy with either dose of ticagrelor vs placebo with a similar percentage increase in bleeding with ticagrelor. Thus, in both trials with different patient populations, we see an approximate equipoise between enhanced efficacy and reduced safety making it difficult to generalize about the routine use of prolonged DAPT as practiced in these two studies.

6. We thought that there should be a little more discussion concerning contrast-induced nephropathy (CIN). Unfortunately, there are little data regarding the risk of CIN in stage 4 or 5 renal insufficiency as these patients are usually excluded from trials. However, multiple studies have been publisher with lesser degrees of insufficiency. First of all, a basic rule of thumb is to avoid contrast with severe

renal insufficiency unless it is absolutely necessary. The patient and family need to be adequately informed of the risks versus benefits if contrast is to be administered. The following are general guidelines we recommend if contrast is to be used in stage 4 or 5 insufficiency although they are not necessarily based on trials with this degree of decrease in function: (1) always hydrate adequately before and after contrast with isotonic saline as long as there are no contra indications to volume expansion. (2) the data on bicarbonate use for hydration is equivocal. (3) Use as little contrast as possible based on the e GFR and separate diagnostic and interventional procedures. The exact safe dose of contrast is unknown in these situations. (4) Iso-osmolar, non-ionic contrast agents may be preferable in these patients. (5) High dose rosuvastatin in statin-naïve patients prior to the procedure may also be protective against contrast-induced damage [7]. (6) The data on acetyl cysteine is, for the most part, negative in reducing CIN and we do not routinely use it.

7. Concerning radial versus femoral access for PCI in acute coronary syndromes, a recent trial has just been published that deserves mention. Valgimigli et al. randomized 8404 patients with an ACS with or without ST-segment elevation to radial vs femoral access for coronary angiography and PCI [8]. 9.8 % of patients with radial access had net adverse CV events (30 day rate of death, myocardial infarction or stroke and serious bleeding) versus 11.7 % with femoral access, p=0.009. Major bleeding (BARC type 3–5) was increased with femoral access. All-cause mortality was also higher with femoral vs radial access (2.2 vs 1.6 %, respectively, p=0.045) [9].

8. Should we be considering advanced therapies in heart disease management even in patients 90 year of age or greater? According to the 2010 US Census Bureau, there were 1.9 million Americans at least 90 years of age and it is predicted that by 2050, they will comprise 10 % of Americans ≥ 65 years of age. This is approximately twice what it was in 2010. There are very little data in the literature for advanced cardiology procedures in this age group. Of course, the answer is complicated and should consider biologic rather than chronologic age along with the patient's co morbidities and wishes. While most of us tend to be more conservative in the very elderly relative to younger patients, anecdotally, percutaneous coronary or peripheral interventions in appropriate candidates, TAVR and pacemaker implantation can be safely performed with an acceptable at least short term success rate. However, bleeding and other complications are increased in the very elderly, so a careful discussion of risks versus benefits should always be carried out prior to the procedure.

References

1. Douglas PS, Hoffman U, Patel MR, et al. Outcomes of anatomical versus functional testing for coronary artery disease. N Engl J Med. 2015;372(14):1291–300. doi:10.1056/NEJMoa1415516.
2. Jolly SS, Cairns S, Yusuf B, et al. Randomized trial of primary PCI with or without routine manual thrombectomy. N Engl J Med. 2015. doi:10.1056/NEJMoa1415098.

3. Ambrose JA. Managing intracoronary thrombus in the catheterization laboratory laboratory during PCI-editorial comment. Curr Cardiol Rev. 2012;8:200.
4. Park S-J, Ahn J-M, Kim Y-H, et al. Trial of everolimus-eluting stents or bypass surgery for coronary disease. N Engl J Med. 2015. doi:10.1056/NEJMoa1415447.
5. Rodriguey AE for the ERACI IV investigators. Second versus first generation DES in multivessel disease and unprotected left main stenosis: insights from ERACI IV study. Minerva Cardioangiol (in press).
6. Mauri L, Kereiakes DJ, Yeh RW, et al. Twelve or 30 months of dual antiplatelet therapy after drug eluting stents. N Engl J Med. 2014;371:2155–66.
7. Bonaca MP, Bhatt DL, Cohen M, et al. Long-term use of ticagrelor in patients with prior myocardial infarction. N Engl J Med. 2015. doi:10.1056/NEJMoa1500857.
8. Hun Y, Zhu G, Han L, et al. Short-term rosuvastatin therapy for prevention of contrast-induced acute kidney injury in patients with diabetes and chronic kidney disease. J Am Coll Cardiol. 2014;63:62–70.
9. Valgimiglia M, Gagnor A, Calabro P, et al. Radial versus femoral access in patients with acute coronary syndromes undergoing invasive management: a randomized multicentre trial. Lancet. 2015;385(9986):2465–76. doi:10.1016/S0140-6736(15)60292-6.

Index

© Springer International Publishing Switzerland 2015
J.A. Ambrose, A.E. Rodríguez (eds.), *Controversies in Cardiology*,
DOI 10.1007/978-3-319-20415-4